SPORTS MEDICINE SECRETS

Second Edition

MORRIS B. MELLION, MD

Senior Vice President, Health Care Policy
and Chief Medical Officer, Blue Cross
 and Blue Shield of Nebraska
Omaha, Nebraska

Clinical Associate Professor
Departments of Family Practice and
 Orthopaedic Surgery (Sports Medicine)
University of Nebraska Medical Center

Adjunct Asssociate Professor
School of Health, Physical Education, and Recreation
University of Nebraska at Omaha

Team Physician
Men's and Women's Sports
University of Nebraska at Omaha

HANLEY & BELFUS, INC./ Philadelphia

Publisher: HANLEY & BELFUS, INC.
                  Medical Publishers
                  210 South 13th Street
                  Philadelphia, PA 19107
                  (215) 546-7293; 800-962-1892
                  FAX (215) 790-9330
                  Web site: http://www.hanleyandbelfus.com

Disclaimer: Although the information in this book has been carefully reviewed for correctness of dosage and indications, neither the authors nor the editor nor the publisher can accept any legal responsibility for any errors or omissions that may be made. Neither the publisher nor the editor makes any warranty, expressed or implied, with respect to the material contained herein. Before prescribing any drug, the reader must review the manufacturer's current production information (package inserts) for accepted indications, absolute dosage recommendations, and other information pertinent to the safe and effective use of the product described.

Library of Congress Cataloging-in-Publication Data

    Sports Medicine Secrets : questions you will be asked in the office, on the
    sidelines, in the training room, on examinations / edited by Morris B. Mellion.
    2nd ed.
         p.   cm. — (The Secrets Series®)
    Includes bibliographical references and index.
    ISBN 1-56053-308-0 (alk. paper)
      1. Sports medicine—Handbooks, manuals, etc.   I. Morris B. Mellion.
    II. Series.
      [DNLM: 1. Sports Medicine—handbooks.   QT 29 S764 1999]
    RC1210.S765   1999
    617.1'027—dc21
    DNLM/DLC
    for Library of Congress   98-43414
                                                                         CIP

SPORTS MEDICINE SECRETS, 2nd edition   ISBN 1-56053-308-0

Last digit is the print number: 9   8   7   6   5   4   3   2   1

DEDICATION

I dedicate this book:

To the memory of my father, Frank Mellion, who taught me how to dream;

To the memory of my mother, Yvette Shaset Mellion, who taught me how to make my dreams into reality;

To the memory of my father-in-law, Gabel Henry Conner, who was a second father to me; and

To my mother-in-law, Thelma Marie Conner, who is a constant source of love and encouragement.

CONTENTS

IX. OVERUSE AND TRAUMA

X. MANAGEMENT APPROACHES AND TECHNIQUES

XI. SPECIFIC SPORTS

CONTRIBUTORS

Jeffrey P. Anthony, D.O.
Team Physician, San Diego State University; Clinical Faculty, Stanford-Sharp Family Practice Residency Program; Clinical Faculty, University of California, San Diego, and Western University Health Services, Department of Family Practice, San Diego, California

Henry C. Barry, M.D., M.S.
Associate Professor, Department of Family Practice, Michigan State University, East Lansing, Michigan

James R. Barrett, M.D., C.A.Q.
Associate Professor, Family and Preventive Medicine, University of Oklahoma, Oklahoma City, Oklahoma

Mark Batt, M.B., B. Chir., MRCGP, Dip. Sport Med.
Senior Lecturer and Honorary Consultant in Sports Medicine, Centre for Sports Medicine, Queen's Medical Centre, Nottingham, United Kingdom

Kenneth B. Batts, D.O.
Department of Family Practice and Community Medicine, Tripler Army Medical Center, Honolulu, Hawaii

Donald R. Bennett, M.D.*
Reynolds Professor of Neurology, University of Nebraska College of Medicine, Omaha, Nebraska

Kris E. Berg, Ed.D.
Isaacson Professor, School of Health, Physical Education, and Recreation, University of Nebraska at Omaha, Omaha, Nebraska

Daniel Blanke, Ph.D.
Director, School of Health, Physical Education, and Recreation, University of Nebraska at Omaha, Omaha, Nebraska

Brent A. Blue, M.D.
Medical Director, Grand Teton Medical Clinic, Grand Teton National Park, Jackson Hole; Private Practice, Jackson Hole, Wyoming

Frank M. Brasile, Ph.D.
Professor, School of Health, Physical Education, and Recreation, University of Nebraska at Omaha, Omaha, Nebraska

David E. Brown, M.D.
Clinical Assistant Professor of Orthopaedic Surgery, Department of Orthopaedic Surgery and Rehabilitation, University of Nebraska Medical Center, Omaha, Nebraska

Douglas G. Browning, M.D., A.T.C.
Assistant Professor of Family Medicine and Associate in Surgical Sciences–Orthopaedics/Sports Medicine, Department of Family and Community Medicine, Wake Forest University School of Medicine, Winston-Salem, North Carolina

Kristine L. Burke, M.D.
Assistant Clinical Professor, Department of Family and Community Medicine, University of California, Davis, School of Medicine, Sacramento, California
* Deceased.

Kevin E. Burroughs, M.D.
Resident Physician, Moses Cone Family Practice, Greensboro; Assistant Team Physician, Elon College, Burlington, North Carolina

Cindy J. Chang, M.D.
Head Team Physician, University Health Services and Department of Intercollegiate Athletics, University of California–Berkeley, Berkeley; Assistant Clinical Professor, Departments of Family and Community Medicine, University of California, San Francisco, and University of California, Davis, Schools of Medicine, San Francisco and Sacramento, California

Chris N. Christakos, M.D., C.A.Q., SpMed.
Private Practice, Family Practice and Sports Medicine, Salem Family Practice; Team Physician, North Forsyth High School, Winston-Salem, North Carolina

Clark H. Cobb, III, M.D.
Staff Physician, The Columbus Clinic, Department of Family Medicine and Sports Medicine, Columbus, Georgia

Ian D. Crabb, M.D.
Attending Physician, Nebraska Methodist Hospital, Omaha, Nebraska

John P. DiFiori, M.D.
Assistant Professor, Department of Family Medicine, Division of Sports Medicine, and Team Physician, Department of Intercollegiate Athletics, University of California, Los Angeles, UCLA School of Medicine, Los Angeles, California

R. Todd Dombroski, D.O., FAAFP
Assistant Professor of Family Medicine, Department of Sports Medicine, Uniformed Services University of the Health Sciences, Madigan Army Medical Center, Fort Lewis, Washington

Edward P. Dominguez
Third-year student, the Ohio State University College of Medicine, Columbus, Ohio

L. Christine Dunn, B.S., L.A.T.C.
Teacher/Athletic Trainer, Millard Public Schools, Department of Physical Education, Millard Public School District, Omaha, Nebraska

Scott W. Eathorne, M.D.
Program Director, Providence Athletic Medicine, Providence Hospital and Medical Centers, Novi, Michigan

E. Randy Eichner, M.D., FACSM
Professor of Medicine, University of Oklahoma Health Sciences Center, University Hospital and VA Medical Center, Oklahoma City; Internal Medicine Consultant, University of Oklahoma varsity athletes, Oklahoma City, Oklahoma

Denise M. Fandel, M.S., ATC
Administrator of Credentialing Programs, NATA Board of Certification, Inc., Omaha, Nebraska

Karl B. Fields, M.D., C.A.Q., SpMed
Professor of Family Medicine, and Associate Chairman, Department of Family Medicine, University of North Carolina at Chapel Hill School of Medicine, Chapel Hill; Director, Family Medicine Residency and Sports Medicine Fellowship, Moses Cone Health System and Greensboro AHEC, Greensboro, North Carolina

Timothy C. Fitzgibbons, M.D.
Assistant Clinical Professor, Department of Orthopaedic Surgery, Creighton University School of Medicine; Clinical Instructor, Department of Orthopaedics, University of Nebraska College of Medicine, Omaha, Nebraska

Thomas A. Frette, M.A., ATC
Head Athletic Trainer and Instructor, Department of Athletic Training, University of Nebraska at Omaha, Omaha, Nebraska

Harry L. Galanty, M.D.
Assistant Professor, Department of Orthopaedics, Texas Tech University Health Science Center; Medical Director, Texas Tech University Athletics, Lubbock, Texas

Elizabeth M. Gallup, M.D., J.D., M.B.A.
Health Care Consultant, William M. Mercer, Inc., Kansas City; Clinical Associate Professor, University of Missouri, Kansas City, Missouri

Robert C. Gambrell, M.D., FACSM
Assistant Professor, Department of Family Medicine, Center for Sports Medicine, Medical College of Georgia, Augusta, Georgia

Mathew C. Gordon, M.D., D.D.S.
Private Practice, San Pedro Facial Surgery, San Antonio, Texas

Ann C. Grandjean, Ed.D.
Director, International Center for Sports Nutrition, Omaha; Clinical Assistant Professor, Sports Medicine Program, Orthopaedic Surgery, University of Nebraska Medical Center, Omaha, Nebraska

Gary A. Green, M.D., FACP
Clinical Associate Professor, Department of Family Medicine, UCLA School of Medicine, Los Angeles, California

Brian C. Halpern, M.D., FAAFP
Clinical Assistant Professor of Sports Medicine, Department of Family Medicine, University of Medicine and Dentistry of New Jersey, Robert Wood Johnson Medical School, New Brunswick, New Jersey; Clinical Instructor of Medicine, Hospital for Special Surgery, New York, New York

Gene A. Hannah, M.D.
Private Practice, Nashville, Tennessee

Robert W. Heck, M.D.
Private Practice, Salt Lake City, Utah

Michele Helzer-Julin, PA-C, M.S.
Physician Assistant and Exercise Physiologist, Sports Medicine Center, Omaha, Nebraska

John M. Henderson, D.O.
Director of Primary Care Sports Medicine, Hughston Sports Medicine Center and Medical Director, Rehabilitation Unit, Hughston Sports Medicine Hospital, Columbus, Georgia

Todd P. Hendrickson, M.D.
Assistant Professor of Psychiatry, Creighton University School of Medicine and University of Nebraska College of Medicine, Omaha, Nebraska

David O. Hough, M.D.*
Professor of Family Practice, Director of Sports Medicine, and Head Team Physician, Michigan State University, East Lansing, Michigan

Warren B. Howe, M.D.
Team Physician/Student Health Physician, Western Washington University Student Health Service, Western Washington University, Bellingham, Washington

Kirk S. Hutton, M.D.
Clinical Assistant Professor, Department of Orthopaedic Surgery, University of Nebraska Medical Center, Omaha, Nebraska

* Deceased.

Rebecca Jaffe, M.D., FAAFP, FACSM
Instructor, Department of Family Medicine, Jefferson Medical College, Philadelphia, Pennsylvania

John B. Jeffers, D.V.M., M.D.
Associate Professor, Department of Ophthalmology, Thomas Jefferson University/Wills Eye Hospital; Attending Surgeon, Director, Emergency Department and Center for Sports Vision, Wills Eye Hospital, Philadelphia, Pennsylvania

Robert J. Johnson, M.D.
Director, Primary Care Sports Medicine, Department of Family Practice, Hennepin County Medical Center, Minneapolis, Minnesota

Brian J. E. Jones, M.S., A.T.C.-R
Teacher and Athletic Trainer, Park Hill High School, Department of Computer Science, Park Hill Public High School District, Kansas City, Missouri

Barry D. Jordan, M.D., M.P.H.
Instructor, Department of Neurology, UCLA School of Medicine, Los Angeles, California

Gary Keogh, M.D., MRCGP, DA(UK)
Resident, Department of Physical Medicine and Rehabilitation, Loma Linda University, Loma Linda University Medical Center, Loma Linda, California

Razib Khaund, M.D.
Clinical Assistant Professor of Medicine, Department of Medicine, Brown University School of Medicine, Providence; Director, Primary Care Sports Medicine, The New England Center for Athletes, Providence, Rhode Island

Roger H. Kobayashi, M.D.
Clinical Professor of Pediatrics, Department of Pediatrics, UCLA School of Medicine, Los Angeles, California; Physician, Allergy, Asthma and Immunology Associates, Omaha, Nebraska

Gregory L. Landry, M.D.
Professor of Pediatrics, University of Wisconsin Medical School; Head, Medical Team Physician, University of Wisconsin athletic teams, Madison, Wisconsin

Walter L. Larimore, M.D., D.A.B.F.P.
Associate Clinical Professor, Department of Family Medicine, University of South Florida College of Medicine, Tampa; Private Practice, Kissimmee, Florida

Richard W. Latin, Ph.D.
Professor of Exercise Science, School of Health, Physical Education, and Recreation, University of Nebraska at Omaha, Omaha, Nebraska

Constance Marie Lebrun, M.D.C.M., M.P.E., C.C.F.P., FACSM, Dip. Sport Med. (CASM)
Director, Primary Care Sport Medicine, Departments of Orthopaedics and Family Medicine, Fowler-Kennedy Sport Medicine Clinic 3M Centre, University of Western Ontario, London, Ontario, Canada

Mark J. Leski, M.D.
Assistant Professor and Director of Sports Medicine, Family and Preventive Medicine, University of South Carolina School of Medicine, Columbia, South Carolina

Richard Levandowski, M.D.
Associate Clinical Professor, Department of Family Medicine, University of Medicine and Dentistry of New Jersey, Robert Wood Johnson Medical School, New Brunswick, and New Jersey Medical School, Newark; Team Physician, USA Track and Field, The College of New Jersey, Mercer County Community College, Newark, New Jersey

Benjamin D. Levine, M.D.
Director, Institute for Exercise and Environmental Medicine, Presbyterian Hospital, Dallas; Associate Professor of Medicine, University of Texas Southwestern Medical Center, Dallas, Texas

Wade A. Lillegard, M.D.
Assistant Professor, Department of Family Practice, University of Minnesota—Duluth; Co-Director, Department of Sports Medicine and Orthopedics, St. Mary's/Duluth Clinic, Duluth, Minnesota

John A. Lombardo, M.D.
Professor, Department of Family Medicine; Medical Director, Ohio State University Sports Medicine Center; Head Team Physician, Ohio State University, Columbus, Ohio

Mark E. Longacre, M.P.T.
Manager, Physical and Occupational Therapy, University Hospital, University of Nebraska Medical Center, Omaha, Nebraska

James M. Lynch, M.D.
Assistant Professor, Department of Education, Quincy University, Quincy, Illinois

John W. McClellan III, M.D.
Spine Fellow, Queens Medical Centre–Spinal Unit, Nottingham, United Kingdom

Christopher A. McGrew, M.D.
Associate Professor, Departments of Orthopaedics and Rehabilitation and Family and Community Medicine, University of New Mexico Health Sciences Center, Albuquerque, New Mexico

Douglas B. McKeag, M.D., M.S.
Arthur J. Rooney Sr. Professor of Sports Medicine, and Professor and Vice-Chair, Department of Family Medicine, University of Pittsburgh; Director, Sports Medicine, University of Pittsburgh Medical Center (UPMC) St. Margaret Hospital and UPMC Shadyside Hospital, Pittsburgh, Pennsylvania

Matthew A. McQueen, M.D.
Clinical Instructor, Family Medicine/Sports Medicine, Department of Family Medicine, Ochsner Clinic, New Orleans, Louisiana

Morris B. Mellion, M.D.
Senior Vice President, Health Care Policy and Chief Medical Officer, Blue Cross and Blue Shield of Nebraska, Omaha; Clinical Associate Professor, Departments of Family Practice and Orthopaedic Surgery (Sports Medicine), University of Nebraska Medical Center, Omaha; Adjunct Associate Professor, School of Health, Physical Education, and Recreation, University of Nebraska at Omaha; Team Physician, Men's and Women's Sports, University of Nebraska at Omaha, Nebraska

Alexander K. Morley, M.D., FAAFP, FACEP
Private Practice, Eugene, Oregon

Dianne T. Morley, P.T.
Private Practice, Eugene, Oregon

Joseph P. Mullane, M.D.
Clinical Instructor, Department of Family Medicine, University of Medicine and Dentistry of New Jersey, New Brunswick; Medical Director, Princeton Occupational Health and Family Medicine, Hamilton, New Jersey

Scott Naftulin, D.O.
Attending Physiatrist, Department of Physical Medicine and Rehabilitation, Lehigh Valley Hospital Center, Bethlehem, Pennsylvania

Aurelia Nattiv, M.D.
Assistant Professor, Departments of Family Medicine and Orthopaedic Surgery, UCLA School of Medicine, and Team Physician, UCLA Department of Intercollegiate Athletics, Los Angeles, California

Randall D. Neumann, M.D.
Orthopedic Surgeon, Sports Medicine Center, Omaha, Nebraska

Terry L. Nicola, M.D.
Assistant Professor, Director of Sports Medicine Rehabilitation, Department of Rehabilitation Medicine and Restorative Sciences, University of Illinois College of Medicine, Chicago, Illinois; Associate Team Physician, University of Illinois Flames

Richard A. Parker, D.O., FAOASM
Assistant Clinical Professor, Department of Family Preventive Medicine, University of California, San Diego, School of Medicine, San Diego; Team Physician, San Diego State University Department of Intercollegiate Athletics, San Diego, California

Lucy Patti, M.D.
Staff Physician, House of the Good Samaritan Hospital, Watertown, New York

Ross M. Patton, M.D.
Associate Professor, Department of Family and Community Health, Marshall University School of Medicine, Huntington, West Virginia

Kirk M. Peck, M.S., P.T.
Director/Instructor, Physical Therapist Assistant Program, Clarkson College, Omaha, Nebraska

David J. Petron, M.D.
Assistant Professor of Family Practice, Assistant Professor of Orthopaedics–Sports Medicine, University of Utah School of Medicine, Salt Lake City, Utah

John L. Pfenninger, M.D., FAAFP
Director, The National Procedures Institute, Midland; Clinical Professor of Family Practice, Michigan State College of Human Medicine, East Lansing, Michigan

Laurence D. Powell, M.D.
Assistant Professor, Primary Care Sports Medicine Director, Department of Family Medicine, Morehouse School of Medicine, Atlanta, Georgia

Joel M. Press, M.D.
Associate Professor of Physical Medicine and Rehabilitation, Department of Physical Medicine and Rehabilitation, Northwestern University Medical School, Chicago; Medical Director, Center for Spine, Sports, and Occupational Rehabilitation, Rehabilitation Institute of Chicago, Chicago, Illinois

James C. Puffer, M.D.
Professor and Interim Chair, Department of Family Medicine, UCLA School of Medicine, Los Angeles, California

Margot Putukian, M.D., FACSM
Team Physician, Assistant Professor, Departments of Internal Medicine, Orthopaedics, and Rehabilitation, Penn State University, University Park, Pennsylvania

Curtis D. Reimer, M.D.
Team Physician, Hastings College and Hastings Senior High School, Hastings, Nebraska

E. Lee Rice, D.O., FAAFP
Associate Clinical Professor of Family Practice and Preventive Medicine, University of California, San Diego; Clinical Professor, Department of Family Practice and Sports Medicine, Western University of Health Sciences, Pomona, California

Stephen G. Rice, M.D., Ph.D., M.P.H., FAAP, FACSM
Director, Primary Care Sports Medicine Fellowship; Director, Athletic Health Care System; Co-Director, Jersey Shore Sports Medicine Center; Department of Pediatrics, Jersey Shore Medical Center, Neptune, New Jersey

Tony C. Roisum, M.D.
American Sports Medicine Institute, Birmingham, Alabama

Matthew H. Rosen, M.D.
Primary Care Sports Medicine Fellow, Department of Family Medicine, University of Medicine and Dentistry of New Jersey, Robert Wood Johnson Medical School, New Brunswick, New Jersey

Jaime S. Ruud, M.S., R.D.
Sports Nutritionist, International Center for Sports Nutrition, Omaha, Nebraska

Thomas R. Sachtleben, M.D.
Private Practice, Colorado Springs, Colorado

Marie D. Schafle, M.D.
Director, Sports and Performing Arts, Student Health Services, San Francisco State University, San Francisco, California

Robert B. Schoene, M.D.
Professor of Medicine, Division of Pulmonary and Critical Care Medicine, University of Washington, Seattle; Director, Pulmonary Function Laboratory, Harborview Medical Center, Seattle, Washington

Donald Shell, M.D.
Assistant Professor, Department of Family Medicine, and Team Physician, The Ohio State University, Columbus, Ohio

Guy L. Shelton, M.A., P.T., A.T.C.
Sports Physical Therapist and Administrator, HealthSouth Sports Medicine and Rehabilitation Center of Omaha; Clinical Instructor, Division of Physical Therapy Education, School of Allied Health, University of Nebraska Medical Center, Omaha, Nebraska

Mark E. Shirley, D.O.
Staff Physician, Department of Family Practice, Physicians Clinic, Omaha; Associate Team Physician, All Men's and Women's Sports, University of Nebraska at Omaha, Omaha, Nebraska

R. Trent Sickles, M.D., FACSM
Associate Professor of Clinical Family Medicine, Department of Family Medicine, The Ohio State University, Columbus, Ohio

Reuben Sloan, M.D.
Private Practice, Physical Medicine and Rehabilitation, The Hughston Clinic, P.C.; Team Physician, Columbus Cottonmouths Hockey, Columbus, Georgia

Deborah L. Squire, M.D.
Assistant Professor of Pediatrics, Community and Family Medicine, Duke University Medical Center, Durham, North Carolina

Keith L. Stanley, M.D.
Private Practice, Eastern Oklahoma Orthopedic Center, Tulsa; Affiliate Professor, University of Oklahoma College of Medicine, Department of Family Medicine, Tulsa, Oklahoma

Stephen R. Steele, D.O.
Private Practice, Bermuda Dunes, California

James Stray-Gundersen, M.D.
Visiting Professor, Physiology, Norwegian University of Sports and Physical Education, Oslo, Norway

Paul R. Stricker, M.D.
Assistant Professor, Department of Pediatrics and Department of Orthopaedics and Rehabilitation, and Team Physician, Vanderbilt University Medical Center, Vanderbilt University, Nashville, Tennessee

Ravi S. Tak, M.D.
Fellow, Sports Medicine, Family Practice Residency, Bayfront Medical Center, St. Petersburg, Florida

Jeffrey L. Tanji, M.D.
Associate Professor of Family Practice, University of California, Davis, School of Medicine, Sacramento, California

Suzanne M. Tanner, M.D.
Resident, Division of Orthopaedics, University of Alabama School of Medicine, Birmingham, Alabama

L. Kay Thigpen, Ph.D.
Executive Director, Texas Orthopaedic and Sports Medicine Institute, San Antonio, Texas

David Thorson, M.D.
Private Practice, MinnHealth, P.A., White Bear Lake, Minnesota

Joseph L. Torres, M.D.
Private Practice, Kissimmee, Florida

Harold Kai Tu, M.D., D.M.D., FACS
Private Practice, Omaha, Nebraska

Andrew M. Tucker, M.D.
Assistant Professor, Department of Family Medicine, University of Maryland School of Medicine; Director, Primary Care Sports Medicine, University of Maryland Medical Center, Baltimore, Maryland

Robert O. Voy, M.D., FACSM
Private Practitioner, Family Physician/Sports Medicine Specialist, Las Vegas, Nevada

W. Michael Walsh, M.D.
Clinical Associate Professor of Orthopaedic Surgery, University of Nebraska Medical Center; Adjunct Graduate Associate Professor, School of Health, Physical Education, and Recreation, University of Nebraska at Omaha, Omaha, Nebraska

Kevin N. Waninger, M.D.
Assistant Professor of Family Medicine, Robert Wood Johnson Medical School, Camden, New Jersey; Team Physician, University of Delaware, Newark, Delaware

Stuart M. Weinstein, M.D.
Clinical Associate Professor, Department of Rehabilitation Medicine, University of Washington, Seattle; Physician, Puget Sound Sports and Spine Physicians, Seattle, Washington

Russell D. White, M.D., FAAFP
Associate Director, Family Practice Residency and Director, Sports Medicine Fellowship Program, Bayfront Medical Center, St. Petersburg; Clinical Associate Professor, Department of Family Medicine, University of South Florida College of Medicine, Tampa, Florida; Crew Chief, U.S. Olympic Committee

James A. Whiteside, M.D.
Eminent Scholar in Sports Medicine and Team Physician, and Professor of Health and Human Services, Troy State University, Troy, Alabama

Leonard A. Wilkerson, D.O., M.B.A., FAAFP, FAOASM
Medical Director, Cigna Healthcare of Tennessee, Memphis, Tennessee; Chair, Joint Commission on Sports Medicine and Science; Event Physician, U.S. National TaeKwon-Do Team Trials and Junior Olympic TaeKwon-Do Championships

Mark S. Williams, D.O.
Assistant Director of Primary Care Sports Medicine, Department of Family Practice and Community Medicine, Tripler Army Medical Center, Honolulu, Hawaii

Jeffrey L. Young, M.D., M.A.
Assistant Professor, Physical Medicine and Rehabilitation, Northwestern University Medical School, Chicago; Sports Rehabilitation Program, Rehabilitation Institute of Chicago, Chicago, Illinois

PREFACE TO THE FIRST EDITION

I want to thank Linda Belfus for asking me to edit *Sports Medicine Secrets*. I initially responded reluctantly, but with her urging, I agreed for two reasons. First, *Sports Medicine Secrets* would provide the opportunity for many sports medicine fellows and recently trained physicians to publish in the same volume with established teachers and clinicians. As a result, many of the chapters are a "fresh look," featuring new information and crisp insights. Many of these new authors represent the future leadership of primary care sports medicine in North America.

Second, the question-and-answer format of The Secrets Series® captures the interaction between athlete and team physician, student and teacher. As physicians and educators, we try to respond to the needs of our patients and students. As Socrates demonstrated, important fundamentals become clear when they are stated in response to a series of questions.

I want to thank several very special people:

> My partners, Mike Walsh, Dave Brown, and Randy Neumann, for tolerating my penchant for publication and for supporting me over three years while I traveled frequently in service to the American Academy of Family Physicians.

> Pat Fahey, our Administrator, who shares our interest in scholarship as well as patient care, and who recruits fine people like:

> Mary Parnick and Marilyn Novak, without whom the manuscript organization and preparation would have been impossible.

Morris B. Mellion, M.D.
Omaha, Nebraska
December 1993

PREFACE TO THE SECOND EDITION

The first edition of *Sports Medicine Secrets* was well received in the United States and abroad. This second edition is both updated and expanded. The chapters from the first edition have been revised and upgraded by a mix of original and new authors, and eight new chapters are introduced: Sudden Death in High School and College Athletes, Electromyography and Nerve Conduction Studies, Functional Bracing in Athletes, Springboard and Platform Diving, Weightlifting and Powerlifting, In-line Skating, Cheerleading, and Mass Participation Sports and Events.

This edition would not have been possible without the efforts of my teenage son, Frank Bruce Mellion, who performed all of the administrative work in a fraction of the time it would have taken his father.

Sports Medicine Secrets, 2nd edition is a tribute to the athletes, coaches, athletic trainers, and athletic directors at the University of Nebraska at Omaha, who constantly challenge and reward me.

Morris B. Mellion, M.D.
Omaha, Nebraska

I. Medical Supervision of the Athlete

1. THE TEAM PHYSICIAN

Morris B. Mellion, M.D., and W. Michael Walsh, M.D.

1. What is the role of the team physician?

The team physician should address the physical, emotional, and spiritual needs of the athlete in the context of the sport and the needs of the team. Regardless of training, the team physician should function as a generalist. When specialists or subspecialists are team physicians, their overall success depends not on their technical skills, but on their ability and supplemental training to meet the athlete's broad range of medical and psychosocial needs.

2. What are the team physician's responsibilities to the athlete?

1. The team physician has an ethical responsibility to allow the athlete to participate. The physician should not arbitrarily disqualify athletes from participation for insignificant reasons. Because athletes in school-based programs have a right to participate if there is no valid medical contraindication, the team physician must know the current valid medical contraindications in detail.

2. The team physician should protect the athlete from injury, reinjury, and permanent disability. This responsibility entails protecting athletes from themselves by keeping them out of play until they are adequately rehabilitated from an injury, which may be challenging when an athlete has a "play at any cost" mentality.

3. The team physician must provide optimal health care.

4. The team physician must maintain confidentiality and be sensitive to how widely information about an athlete is disseminated. In organized athletics, information is seldom held in the strict doctor-patient confidentiality. That confidentiality is often compromised by the physician's relationship with the school or professional athletic organization. However, the athletic patient may have medical conditions affecting ability to play that he or she does not want to share with the rest of the team; the athlete's privacy should be respected whenever it is not in direct conflict with explicit agreement by the athlete to provide medical information to the team.

3. What are the team physician's responsibilities to the team?

To facilitate the success of the team without sacrificing the care of the individual athlete.

4. What are the team physician's responsibilities to the coach?

The team physician is responsible for facilitating success. The physician is responsible for educating the coach about improvements in medical and preventive care. The physician can provide continuing education to the coaching staff and thereby eliminate outdated and occasionally harmful techniques. This education process often protects the coaches from potential future liability.

5. What are the team physician's responsibilities to the institution?

To provide optimal health care for athletes, to prescreen scholarship and professional athletes, and to protect the institution from liability.

6. What is the cornerstone for success as a team physician?

In all medical practices the cornerstone for success is availability. In sports, the physician should be available at appropriate times on the sidelines, in the training rooms, in the office, and after hours. You cannot be an effective team physician if you are not willing to make arrangements to see athletes when they need to see you, rather than when you are available. The team physician also needs to spend unstructured time with the athletic trainer and/or coach.

7. Who serves as team physician?

Family physicians, general practitioners, and orthopedists make up over half of team physicians. The rest consist of a wide variety of specialists. Some physicians share the responsibility for a team (often a generalist and a specialist). In many settings, there is a team physician and a team orthopedist. This combination may provide a broad range of expertise along with high-quality surgical talent.

8. What rewards can an individual expect from serving as a team physician?

The greatest reward is the immense personal satisfaction of working with young motivated patients while, at the same time, providing a community service. Affiliation with athletic teams at the high school, college, and professional level may enhance a physician's reputation in the community and contribute to practice building. Remuneration is generally secondary at anything less than a professional team level. Some high schools pay a small stipend for football game coverage. Above the high school level, there may be compensation, but the amount is extremely variable. In professional sports, there may be a significant retainer. Surgeons may receive payment for surgical procedures performed, but these services may also be provided on a discount basis as well.

9. Should the team physician have a formal relationship with the institution?

Yes. If a formal contract is not appropriate or possible, there should be a detailed verbal agreement before the season begins. It should include job description, fiscal arrangements, and a statement of mutual expectations. If monetary arrangements are involved, a written document is essential. A team physician may be secured or hired by the athletic director, athletic trainer, coach, business manager, or other officer of a professional team. The job description of the team physician should include to whom the physician reports, services provided both at home and away, remuneration and benefits, including reimbursement for travel, and any other expectations of the institution or of the physician.

10. Which role of the team physician occupies the most time and effort?

The major effort is medical supervision of athletes. This traditional function has been greatly expanded to include prevention, supervision, evaluation, and management. Prevention starts with the preparticipation evaluation, which helps athletes to receive counseling about appropriate sports in which to participate, advanced treatment of injuries, or rehabilitation of deficits before the season starts. The team physician also provides advice on proper conditioning techniques, injury prevention, and selection and fit of protective equipment.

The team physician provides on-site coverage. For high-risk situations and high-risk sports, the team physician should be present. If the physician is not on-site, then coverage should be provided by athletic trainers or other highly trained personnel.

The team physician evaluates illness and injury on the field, in the training room, in the office, and in the emergency room. Finally, the team physician manages the athlete's care and seeks appropriate consultation and referral when necessary.

11. Who makes up the sports medicine team?

The key players in the sports medicine team are the athlete, the team physician, the coach, and the athletic trainer. The athletic trainer occupies a unique position at the center of the athletic health care triangle. The athletic trainer is a therapist and counselor for the athlete, advisor and friend to the coach, and an extra pair of eyes and ears for the team physician. Every athletic program at the high school level and above should have a certified athletic trainer.

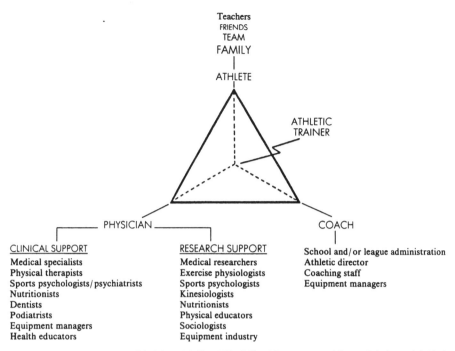

The sports medicine team. (Modified from Mellion MB: Office Management of Sports Injuries and Athletic Problems. Philadelphia, Hanley & Belfus, 1988.)

12. What is the team physician's administrative role?

The team physician is responsible for developing a general system of care for the team. When an athletic trainer is available, this should be a joint project. Important planning areas include guidelines for consultation, organization and planning for the preparticipation evaluation, and development of a prearranged system of emergency care.

13. What are the main legal and medicolegal issues for the team physician?

The team physician should act ethically to protect the institution and himself or herself from professional and institutional liability. The physician may be called upon to advice the institution in a variety of areas to prevent liability. Examples include recognizing the athlete's right to participate and ensuring that proper permission has been obtained to treat minors.

A gray area in the treatment of athletes involves out-of-state trips. For routine competitions and tournaments, it is advisable to work through the host team or tournament physician or through a local physician in the host town. If a physician is not obtaining a fee for service, "good samaritan" laws generally cover treatment of emergencies on road trips.

14. What are some of the other roles that a team physician may play?

1. The team physician may help with logistics, particularly in planning how to handle potential emergencies.

2. The team physician coordinates and often supervises medical care by other medical personnel and athletic trainers, perhaps including advice on medical insurance.

3. The team physician must be a good communicator. One one level, this means helping to resolve conflicts or enhance cooperation when thorny issues arise between the athlete and the coach, parents, other physicians, or the press.

4. The other side of communication is education. Here, the team physician should function as an educator at many levels. Using a wide variety of instructional tools, the team physician

should be prepared to educate athletes, coaches, athletic trainers, administrators, medical personnel, paramedical personnel, students, parents, and the general public.

5. The team physician must be a student as well as an educator. The physician is responsible for keeping current with a body of knowledge that changes rapidly.

15. What about "the laying on of hands"?

The athlete deserves a personal physician who understands both the demands of and commitment to the sport. In this highly technical medical environment, it is important not to underestimate the intangible effect of the physician as healer. Supportive care is often essential to the athlete's recovery and participation.

BIBLIOGRAPHY

1. Dick AD: Chalktalk for the team physician. Am Fam Physician 28(3):231–236, 1983.
2. Dyment PG (ed): Sports Medicine: Health Care for Young Athletes, 2nd ed. Evanston, American Academy of Pediatrics, 1991, pp 188–195.
3. Howe WB: Primary care sports medicine: A part-timer's perspective. Phys Sportsmed 16(1):103–114, 1988.
4. Karofsky PS: Death of a high school hockey player. Phys Sportsmed 18(2):99–103, 1990.
5. Lombardo JA: Sports medicine: A team effort. Phys Sportsmed 13(4):72–81, 1985.
6. Mellion MB, Walsh WM: The team physician. In Mellion MB, Walsh WM, Shelton GL (eds): The Team Physician's Handbook, 2nd ed. Philadelphia, Hanley & Belfus, 1997.
7. Redfearn RW: The physician's role in school sports programs. Phys Sportsmed 8(9):67–71, 1980.
8. Samples P: The team physician: No official job description. Phys Sportsmed 16(1):169–175, 1988.
9. Scheiderer LL: A survey of the practices of appointing and utilizing intercollegiate athletic team physicians. Athletic Training 22(3):211–218, 1987.
10. Shaffer TE: So you've been asked to be the team physician. Phys Sportsmed 4(12):57–63, 1976.
11. Walsh WM, Mellion MB: The team physician. In DeLee JC, Drez D Jr (eds): Orthopaedic Sports Medicine: Principles and Practice. Philadelphia, W.B. Saunders, 1994, pp 346–355.

2. THE ATHLETIC TRAINER AND THE TRAINING ROOM

Denise M. Fandel, M.S., ATC

1. What is the role of the athletic trainer?

Athletic trainers are responsible for the prevention, emergency care, first aid, evaluation, and rehabilitation of injuries to athletes under their care. Athletic trainers are often consulted by the coaching staff about conditioning and nutrition programs. At some institutions they participate in decision making about the purchase of protective equipment. They also serve as liaison between team physician, athlete, parents, coaches, and other health professionals. The athletic trainer certified by the National Athletic Trainers' Association, Board of Certification (NATABOC) is an allied health professional. The initials ATC signify board certification. An athletic trainer must have a minimum of a bachelor's degree, although almost 70% of all certified athletic trainers have a master's degree. In over 25 states, athletic trainers are licensed health care practitioners.

2. What educational training does an athletic trainer have?

NATABOC identifies five domains of the athletic trainer's skills and knowledge: (1) prevention of athletic injuries; (2) recognition, evaluation, and immediate care of athletic injuries; (3) rehabilitation and reconditioning of athletic injuries; (4) health care administration; and (5) professional development and responsibility.

Currently an athletic trainer may become eligible for NATABOC certification examination by completion of an approved or accredited curriculum or by completion of internship requirements. Students applying under the approved or accredited curriculum route must have spent at least 800 clinical hours under the supervision of a NATABOC-certified athletic trainer. In addition, they must have successfully completed a full curriculum of courses that match the five domains outlined by NATABOC. Much of the their course work precedes clinical exposure.

Students who apply for national boards through the internship route must have been supervised for a minimum of 1,500 clinical hours by a NATABOC-certified athletic trainer. Supervision and mentorship must occur over a minimum of two to a maximum of five calendar years before the candidate takes the national boards. Internship candidates must have taken one course in each of the following areas in preparation for the boards: (1) human anatomy, (2) human physiology, (3) kinesiology/biomechanics, (4) personal health, (5) exercise physiology, (6) basic athletic training, and (7) advanced athletic training.

3. Where do athletic trainers practice?

Athletic trainers are employed in various practice settings: high schools, colleges or universities, hospitals or clinics, and professional, amateur, or Olympic sports organizations.

In the high school setting the athletic trainer may be employed as a full-time trainer or more commonly as a teacher-trainer. Most colleges and universities employ one or more athletic trainers to work with all athletes. They also may teach classes or supervise student athletic trainers.

Athletic trainers may be employed by clinics or hospitals. Some athletic trainers work in the clinic in the morning and then at one or more high schools in the afternoon. The athletic trainer may provide game coverage for high schools.

At the professional and semiprofessional level, athletic trainers are employed by each club or team, and their duties may extend beyond medical care of the athletes. It is not uncommon for athletic trainers to assist in planning team travel, meals, and lodging. Athletic trainers also may be responsible for the team and players' equipment.

Athletic trainers work with amateur athletes at various levels. The United States Olympic Committee has a structured learning and evaluation process for athletic trainers.

4. What is the role of athletic trainers on the health care team?

Athletic trainers provide the first line of health care when an injury occurs. Their education and training enable them to recognize the injury, assess the athlete, initiate appropriate first-aid care, and refer the athlete to the appropriate next step in the health care process. When the athlete returns to the athletic trainer, the athletic trainer assesses whether rehabilitation is complete and whether the athlete is ready to return to practice and competition through a sport-specific testing procedure.

5. What sets an athletic trainer apart from other sports medicine personnel?

In the traditional setting, athletic trainers are in contact with the athlete daily. They learn the idiosyncrasies of each athlete and are able to identify possible injury-causing situations, to recognize improper or potentially hazardous equipment, and to prevent injuries. The athletic trainer is skilled in on-field injury recognition and evaluation. Athletic trainers are available to examine the injury immediately before swelling and pain make it difficult to assess. Athletic trainers are also confidantes of the coach and often serve as liaisons for the physician. Athletic trainers understand the demands of the athlete's sport and playing position. This understanding allows them to design a functional progression of flexibility, strength, proprioception, and sport-specific workouts for each athlete. They are frequently confidantes of the athletes as well and often provide a sympathetic and understanding ear. The athletic trainer treats the entire athlete.

6. What is the function of the athletic training room?

The athletic training room is a medical facility for the care, treatment, and rehabilitation of athletic injuries. It is the domain of the athletic trainer and is most often coeducational. It is also an educational facility for athletic training students. Regulations of the Occupational Safety and Health Administration (OSHA) and universal precautions should be observed for all procedures in the athletic training room.

7. Who is responsible for referral of athletes to the team physician?

The athletic trainer controls referral of athletes to the team physician. By adhering to this chain of communication and authority, the smooth, orderly operation of the athletic training room is maintained. It is important to emphasize to coaches and athletes that the proper communication of each athlete's injuries to the team physician is through the athletic trainer.

8. Which medical records should be kept in the athletic training room?

A medical history for each athlete must be maintained. Injury report forms, progress notes, physician evaluations, referrals, laboratory reports, surgical reports, and physical therapy notes and follow-ups must be included in the medical record. Safeguarding each athlete's medical records is as important in the athletic training room as it is in the physician's office or department of medical records. Because many different professionals work with athletes in the course of their years of competition, the medical record must be complete. The physician should know which records are kept in the athletic training room and ensure their completeness.

9. What is the role of the physician on the sidelines and in the athletic training room?

The athletic trainer and physician predetermine how injuries will be evaluated and treated during competition and practices. The athletic trainer is generally the first to question the athlete about the mechanism of injury and location of pain. After the athletic trainer has made the initial evaluation, the team physician may be called upon for further evaluation. The physician and athletic trainer should have predetermined roles and responsibilities for both on-field and off-field assessment of athletes, and they should practice or drill for emergency situations.

10. Why is communication vital to the athletic trainer–team physician relationship?

Effective communication between members of the entire sports medicine team is crucial for the efficient, prompt, and complete return of the athlete to practice or competition. Coordination of this communication is often the role of the athletic trainer. The athletic trainer functions as an integral part of the team of allied health professionals.

Whenever possible, the athletic trainer should function under standard operating procedures, which preferably are written. The athletic trainer coordinates referrals for the physician. Any professional disagreements that may arise between the physician and athletic trainer should not be communicated to coaches or student athletes. Team physicians should allow athletic trainers to do the tasks that they are trained to do and that they do best. Because athletic trainers work with student athletes and coaches daily, they can be the physician's eyes and ears and provide information important for the decision-making process. Conversely, the athletic trainer must confide in the physician and help the physician to understand the complete athlete. A good relationship between the team physician and athletic trainer enhances the quality of care for athletes.

BIBLIOGRAPHY

1. National Collegiate Athletic Association: NCAA Sports Medicine Handbook. Kansas City, NCAA, 1997.
2. Ray R: Management Strategies in Athletic Training. Champaign, IL, Human Kinetics, 1995.
3. Ingersol C: Management in Athletic Training. St. Louis, Mosby, 1995.
4. National Athletic Trainers' Association, Board of Certification: NATABOC Role Delineation. Philadelphia, F.A. Davis, 1995.

3. THE PREPARTICIPATION EVALUATION

Andrew M. Tucker, M.D.

OBJECTIVES

1. What are the objectives of the preparticipation physical examination (PPE)?

One primary objective of the PPE is detection of underlying medical problems that may limit competition or place a person at "increased risk": for example, exercise-induced bronchospasm, trauma-induced headaches, or hypertrophic cardiomyopathy. Another primary objective is detection of physical deficiencies that may place the participant at increased risk for injury: for example, unrehabilitated ankle sprain or ligament instability of the knee or shoulder. Completion of the PPE fulfills state and local legal requirements.

Other potential objectives include assessment of general health, assessment of fitness so performance can be maximized, and counseling on health-related issues. Finally, the PPE may serve as the athlete's entry into the local health care or sports medicine system, providing for a relationship with the physician, trainer, and/or therapist. Assessment of maturity by Tanner staging or any other means is not an objective of the PPE.

Objectives of the PPE

PRIMARY OBJECTIVES	SECONDARY OBJECTIVES
Detect conditions that may limit participation	Determine general health
Detect conditions that may predispose to injury·	Counsel on health-related issues
Meet legal and insurance requirements	Assess fitness level and performance

From Preparticipation Physical Evaluation,[10] with permission.

METHODS OF PREPARTICIPATION SCREENING

2. What are the methods of preparticipation screening?

PPE can be accomplished by office-based evaluations or mass screening "station" evaluations.

3. What are the advantages and disadvantages of office-based evaluations? Of mass screening evaluations?

Potential Advantages and Disadvantages of Office-based and Station Screening PPEs

OFFICE-BASED PPE	STATION SCREENING PPE
Advantages	*Advantages*
Physician-patient familiarity	Specialized personnel
Continuity of care	Efficient and cost-effective
Opportunity for counseling	Good communication with school athletic staff
	Opportunity for performance testing
Disadvantages	*Disadvantages*
Many athletes don't have a primary care physician	Noisy, hurried environment
Limited time for appointments	Lack of privacy
Varying knowledge of and interest in sports medicine problems	Difficulty following up on medical problems and concerns
Greater cost	Lack of communication with parents
Lack of communication with school athletic staff	

From Preparticipation Physical Evaluation,[10] with permission.

4. What is the recommended frequency of the PPE?

Over three-fourths of the states require annual evaluations for sports participation. Some schools engage in screening evaluations before each new sports season. Many authorities now recommend complete screening examinations at the beginning of a new level of competition (for example, junior high, high school, college), with intercurrent interviews at the start of each new sports season to screen for new problems or evaluate rehabilitation of old injuries. Considerations for choosing the appropriate frequency of examination include requirements of the school or state, degree of risk of the sport, cost, and availability of qualified personnel.

5. What is the ideal timing of the evaluation?

The timing of the PPE must allow sufficient time for adequate rehabilitation/treatment of injuries or further investigation of new findings. However, the evaluation should not take place so far in advance of a season or school year that the development of new problems might become a significant factor. A time frame of 4–6 weeks before a season seems to satisfy both considerations.

CONTENT OF EVALUATION

History

6. Which organ systems should the PPE history focus on?

The history should focus primarily on the cardiovascular, musculoskeletal, and neurologic systems as well as adequately cover questions of general health. If history forms are used, it is important that they be brief, easy to read, understandable by athletes and parents, and allow adequate space for elaboration of positive findings.

7. What are the most important questions for the cardiovascular review of systems?

Certain symptoms can identify at-risk individuals with underlying cardiac abnormalities. The examiner should ask about syncope/near-syncope with exercise, chest pain associated with exercise, easy fatigability, history of palpitations or "racing heart," history of a heart murmur or hypertension or any history of deferred clearance because of cardiac reasons, and family history of sudden cardiac death before age 50. A history of recent severe viral infection may indicate a risk for myocarditis.

8. Asthma is a common condition that limits participation in sports and may go undiagnosed for many years. What questions help identify this condition?

The examiner should inquire about difficulty breathing or wheezing during or after exercise. However, the only complaint may be a persistent cough during or after exercise.

9. What questions adequately cover the neurologic review of systems?

The athlete is questioned about a history of head injuries/concussions, brachial plexus injuries or so-called burners or stingers, transient quadriparesis/quadriparesthesias, seizures, or recurrent headaches.

10. List the questions that are most pertinent for the musculoskeletal review of systems.

The examiner should inquire about previous fractures, dislocations, subluxations, sprains, strains, and tendinitis. Other useful information includes regular use of braces, sleeves, or padding.

11. Why is it important to inquire about a history of heat illness?

Those with a history of a heat-related illness may have an increased likelihood of recurrence.

12. What questions are important to ask the female athlete?

The examiner should ask about the participant's ideal weight, history of weight loss or gain, and menstrual history to screen for indicators of eating disorders, inadequate nutrition, and menstrual abnormalities. Problems in these areas may predispose to injuries such as stress fracture or indicate a significant underlying condition, such as anorexia or bulimia, that may be life-threatening.

The Physical Examination

13. What parts of the physical exam should be emphasized in the PPE?

The physical exam can be relatively brief and focus on areas that are most pertinent to safe participation, specifically the cardiopulmonary and musculoskeletal exams. The examiner must be prepared to pursue other areas of the exam should the patient's history dictate. The physical exam should be performed with the examiner's awareness of the intended sport or sports of participation.

14. Why should height and weight be routinely measured during the PPE and monitored from year to year?

Significantly underweight athletes may arouse concern about malnutrition or eating disorders. Special awareness is needed for those involved in sports in which weight control is especially important (for example, wrestling and gymnastics). Rapid weight gains in a short period of time may raise suspicion about use of anabolic steroids. In addition to height and weight, visual acuity and blood pressure must be checked during each PPE.

15. Is a head and neck exam important for safe participation?

Assuming the history is negative for neurologic problems, the head and neck exam is of little utility in the PPE, except in swimmers and divers. It is also worthwhile to check for pupil equality. In cases of head injury, it is beneficial to have prior documentation of unequal pupils on the screening examination.

16. Differentiating a benign (innocent) murmur from a pathologic murmur is critical. Will the murmur of hypertrophic cardiomyopathy (HCM) increase or decrease with a Valsalva maneuver?

The murmur of HCM should increase with the Valsalva maneuver because the functional outflow tract obstruction increases with a decrease in venous return. It should be noted that some patients with HCM will not have a detectable murmur.

17. If the physical exam or history is worrisome for a significant cardiac abnormality, what is/are the appropriate next step(s) in the evaluation?

Chest x-ray and electrocardiogram (EKG) are appropriate. Authorities have noted if the chest x-ray and EKG are entirely normal, it is unlikely that a young athlete has a significant cardiac abnormality that would put him or her at high risk for sudden death. Cardiac consultation should be sought in cases of indecision. Other tests that may be necessary to clarify the participant's status include stress testing, echocardiography, Holter monitoring, stress echocardiography, and cardiac catheterization.

18. Is an abdominal exam necessary?

Abdominal examination is necessary to rule out hepatic or splenic enlargement. These conditions can accompany mononucleosis, a common infection in the scholastic age group, and may require deferred clearance for sports activities, because the enlarged organ carries an increased risk of rupture.

19. Are genitourinary exams necessary?

The male genitourinary exam is worthwhile because it may detect an undescended testicle, which will affect the young athlete who desires to participate in a collision or contact sport. This simple and quick exam may also uncover an undiagnosed testicular mass. Inguinal hernia may require further consultation to assess the risk of possible complications of this condition.

Pelvic exams in female athletes are indicated if the history reveals abnormalities of the menstrual cycle.

20. Why is the skin exam important in the PPE?

The skin exam is important in contact or collision sports because of risk of contagion to others. A number of dermatologic infections require deferred clearance, including herpes, impetigo, and louse or scabies infestation.

21. What constitutes a good musculoskeletal screening exam for the PPE?

The musculoskeletal exam can be accomplished in a short period of time and emphasizes the documentation of full range of motion and symmetric strength about the major joints. Special attention and further evaluation focus on joints that (a) have been previously injured, or (b) are of particular importance for the sport(s) to be played.

Musculoskeletal Physical Examination

ATHLETIC ACTIVITY (INSTRUCTIONS)	OBSERVATIONS
1. Stand facing examiner	AC joints, general habitus
2. Look at ceiling, floor, over both shoulders, touch ears to shoulder	Cervical spine motion
3. Shrug shoulders (examiner resists)	Trapezius strength
4. Abduct shoulders 90° (examiner resists at 90°)	Deltoid strength
5. Full external rotation of arms	Shoulder motion
6. Flex and extend elbows	Elbow motion
7. Arms at sides, elbows at 90° flexed; pronate and supinate wrists	Elbow and wrist motion
8. Spread fingers; make fist	Hand and finger motion and deformities
9. Tighten (contract) quadriceps; relax quadriceps	Symmetry and knee effusion, ankle effusion
10. "Duck walk" 4 steps (away from examiner)	Hip, knee, and ankle motion
11. Back to examiner	Shoulder symmetry, scoliosis
12. Knees straight, touch toes	Scoliosis, hip motion, hamstring tightness
13. Raise up on toes, heels	Calf symmetry, leg strength

From McKeag DB: Preparticipation screening of the potential athlete. Clin Sports Med 8:373–397, 1989, with permission.

SPECIAL TESTS

22. List some common laboratory tests and discuss their utility in the PPE.

Although urinalyses have been required as part of the PPE in many communities, the literature has shown that it is not a cost-effective screening test in the young population and results in numerous unnecessary referrals. Many authorities are recommending that this test not be done in the screening setting.

Hemoglobin/hematocrit determination is also of questionable benefit in the screening setting. The use of other tests such as ferritin, sickle cell test, blood chemistries, and lipid assays are also not recommended for the screening PPE. The use of EKG, echocardiogram, and exercise stress testing are indicated only when findings on history and physical examination warrant further testing.

CLEARANCE FOR PARTICIPATION

23. List several factors that an examiner might consider when determining a participant's potential clearance for sports.

When considering a participant's potential clearance for an activity, the examiner must consider: (1) Does the problem place the athlete or any other participant at increased risk of injury? (2) Can the athlete safely participate with treatment? (3) Can limited participation be allowed while treatment is being initiated? (4) If clearance is denied for certain activities, are there other activities in which the person may participate?

BIBLIOGRAPHY

1. Ades PA: Preventing sudden death: Cardiovascular screening of young athletes. Phys Sportsmed 20(9):75–89, 1992.
2. Fahrenbach MC, Thompson PD: The preparticipation sports examination: Cardiovascular considerations for screening. Cardiol Clin 10:319–328, 1992.
3. Feinstein RA, Soileau EJ, Daniel WA: A national survey of preparticipation physical examination requirements. Phys Sportsmed 16(5):51–59, 1988.
4. Goldberg B, et al: Pre-participation sports assessment—an objective evaluation. Pediatrics 66:736–745, 1980.
5. Kreipe RE, Gewanter HL: Physical maturity screening for participation in sports. Pediatrics 75:1076–1080, 1985.
6. Linder CW, et al: Preparticipation health screening of young athletes. Results of 1268 examinations. Am J Sports Med 9:187–193, 1981.
7. Lombardo JA: Preparticipation physical examination. Prim Care Clin 11:3–21, 1984.
8. McKeag DB: Preseason physical examination for the prevention of sports injuries. Sports Med 2:413–431, 1985.
9. Peggs JF, Reinhardt RW, O'Brien JM: Proteinuria in adolescent sports physical examinations. J Fam Pract 22:80–81, 1986.
10. Preparticipation Physical Evaluation, 2nd ed [monograph]. Kansas City, MO: American Academy of Family Physicians, American Academy of Pediatrics, American Medical Society for Sports Medicine, American Orthopaedic Society for Sports Medicine, American Osteopathic Academy of Sports Medicine, 1996.
11. Risser WL, Hoffman HM, Bellah GG: Frequency of preparticipation sports examinations in secondary school athletes: Are the university interscholastic league guidelines appropriate? Texas Med 81:35–39, 1985.
12. Thompson TR, Andrish JT, Bergfeld JA: A prospective study of preparticipation sports examinations of 4670 young athletes: Method and results. Cleve Clin 49:225–233, 1982.
13. VanCamp SP: Sudden death in athletes. In Grana WA, Lombardo JA (eds): Advances in Sports Medicine and Fitness 1:121–142, 1988.

4. LIMITING CONDITIONS FOR SPORTS PARTICIPATION

Andrew M. Tucker, M.D.

The vast majority of those presenting for participation in sports will be cleared to participate without any restrictions. Numerous studies have reinforced the low incidence of disqualification from sports as a result of preparticipation evaluations. Although they are relatively infrequent, a variety of conditions may limit participation in sports activities. These conditions may be uncovered during the preparticipation physical examination (PPE) or may arise during participation. The recommendations presented here and in the bibliography are guidelines; each case in practice must be individualized. A widely accepted classification of sports and guidelines for participation in competitive sports are summarized in the tables below.

Classification of Sports

CONTACT		NONCONTACT		
Contact/ Collision	*Limited Contact/Impact*	*Strenuous*	*Moderately Strenuous*	*Nonstrenuous*
Boxing	Baseball	Aerobic dance	Badminton	Archery
Field hockey	Basketball	Crew	Curling	Golf
Football	Bicycling	Fencing	Table tennis	Riflery

(Table continued on following page.)

Classification of Sports (Continued)

CONTACT		NONCONTACT		
Contact/ Collision	*Limited Contact/Impact*	*Strenuous*	*Moderately Strenuous*	*Nonstrenuous*
Ice hockey	Diving	Field (discus,		
Lacrosse	Field (high jump,	javelin, shot put)		
Martial arts	pole vault)	Running/track		
Rodeo	Gymnastics	Swimming		
Soccer	Horseback riding	Tennis		
Wrestling	Skating (ice, roller)	Weightlifting		
	Skiing (cross country,			
	downhill, water)			
	Softball			
	Squash/handball			
	Volleyball			

From Committee on Sports Medicine. Pediatrics 81:737, 1988, with permission.

Recommendations for Participation in Competitive Sports

	CONTACT		NONCONTACT		
	Contact/ Collision	*Limited Contact/ Collision*	*Strenuous*	*Moderately Strenuous*	*Non-strenuous*
Atlantoaxial instability * Swimming: no butterfly, breast stroke, or diving starts	No	No	Yes*	Yes	Yes
Acute illnesses * Needs individual assessment, e.g., contagiousness to others, risk of worsening illness	*	*	*	*	*
Cardiovascular					
Carditis	No	No	No	No	No
Hypertension					
Mild	Yes	Yes	Yes	Yes	Yes
Moderate	*	*	*	*	*
Severe	*	*	*	*	*
Congenital heart disease * Needs individual assessment † Patients with mild forms can be allowed a full range of physical activities; patients with moderate or severe forms, or who are postoperative should be evaluated by a cardiologist before athletic participation.	†	†	†	†	†
Eyes					
Absence or loss of function of eye	*	*	*	*	*
Detached retina * Availability of American Society for Testing and Materials (ASTM)-approved eye guards may allow competitor to participate in most sports, but this must be judged on an individual basis. † Consult ophthalmologist	†	†	†	†	†
Inguinal hernia	Yes	Yes	Yes	Yes	Yes
Kidney: Absence of one	No	Yes	Yes	Yes	Yes
Liver: Enlarged	No	No	Yes	Yes	Yes

(Table continued on following page.)

Recommendations for Participation in Competitive Sports (Continued)

	CONTACT		NONCONTACT		
	Contact/ Collision	Limited Contact/ Collision	Strenuous	Moderately Strenuous	Non-strenuous
Musculoskeletal disorders * Needs individual assessment	*	*	*	*	*
Neurologic					
History of serious head or spine trauma, repeated concussions, or craniotomy	*	*	Yes	Yes	Yes
Convulsive disorder					
Well controlled	Yes	Yes	Yes	Yes	Yes
Poorly controlled * Needs individual assessment † No swimming or weightlifting ‡ No archery or riflery	No	No	Yes†	Yes	Yes‡
Ovary: Absence of one	Yes	Yes	Yes	Yes	Yes
Respiratory					
Pulmonary insufficiency	*	*	*	*	Yes
Asthma * May be allowed to compete if oxygenation remains satisfactory during a graded stress test	Yes	Yes	Yes	Yes	Yes
Sickle cell trait	Yes	Yes	Yes	Yes	Yes
Skin: Boils, herpes, impetigo, scabies * No gymnastics with mats, martial arts, wrestling, or contact sports until not contagious	*	*	Yes	Yes	Yes
Spleen: Enlarged	No	No	No	Yes	Yes
Testicle: Absent or undescended * Certain sports may require protective cup.	Yes*	Yes*	Yes	Yes	Yes

From Committee on Sports Medicine: Pediatrics 81:738, 1988, with permission.

CARDIOVASCULAR CONDITIONS

1. In the young athletic population (less than 35 years of age), list the most common cardiac abnormalities that predispose to sudden death.

Hypertrophic cardiomyopathy, idiopathic left ventricular hypertrophy, anomalous left coronary artery, Marfan's syndrome, myocarditis, congenital valvular disorders, and conduction system disorders (e.g., idiopathic long QT syndrome).

2. What questions would you ask a prospective high school athlete to screen for underlying cardiac abnormality?

Important historical features include a history of passing out during or immediately after exercise (possible underlying hypertrophic cardiomyopathy, conduction abnormality, arrhythmia, or valve problem), chest pain with exercise (possible congenital abnormality of the coronary arteries, advanced premature atherosclerotic disease), unusually easy fatigability (valvular disorder or underlying lung pathology), history of a "racing heart" or skipped beats (arrhythmias or conduction abnormalities), history of high blood pressure, history of a known heart murmur or a family history of sudden cardiac death in a family member under age 50 (hypertrophic cardiomyopathy, Marfan's syndrome, or prolonged QT syndrome, all of which have a familial component. A history of a recent severe viral illness may be a clue for myocarditis.

3. You are examining a prospective high school athlete and you hear a soft systolic murmur at the left lower sternal border during physical examination. What characteristics of the murmur would alert you to the possibility that this murmur may represent an underlying hypertrophic cardiomyopathy?

The murmur of hypertrophic cardiomyopathy may be amplified by having the patient perform a Valsalva maneuver or assume a standing position. These maneuvers decrease the venous return to the heart and subsequently the left ventricular end-diastolic volume, thus functionally increasing the outflow tract obstruction and increasing the murmur.

4. Should any restrictions be placed on a young athlete diagnosed with mild-to-moderate hypertension?

According to the guidelines of the 26th Bethesda Conference, the presence of mild-to-moderate hypertension in the absence of target organ damage or other heart disease should not limit participation in any competitive sports. For athletes with severe hypertension, participation should be restricted until the hypertension is controlled either by lifestyle modification or medication, particularly athletes engaged in high static sports (see classification in the 26th Bethesda Conference document).

5. List the classification of sports in which participation would be allowed in an athlete with a diagnosis of myocarditis.

Myocarditis is an acute illness, usually of viral etiology, that can potentially cause sudden death or chronic cardiac dysfunction. According to the AAP Policy Statement, myocarditis should disallow participation in any of the categories of sports. These athletes should be followed by a cardiologist and undergo thorough cardiac evaluation at rest and with exercise before determining return to any form of competition.

6. Marfan syndrome can cause sudden death in a young athlete, and, depending on the manifestations of the disease, may be a limiting condition for sports. List some common characteristics of Marfan syndrome.

Marfan syndrome is an inherited connective tissue disorder that may affect several organ systems. Manifestations may involve the cardiovascular, musculoskeletal, and ophthalmologic systems. Cardiovascular manifestations may include dilated aortic root secondary to cystic medial necrosis. Complications include severe aortic insufficiency, ruptured aortic aneurysm, or aortic dissection. Musculoskeletal manifestations may include disproportionately long limbs, arachnodactyly, and deformities of the thorax and vertebral column, including pectus excavatum, pectus carinatum, and kyphoscoliosis. Ocular manifestations, present in 70% of patients, may include ectopia lentis, a dislocation of the lens. Dermatologic manifestations of Marfan syndrome occur in only about one-fourth of patients. Striae distensae is the most common skin manifestation and occurs most frequently on the abdomen, buttocks, and upper thorax. Family history is very important, with 85% of cases occurring in people who have a family member diagnosed with the disorder.

NEUROLOGIC CONDITIONS

7. What are the considerations in limitation of participation of an athlete with a history of seizures?

A person with a history of seizures should not participate in scuba diving, rope and rock climbing, gymnastics on high apparatus, parachuting, hang gliding, or high diving. In persons with well-controlled seizures, participation in any other sports should not be limited provided that seizures are not precipitated by contact and/or collision sports. In athletes with poorly controlled seizures, clearance for most other sports is deferred until a 1-month seizure-free interval is obtained and the neurologic exam is normal. Consultation with a neurologist may be necessary.

Athletes may still participate in several noncontact sports if there is no risk to themselves or other participants. Examples of noncontact sports that would be contraindicated if seizures are not well controlled are swimming, weightlifting, javelin, shot put, discus, archery, and riflery.

8. Brachial plexus neurapraxia (so-called burner or stinger) is a common injury in contact and collision sports such as football and wrestling. Describe the clinical manifestations and discuss the parameters for return to play.

A brachial plexus neurapraxia is usually a stretch or compression injury to the brachial plexus that results in pain and paresthesias down the affected arm with associated weakness. Symptoms are usually transient, with resolution within a few to several minutes. The examiner must differentiate the more serious cervical spine injury from the common stinger. Athletes with symptoms involving both arms or transient quadriparesis must be thoroughly evaluated, including a referral to an orthopedic or neurosurgeon. Following the simple burner, the participant may return to play when asymptomatic and when the exam is normal. Recurrent burners may require further evaluation, including cervical spine films and MRI.

9. A high school football player sustains a concussion in a game on Friday night. He apparently did not lose consciousness but was disoriented for several minutes and had posttraumatic amnesia for 15 minutes. He had a persistent headache following the head injury and was not allowed to return to play. He presents to your office on Monday morning, desiring clearance to return to practice that day. Neurologic exam is normal. He does continue to have a frontal headache with some inability to concentrate in the classroom. What are your recommendations for return to play?

Guidelines for return to participation and competition following a head injury are somewhat controversial. Existing guidelines have been published and are referenced at the end of the chapter. Concerning this case, the player is still symptomatic, given the headache and decreased ability to concentrate. As long as these postconcussive symptoms are present, his activity should be limited. Recommendations for return to competition vary, but almost all would agree that the athlete must be without symptoms for a few to several days before gradually increasing activities and returning to participation. Many team physicians recommend that when an athlete is without symptoms, aerobic and strength training may be started for 1–2 days. If no symptoms recur with activities, resumption of contact activity may then be considered.

DERMATOLOGIC CONDITIONS

10. List examples of skin infections that preclude participation in contact or collision sports.

Impetigo, herpes, scabies, louse infestation, molluscum contagiosum, furuncles, and carbuncles. The patient would be cleared to return to contact/collision sports when the infection resolves or is no longer contagious.

MUSCULOSKELETAL CONDITIONS

11. Explain the considerations for allowing a volleyball player to return to competition after a moderate ankle sprain.

Before the athlete is returned to vigorous activities or competition, the injured ankle should demonstrate minimal pain, swelling, and tenderness on exam. Range of motion of the ankle should be almost equal to that of the opposite side. Strength of the muscle groups responsible for ankle motion should be essentially symmetrical with the unaffected side. The participant should be able to demonstrate basic functional tests such as running, jumping, and cutting activities without problems before being returned to play.

ABDOMINAL CONDITIONS

12. A competitive swimmer is found to have splenomegaly secondary to mononucleosis. Her acute symptoms have improved significantly but the splenomegaly has yet to resolve. She is anxious to return to swimming. What are your recommendations?

The risk of splenic rupture is small and is usually associated with contact or collision sports. However, there have been case reports of splenic rupture in strenuous noncontact sports. It is advised to withhold an athlete from contact and collision sports and strenuous noncontact sports such as swimming until resolution of splenomegaly. If the examination is unclear, an ultrasound scan may be obtained to document resolution.

13. Should an athlete with an inguinal hernia be limited from contact/collision sports?

In the past, a participant with an inguinal hernia was precluded from all but noncontact activities. Currently the recommendation is that an athlete with such a finding should not be withheld from any activity unless the hernia is symptomatic. Athletes with symptomatic hernias will require treatment at some time. Each case is evaluated individually and recommendations depend on the desired sport.

SINGLE PAIRED ORGANS

14. Discuss the factors involved in allowing an athlete with a single functional eye to participate in sports.

Defining loss of function of an eye is controversial and should be made in consultation with an ophthalmologist. According to the new edition of the Preparticipation Evaluation monograph, the functionally one-eyed athlete will now be defined by the American Academy of Ophthalmology as one who has the best corrected vision in one eye poorer than 20/40. In general, for sports in which no eye protection can be worn, such as boxing, martial arts or wrestling, participation should be contraindicated for single-eyed participants. In other sports involving a high risk of injury, including racquetball, baseball, and football, consideration for clearance of participation involves the availability and effectiveness of protective eye guards. The sports physician and the consulting ophthalmologist should discuss the issues with the athlete, his or her parents, school administrators, and coaches. The discussion should include the risk of injury to the uninvolved eye, the level of protection available, and the long-term consequences of injury to the uninvolved eye.

Similarly, risk of injury, availability of protective devices, and ramifications of injury should be considered when athletes with any single paired organ such as kidney or testicle desire to participate in a contact/collision sport. Oftentimes the athlete and parents are asked to sign a special consent form acknowledging awareness and understanding of the risk involved and acceptance of that risk. Although an exculpatory waiver or risk release should be signed by the athlete or parents, some experts question the adequacy of protection for a physician against lawsuits.

BIBLIOGRAPHY

1. Ades PA: Preventing sudden death: Cardiovascular screening of young athlete. Phys Sportsmed 20(9): 75–89, 1992.
2. American Academy of Pediatrics Committee on Sports Medicine: Atlantoaxial instability in Down's syndrome. Pediatrics 74:152–154, 1984.
3. Cantu RC: Functional cervical spinal stenosis: A contraindication to participation in contact sports. Med Sci Sports Exerc 25:315–317, 1993.
4. Cantu RC: Guidelines for return to contact sports after a cerebral concussion. Phys Sportsmed 14(10):75–83, 1986.
5. Colorado Medical Society. Report of the Sports Medicine Committee: Guidelines for the management of concussions in sports (revised). Denver, Colorado Medical Society, 1991.
6. Fahrenbach MC, Thompson PD: The preparticipation sports examination: Cardiovascular considerations for screening. Cardiol Clin 10:319–328, 1992.

7. Maron BJ, Mitchell JH: 26th Bethesda Conference: Recommendations for determining eligibility for competition in athletes with cardiovascular abnormalities. J Am Coll Cardiol 24:846–899, 1994.
8. National Heart, Lung and Blood Institute: Report of the Second Task Force on Blood Pressure Control in Children—1987. Pediatrics 79:1–25, 1987.
9. Nelson MA: Medical exclusion from participation in sports. Pediatr Ann 21:149–155, 1992.
10. Nelson WE, Jane JA, Gieck JH: Minor head injury in sports: A new system of classification and management. Phys Sportsmed 12:103–107, 1984.
11. Practice Parameter: The management of concussion in sports. Neurology 48:581–585, 1997.
12. Preparticipation Physical Evaluation, 2nd ed [monograph]. Kansas City, MO: American Academy of Family Physicians, American Academy of Pediatrics, American Medical Society for Sports Medicine, American Orthopaedic Society for Sports Medicine, American Osteopathic Academy of Sports Medicine, 1996.
13. Torg JS, Glasco SG: Criteria for return to contact activities following cervical spine injury. Clin J Sports Med 1:12–26, 1991.

5. EVALUATING THE SEVERELY INJURED ATHLETE

Brian C. Halpern, M.D., FAAFP, and Matthew H. Rosen, M.D.

1. Who is responsible for the care of the injured athlete on the field?

This question is answered by first identifying the medical personnel on the field. If there is a team physician, that person is responsible for all of the medical care that is administered on the field. If the team physician is not present, the athletic trainer assumes the ultimate responsibility for the treatment of athletes on the field.

2. What are the components of adequate preparation for an on-field emergency?

- Someone must be designated as the team leader, responsible for supervising on the field care.
- Appropriate health care personnel should be on or readily accessible to the field to assist the team leader.
- All the necessary emergency equipment should be at the site of the potential injury.
- Ambulance transportation to a hospital or neurosurgical center must be immediately available for high-risk sports and on call for other sports.
- Telephone link-up should be available to the emergency room, ambulance, or trauma center.
- Various injury scenarios should be worked through before the actual occurrence.

3. What equipment should be available for an emergency?

Equipment List for Emergencies

Mandatory for head, neck, and other neurologic and orthopedic trauma		
Spine board	Bolt cutters/knife/screwdriver	Sand bags
Stretcher	Rigid cervical collar	
Mandatory for cardiac basic CPR and ACLS (usually supplied by the ambulance)		
Oral and nasal airway	Intravenous D5/Ringer's lactate	BP cuff
Oxygen w/mask	Military antishock trousers	18- and 14-gauge catheters
Suction	Cardiac monitor/defibrillator	Crash cart with cardiac and
Endotracheal tube	Stethoscope	anaphylactic medications

(Table continued on following page.)

Equipment List for Emergencies (Continued)

For general care			
Scissors	Blankets	Tongue depressors	Eye kit with eye chart
Foil	Ace bandages	Gauze	Irrigation kit
Tape	Splints	Adhesive bandages	Scalpel
Bandages	Crutches	Hemostats	Syringes and needles
Penlight	Slings	Suture kits	Thermometer
Otoscope/ophthalmoscope	Ice	Alcohol & Betadine swabs	Sterile gloves

4. Do you need all of the items on the equipment list for every possible sports event?

No. The equipment listed is for coverage of football games. Other, less contact-oriented events require fewer materials at the site. Ambulance coverage at the sporting event can usually be arranged; the ambulance should be equipped with all items that may be needed.

5. Are bolt cutters still the best method to remove face masks?

Face masks have been redesigned such that it is much easier to use a knife or pruning shears or even a screwdriver to remove the face mask. However, bolt cutters are still appropriate if they are available.

6. Should you continue to have an esophageal obturator airway available in your doctor's bag?

The esophageal obturator airway is no longer in vogue because of the complications related to its insertion. If you need to advance beyond an airway for artificial ventilation, intubation is more appropriate.

7. Describe the initial assessment of the downed athlete on the field.

During initial assessment, maintain close and continuous observation and take all the time necessary to evaluate the athlete. Use the letters ABCDE as a guide for a step-by-step assessment.

A   Airway and cervical spine
B   Breathing
C   Circulation
D   Disability
E   Exposure

8. How do you assess the airway?

Look and listen for spontaneous breathing. If the athlete is face down, the airway cannot be assessed; he or she must be brought to the face-up position by the "log roll" (see figure, top of next page). The body must be maintained in line with the head and spine during the roll. Then airway access is established by removing the face mask. Because a cervical spine injury should be suspected the airway should be opened using the chin lift or the jaw thrust techniques (while someone maintains in-line traction). The airway can then be cleared with a finger sweep or suction. If the airway remains obstructed, only then should a slow, gentle head tilt be added until the airway is open.

9. When should a cervical spine injury be suspected?

When a player sustains an injury above the clavicle or a head injury that results in an unconscious state, an associated cervical spine injury should be suspected.

10. How quickly should the helmet be removed when a cervical spine injury is suspected?

Do not remove the helmet at all when you suspect a cervical spine injury until the patient has been cleared with a cross-table lateral x-ray of the cervical spine. If the EMT personnel attending the game try to remove the helmet, the team leader should intervene and explain that helmet removal on the field is different from removal of a motorcycle helmet; motorcycle riders do not wear shoulder pads.

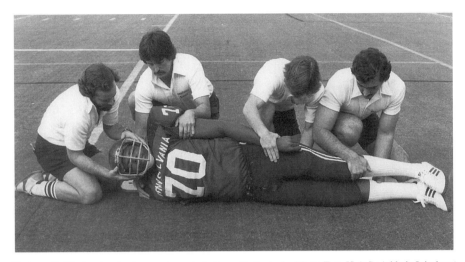

The log roll. The head and spine must remain in line with the body. (From Torg JS (ed): Athletic Injuries to the Head, Neck and Face. Philadelphia, Lea & Febiger, 1982, with permission.)

11. When should a laryngeal fracture or marked laryngeal edema be suspected?

Stridor, hoarseness, anterior neck pain, bony crepitus, or subcutaneous emphysema may be signs of laryngeal fracture. In such instances, needle cricothyroidotomy might need to be considered. It is performed by palpating the cricothyroid membrane and puncturing the skin with a 14-gauge catheter over-needle directed at a 45° angle caudad. Aspiration signifies entry into the tracheal lumen and ventilation is possible through the catheter.

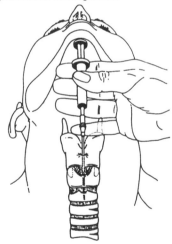

Needle cricothyroidotomy.

12. How do you assess circulation?

Check the carotid pulse for quality, rate, and regularity. If the pulse is absent, begin CPR.

13. When assessing disability, what is an easy way to grade a limited neurologic examination? What is a more extensive examination?

A limited neurologic examination may be graded with the letters AVPU:

A   Alert
V   Response to vocal stimuli
P   Response to painful stimuli
U   Unresponsive

A more extensive examination is the Glasgow Coma Scale:

The Glasgow Coma Scale

INDICATION	RESPONSE	SCORE
Eyes open	Spontaneously	4
	To verbal command	3
	To pain	2
	No response	1
Best motor response:		
To verbal command:	Obeys	6
To painful stimulus:	Localizes pain	5
	Flexion—withdraws	4
	Flexion—abnormal (decorticate rigidity)	3
	Extension (decerebrate rigidity)	2
	No response	1
Best verbal response:		
Arouse patient with	Oriented and converses	5
painful stimulus, if	Disoriented and converses	4
necessary	Inappropriate words	3
	Incomprehensible sounds	2
	No response	1
	Total	3–15

From Friedman WA: Head injuries. CIBA Clinical Symposia 34(4), 1983, with permission.

14. What is meant by assessing exposure?
The extremities and other body parts should be inspected for bleeding, fractures, and contusions.

15. Which system complexes must be evaluated in every significant extremity injury?

Vascular	Osseous	Muscular	Skin and subcutaneous
Neural	Ligamentous	Tendinous	tissue

BIBLIOGRAPHY

1. American Heart Association: Textbook of Advanced Cardiac Life Support. 1994.
2. Cantu RC, Micheli LJ (eds): ACSM's Guidelines for the Team Physician. Philadelphia, Lea & Febiger, 1991.
3. Friedman WA: Head Injuries. CIBA Clinical Symposia 34(4):1, 1983.
4. Halpern BC: Injuries and emergencies on the field. In Mellion MB, Walsh WM, Shelton GL (eds): The Team Physician's Handbook, 2nd ed. Hanley & Belfus, 1997, pp 36–52.
5. Halpern BC: Down man on the field. Prim Care 18:833–849, 1991.

6. INJURIES AND EMERGENCIES ON THE FIELD

Brian C. Halpern, M.D., FAAFP, and Matthew H. Rosen, M.D.

CARDIOVASCULAR EMERGENCIES

1. What is the most common cause of death on the playing field?
Cardiovascular death. Hypertrophic cardiomyopathy (idiopathic hypertrophic subaortic stenosis) is the most common cause in athletes under 35 years of age. Coronary artery disease is the most common cause in athletes over 35 years of age.

2. What is the best way to identify the athlete at risk for a cardiovascular death?

Preparticipation history is the most important factor in identifying the athlete at risk for cardiovascular death. Two questions that are vital to ask are (1) "Has there been any history of syncope or near syncope with exercise?"; and (2) "Has anyone in your immediate family died under the age of 50 from cardiac death?" These two questions alert the team physician to investigate the player's history further and to pay close attention to the athlete's cardiovascular status.

3. If an athlete has hypertrophic cardiomyopathy (idiopathic hypertrophic subaortic stenosis), is a murmur always audible?

Probably not. Often the murmur is not audible, but detection may depend on the ability and expertise of the physician. Provocative maneuvers are important in distinguishing this murmur from other murmurs. The murmur of hypertrophic cardiomyopathy increases with the Valsalva maneuver and decreases with squatting.

4. In the athlete with a history of anaphylaxis to bee stings, should administration of epinephrine after a bee sting be delayed until manifestations appear?

No. An athlete with a history of allergic reaction to a bee sting should be given epinephrine immediately. The adult dose is 0.3 mg of a 1:1000 solution.

HEAD INJURIES

5. What types of head injuries occur on the playing field?

Diffuse brain injuries, which are concussive-type syndromes, are the most common, but other more focal syndromes, such as epidural, subdural, or intracerebral hematoma, also occur. Concussion is a clinical syndrome characterized by immediate and transient posttraumatic impairment of neural function, such as alteration of consciousness, vision, or equilibrium, caused by brainstem involvement.

6. How is a head injury evaluated on the field?

When evaluating a head injury, one should look for these signs: Did loss of consciousness occur? Is there any element of amnesia, specifically posttraumatic amnesia? Was there a history of paresthesia or weakness in any of the extremities or obvious neurologic abnormalities?

7. How do you treat the athlete who is decompensating from a closed head injury?

1. Consider hyperventilation, trying to bring $PaCO_2$ down to 22–30 mmHg. This will decrease cerebral edema.
2. Consider intravenous dexamethasone.
3. Use mannitol as a diuretic, and try to keep the serum osmolarity less than 320 mOsm/L.
4. Monitor intracranial pressure and try to keep it less than 15 mmHg.

8. What vital sign changes after a head trauma are an ominous finding?

Hypertension and bradycardia, referred to as the Cushing reflex, are signs of increasing intracranial pressure. A rapid change from bradycardia to tachycardia and hypertension to hypotension is usually a sign of brain stem herniation.[7]

9. Is there one standard classification of concussive syndrome?

No. There are many classifications. My classification combines two of these. I divide the mild head injuries into three grades—I, II, III—and depend on the grading system to determine when the athlete can return to play. The only athlete permitted to return to play the same day of injury is one who has a mild, grade 1 concussion with no loss of consciousness and no amnesia. The injured athlete should be observed frequently on the sidelines and probably allowed to return after about 10–20 minutes if he or she demonstrates no sequelae of head injury and no postconcussive syndrome (see question 10). It is important to have the athlete exercise on the sidelines, running back and forth, to try to elicit symptoms before return to play is allowed. If exercise reproduces the symptoms, the athlete is restricted from play.

Assessment of a Head Injury

	MILD			MODERATE	SEVERE
DIAGNOSIS	I	II	III		
Loss of consciousness	—	—	—	< 5 min	> 5 min
Amnesia	—	+ retrograde	+ retrograde and post-traumatic	+ retrograde and post-traumatic	+ retrograde and post-traumatic
Confusion	Slight	Increased	More pronounced	Obvious	For 5 or more min
TREATMENT					
ABCDE	+	+	+	+	+
Immobilize cervical spine and transport to hospital for radiographic and further evaluation	–/+ if also have neck pain or abnormal neurologic or cervical examination			+	+
Observation out of hospital	+	+	+	–	–
Transportation to hospital for neurosurgical consultation, CT scan/MRI, and close observation	–	–	–	+	+
Consider hyperventilation to Pco 22–30 mmHg, dexamethasone 1 mg/kg, and maintain serum osmolarity at less than 320 mOsm/L	–	–	–	–	+
Return to play the same day if: appropriate evaluation on sidelines is negative: no headache, irritability, inability to concentrate, or obvious changes in functions (as in normal dexterity, strength, and speed), no photophobia, is first concussion	+	–	–	–	–

Data from Cantu RC: Guidelines for return to contact sports after a cerebral concussion. Phys Sportsmed 14(10):75, 1986.

10. What are the signs of postconcussive syndrome?
1. Headache
2. Irritability
3. Inability to concentrate
4. Any obvious changes in functions, such as dexterity, strength, and speed
5. Any psychomotor abnormalities.

Athletes should not be allowed to return to participation when they are demonstrating any of these postconcussive signs because they are more susceptible to more severe injury at this time.

NECK INJURY

11. What is the approach to an athlete with a potential neck injury?
First, find out if the athlete has had paresthesia in any of the extremities. If there have been paresthesias or dysesthesias in both the arm and the leg on one side, you must immobilize the athlete on the field. Likewise, an injured athlete should be immobilized immediately if he or she has bilateral symptoms in the arms or legs. If the symptoms are unilateral in one arm, one might consider this a brachial plexus type of injury but continue to evaluate the cervical spine.

With the helmet still on the athlete, palpate the posterior cervical spine for any tenderness. If there is significant tenderness or guarding, the athlete should be immobilized on the field and transported. If the history is negative for paresthesias or dysesthesias and the initial palpation of the cervical spine reveals no tenderness or spasm, then ask the athlete actively to flex and extend the neck slowly and gently to see if there is pain or guarding. If there is pain or guarding, then the athlete should be immobilized and transported for radiographic evaluation of the cervical spine. Passive motion is not appropriate—only active motion determines injury at this time. If the athlete has no history of dysesthesias or paresthesias in any extremities, has no tenderness to palpation on physical examination, has full range of motion without discomfort in the neck, and has not suffered additional head injury with this trauma, return to play should be allowed.

12. Radiographically, what is a significant finding for instability of the cervical spine?

1. Greater than 3.5 mm of displacement of one vertebral body on another.
2. Greater than 11° interspace angle in lateral or flexion and extension radiographs.

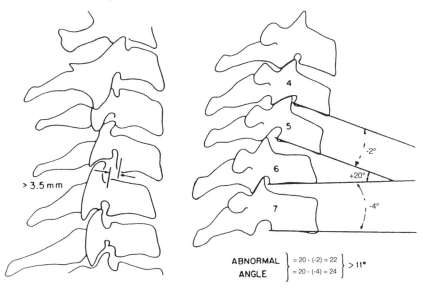

The method for determining translatory displacement, as described by White et al. Using the posteroinferior angle of the superior vertebral body as one point of reference and the posterosuperior angle of the vertebral body below, the distance between the two in the sagittal plane is measured. A distance of 3.5 mm or greater is suggestive of clinical instability. (From Torg JS, Glasgow SG: Clin J Sports Med 1:14, 1991, with permission.)

Abnormal angulation between two vertebrae at any one interspace is determined by comparing the angle formed by the projection of the inferior vertebral body borders with that of either the vertebral body above and/or the vertebral body below. If the angle at the interspace in question is 11° or greater than either adjacent interspace, this is considered by White et al. as clinical instability. (From Torg JS, Glasgow SG: Clin J Sports Med 1:14, 1991, with permission.)

13. Besides head injury and cervical spine injury, what is another potential cause of neurologic deficits resulting from blunt trauma to the head and neck?

Injury to the carotid artery can result from a stretch, traction, or rotation injury, from compression between the mandible and upper cervical transverse processes, or from a direct blow to the neck. Symptoms may appear immediately, within 24 hours, or up to 6 months after the injury. Signs and symptoms may include unilateral headache, aphasia, Horner's syndrome, transient ischemic attack, bruit, hemiparesis in an alert patient, hemianesthesia, neck hematoma, and unilateral facial weakness. Angiography is the test of choice for evaluating carotid artery injury.[3]

EYE INJURY

14, What are some danger signs associated with blunt eye injuries?

Sudden loss of vision	Protrusion of one eye
Loss of field of vision	Blood in the anterior chamber
Photophobia	Irregularly shaped pupil
Diplopia	Foreign body sensation
The patient sees flashing lights	Red eyes

15. How are eye injuries managed?
- For eyelid edema, use crushed ice in a baggie.
- Shield an injured eye.
- Do not allow the athlete to blow his or her nose, because this may cause subcutaneous emphysema with concomitant orbital fracture.

ABDOMINAL AND PELVIC INJURIES

16. With trauma to the abdomen and pelvis, what sequelae should the physician be thinking about?

Trauma to the abdomen can result in injury to, for example, the spleen, pancreas, liver, bowel, kidney, urethra, testicles, aorta, and vena cava. The key to successful management is rapid detection of a vascular or visceral injury and control of hemorrhage and abdominal contamination.

17. When should a spleen injury be suspected? What is the appropriate diagnostic work-up?

Left shoulder or neck pain, abdominal pain in the left upper quadrant, and left lower rib fracture are all associated with spleen injury. CT with a contrast agent is probably the best evaluation, although ultrasound and a spleen scan also are useful.

18. If someone presents with an abdominal injury and right shoulder pain, should you be thinking of a rotator cuff problem?

No. The liver and subphrenic irritation from a possible liver laceration or liver contusion should be considered. Appropriate assessment of the abdomen is important at this time.

19. If an athlete has an abdominal injury with an expanding lesion within the rectus abdominis, what would be the initial diagnosis?

An expanding rectus hematoma would cause a somewhat rigid abdomen, a lot of tenderness over the rectus, and this expanding lesion. The treatment is appropriate assessment with either CT or MRI. If the lesion continues to expand rapidly, aspiration may be indicated.

20. Does hematuria in an athlete always signify renal, bladder, or urethral trauma?

No. Microscopic and frank hematuria may result just from strenuous exercise. But in the face of trauma to the flank or abdomen, injuries to these areas should be considered. Appropriate work-up would be rapid-sequence intravenous pyelogram, CT scan with a contrast agent, or both.

EXTREMITY INJURY

21. What initial treatment is most appropriate for extremity injuries?
1. Splint the injury.
2. Cover any wound with a moist dressing.
3. Reduce any dislocation after a neurovascular check.
4. Transport the patient immediately, especially after a neurovascular injury.
5. Rest, ice, compression, and elevation (RICE).

BIBLIOGRAPHY

1. Cantu RC: Guidelines for return to contact sports after a cerebral concussion. Phys Sportsmed 14(10):75–83, 1986.
2. Cantu RC, Micheli LJ (eds): ACSM's Guidelines for the Team Physician. Philadelphia, Lea & Febiger, 1991.
3. Carr S, Troop B, Hurley J, Pennell R: Blunt-trauma carotid artery injury: Mild symptoms may disguise serious trouble. Phys Sportsmed 24(2): 1996.
4. Halpern BC: Injuries and emergencies on the field. In Mellion MB, Walsh WM, Shelton GL (eds): The Team Physician's Handbook, 2nd ed. Philadelphia, Hanley & Belfus, 1997, pp 36–52.
5. Halpern BC: Down man on the field. Prim Care 18:833–849, 1991.
6. Haycock CE: How I manage abdominal injuries. Phys Sportsmed 14(6):86–99, 1986.
7. Lawrence PF (ed): Essentials of General Surgery. Baltimore, Williams & Wilkins, 1988, p 147.

7. SPORTS MEDICINE AND THE LAW*

Elizabeth M. Gallup, M.D., J.D., M.B.A.

1. What types of physicians are team physicians?

Team physicians hail from all areas of medicine. In the recent past, the majority of team physicians were orthopedic surgeons. However, in the 1990s, many team physicians are primary care physicians, most often family physicians, internists, pediatricians, and emergency physicians.

2. How often are team physicians sued?

Fortunately, team physicians are sued infrequently. Most team physicians who have been sued in the past are those who care for professional athletes. A handful of team physicians have been sued on the collegiate level.

3. What is the legal theory by which team physicians are sued?

Team physicians are sued on the same basis, in general, as any other type of physician—the laws of negligence. To sue a team physician successfully under the laws of negligence, the plaintiff (athlete) must prove all four elements of negligence: (1) the team physician had **a duty** to act in a certain manner; (2) the team physician **breached** that duty; (3) the breach of the duty **caused damages** to the athlete; and (4) the damages are **identifiable** in some way. Without proving all four elements, the plaintiff will not be successful in suing a team physician.

4. Are team physicians every protected from liability?

Team physicians may be protected from liability under a Good Samaritan statute. Good Samaritan statutes have been enacted by state legislators to encourage physicians and others to provide care to those who are in an emergency situation. Generally, if a physician's actions are governed by a Good Samaritan statute, the team physician is liable only if his or her actions would be considered wantonly or willfully reckless, which is a more difficult standard to prove than the standard for negligence. Thus, in effect, Good Samaritan statutes help to protect team physicians from lawsuits.

5. Are all Good Samaritan statutes alike?

Absolutely not. Good Samaritan statutes vary from state to state in language and degree of protection. Therefore, it is essential for team physicians to ascertain the specific language and coverage of the Good Samaritan statutes in their state.

* Extracted from Gallup EM: Law and the Team Physician. Champaign, IL, Human Kinetics, 1995.

6. What are the usual elements of a Good Samaritan statute?

Most Good Samaritan statutes provide protection for team physicians while they are caring for athletes under these conditions:

• At the scene of the athletic event (therefore, they are not operational for care rendered in the office or hospital)
• The team physician receives no remuneration for the care rendered
• There is an emergency

7. What is the standard of care to which team physicians are held?

Team physicians have a duty to act according to an accepted standard of care. This standard of care is determined in a court of law by the testimony of expert witnesses. Both the plaintiff and the defendant (the team physician) have experts who testify on their behalf as to what they believe would have been appropriate conduct in the case at trial. This testimony then helps to define what they believe should have been the standard of care against which the physician's conduct is measured. The experts may be required to be in the same specialty as the team physician (e.g., a family physician testifies as an expert in a lawsuit against a family physician) or they may have to be only in the same specialty area (e.g., an orthopedic surgeon may testify against a family physician in a case involving a knee injury).

DRUG USE AND THE ATHLETE

8. What should a team physician do if he or she knows an athlete is taking steroids or growth hormone?

The team physician should counsel the athlete with a balanced discussion that addresses not only the potential harms of using steroids and/or growth hormone but also the potential benefits such as increased muscle mass. In most states, it is a crime for physicians to prescribe steroids to athletes except in exceptional circumstances. However, just because an athlete is on steroids does not mean that the team physician should abandon the athlete. Rather, the team physician should be available for counseling the athlete regarding tapering of the steroids. Some team physicians even monitor known steroid-abusing athletes for potential side effects, including elevations of blood pressure and lipoproteins.

9. Is it appropriate for team physicians to be involved in drug testing programs?

I would recommend against involvement by team physicians in the administration of drug testing programs. Team physicians may want to be involved in setting policies and procedures, but if a team physician is involved in choosing the athletes to be tested and testing them, there is a serious risk of damage to the physician/athlete relationship. Athletes might not seek counseling from a team physician who they feel may violate their right to confidentiality.

CONTROVERSIES

10. What is the most legally valid preparticipation examination—the short, focused preparticipation examination or the all-inclusive lengthy preparticipation examination?

This depends on whom you ask. The advocates of a lengthy all-inclusive preparticipation examination note, probably correctly, that the preparticipation examinations are often the only contact that athletes have with physicians. Therefore, this interaction must be detailed and include a thorough evaluation and counseling about not only the athlete's participation in sports but also other topics such as birth control and drug use. Advocates of the short, focused exam note that it often is impractical to perform a lengthy exam on every athlete and that the purpose of the preparticipation examination is to identify athletes who are at risk for injury or illness if they participate in sports. Regardless of which examination format is chosen, it is essential that the athlete be evaluated in a quiet environment and be given individualized attention by the physician and that special attention be given to the cardiac examination and the musculoskeletal system. It is also essential to obtain a thorough history.

11. Should athletes with one kidney or one eye be allowed to participate in contact sports such as football or hockey?

In the past, such athletes were routinely denied clearance to participate in contact sports. Several lawsuits against school systems, however, have compelled them to allow athletes with one kidney or one eye to participate in the sport of their choice. If the athlete is a minor, it is recommended that he or she be denied clearance and that the parents of the athlete pursue participation through the court system. If the courts compel participation and something untoward occurs, the team physician will, more likely than not, be shielded from liability.

12. Should the athlete who is denied clearance be allowed to execute an exculpatory waiver and then be allowed to participate?

An exculpatory waiver is a document that has elements of informed consent, assumption of risk, and a release of liability. In the recent past, exculpatory waivers were not widely used because courts generally found them invalid against public policy. However, their use is becoming increasingly widespread. It is important to remember that an exculpatory waiver is a contract and as such can be executed only by adult athletes (generally those older than 18 years of age). Parents usually are not allowed to execute an exculpatory waiver on behalf of their minor child. Before a team physician considers executing an exculpatory waiver, he or she should seek legal advice regarding state law that governs the use of exculpatory waivers and the language that should be contained therein.

13. Should athletes with human immunodeficiency virus (HIV) infection be denied participation in athletics?

Both the World Health Organization and the American Academy of Pediatrics (AAP) have issued guidelines regarding athletes infected with HIV. Neither set of guidelines precludes athletes from participating in any sport they desire. The AAP's guidelines state that physicians should strongly encourage HIV-positive patients to participate in sports other than those that may involve blood exposure.

II. *Special Populations*

8. QUESTIONS PARENTS ASK ABOUT THE YOUNG ATHLETE

Morris B. Mellion, M.D.

1. "Should my child play competitive sports?"
Properly organized youth sports programs can offer a positive growth experience for children. Children are not merely small adults. Their needs are quite different. The quality of their experience depends on effective coaching and effective parenting.

2. Are there enough youth sports coaches?
Over 20 million children participate in non-school youth sports programs. Over 2.5 million volunteer coaches are necessary to meet their needs. An estimated 800,000 new coaches are needed each year. Most of these are volunteers. They have little or no formal training and tend to fall back on their own personal past athletic experience, which is usually at a higher level of participation than they are coaching.

3. What resources are available to train youth sports coaches?
The American Coaches Effectiveness Program (ACEP) was developed by Rainer Martens, PhD, a leading sports psychologist, as a system for training entry-level coaches, as well as for providing ongoing higher-level training for those with more experience. The text for ACEP Level I courses, *Coaching Young Athletes*, is available to the public. The addresses of ACEP and three other major organizations concerned with the training and competency of youth coaches are given below.

Organizations Concerned with the Training and Competency of Youth Coaches

American Coaching Effectiveness Program PO Box 5076 Champaign, IL 61820	Little League Baseball, Inc. PO Box 3485 Williamsport, PA 17701
Canadian National Certification Program Coaching Association of Canada 333 River Road Ottawa K1L 8H9 Canada	National Youth Sports Coaches Association 2611 Okeechobee Road West Palm Beach, FL 33409

4. What is the central issue in coaching young athletes?
The value of youth sports is proportional to the child's opportunity to grow as a person while also having fun. "Winning" is clearly secondary. The exaggerated emphasis on winning that characterizes so many sports on television should not be carried over to youngsters.

Effective coaches teach children the proper balance between competition and cooperation. In sports for the youngest children, it is not even necessary to keep score. As the children get a little older and their skill and interest increase, the intensity of competition should rise in proportion.

5. What is the role of self-esteem?

Well-trained coaches boost children's self-esteem more than those without experience. Moreover, children with low self-esteem are the most vulnerable. They have the greatest need for good athletic experience. They can gain more from good coaching and suffer more from bad coaching than children with high self-esteem.

6. What is the ideal relationship between parents and coach?

Parents, too, play a major role in the athlete's experience. This is represented graphically by the athletic triangle below. Note that with skillful parenting and effective coaching, the triangle is filled with fun and growth. When one or both is absent, the triangle and the athletic experience may be hollow.

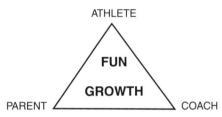

The athletic triangle. (From Mellion MB: Office Management of Sports Injuries & Athletic Problems. Philadelphia, Hanley & Belfus, 1988.)

7. What is the key issue in effective parenting of the young athlete?

Here again the issue is self-esteem. Positive reinforcement by the parents is critical. To paraphrase Blanchard and Johnson[2] in *The One Minute Manager*, "Walk around looking for your child to do something right." Repeated praise for gradually increasing skills enhances self-esteem and motivation to participate.

8. What is the parents' role on the sideline?

On the sideline, the parents should encourage and support. Young children find it difficult to understand or appreciate their parents arguing with the coach or with an official.

9. What is "the vicarious athlete"?

The vicarious athlete is a parent who pressures a child to excel in athletics so that the parent can experience the child's success vicariously. A common pattern is that the vicarious athlete, who may be either the father or the mother, recruits the spouse into an alliance that continues this behavior. The result is an extremely confining and bizarre form of support and encouragement.

The parents place an ever-increasing set of expectations on their child, and the child begins to narrow athletic participation to a single year-around sport. Any success is met immediately with a new set of higher performance expectations. The child may feel trapped. The only way out of the sport without disappointing the parent(s) is to become injured. These children develop injuries that are typical of their sport: gymnasts have back pain, skiers have knee pain, and swimmers have sore shoulders. These situations are clearly major diagnostic challenges for physicians, and they demand well-honed communications skills to change the painful pattern.

10. What is the key characteristic of effective parents?

Their children know that they are loved for who they are and not for how they perform, either on the playing field or in the classroom.

11. "Should I coach my own child?"

It is estimated that one coach is necessary for eight children participating in youth sports. Consequently, in many cases, if the parent does not coach, there will be no team for the child. Coaching effectiveness training becomes a tremendous asset in this situation.

12. "How do I treat my own child when I am coaching?"

Focus approval or criticism to the specific effort made or skill demonstrated. Avoid global criticism with children. Praise your own child's effort moderately on the field and more generously on the way home.

13. Are there age guidelines for youth sports participation?

Many physical educators accept the following guidelines, but the greatest consideration is the level of the child's emotional and physical maturity.

Age Guidelines for Beginning Participation in Competitive Youth Sports

AGE	TYPE OF SPORT	EXAMPLES
6	Noncontact	Swimming Tennis Track and field
8	Contact	Basketball Soccer Wrestling
10	Collision	Tackle football Ice hockey

14. What is the best way of organizing youth sports into different levels of participation in the peripubertal years?

Because the onset of puberty varies normally from 8.5 to 13.0 years in girls and 9.5 to 13.5 years in boys, age-based athletic classifications may lead to marked mismatches in strength, coordination, and size. Whenever it is possible, match participants using the generally accepted Tanner levels of sexual maturation. This approach requires a great deal of tact and sensitivity. It is not used widely because it often cuts across school grades and other social patterns.

15. Should boys and girls play together?

There is general consensus that boys and girls can play safely together before puberty. After puberty, the situation has been controlled by litigation. When girls have sued for the right to participate in football, wrestling, and other contact and collision sports with boys, they have consistently won.

16. Would children rather *play* on a losing team than *sit* on the bench of a winning team?

When sports psychologist Rainer Martens asked this question in a survey, more than 90% indicated they would rather play on a losing team than sit on the bench of a winning team. Youth sports should involve a commitment that every child plays at least half of every game.

17. Are there dangerous sports that children should avoid?

Boxing and trampoline may present extreme risks. The American Medical Association, the American Academy of Family Physicians, and the American Academy of Pediatrics have all issued statements opposing boxing for children because of a perceived high risk of head injury and chronic brain damage. There is some debate about whether this risk is as high as assumed in amateur boxing. On the other hand, there also is a concern about sports in which the goal of the sport may be hitting and intimidating another child. A major inconsistency in this argument is that the same concern is not expressed as intensively about football and hockey.

The trampoline has a valid role in youth sports, but it should be used *only* under the immediate supervision of highly trained instructors; therefore, the trampoline should be secured in a locked space when a qualified instructor is not present.

18. Is there a recognized set of guidelines for youth sports?

The American Alliance for Health, Physical Education, Recreation and Dance has developed the Bill of Rights for Young Athletes.

The Bill of Rights for Young Athletes

Right to participate in sports
Right to participate at a level commensurate with each child's maturity and ability
Right to have qualified adult leadership
Right to play as a child and not as an adult
Right of children to share in the leadership and decision-making of their sport participation
Right to participate in safe and healthy environments
Right to proper preparation for participation in sports
Right to an equal opportunity to strive for success
Right to be treated with dignity
Right to have fun in sports

Reprinted with permission of the American Alliance, for Health, Physical Education, Recreation and Dance, 1990 Association Drive, Reston, VA 22091.

19. Can prepubertal and pubertal athletes gain significant strength through weight training?

Yes. Young athletes can make significant gains in strength through weight training. The greatest component of their improvement is from skill development, but an increment of actual strength increase is present. The major gains in pure strength come after the hormonal changes of puberty.

20. Is strength training safe for children?

Many opinions and concerns exist about the safety of strength training for children, but there is a paucity of data available. There is a growing consensus that strength training supervised by a coach trained to teach age-specific strength training is relatively safe.

21. Are there some guidelines for strength training in young athletes?

In 1985, the American Orthopaedic Society for Sports Medicine (AOSSM) and the National Strength Coaches Association each developed sets of guidelines. The common guidelines suggested by both groups include (1) the need for preparticipation physical examination; (2) the requirement that the child have adequate emotional maturity to accept coaching; (3) supervision by competent coaches trained in strength training specifically for the age group; (4) strength training only as part of a broader program designed to increase other motor skills and fitness levels; (5) adequate warm-up and cool-down; (6) all exercises performed through full joint range of motion; (7) no lifting to attain the individual's maximum single repetition capacity; (8) initial training without resistance to learn proper techniques; (9) 6–15 repetitions per set; (10) small load increments (maximum 3 pounds) when building up resistance levels; (11) 20–30-minute strength training sessions up to three times per week. The AOSSM guidelines also prohibit competition and call for emphasis on concentric lifting rather than eccentric lifting. (In concentric lifting, the major resistance occurs while the muscles are shortening and tightening, whereas in eccentric lifting resistance occurs while the muscles are lengthening and releasing.)

22. Are young children more susceptible to injury than older children?

In fact, younger children have many fewer injuries than older children and the rate of injury increases with age until the high school years. The increase is probably related to the fact that high school athletes are generally postpubertal and, consequently, stronger, larger, and faster. The injury incidence rises in proportion to the intensity of the contact involved in the sport and to the increased moment of force of a faster, larger body in noncontact injuries.

23. Are girls more likely to be injured than boys?

In sports in which both boys and girls participate, the injury rates are the same. Overall, boys have a higher total injury rate because they tend to play in more contact and collision sports.

BIBLIOGRAPHY

1. American Academy of Pediatrics: Committee on Sports Medicine: Weight training and weight lifting: Information for the pediatrician. Pediatrics 86:801–803, 1990.
2. Berg K: Youth sports issues. In Mellion MB, Walsh WM, Shelton GL (eds): Team Physician's Handbook, 2nd ed. Philadelphia, Hanley & Belfus, 1997, pp 67–72.
3. Blanchard K, Johnson S: The One Minute Manager. New York, Berkley Publishing Group, 1983.
4. Cahill BR, Griffith EH: Effect of preseason conditioning on the incidence and severity of high school football knee injuries. Am J Sports Med 6:180–184, 1978.
5. Garrick JG, Requa RK: Injuries in high school sports. Pediatrics 61:465–469, 1978.
6. Goldberg B, Witman PA, Gleim GW, Nicholas JA: Children's sports injuries: Are they avoidable? Phys Sportsmed 7(9):93–101, 1979.
7. Jackson DW, Wiltse LL, Dingeman RD, Hayes M: Stress reactions involving the pars interarticularis in young athletes. Am J Sports Med 9:304–312, 1981.
8. Lillegard WA: Strength training for the young athlete. J Back Musculoskel Rehabil 1:29–37, 1991.
9. Maffulli N, Pintore E: Intensive training in young athletes. Br J Sports Med 24:237–239, 1990.
10. Martens R: The uniqueness of the young athlete: Psychological considerations. Am J Sports Med 8:382–385, 1980.
11. Martens R, Christina RW, Harvey JS, Sharkey BJ: Coaching Young Athletes. Champaign, IL, Human Kinetics Publishers, 1981.
12. Mellion MB: Special issues in youth sports. In Mellion MB (ed): Office Sports Medicine, 2nd ed. Philadelphia, Hanley & Belfus, 1996, pp 65–79.
13. National Strength and Conditioning Association: Position paper on prepubescent strength training. Natl Strength Condit Assoc J 7:27–31, 1985.
14. Smith RE, Smoll FL, Curtis B: Coach effectiveness training: A cognitive-behavioral approach to enhancing relationship skills in youth sport coaches. J Sports Psychol 1:59–75, 1979.
15. Smoll FL, Smith RE: Psychology of the young athlete—stress-related maladies and remedial approaches. Pediatr Clin North Am 37:1021–1046, 1990.
16. Tursz A, Crost M: Sports-related injuries in children: A study of their characteristics, frequency, and severity, with comparison to other types of accidental injuries. Am J Sports Med 14:294–299, 1986.
17. U.S. Public Health Service: Physical activity in children. Am Fam Physician 50:1285–1288, 1994.
18. Wilkins KE: The uniqueness of the young athlete: Musculoskeletal injuries. Am J Sports Med 8:377–382, 1980.
19. Zaricznyj B, Shattuck LJM, Mast TA, et al: Sports-related injuries in school-aged children. Am J Sports Med 8:318–324, 1980.

9. THE FEMALE ATHLETE: PERFORMANCE EXPECTATIONS

Rebecca Jaffe, M.D., FAAFP, FACSM

1. Why is a chapter about female athletes so difficult to write?

Because there are not many well-done, conclusive studies of female athletes of varying ages to derive generalizations about their performances.

2. Can boys and girls safely compete together on the playing field?

Before puberty, as long as children are "sized up," they can compete side by side.

3. Can young girls participate in 5-K and 10-K runs?

According to the American Academy of Pediatrics Committee on Sports Medicine, "provided the child is enjoying the activity and is without symptoms, there is no reason to preclude (him or) her from training for the participating in such events."

4. What are the main goals in youth sports?

That the child have fun, improve skills, stay in shape, and learn to compete.

5. What determines how high a VO_2max a child can attain?

The amount and intensity of training seem to determine the VO_2max.

6. Are there performance differences in different phases of the menstrual cycle?

Physically, women have broken world records in phases of the menstrual cycle; however, when surveyed, female athletes state that their performance declines during menses.

7. Why have women's performances improved so dramatically over the past 20 years?

1. More women participate (bigger talent pool).
2. Women receive better coaching.
3. Women have more opportunities to compete at higher levels.

8. Does exercise affect estrogen?

Strenuous exercise lowers estrogen levels but does not necessarily affect performance.

9. Why is performance altered at higher altitudes? How long does it take to adapt?

Because there is less oxygen at higher altitudes, the body must make more red blood cells to compensate. A well-trained athlete takes 12–32 days to adapt; however, faster results have been obtained using a hypobaric chamber.

10. What is periodization? How does it work?

Periodization is a training method, developed by the Soviets, to maximize performance. It divides the workout period into five phases, each about 4–6 weeks in length: preparation (overall conditioning), strength phase, strength/power phase (fine-tune strength and work on power and speed), maintenance, and active rest (recovery). The athlete works to excel throughout the schedule to peak during the maintenance phase.

11. Does athletic performance decline after adolescence?

Not necessarily. With proper training and motivation, many athletes continue to improve their performance. Over half the 8,000 entrants in the 1989 Boston marathon were over 40 years of age.

12. What is the best way to improve performance in distance running?

In distances longer than 1,500 meters, maximal oxygen uptake is the most important variable and can be improved through training techniques. Also of importance are stride length and anaerobic capacity and power, which also can be improved with training.

13. Can women strength-train without developing gross muscle hypertrophy?

Definitely. Women can gain great improvements with strength training without gaining noticeable muscle mass, probably because of lower androgen levels.

14. Are female athletes more prone to injury?

No. With equal training, there appears to be no increase in injury.

15. What is the one determinant of structural and physiologic characteristics?

Genetic endowment.

16. Is there an optimal body fat percentage for top performance?

No. There is wide variation in body fat percentage among competitive athletes. For example, body fat among elite runners ranges from 10–20%.

17. Which female athletes have the highest VO$_2$max?

Cross-country skiers, rowers, Alpine skiers, cyclists, and distance runners.

18. Will women ever be able to run faster than men?

We do not know yet. We do know that women have improved their running by 14 meters per minute per decade compared with men at 7 meters per minute. However, because of physical differences, it is unlikely that women will surpass men in short distances, but some will become competitive. In long distances and ultradistances (longer than a marathon), women have a good chance to surpass men. It is thought that women's naturally higher body fat may act as a back-up energy supply. In addition, women initiate sweating at higher body temperatures, which may conserve water.

19. Do women currently excel in any particular sport?

Yes. Women outperform men in long-distance swimming. A good example is the swim across the English Channel.

20. How well do women compete in international competition?

It depends on the competition. During the 1992 Winter Olympics, all five U.S. gold medals were won by women. Women accounted for 34% of the U.S. team, yet won 82% of the medals.

Medals Won in the Last 10 Winter Olympic Games

	WOMEN	MEN	SHARED (PAIR SKATE)
Albertville, 1992	9	2	
Calgary, 1988	3	2	1
Sarajevo, 1984	3	4	1
Lake Placid, 1980	4	8	
Innsbruck, 1976	6	3	1
Sapporo, 1972	7	1	
Grenoble, 1968	3	2	
Innsbruck, 1964	2	4	
Squaw Valley, 1960	6	3	1
Cortina, 1956	2	5	

21. Do oral contraceptives affect women's athletic performance?

Few studies address this issue. The literature suggests that there may be subtle physiologic changes, but none that greatly affect performance.

22. Do iron supplements enhance performance?

They enhance performance in athletes who are iron-deficient.

23. Are special foods or vitamins necessary for optimal performance?

A balanced diet of adequate calories is the best performance enhancer. Athletes who restrict calories or do not vary foods need diet counseling or supplements. Vegetarians may lack vitamin B12 and require supplements. Vitamin E is popular; however, its proven benefits are few and are seen only at higher altitudes.

24. Does pregnancy affect athletic performance?

Up to the first 2 or 3 months, pregnancy appears to have no negative effects on performance. In the 1956 Melbourne Olympics, reportedly three gold medal winners were known to be pregnant.

There were also reports of an ergogenic benefit of early pregnancy and of purposeful insemination for optimal performance by Eastern European women competitors; however, no scientific research corroborated the reports.

25. Does pregnancy alter postpregnancy performance?

No. If the athlete gets back in shape, she should have no difficulty in competing. One study indicates that there is a small but significant increase in VO_2max immediately after delivery in women who maintain moderate-to-high levels of exercise during and after pregnancy.

26. Does exercise improve bone density in women?

No. Exercise only maintains density. It probably is helpful in building stronger bones in adolescents who take adequate calcium.

27. How long can one continue to compete in endurance events?

There is no age limit. Women over the age of 80 run marathons regularly. Their times are slower (5 hr), but they can complete the course.

28. When does the aging process begin? How is it affected by exercise?

People who exercise on a regular basis and maintain healthy lifestyles (e.g., healthy diet, no smoking) appear to delay the morbidity and disability associated with an inactive lifestyle. A modest increase in life span and a higher quality of life are noted by people who exercise regularly. Lean body tissue is gradually lost, eventually leading to a decrease in maximal cardiac output, maximal oxygen consumption, strength, and performance. This loss happens at different ages for different individuals.

29. Is the decline in physical working capacity and the increase in body fat in the elderly due to advancing age?

Only to a limited extent; it is more likely due to decrease in daily physical activity than to age.

30. What parameter has shown that an active 50-year-old woman is physiologically two decades younger than a sedentary woman of the same age?

VO_2max.

BIBLIOGRAPHY

1. Agostini R (ed): The athletic female. Clin Sports Med 13(2), 1994 [special issue].
2. Blair S, Kohl HW III, Paffenbarger RS Jr, et al: Physical fitness and all causes of mortality: A prospective study of healthy men and women JAMA 262:2395–2401, 1989.
3. Brandon LJ, Boileau RA: Influence of metabolic, mechanical and physique variables in middle distance running. J Sports Med Phys Fitness 32:1–9, 1992.
4. Clapp JF, Capeless E: The VO_2max of recreational athletes before and after pregnancy. Med Sci Sports Exerc 23:1128–1133, 1991.
5. Moller-Nielsen J, Hammar M: Sports injuries and oral contraceptive use: Is there a relationship? Sports Med 12:153–160, 1991.
6. Richalet P, et al: Use of a hypobaric chamber for pre-acclimatization before climbing Mount Everest. Int J Sports Med 13(Suppl 1):S216–220, 1992.
7. Risser WL, et al: Iron deficiency in female athletes: Its prevalence and impact on performance. Med Sci Sports Exerc 20:116–121, 1988.
8. Robinson BE: The changing scope of prevention in late life. Clin Rep Aging 2:1–21, 1988.
9. Shangold MM, Mirkin G (eds): Women and Exercise: Physiology and Sports Medicine. Philadelphia, F.A. Davis, 1988.
10. Simon-Schnass I, Kornizewski L: The influence of vitamin E on rheological parameters in high-altitude mountaineers. Int J Vitam Nutr Res 60:26–34, 1990.
11. Simon-Schnass I, Pabst H: Influence of vitamin E on physical performance. Int J Vitam Nutr Res 68:49–54, 1988.
12. Wells C: Women, Sports and Performance, 2nd ed. Champaign, IL, Human Kinetics, 1991.

10. THE FEMALE ATHLETE: EXERCISE, OSTEOPOROSIS, AND BIRTH CONTROL

Constance Marie Lebrun, B.Sc., M.D.C.M., M.P.E., C.C.F.P., FACSM, Dip. Sport Med. (CASM)

GENERAL QUESTIONS

1. Are there physiologic differences between male and female athletes?
There are biomechanical factors and skeletal system differences. The female athlete is usually (but not always) smaller and shorter, with a wider pelvis, as compared with the male. Her knees slant inward and her legs are less bowed. She also may have shorter limbs relative to her leg length, narrower shoulders with more slope, and a greater "carrying angle" of the elbows. These characteristics may lead to an increased incidence of certain injuries such as patellofemoral pain syndrome. In addition, female athletes generally have a higher percentage of body fat and about 30% less muscle strength than males, primarily in the upper extremities. Nevertheless, the majority of sports injuries are sport-specific rather than gender-specific.

2. Describe some of the significant differences in the cardiovascular system of female and male athletes.
The female athlete has a smaller heart, with a faster heart rate and a lower blood volume than the male. She has approximately 15% less hemoglobin and about 6% fewer red blood cells. These differences all combine to give a lower maximal aerobic capacity ($\dot{V}O_2$max) as compared with a similarly trained male. This capacity is typically up to 50% less, but when corrected for percentage body fat, the difference shrinks to 16%. If $\dot{V}O_2$max is calculated per kilogram of lean body mass, elite female athletes are only about 9% behind their male counterparts.

3. Is exercising beneficial for women?
Regular physical exercise has similar training effects in both men and women: decreased blood pressure, lowered heart rate, and improved aerobic capacity, as well as a decrease in percentage of body fat. All of these changes help to protect against atherosclerosis and heart disease. In addition, weight-bearing exercise promotes the deposition of strong and healthy bone to prevent osteoporosis.

4. Are there any contraindications for women who exercise?
Previous superstitions about athletic participation, particularly during menstruation, have largely been eliminated with better education and with modern conveniences such as tampons. It also used to be thought that women might somehow damage their reproductive systems with vigorous exercise, but this has been shown to be a myth as well. In actual fact, the male testes are much more vulnerable to injury and in need of protection during certain sporting activities!

THE MENSES

5. Describe the different phases of a regular ovulatory menstrual cycle.
Normal menstrual cycles can vary from 23 to 35 days in length, with an average of about 28 days. The first 3–5 days, when menstrual flow is occurring, is called the *menstrual* phase. The *follicular*, or *proliferative*, phase extends from the first day of menstruation until ovulation. During this time, both estrogen and progesterone levels are low. Throughout the cycle, the hypothalamus secretes gonadotropin-releasing hormone (GnRH), which in turn stimulates production

36

of the pituitary gonadotropins luteinizing hormone (LH) and follicle-stimulating hormone (FSH). Ovulation is preceded by a surge in LH through a positive feedback mechanism of the rising levels of estradiol from the developing follicle. Although these events generally occur between days 13 and 15, stress and a variety of other factors can cause ovulation to be delayed. The *luteal*, or *secretory*, phase lasts from ovulation until the onset of the next menses. During this phase, estrogen and progesterone levels remain high due to secretion by the corpus luteum. If conception does not occur, then the decline in the concentrations of the steroid hormones results in menstruation, which is the desquamation of the endometrium. The complex hormonal changes that take place during the course of an ovulatory cycle are shown schematically below.

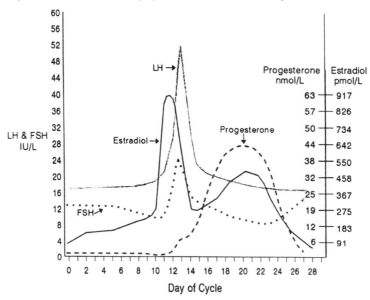

Adapted by Dr. J. C. Prior from Speroff L, Van de Wiele RL: Regulation of the human menstrual cycle. Am J Obstet Gynecol 109:234–247, 1971, with permission.

6. How might a woman be able to tell if she is ovulating?

Symptoms suggestive of ovulation include lateral breast tenderness, fluid retention, appetite changes, and mood changes during the second half of the cycle. Collectively, these symptoms are called *molimina*. In moderation, they signal that the neuroendocrine axis is functioning adequately and that regular ovulation is occurring. In excess, they can become troublesome as the constellation known as *premenstrual syndrome* (PMS). Other methods of detecting ovulation include measurement of *basal body temperature* (BBT). During the second phase of the cycle, the increased progesterone causes a rise in the core body temperature and, therefore, a biphasic curve. The newer urinary ovulation detection kits can also be used to determine the time of the maximal LH surge (ovulation takes place shortly afterward). Accurate determination of the menstrual cycle phase, however, requires measurement of the female sex steroids, estradiol and progesterone.

7. Can the phase of the menstrual cycle affect athletic performance?

During an ovulatory menstrual cycle, changing concentrations and ratios of estrogen and progesterone can cause alterations in vascular volume dynamics, temperature, ventilation, and substrate metabolism. Nevertheless, there are no conclusive studies showing variations in performance during the menstrual cycle. Individual athletes may be adversely affected by weight gain and fluid retention or by severe menstrual cramping (*dysmenorrhea*). Regular physical exercise has been shown to be beneficial in reducing premenstrual symptoms. Antiprostaglandin medications may be used to treat dysmenorrhea.

8. Can the menstrual cycle be affected by exercise?

Exercising female athletes can be subject to a variety of menstrual cycle disorders, including delayed menarche, primary amenorrhea, oligomenorrhea, secondary amenorrhea, shortened luteal phase, and anovulation. There can be significant health concerns with any form of menstrual dysfunction.

9. At what age does menarche usually occur?

Normal onset of menstrual cycles (*menarche*) generally begins at about 12.8 years of age, with the development of secondary sex characteristics (*thelarche*) occurring 1–2 years earlier. A girl is considered to have *primary amenorrhea* if she has not started menstruating by age 16, or has not yet begun to develop breasts or pubic hair by the age of 14. In some girls, there may be a constitutional delay in menarche. *Secondary amenorrhea* refers to the cessation of periods once regular menstruation has already been established.

10. What is the difference between amenorrhea and oligomenorrhea?

Amenorrhea has had many definitions, but the currently accepted one is no menstrual cycles for at least 3 months, or less than 2 periods in a year. *Oligomenorrhea* is defined as 3–6 menstrual cycles per year, or cycles at intervals greater than 38 days.

11. What are the other menstrual cycle changes that can be seen?

Athletic women may also have a *shortened luteal phase* (less than 10 days in duration) or *anovulatory cycles*. With these menstrual variations, a woman may still appear to be having regular menstrual bleeding. In many cases, a difficulty in conceiving can be the first indication to the athlete and her physician that these disorders may be present.

12. How common are these menstrual cycle changes in female athletes?

Amenorrhea occurs in about 3–5% of the general population, but can be found in between 15 and 60% of exercising women. The other disorders, such as oligomenorrhea, short luteal phase, and anovulation are also more common in athletic females, but are more difficult to detect, and therefore the real incidence is not known.

13. What is the pathophysiology of athletic amenorrhea?

The etiology is currently postulated to be multifactorial and includes low body weight, rapid weight loss, sudden onset of vigorous exercise, inadequate nutrition for the energy needs, and psychological and physical stress. A current hypothesis is that there is a reduction in the gonadotropin-releasing hormone (GnRH)-generated pulsatile surges of LH that normally would lead to ovulation, but elevated endorphins, melatonin, and cortisol may also play a role. Some researchers espouse the theory of "energy drain," whereby athletic amenorrhea is a physiologic adaptation to the negative energy balance caused by the combination of inadequate caloric intake and increased daily energy expenditure.

14. How should a physician evaluate an athlete presenting with amenorrhea?

Athletic amenorrhea is a diagnosis of exclusion. The physician must first exclude other causes, including pregnancy, thyroid and other endocrine disorders, androgen excess, prolactinoma, polycystic ovarian syndrome, and genetic abnormalities. A good history and physical examination should suggest possible diagnoses and can be followed with appropriate laboratory tests (see table, top of next page).

15. How should an athlete with these problems be managed?

Once other pathologies have been excluded, administration of a 5-day course of medroxyprogesterone acetate (10 mg/day) can be used to evaluate the uterine tract. Any withdrawal bleeding can be taken as evidence that the pituitary axis is intact and the endometrium is functioning normally. Treatment solutions can then include a slight reduction in the amount of training (5–10%), a slight increase in weight (5%), and proper attention to such factors as nutrition, stress,

Evaluation of Amenorrhea

History
 Menstrual history (including moliminal symptoms)
 Development of secondary sexual characteristics
 Physical activity—frequency, intensity, duration, recent changes
 Gynecologic and sexual history—age of menarche, pregnancies, contraception
 Nutritional history, including weight gain/loss, potential eating disorders
 Conflicts and support systems—home, work, social, coping skills
 Symptoms of estrogen deficiency (dyspareunia, hot flushes) or androgen excess
 Galactorrhea, headaches, sense of smell, visual disturbances
 Medications
 Family history

Physical Examination
 General examination—height, weight, stigmata of syndromes such as Turner's
 Fundi, visual fields (by confrontation)
 Tanner stage—breast development, axillary and pubic hair
 Thyroid
 Breasts—galactorrhea
 Pelvic examination—normal sexual organs, polycystic ovaries, vaginal dryness, clitoromegaly
 Acne and hirsutism (symptoms of androgen excess)

Investigations
 Pregnancy test
 Thyroxine (T_4), thyroid-stimulating hormone (TSH)
 Prolactin
 Follicle-stimulating hormone (FSH), luteinizing hormone (LH)
 Karyotype (women under age 30 with elevated FSH and amenorrhea, or absent uterus)
 Testosterone and dehydroepiandrosterone sulfate (DHEAS) (if signs of androgen excess)
 Consider imaging of pituitary, pelvis, bone age, depending on other findings

---

and sleep. If the menstrual cycles do not resume spontaneously after 6 months, then it may be necessary to stimulate them with clomiphene (if pregnancy is desired) or to give replacement hormones. In a young woman who is sexually active, this can be accomplished by giving oral contraceptives, although some concerns remain about the potential for further suppression of the neuroendocrine axis. In other women, estrogen and/or progesterone therapy may be required, usually estrogen, 0.625 mg daily on days 1–25, and medroxyprogesterone, 10 mg daily on days 16–25.

16. Why is it so important to treat amenorrhea in women, athletic or otherwise?
 In some women, the biggest problem is infertility. An increased incidence of scoliosis and stress fractures has been demonstrated in amenorrheic dancers, and other athletes have been shown to have more musculoskeletal injuries. The greatest unseen risk from a prolonged period of amenorrhea, however, is a loss of bone density, or premature osteoporosis. It is thought that other types of menstrual dysfunction (such as oligomenorrhea, shortened luteal phase, and anovulation) also lead to a decreased bone density. Estrogen, and possibly progesterone as well, has a protective effect on bone by increasing the absorption of calcium and its uptake and deposition into bone. The loss of estrogen may also theoretically increase blood lipid levels and lead to premature atherosclerosis. There may also be a higher incidence of cancer of the reproductive organs.

OSTEOPOROSIS

17. Exactly what is osteoporosis?
 Osteoporosis is a systemic skeletal disease characterized by low bone mass and microarchitectural deterioration of bone tissue, with a consequent increase in bone fragility and susceptibility

to fracture risk. It may result from the loss of bone that was already present, a failure to lay down adequate amounts of bone during a critical time of life, or a combination of both.

18. How is bone formed?

Bone is constantly being remodeled by cells that resorb bone (*osteoclasts*) and by other cells that lay down or deposit bone (*osteoblasts*). There are two types of bone: *cortical bone*, which makes up two-thirds of the skeleton (present in the shafts of long bones), and *trabecular bone*, which traverses the internal cavities (found in the vertebrae and pelvis, flat bones, and the ends of long bones). The latter type of bone is more metabolically active, with a greater rate of turnover.

19. Why should I worry about osteoporosis in my patients?

Osteoporosis can lead to painful compression fractures of the vertebrae (causing progressive kyphosis and "dowager's hump"), but it also may lead to fractures of the wrist, humerus, and proximal femur. Hip fractures in elderly women cause significant morbidity and are often "the beginning of the end," with loss of independence and the ability to carry out the activities of daily living. The health care costs for these ailments can add up to billions of dollars per year.

20. Are there any tests to predict or detect osteoporosis?

By the time osteoporosis is evident on plain radiographs, there has already been at least a 20–30% loss in bone density. Other tests such as single photon absorptiometry (SPA), dual energy x-ray absorptiometry (DEXA), or quantitative computed tomographic (CT) scanning can be used to measure bone density, but these tests are expensive and not suitable for mass screening. There are a number of risk factors for osteoporosis (see below), but these predict only about 70% of women who will develop osteoporosis.

Risk Factors for Osteoporosis

Slender body habitus and fair skin
Race (European/Asian descent)
Family history of premature osteoporosis
Early menopause (including oophorectomy and possibly athletic amenorrhea)
Advanced age
Nulliparity
Sedentary lifestyle
High consumption of cigarettes, alcohol, caffeine
Corticosteroid use

21. Isn't osteoporosis a disease of postmenopausal women?

Osteoporosis usually occurs in older women but may occur much earlier in life under certain circumstances. It is now thought that 60–70% of a woman's peak bone mass is laid down during the adolescent growth spurt and that bone mass declines gradually after age 35 until the menopause, when the lack of the female reproductive hormones, estrogen and progesterone, causes a much more rapid bone loss. The amenorrheic athlete is analogous to the postmenopausal woman in that she also has lowered levels of the reproductive hormones. This has been shown to have a detrimental effect on bone density, which is at least partly irreversible. In a young athlete with either prolonged amenorrhea or recurrent stress fractures, decreased bone density must be ruled out. These problems may be initially detected on a screening preparticipation physical examination.

22. How can premature osteoporosis be treated?

The best treatment is prevention, and reduction of risk factors. There is a critical "window of opportunity" for establishment of strong and healthy bone in the adolescent and young adult. In athletes with altered menstrual cycles, an adequate calcium intake (at least 1500 mg of elemental calcium per day) also is essential. Food sources include milk and milk products, canned salmon with bones, and dark green leafy vegetables. Additional supplementation may be necessary, with calcium carbonate and calcium citrate preparations giving the best absorption. Restoration of normal menses is ideal, but if this does not occur with the strategies already outlined, then serious consideration should be given to hormonal replacement, either with estrogen and/or progesterone. In sexually active women desiring contraception, the combination oral contraceptive pill may be prescribed. There has been a recent surge of interest in the "osteoprotective properties" of oral contraceptives. Other treatments that are used in postmenopausal women, such as etidronate, alendronate, or calcitonin, have not been tested extensively in young female athletes. Regular weight-bearing exercise also is important in athletes of all ages, but in women with established osteoporosis, flexion exercises of the spine (i.e., situps) should be avoided because of the risk of vertebral compression fractures.

BIRTH CONTROL

23. What are the contraceptive options for female athletes?

Sexually active female athletes must consider birth control, even if they are amenorrheic, as ovulation can occur irregularly and unpredictably. Options include abstinence (not acceptable for many!); barrier methods, such as the condom and spermicidal jelly, or a diaphragm, or cervical cap, and spermicidal jelly; intrauterine devices (IUD); and the oral contraceptive pill. Long-acting injectable or implantable forms of progesterone are available for women who cannot tolerate estrogen. The vaginal sponge has been taken off the market because of complications related to infection and disintegration of the material and an unacceptably high pregnancy rate. The barrier methods, especially the condom, have an advantage in decreasing the incidence of sexually transmitted diseases and, in addition, do not interfere with the hypothalamic pituitary axis. Effectiveness rates of these methods depend on the motivation of the user and on correct usage. The IUD is more reliable in terms of pregnancy prevention than barrier methods, but there is a greater potential for pelvic inflammatory diseases. The increase in menstrual flow (menorrhagia) and cramps (dysmenorrhea) associated with use of IUDs may be disruptive for many female athletes and may also cause iron deficiency anemia, all of which may have a negative effect on performance.

24. What about oral contraceptives in the athlete?

The newer low-dose triphasic oral contraceptives contain much lower total hormone concentrations than the older formulations, so their corresponding side effects (weight gain, fluid retention, detrimental effects on serum lipids and hemostatic mechanisms) have been greatly decreased. Combination pills containing the newer third-generation progestins (desogestrel, gestodene, and norgestionate) have even fewer androgenic side effects because of an enhanced selectivity for the progestin receptors. Beneficial effects of oral contraceptives include elimination of dysmenorrhea and reduction in iron deficiency anemia, benign breast lesions, pelvic inflammatory disease, ovarian cysts, and rheumatoid arthritis. In addition, pill users have a decreased risk of both ovarian and endometrial cancer. These medications can now be safely used in nonsmoking women from age 16 (or 3 years past menarche) until the perimenopausal years (with no medical contraindications). Nevertheless, many female athletes are still reluctant to "put chemicals into their bodies." Current research has not conclusively demonstrated a substantial impact on any aspect of performance, but for many athletes, this remains a potential concern.

25. Can the pill be used to manipulate the menstrual cycle around competitions?

Some women try to manipulate their cycles around major competitions. The onset of a period can be delayed for up to 10 days by continuing to administer a monophasic oral contraceptive or the highest dosage of a triphasic preparation, but after this length of time, breakthrough bleeding invariably occurs. The potential health risks of this practice are not known, and it is not recommended that a woman engage in this hormonal manipulation repeatedly throughout the year. It may be more suitable progressively to shorten the cycle by starting the pill sooner in each successive cycle or stopping it 10 days or so prior to competition to allow withdrawal bleeding to occur.

BIBLIOGRAPHY

1. Burkman RT Jr: Noncontraceptive effects of hormonal contraceptives: Bone mass, sexually transmitted disease, pelvic inflammatory disease, cardiovascular disease, menstrual function and future fertility. Am J Obstet Gynecol 170(5 Pt 2):1569–1575, 1994.
2. Cann CE, Martin MC, Genant HK, et al: Decreased spinal mineral content in amenorrheic women. JAMA 251:626–629, 1984.
3. DeCherney A: Physiologic and pharmacologic effects of estrogen and progestins on bone. J Reprod Med 38(Suppl 12): 1007–1014, 1993.
4. Drinkwater BL, Nilson K, Chesnut CH III: Bone mineral content of amenorrheic and eumenorrheic athletes. N Engl J Med 311:277–281, 1984.
5. Drinkwater BL, Nilson K, Ott S, Chesnut CH III: Bone mineral density after resumption of menses in amenorrheic athletes. JAMA 263:380–382, 1986.
6. Drinkwater BL, Bruemner B, Chestnut CH III: Menstrual history as a determinant of current bone density in young athletes. JAMA 263:545–548, 1990.
7. Hale RW (ed): Current Topics in Obstetrics and Gynecology: Caring for the Exercising Woman. New York, Elsevier Science, 1991.
8. Hergenroeder AC: Bone mineralization, hypothalamic amenorrhea and sex steroid therapy in female adolescents and young adults. J Pediatr 126(5 Pt 1):683–689, 1995.
9. Johnson MD: Tailoring the preparticipation exam to female athletes. Phys Sportsmed 20(7):61–72, 1992.
10. Jonnavithula S, Warren MP, Fox RP, Laxaro MI: Bone density is compromised in amenorrheic women despite return of menses: A 2-year study. Obstet Gynecol 81:669–674, 1993.
11. Lloyd T, Triantafyllou SJ, Baker ER, et al: Women athletes with menstrual irregularity have increased musculoskeletal injuries. Med Sci Sports Exerc 18:374–379, 1986.
12. Loucks AB: Effects of exercise training on the menstrual cycle: Existence and mechanisms. Med Sci Sports Exerc 22:275–280, 1990.
13. Marcus R, Cann C, Madvig P, et al: Menstrual function and bone mass in elite women distance runners. Ann Intern Med 102:158–163, 1985.
14. Mishell DR: Noncontraceptive health benefits of oral steroidal contraceptives. Am J Obstet Gynecol 142:809–816, 1982.
15. Naessen T, Olsson S-E, Gudmundson J: Differential effects on bone density of progestogen-only methods for contraception in premenopausal women. Contraception 52:35–39, 1995.
16. Otis CL: Exercise-associated amenorrhea. Clin Sports Med 11:351–362, 1992.
17. Prior JC, Vigna YM, Schechter MT, Burgess AE: Spinal bone loss and ovulatory disturbances. N Engl J Med 323:1221–1227, 1990.
18. Prior JC: Progesterone as a bone-trophic hormone. Endocrinol Rev 11:386–398, 1990.
19. Prior JC, Vigna YM, McKay DW: Reproduction for the athletic woman: New understandings of physiology and management. Sports Med 14:190, 1992.
20. Puhl JL, Brown CH (eds): The Menstrual Cycle and Physical Activity. Champaign, IL, Human Kinetics, 1986.
21. Shangold MM, Mirkin G (eds): Women and Exercise: Physiology and Sports Medicine. Philadelphia, F.A. Davis, 1988.
22. Speroff L, Van de Wiele RL: Regulation of the human menstrual cycle. Am J Obstet Gynecol 109:234–247, 1971.
23. Tuppurainen M, Kroger H, Saarikoski S, Honkanen AE: The effect of previous oral contraceptive use on bone mineral density in perimenopausal women. Osteoporos Int 4(2):93–98, 1994.
24. Volpe A, Sifferi M, Genazzani AD: Contraception in the older woman. Contraception 47(3):229–239, 1993.
25. Wells CL (ed): Women, Sport & Performance: A Physiological Perspective, 2nd ed. Champaign, IL, Human Kinetics, 1991.

11. GUIDELINES FOR EXERCISE DURING PREGNANCY

Suzanne M. Tanner, M.D.

1. What are the potential benefits of exercise during pregnancy?
- Maintenance of maternal physical fitness
- Avoidance of excessive maternal weight
- Decreased backache and varicose veins
- Improved sleep
- Heightened self-esteem
- Possible easier labor, delivery, and postpartum recovery

2. Is fetal outcome better in women who exercise during pregnancy?
This is unknown. Large, well-controlled, prospective studies are needed to differentiate the effect of one variable, such as exercise, from genetic, nutritional, environmental, and socioeconomic factors that affect fetal outcome.

3. What are the theoretical risks of exercise during pregnancy?
Reduced uterine blood flow. Intense exercise may potentially shunt blood from the uterus to exercising muscles. However, maternal cardiac output increases of 30–50% and a 40% increase of blood volume during pregnancy lessen this risk. Also, several studies reveal no evidence of fetal hypoxia or distress, such as fetal bradycardia or tachycardia, in pregnant women exercising at 70–80% of maximum heart rate.

Fetal hyperthermia. Maternal hyperthermia has been shown to increase the risk of fetal abnormalities, including neural tube defects, in animal and human studies. Fortunately, thermoregulatory mechanisms during pregnancy reduce this risk when exercise is not performed in hot, humid environments.

Microtrauma to the fetus. Amniotic fluid is thought to provide adequate fetal cushioning during most exercise.

Maternal musculoskeletal injury

4. What are the American College of Obstetricians and Gynecologists (ACOG) guidelines for exercise during pregnancy?

American College of Obstetricians and Gynecologists Recommendations for Exercise in Pregnancy and Postpartum

There are no data in humans to indicate that pregnant women should limit exercise intensity and lower target heart rates because of potential adverse effects. For women who do not have any additional risk factors for adverse maternal or perinatal outcome, the following recommendations may be made:

1. During pregnancy, women can continue to exercise and derive health benefits even from mild-to-moderate exercise routines. Regular exercise (at least three times per week) is preferable to intermittent activity.

2. Women should avoid exercise in the supine position after the first trimester. Such a position is associated with decreased cardiac output in most pregnant women: because the remaining cardiac output will be preferentially distributed away from splanchnic beds (including the uterus) during vigorous exercise, such regimens are best avoided during pregnancy. Prolonged periods of motionless standing should also be avoided.

(Table continued on following page.)

*American College of Obstetricians and Gynecologists Recommendations
for Exercise in Pregnancy and Postpartum (Continued)*

3. Women should be aware of the decreased oxygen available for aerobic exercise during pregnancy. They should be encouraged to modify the intensity of their exercise according to maternal symptoms. Pregnant women should stop exercising when fatigued and not exercise to exhaustion. Weight-bearing exercises may under some circumstances be continued at intensities similar to those prior to pregnancy throughout pregnancy. Non-weight-bearing exercises such as cycling or swimming will minimize the risk of injury and facilitate the continuation of exercise during pregnancy.

4. Morphologic changes in pregnancy should serve as a relative contraindication to types of exercise in which loss of balance could be detrimental to maternal or fetal well-being, especially in the third trimester. Further, any type of exercise involving the potential for even mild abdominal trauma should be avoided.

5. Pregnancy requires an additional 300 kcal/day in order to maintain metabolic homeostasis. Thus, women who exercise during pregnancy should be particularly careful to ensure an adequate diet.

6. Pregnant women who exercise in the first trimester should augment heat dissipation by ensuring adequate hydration, appropriate clothing, and optimal environmental surroundings during exercise.

7. Many of the physiologic and morphologic changes of pregnancy persist 4–6 weeks postpartum. Thus, prepregnancy exercise routines should be resumed gradually based on a woman's physical capability.

From American College of Obstetricians and Gynecologists: Exercise during pregnancy and the postpartum period. ACOG Technical Bulletin 189. Washington, DC, ACOG, 1994, with permission.

5. What is considered the safe upper limit for maternal heart rate during exercise?
140–160 beats per minute. This heart rate occurs at approximately 70–80% of maximum heart rate in women of childbearing age.

6. Should a premedical screen be conducted before a prenatal exercise program is begun?
Yes. Exercise prescriptions during pregnancy should be individualized and take into account a woman's previous fitness level, medical status, activity interests, and availability of exercise equipment.

7. Is there a safe, maximum level of exercise for female elite athletes who become pregnant?
The answer is unknown. Anecdotal evidence suggests these women can tolerate more exercise stress than outlined in the ACOG guidelines. There are no scientific studies involving large groups of women, however, to validate this position.

8. List the general and relative contraindications for exercise during pregnancy.

Contraindications to Exercise During Pregnancy

General Contraindications	Relative Contraindications
Hemodynamically significant heart disease	Essential hypertension
Recurrent cervical incompetence	Controlled diabetes mellitus
Current uterine bleeding	Excessive obesity
Current ruptured membranes	Malnutrition
Intrauterine growth retardation	Multiple gestations
Fetal distress	Thyroid disease
Previous miscarriage (more than one)	Anemia
Previous premature labor (more than one)	
Pregnancy-induced hypertension	
Uncontrolled diabetes mellitus	
Uncontrolled renal disease	
Hemodynamically significant anemia	
Intrauterine growth retardation	

Modified from Paisley JE, Mellion MG: Exercise during pregnancy. Am Fam Physician 38(5):147, 1988, with permission.

9. Should an exercise program be started during pregnancy?

Previously sedentary women may begin an exercise program during pregnancy if exercise begins at low intensity, and strength and endurance are built up gradually. Low-intensity exercise may include walking and aquatic exercise. ACOG has developed a video demonstrating mild to moderate activities for pregnant women.

10. What are the signals suggesting that exercise should be stopped?

Signals to Stop Exercising

Breathlessness	Fatigue	Generalized edema
Dizziness	Chest pain or tightness	Decreased fetal activity
Headache	Back pain	Uterine contractions
Muscle weakness	Hip or pubic pain	Vaginal bleeding
Nausea	Difficulty walking	Amniotic fluid leakage

Modified from Paisley JE, Mellion MB: Exercise during pregnancy. Am Fam Physician 38(5):148, 1988, with permission.

11. Do musculoskeletal changes occur during pregnancy?

Pregnancy causes lordosis and shifting of a woman's center of gravity. Altered balance and back pain may develop.

Progesterone and relaxin induce ligamentous laxity. Separation of the symphysis pubis, osteitis pubis, and perhaps ligamentous injuries may develop.

Increased weight and lack of exercise may potentiate patellofemoral pain.

Nerve compression, such as carpal tunnel syndrome, may develop from fluid retention.

12. Is weight training safe during pregnancy?

Opinions vary about whether a woman who has not participated in a weightlifting program should begin weightlifting during pregnancy. Although the safety of weight training during pregnancy has not been definitively studied, low-intensity weight training probably is not risky for the mother or fetus. A strengthening program may help a pregnant woman tolerate postural changes and weight gain during pregnancy, reduce back pain, and prepare her for carrying an infant after delivery.

Risks from heavy lifting include damaging ligaments and disks and straining the back. Holding one's breath while lifting a heavy weight may elicit a Valsalva maneuver, which diverts blood from internal organs, including the uterus.

Recommendations for continuing a weightlifting program during pregnancy may include performing low-weight, high-repetition exercises. Proper breathing includes exhaling while lifting a weight and not holding one's breath. Lifts that may strain the lower back, such as dead lifts, overhead lifts, bent rows, and squats, should be avoided. Sudden increases in workout intensity should be avoided.

13. When may exercise be resumed after delivery?

It is usually safe to resume exercise 1 week after a vaginal delivery. After a cesarean section, stress should not be put on the wound until approximately 21 days postoperatively. Water sports should not be resumed until bleeding has stopped. A general recommendation is to wait 6–10 weeks after a cesarean section before resuming exercise.

14. Which activities and environmental situations should be avoided during pregnancy?

ACOG guidelines warn against exercise performed in a supine position after the first trimester. Late in pregnancy, the enlarged uterus may theoretically impinge on the aorta and/or inferior vena cava, reducing blood flow to the placenta. This appears to be an uncommon problem, however.

If jogging is continued during pregnancy, monitoring for symptoms listed in question 10 should be done, and as pregnancy progresses, speed and distance may be gradually reduced while maintaining the same perceived level of exertion.

Outdoor bicycling may be risky owing to changes in balance during pregnancy. If outdoor riding is continued during pregnancy, a touring or mountain bike with wide tires and elevated handlebars may be safest.

Activities with high risk of abdominal trauma include ice skating, football, and field hockey. Other sports with moderate risk of abdominal trauma include outdoor bicycling (see above), downhill and cross-country skiing, horseback riding, basketball, volleyball, and gymnastics.

Water skiing is contraindicated during pregnancy because high-speed falls have caused forceful entry of water into the uterus and subsequent miscarriage.

Risks from scuba diving include decompression sickness in the mother and fetal intravascular air embolism. Diving by inexperienced divers should be avoided. Experienced pregnant divers should limit dives to 30 minutes and 1 atmosphere in pressure (= 10 m, 33 ft). There are no medical contraindications to snorkeling at the surface of the water.

Avoid high-altitude, low-oxygen situations. The exact altitude at which hypoxia becomes risky is unknown.

Swimming in excessively cold or hot water should be avoided. The pregnant woman's body temperature should never exceed 100.4° F. Prolonged exercise should be avoided in hot, humid environments. Hot tubs and saunas should not be used.

15. Which activities are usually well tolerated during pregnancy?

Swimming and other exercise in a pool provide good aerobic exercise. Water accelerates heat transfer and buoyancy decreases stress on joints. Excessively hot or cold water should be avoided.

Riding a stationary bicycle.

Low-impact aerobics.

Racquet sports such as tennis, racquetball, and squash. The intensity of play should be decreased as pregnancy progresses to avoid falls from impaired coordination and heat stress.

Stretching exercises except while supine.

The obvious simplest form of exercise should not be overlooked; in a word, walking.

BIBLIOGRAPHY

1. American College of Obstetrics and Gynecology Guidelines for Exercise During Pregnancy and the Postpartum Period: ACOG Technical Bulletin 189. Washington, DC, ACOG, 1994.
2. Artal R, Friedman MJ, McNitt-Gray JL: Orthopedic problems in pregnancy. Phys Sportsmed 18(9):93–105, 1990.
3. Jarski RW, Trippett DL: The risks and benefits of exercise during pregnancy. J Fam Pract 30:185–189, 1990.
4. Lotgering FK: Pregnancy. In Shangold MM, Mirkin G (eds): Women and Exercise: Physiology and Sports Medicine. Philadelphia, F.A. Davis, 1988, pp 145–155.
5. McMurray RG, Mottola MF, Wolff LA, et al: Recent advances in understanding maternal and fetal responses to exercise. Med Sci Sports Exerc 25:1305–1321, 1993.
6. Mullinax KM, Dale E: Some considerations of exercise during pregnancy. Clin Sports Med 5:559–570, 1986.
7. Paisley JE, Mellion MB: Exercise during pregnancy. Am Fam Physician 38:143–150, 1988.
8. Warren MP: Exercise in women: Effects on reproductive system and pregnancy. Clin Sports Med 10:131–139, 1991.
9. Wolfe LA, Hall P, Webb KA, et al: Prescription of aerobic exercise during pregnancy. Sports Med 8:273–301, 1989.
10. Work JA: Is weight training safe during pregnancy? Phys Sportsmed 17(3):257–259, 1989.

12. THE MATURE ATHLETE

David O. Hough, M.D., Henry C. Barry, M.D., and Scott W. Eathorne, M.D.

1. Why is there increasing emphasis on physical activity in the elderly?

The proportion of the elderly in the U.S. population is increasing with each census. The percentage of the U.S. population 65 years of age and older increased from 11.2% in the 1980 census to 12.5% in the 1990 census. There has been a disproportionate rise (3.5%) during the 1980s among the group aged 85 and over. Generally, the elderly are more sedentary than their younger colleagues. They tend to suffer from medical problems that result in functional impairment, less independence, and greater utilization of health care services.

2. At what age do individuals begin to have significant disabilities affecting their activities?

Even though there continues to be a difference in the average life expectancy between men and women, the age at which significant disability begins appears to be relatively constant. In general, women tend to live nearly a decade longer than men; however, the onset of disability generally begins around age 60 for both sexes. Nearly one-third of people over age 65 have some impairment in performing activities such as walking. There is growing evidence that physical activity may have a beneficial influence in these areas.

3. What are some of the physiologic changes associated with aging?

There are five major areas to consider: the cardiovascular, respiratory, musculoskeletal, central nervous systems, and metabolism. Perhaps the greatest area of concern regarding functional capacity and mobility is the changes seen in the musculoskeletal system.

Age-related Decreases in Functional Status

Cardiovascular system	↓ Max. heart rate	10 beats/minute/decade
	↓ Resting stroke vol.	30% by age 85
	↓ Max. cardiac output	20–30% by age 65
	↓ Vessel compliance	↑ bp 10–40 mmHg
Respiratory system	↑ Residual vol.	30–50% by age 70
	↓ Vital capacity	40–50% by age 70
Nervous system	↓ Nerve conduction	1–15% by age 60
	↓ Proprioception and balance	Falls 35–40% by age 60
Musculoskeletal system	↑ Bone loss > 35 yo	1%/year
	> 55 yo	3–5%/year
	↓ Muscle strength	20% by age 65
	↓ Flexibility	Degenerative disease or inactivity
Metabolism	↓ Max. O_2 uptake	9%/decade

Aging is marked by progressive impairment of control mechanisms that allow normal physiologic function. This results in a loss of normal dynamic range of physiologic function and a reduced capacity to adapt. One must raise the question, however, whether the physiologic changes often attributed to aging are in fact more likely due to disease and inactivity.

4. Can exercise benefit the elderly?

Exercise generally serves two major purposes: preventive and therapeutic. These purposes may be seen in the young, the healthy elderly, and the frail elderly. One cannot underestimate the importance and benefits derived from a lifetime pattern of physical activity in ameliorating the ravages of aging. A flexibility and strengthening program that assists in maintaining mobility in an older individual may reduce the incidence of falls and bed sores. People who suffer from arthritis, fractures, or strokes may have clear therapeutic benefit from an exercise program.

5. What are some of the specific benefits of regular exercise in the mature athlete?

Among some of the specific adaptations to exercise, one may see improvements in cardiac output, a decline in resting heart rate, improved cholesterol, a decline in blood pressure, and increased cardiovascular fitness. Improvements in minute ventilation and vital capacity but not chest wall compliance also are observed. Bone density, muscle strength, flexibility, and coordination also are improved. Perhaps just as important are improvements in mood and self-esteem with lessened anxiety and depression as a result of regular exercise. Many elderly have limited opportunities for contact with peers. An organized program of regular physical activity may enhance their socialization and decrease their idle time.

6. How should one begin an exercise program?

Before a patient begins an exercise program, the physician should perform an assessment of the patient's needs and goals and complete a thorough medical evaluation. Evaluate the patient's current level of activity and functional capacity and ascertain the individual's personal goals. For some individuals, these goals are likely to be aimed at improving mobility or improving some other functional aspect of their existence. Others may want to perform at the master's level. The physician should be able to outline progressive steps toward achieving these goals. The physician should also refocus unrealistic goals! Performing a thorough history and physical examination can help assess the patient's goals in the context of his or her current status. If the goals seem disproportionate to the physical capabilities, the physician may need to redirect the goals or set more modest, attainable, short-term goals.

7. What are the specifics of the preexercise evaluation?

The history should include past and current illnesses, previous injuries, and current medication use. For preexisting injuries, the degree of rehabilitation of these injuries should be determined. One should also assess functional capacity. The physical examination should focus on nutritional status, cardiovascular function, and psychoneurologic function. The primary focus, however, should be on the musculoskeletal system. Range of motion, flexibility, strength, and management of prior injuries should be thoroughly evaluated.

8. Should an exercise tolerance test be performed?

Exercise testing is useful when the physician must decide whether closer monitoring of the exercise program is indicated. Patients in this category should undergo a medically supervised test for functional capacity. Patients with the following conditions require supervised stress testing:

Recent myocardial infarction or postcoronary artery bypass surgery
Presence of a pacemaker-fixed rate or demand
Use of chronotropic or inotropic cardiac medications
Presence of morbid obesity combined with multiple coronary risk factors
Occurrence of ST-segment depression at rest
Severe hypertension
Intermittent claudication

Conditions, both medical and environmental, that require moderation of activity or caution in prescribing exercise are listed in the table on the following page. In general, many patients in the mature athlete age group will require some form of exercise testing prior to instituting an exercise program.

Conditions Requiring Caution or Moderation in Exercise Prescription

Caution	Moderation
Viral infection or cold	Extreme heat and high relative humidity
Chest pain	Extreme cold, especially when strong
Irregular heart beat	winds are present
Exercise-induced asthma	Following heavy meals
Prolonged, unaccustomed physical activity	Exposure to high altitudes
Conduction disturbances (left bundle branch block	(greater than 1700 m)
[LBBB], complete atrioventricular [AV] block, or	Significant musculoskeletal injuries
bifascicular block with or without first-degree block)	

9. What are some specific concerns about exercise testing in the elderly?

Even though there are groups recommending exercise tolerance testing, these recommendations are generally intended for people with a high level of function. For the frail elderly, there are significant problems in performing an exercise tolerance test. Access to testing may be limited for many elderly. Functional impairments can hinder one's ability to perform an exercise tolerance test. If an individual's goals are primarily to improve strength and flexibility, the aerobic demands of such a program are relatively low. In this circumstance, a patient's aerobic capacity may in fact exceed the demands of the exercise program. Finally, for those who are interested in beginning a walking program, an exercise tolerance test may not be a useful indicator of limits of intensity.

10. How can compliance with an exercise program be improved?

One needs to keep in mind that the ultimate goal of exercise for most elderly patients is to improve their quality of life. Programs that are enjoyable, emphasize fun, and increase socialization with peers are the most successful. Compliance will be improved if program expense is minimized. Physical therapy in a rehabilitation unit may be appropriate and is often covered by health insurance.

In order to improve compliance, the risk of injury must be minimized. This means that safety measures need to be instituted. The exercise area should be well lit, surfaces should be level, and the temperature should be comfortable. Fluid replacement needs to be encouraged before and during exercise. Appropriate clothing and footwear need to be worn. Finally, to decrease the risk of injury, the physician should emphasize low-impact, low- or moderate-intensity exercise with a slow progression.

11. How can I motivate my elderly patients to exercise?

Many older individuals are self-motivated; however, societal or family expectations tend to promote a sedentary lifestyle. Physicians can educate patients about the benefits of regular exercise. Emphasis should be placed on socialization and the fun aspects of exercise. The goals need to be set in a way that has significance for the patient. These goals need to be attainable and realistic. Because isolation is a common problem for the elderly, the potential for increasing interactions with family and peers can be a powerful motivator. Group activities need to be emphasized and progress toward goal achievement needs to be periodically reassessed. Use of charts, graphs, or diaries can be helpful in plotting improvement. One may need to enlist the aid of spouses, friends, and family to help with motivating the patient to begin a program. In some ways, the physician may need to function as a cheerleader and provide genuine praise and encouragement.

12. What conditions may limit an older person's interest in regular exercise?

Underlying conditions, such as depression and dementia, may impair an individual's interest in exercising. Treatment of the depression and reversible causes of dementia is essential to successful motivation of the patient. The elderly patient may have subtle deficits that do not allow for processing short-term information, yet they may detect frustration in others. In individuals with irreversible causes of dementia, physical activity may continue to provide other benefits.

Demented patients should exercise in supervised group settings in order to increase socialization and provide for safety. Structured activities should be provided. Instructions need to be simple and repeated frequently.

13. What environmental factors should be considered in the exercising elderly?

Elderly individuals involved in exercise programs may be more susceptible to the influence of various environmental factors because of normal age-related changes in thermoregulation and the influence of medications. Exposure to high heat and humidity may predispose to serious injury—including dehydration and heat stroke. Individuals on diuretic therapy may be at greater risk for developing these complications. Prolonged sun exposure can induce both acute skin injury (e.g., sunburn) and chronic changes of premalignant solar keratoses and skin cancer.

14. How does cold exposure affect the older athlete?

Cold exposure can result in common cold injuries such as frostnip, frostbite, and hypothermia. Predisposing factors include alteration of the skin barrier, chronic disease, poor nutrition, inadequate hydration, and the effects of medication used by the patient. Cold-induced angina and bronchospasm are potential environmental problems facing this population. Urban dwellers may be exposed to increased levels of pollution, which may exacerbate such conditions as chronic obstructive pulmonary disease (COPD) and allergic bronchospasm. Local traffic and safety concerns warrant consideration, as they can greatly impact the mature athlete's attempt at enjoyable exercise.

15. What means are available for decreasing the incidence of environmentally related injuries in elderly athletes?

Garments should have adequate insulating capacity against the cold, yet sufficient breathability or ventilation to avoid excessive condensation and overheating. In warmer weather, ventilation is more important in allowing heat dissipation and preventing overheating. Skin coverage to avoid sun-induced skin damage can be achieved with clothing and/or topically applied sun screens. All clothing should fit well with adequate room to avoid restriction of movement and potential injury.

16. What conditions might interfere with exercise performance?

Review of an individual's medical history and medication use can allow for modifications prior to engaging in exercise. Drugs that may contribute to heat illness include tricyclic antidepressants, diuretics, antihistamines, antispasmodics, phenothiazines, and alcohol. Predisposing medical conditions, which alter the body's ability to thermoregulate, include cardiovascular disease, obesity, dehydration, fever, burns, scleroderma, lack of acclimatization, fatigue, and infection. Recognition of such preexisting factors may help prevent an environmentally related injury in the older athlete.

For the urban exerciser, use of mask filters may limit irritation from airborne pollutants. Indoor activities may be required in severely polluted regions, during certain seasons, or in locations where outdoor activities would not be prudent for safety reasons. This could be due to poor road or trail conditions, high traffic volume, or high crime. Exercising with a partner is always encouraged for social and safety reasons.

17. What means of monitoring exercise intensity can be used in the mature athlete?

Intensity becomes an important factor in the older athlete's exercise program. Starting an exercise program at an inappropriately high intensity level may be discouraging to the athlete who is unable to achieve set goals and dangerous for those with preexisting medical conditions such as coronary artery disease or COPD. Elderly patients should exercise within a predetermined intensity range, usually established by exercise stress testing. Intensity can be monitored by measuring the patient's heart rate, perceived exertion level, or by using MET (metabolic equivalent unit) levels (see question 18).

Target heart rates established by the more reliable exercise testing or calculation can be followed directly by taking the pulse during exercise. Individuals should be instructed in proper technique using either the carotid or radial artery, and what to do if pulse rates exceed the target zone (e.g., stop activity or slow pace until within target range). Commercial products are available that allow pulse-rate monitoring and provide a digital readout. Care must be taken, especially in the mature athlete, that the product is reliable, functioning well, and properly calibrated.

18. How are MET levels used to monitor intensity in the mature athlete?

Another method for determining intensity levels uses the MET, or metabolic equivalent unit. This unit represents the amount of energy expended per 1 minute of rest and equals the VO_2 at rest (3.5 ml/kg/min). Exercise testing can provide data about the maximal MET level (MML), which reflects maximum intensity for the patient. Taking a percentage of this establishes the MET intensity range. Using preexisting tables showing the MET levels expended for various activities, the individual can choose an activity appropriate to his or her target MET level. Use of MET levels to monitor intensity may initially require concurrent heart rate monitoring to ensure that exercise intensity is occurring within the target range.

19. What are the guidelines for achieving cardiorespiratory and muscular fitness and how do they relate to the mature athlete?

The American College of Sports Medicine (ACSM) guidelines for developing and maintaining cardiorespiratory and muscular fitness recommend exercise at intensity levels of (1) 50–85% VO_2max; (2) 60–90% HRmax; or (3) 40–85 METS (maximal MET level). Three to five sessions per week (frequency), for 20–60 minutes (duration) completes the prescription. Resistance training recommendations include one set (8–12 repetitions) of 8–10 exercises that condition major muscle groups at least two times each week. The mature athlete may have preexisting medical conditions (e.g., arthritis, coronary artery disease, COPD) or certain age-related changes that limit the ability to achieve the ACSM's guidelines. Starting an older athlete at levels far below those outlined may be indicated. Exercising at lower levels may provide some modest aerobic benefit.

20. How are exercise, aging, and osteoarthritis associated?

Osteoarthritis is diagnosed in almost 85% of people over the age of 85. Most researchers currently believe that osteoarthritis is a multifactorial illness *associated* with aging but not *caused* by aging. Factors associated with the development of osteoarthritis include obesity, congenital anomalies, gender, bone density, biomechanical dysfunction, and previous trauma. There is considerable debate as to whether there is a cause and effect relationship between exercise and arthritis. Clearly, repetitive microtrauma to joint surfaces of people with altered biomechanics increases the propensity to arthritis. This is less clear in individuals who have normal body mechanics. Exercise has been promoted as treatment for osteoarthritis. Some of these benefits are indirect, including weight reduction, improved muscle tone and muscle strength, increased flexibility, and improved biomechanics. Exercise has a direct effect on improving joint fluid viscosity. In the individual who experiences discomfort associated with exercise, non–weight-bearing activity may be helpful. Swimming and water aerobics are popular because the buoyancy of water reduces joint stress, as is biking.

21. What are the possible contributing factors to musculoskeletal injury in the older athlete?

- Decreasing flexibility with aging—primary cause is disuse.
- Decreased nerve conduction and reaction time—15% decrease between age 30 and 70.
- Decreased hearing and/or vision associated with unsteady gait—use of a stationary bicycle may be useful for those with balance problems.
- Degenerative joint disease.
- Rheumatoid arthritis—increased incidence with aging; women > men.
- Gout—increased incidence over age 60; men > women, should curtail activity during acute attack, utilizing adequate rest periods, appropriate splinting and medications.

- Decreased muscle mass—results in decreased strength and shock absorption.
- Osteoporosis—more significant for females, may predispose older individuals to increased fractures. Regular weight-bearing exercise may play an important role in prevention.

BIBLIOGRAPHY

1. American College of Sports Medicine Position Stand: The Recommended Quantity and Quality of Exercise for Developing and Maintaining Cardiorespiratory and Muscular Fitness in Healthy Adults. Med Sci Sports Exerc 22:265–274, 1990.
2. Barry HC, Rich BSE, Carlson RT: How exercise can benefit older patients—A practical approach. Phys Sportsmed 21(2):124–140, 1993.
3. Barry HC: Exercise prescriptions for the elderly. Am Fam Physician 34:155–162, 1986.
4. Belman MJ, Gaesser GA: Exercise training below and above the lactate threshold in the elderly. Med Sci Sports Exerc 23:562–568, 1991.
5. Elia EA: Exercise and the elderly. Clin Sports Med 10:141–155, 1991.
6. Elward K, Larson EB: Benefits of exercise for older adults—A review of existing evidence and current recommendations for the general population. Clin Geriatr Med 8:35–50, 1992.
7. Elward K, Larson EB, Wagner E: Factors associated with regular aerobic exercise in an elderly population. J Am Board Fam Pract 5:467–474, 1992.
8. Franklin BA, et al: Exercise prescription. In Strauss RH (ed): Sports Medicine, 2nd ed. Philadelphia, W.B. Saunders, 1991, pp 48–71.
9. Hough DO, Lillegaard W, McGrew C: The mature athlete. In Mellion M (ed): The Team Physician's Handbook. Philadelphia, Hanley & Belfus, 1997, pp 150–159.
10. Kasch FW, Boyer JL, Van Camp SP, et al: The effect of physical activity and inactivity on aerobic power in older men (a longitudinal study). Phys Sportsmed 18(4):73–83, 1990.
11. Kerland RK (ed): Sports medicine in the older athlete. Clin Sports Med 10:1991.
12. Kipsitz LA, Goldberger AL: Loss of "complexity" and aging—Potential applications of fractals and chaos theory to senescence. JAMA 267:1806–1809, 1992.
13. McKeag DB: The relationship of osteoarthritis and exercise. Clin Sports Med 11(2):471–487, 1992.
14. Paffenbarger RS et al: The association of changes in physical-activity level and other lifestyle characteristics with mortality among men. N Engl J Med 238:538–546, 1993.
15. Rousseau P: Exercise prescription for the elderly patient. Fam Pract Recert 13:58–76, 1991.
16. Sandvik RC: Physical fitness as a predictor of mortality among healthy, middle-aged Norwegian men. N Engl J Med 328:533–538, 1993.
17. Tinetti ME, Liu W-L, Claus EB: Predictors and prognosis of inability to get up after falls among elderly persons. JAMA 296(1):65–70, 1993.
18. Wei JY: Age and the cardiovascular system. N Engl J Med 327(24):1735–1739, 1992.

13. THE WHEELCHAIR ATHLETE AND OTHER FORMS OF ADAPTIVE EXERCISE

Frank M. Brasile, Ph.D.

1. Who is the wheelchair athlete?
Wheelchair sports opportunities, for the most part, are competitive activities for people who have a permanent physical disability (e.g., amputations, spinal cord injuries, poliomyelitis) and who would not be able to participate in the activity without the use of a wheelchair. These activities have been developed to allow people with disabilities to have the opportunity to benefit from sport participation like their peers without permanent physical limitations.

2. What are the most popular wheelchair sports?
The most popular wheelchair sports today are road racing, tennis, basketball, archery, softball, and track and field. These activities usually incorporate a classification system to allow for fair and

equitable competition among participants with varying degrees of disabilities. However, some activities such as quad rugby, are limited to specific participants (e.g., quadriplegics).

3. Describe the classification system for participants in wheelchair sports.

Most wheelchair sport organizations require that participants have a medical examination by an appropriate specialist before participating in the activities. One of the reasons for this examination is to determine the degree or level of disability. On the basis of this examination, the person usually is assigned a classification level for participation in some of the sports. For example, according to the National Wheelchair Basketball Association rules, each individual is placed in one of three participation categories. A class I athlete has a spinal cord injury or similar disability at the T7 level or above; a class II athlete has a spinal cord injury or similar impairment between the T8 and L2 area; and a class III athlete manifests impairment below the L2 level. The class I athlete is the most severely disabled; the class II athlete manifests a moderate level of impairment; and the class III athlete is the least severely disabled.

For other sports participants are placed in competitive categories based on their level of skill or achievement in the sport. Wheelchair tennis has an open division in which any individual can choose to participate. In addition, athletes are classified according to level of performance in different divisions. There are also divisions for quadriplegic and junior (youth) participants.

4. What is quad rugby?

Wheelchair rugby or quad rugby is a unique, competitive sport for quadriplegics. The sport is played on a basketball court, and four players from one team are allowed on the court at a time. The objective is to carry the ball across the opponent's goal line. It is one of the fastest growing wheelchair sports in the world and will be incorporated into the Paralympics in the year 2000.

5. What are Paralympic competitions?

The Paralympics are the Olympic-equivalent competitions for athletes with permanent physical disabilities. The first Paralympic Games were held in Rome in 1960; games have been held every Olympic year since, usually in the city or country hosting the Olympic Games. The Paralympics are governed by the International Paralympic Committee (IPC), a federation of the International Sports Associations serving athletes with physical disabilities. The IPC is formally recognized and partially funded by the International Olympic Committee. The next Paralympic games will be hosted by the city of Sydney, Australia, in the year 2000.

Paralympic activities include athletics (track and field), basketball, boccia, cycling, fencing, soccer, goal ball, weightlifting, judo, swimming, tennis, table tennis, archery, shooting, and volleyball. Not all activities at the Paralympics are wheelchair activities. Amputees and blind, cerebral palsied, and other physically impaired people participate as stand-up athletes in many of the events. Winter Paralympic competitions include skiing and sledge (luge) hockey. The 1998 winter Paralympic competitions were held in Nagano, Japan.

6. Describe the philosophical concepts of modification in relationship to wheelchair sports.

For the most part, even the most knowledgeable observer will notice little to no difference in wheelchair activities except for the use of the wheelchair. In most activities, the rules for participation vary from the regular stand-up rules because of the wheelchair and do not depend on the level of impairment. For example, the rules of wheelchair basketball are similar to the rules that govern participation in basketball by the National Collegiate Athletic Association. One modification in the rules pertains to the dribble:

> A player in possession of the ball may not push more than twice in succession with one or both hands in either direction without tapping the ball to the floor again. Taking more than two consecutive pushes constitutes a traveling violation. A player may, however, wheel the chair and bounce the ball simultaneously just as a stand-up player runs and bounces the ball simultaneously.

The major rule modification in the sport of tennis allows the participant to have two bounces before he or she must return the opponent's volley. Most wheelchair sports maintain the integrity of the sport so that participants are, in a sense, participating in a similar or comparable experience to their stand-up counterpart. Any judgments related to skill levels can be transferred from the specific sport (basketball) to its wheelchair equivalent.

7. How does one train to be a wheelchair athlete?

As in most recreational or sport competitions, the training regimen for competition is up to the athlete. Many wheelchair athletes train on a daily basis to reach the ultimate elite levels of participation. Training includes weight training, wheelchair pushing (sprinting and distance work), and skills development (specific sport-related skills, such as shooting and dribbling for basketball, serving and volleying for tennis). The more competitive wheelchair athlete is likely to be involved in a program that includes general conditioning, sport-specific conditioning, strength training, power training, endurance, flexibility, and technique. The athlete also incorporates personal experimentation necessary for best results based on ability in relationship to specific level of impairment.

8. Describe the elite wheelchair athlete.

As in all sports competitions, certain participants choose to take themselves to the highest level of individual achievement. The elite wheelchair athlete is not born. People who achieve the accolades of their peers as the best in these activities must work hard and train hard. The elite wheelchair athlete is usually the person who is recognized as the best or one of the best in the particular activity. One method for judgment is recognition as the most valuable player, champion, or first-place finisher in sanctioned regional, national, and international competitions. Many elite wheelchair athletes have been selected to represent their country and their sport in Olympic/Paralympic or Gold Cup competitions. One of the most prominent elite wheelchair athletes is Jean Driscoll, who has won the women's wheelchair division of the Boston Marathon 7 of the past 8 years.

9. Discuss some of the benefits of participating in wheelchair sport and recreation activities.

Sport participation by people with disabilities has been promoted for its physical and therapeutic effects and also as a primary therapy to assist renewal of the drive for competence. Sir Ludwig Guttmann, famed neurosurgeon and leader in the development of sports participation for people with physical disabilities stated that "the aims of sport embody the same principles for the disabled as they do for the able-bodied; in addition, however, sport is of immense therapeutic value and plays an essential part in the physical, psychological, and social rehabilitation of the disabled."[4]

Brasile, Kleiber, and Harnisch indicate a general similarity between competitors with disabilities and peers without disabilities with respect to incentives for participation. Results indicated that task incentives were most important to both groups of athletes; however, fitness incentives appeared to be of somewhat more importance to traumatically disabled wheelchair participants. This result may indicate that sport participation offers disabled people a primary source for fitness opportunities; as such, these incentives become more important.

10. What are some of the common sports medicine issues related to wheelchair sports participation?

Curtis and Dillon reported that the most common injuries incurred by athletes with disabilities were soft tissue injuries (sprains, strains, muscle pulls, tendinitis, and bursitis), blisters, and lacerations, abrasions, and cuts (skin infections and other complications). They also found that these injuries were related to activities that required high-risk repetitive wheelchair pushing (road racing, basketball, track, and tennis). Thus, it is imperative that wheelchair athletes have good training patterns, participate in stretching exercises before activity, get proper rest, and pay good attention to the equipment that they are using. Proper medical supervision and nutrition are also important.

11. For the disabled who are not interested in competitive sports, what other forms of adapted exercise are available?

Most people with physical limitations do not participate in organized wheelchair sports; however, there are many other activities that they can choose to acquire benefits from physical leisure pursuits. These pursuits range from individual low-risk activities (wheelchair aerobics) to individual and group organized high-risk activities (skydiving, mountain climbing). Even the sky is no limit to what the individual can do.

12. What group of professionals provides leadership in wheelchair sports and adapted activities?

The initial rehabilitation (treatment-oriented) programs related to sport or adaptive activities for people with physical disabilities are usually conducted under the guidance of a physiatrist. In addition, physical and recreational therapists are involved in providing the day-to-day activities and training for people interested in wheelchair sports and adapted activities. In the school systems instructors with a background in adapted physical education are usually in charge of similar services for children with disabilities.

13. What is the focus of the treatment program in relationship to wheelchair sports in a rehabilitation setting?

The development of skills and strength for future independent leisure involvement is the focus of the treatment-oriented participation program under the recreational therapy service. The cognitive elements of participation (i.e., understanding rules and strategies) also may be introduced. Examples of intervention include motivation of patient involvement in programs that focus on the development of skills related to participation in wheelchair sports (e.g., track and field, basketball, and tennis). Activities may range from initial skill training, which, may include learning how to control a wheelchair while dribbling a basketball or holding a tennis racket, to advanced skill development necessary for successful participation in the activity on a consistent basis (more complicated participation such as team drills or initial one-on-one or team competition).

14. What is recreational therapy?

According to the American Therapeutic Recreation Association, recreational therapy is the provision of treatment services and recreation services to persons with illnesses or disabling conditions. The primary purposes of treatment services are to restore, remediate, or rehabilitate in order to improve functioning and independence as well as to reduce or eliminate the effects of illness or disability. The primary purpose of recreation services is to provide recreation resources and opportunities to improve health and well-being. A certified therapeutic recreation specialist is recognized as the most appropriately prepared person to provide these services.

15. What are the most controversial issues in relationship to wheelchair sports?

Currently, the three most controversial issues in relationship to wheelchair sports continue to be inclusion of people without disabilities in wheelchair sports participation, elimination of disability-related classification systems, and inclusion of select wheelchair sports activities in Olympic competitions. These issues are the subject of debate among many professionals involved in the administration of the sports as well as among the athletes themselves.

16. Where can I acquire additional information related to wheelchair sport/recreation participation?

Visit the following web sites for wheelchair sports:
Comprehensive site on sports for the disabled and the Paralympics:
    http://info.lut.ac.uk/research/paad/ipc/ipc.html
Site of national organization for disabled sports: http://dsusa.org/~dsusa/
Site related to women in wheelchair basketball:
    http://www.unomaha.edu/~brasile/usawomen.htm
Site related to quad rugby: http://www.quadrugby.com
Site related to wheelchair tennis: http://www.nfwt.org
Site related to wheelchair basketball in the United States: http://www.nwba.org

Site related to the 1998 Winter Paralympic Games:
  http://www.nagano.paralympic.org/index_e.html
For additional information on wheelchair sports contact:

Executive Director	Bruce Scott, Director
Wheelchair Sports USA	Recreation and Sports
3595 E. Fountain Blvd.	Paralyzed Veterans of America
Suite L-1	900 17th St. NW, Suite 400
Colorado Springs, CO 80910	Washington, DC 20006

Periodicals that are concerned with sports activities for the disabled include *Adapted Physical Activity Quarterly* (Human Kinetics Publishers, Champaign, IL), *Palaestra* (Challenge Publications, Macomb, IL), and *Therapeutic Recreation Journal* (National Recreation and Parks Association, Arlington, VA).

BIBLIOGRAPHY

1. Brasile F, Kleiber D, Harnisch D: Analysis of participation incentives among athletes with and without disabilities. Ther Recreat J, 1st Quarter, 1991, pp 18–33.
2. Curtis K, Dillon D: Survey of wheelchair athletic injuries: Common patterns and prevention. In Sherrill C (ed): Sport and Disabled Athletes: The 1984 Olympic Scientific Congress Proceedings, vol 9. Champaign, IL, Human Kinetics, 1984, pp 211–216.
3. DePauw K: Disability and Sport. Champaign, IL, Human Kinetics, 1996.
4. Guttmann L: Textbook of Sport for the Disabled. Aylesbury, Bucks, England, HM&M Publishers, 1976.
5. Hedrick B, Morse N: A Guide for Wheelchair Sports Training. Colorado Springs, CO, National Wheelchair Athletic Association, 1989.
6. Paciorek M, Jones J: Sports and Recreation for the Disabled: A Resource Manual. Indianapolis, IN, Benchmark Press, 1995.
7. Sherrill C (ed): Sport and Disabled Athletes: The 1984 Olympic Scientific Congress Proceedings, vol 9. Champaign, IL, Human Kinetics, 1984.
8. Strohkendl H: The Fiftieth Anniversary of Wheelchair Basketball: A History. New York, Waxmann, 1996.

III. Conditioning

14. BUILDING AEROBIC POWER

Richard W. Latin, Ph.D.

1. What is aerobic power?

Aerobic power or capacity is the maximal capability to transport and utilize oxygen. Aerobic power is considered an important index of cardiovascular physical fitness. Training programs for aerobic improvement need to stress the physiologic components of the oxygen transport system.

2. What are the components of oxygen uptake?

Oxygen uptake or VO_2 may be physiologically and mathematically defined as $VO_2 = HR \times SV \times a - \bar{v} \, O_2$ difference. The oxygen uptake system has a central and peripheral component. The central component is cardiac output (Q), which is equivalent to heart rate (HR) multiplied by stroke volume (SV). The peripheral component is the difference between arterial (a) and mixed venous ($\bar{v}$) blood. Therefore, VO_2 depends on the heart's pumping of blood and the tissues' extraction of oxygen from the blood. Ultimately, the oxygen delivered to tissues is used in the resynthesis of adenosine triphosphate (ATP).

3. How is aerobic power measured?

Maximal oxygen uptake is also known as VO_2max. The measure of VO_2max represents the maximal capabilities of the oxygen transport system and aerobic ATP resynthesis. VO_2max is usually expressed in ml of oxygen per kg of body weight per minute (ml/kg/min). It also may be expressed in liters per minute (L/min). Precise assessments of VO_2max require the metabolic analysis of expired gases while an individual is performing a maximal, incremental exercise test. However, many less accurate but simpler tests exist.

4. What are the principles related to an aerobic training program?

The general principles related to an aerobic training program are specificity of training, overload, progression, and individuality. **Specificity of training** has two components: metabolic and neuromuscular specificity. Metabolic specificity relates to stressing the key metabolic pathways responsible for bioenergetics of a specific exercise task. Neuromuscular specificity implies recruiting the motor units that are similarly recruited for a given type of exercise. Therefore, the best results occur when training makes use of movement patterns and speeds similar to a given form of exercise. For instance, a marathoner trains by performing long-endurance runs as opposed to short, high-intensity sprints, and a cyclist trains by cycling rather than running. Both types of exercise use leg muscles but different recruitment patterns. **Overload** relates to exercise workloads that are greater than what one normally encounters. **Progression** occurs when one systematically increases the volume or intensity of training. **Individuality** relates to the fact that no two individuals respond or adapt similarly to the same training program. All of these principles need to be addressed for training to be effective.

5. What are the guidelines related to an aerobic exercise program?

Guidelines proposed by the American College of Sports Medicine[1,3] may be used to train successfully athletes or individuals interested in health-related aerobic fitness. These guidelines address aerobic exercise intensity, frequency, duration, and mode. A summary follows:

Summary of ACSM Guidelines for the Quantity and Quality
of Exercise Programs for Healthy Adults

COMPONENT	RECOMMENDATION
Frequency	3–5 day/wk
Duration	20–60 min
Intensity	60–90% HRmax
	50–85% VO$_2$max
	or
	50–85% HRRmax
Mode	Any exercise using large muscle groups
	that is continuous and rhythmic in nature

HR = heart rate; HRR = heart rate reserve.

6. How does one determine exercise intensity?

Intensity may be established by heart rate or exercise that corresponds to a certain oxygen cost. One guideline is 60–90% of maximal heart rate, which may be predicted by the equation 220 – age. Another guideline is heart rate that corresponds to 50–85% of the heart rate reserve maximum (HRRmax). The HRRmax is the difference between resting heart rate and maximal heart rate. Examples of these calculations are given below.

Calculation of Aerobic Training Heart Rate by HRRmax

STEP	CALCULATION
1. Compute age-predicted HR	220 – 20 = 200
2. Compute heart rate reserve	200 – 60 = 140
3. Select training intensity	80%
4. Calculate percent of reserve	140 × 0.80 = 112
5. Add resting heart rate	112 + 60 = 172
6. Target heart rate	172 beats/min

Note: Example is a 20-year-old with a resting HR = 60 beats/min. A corresponding target HR by the HRmax method is 200 × 0.80 = 160 beats/min.

Another method is based on exercise workloads that correspond with 50–85% of VO$_2$max. This method requires measurement of VO$_2$max and plotting of data based on the exercise intensity/VO$_2$ relationship. Although this is an excellent method, a more complete description is beyond the scope of this discussion. Finally, no exact method exists to determine initial exercise intensities. Refer to the following suggested training guidelines.

Suggested Initial Training Intensities

FITNESS LEVEL	HRmax (%)	HR RESERVE (%)	% VO$_2$max
Beginner (unconditioned)	60–70	50–65	50–65
Intermediate (recreational athlete)	70–80	65–75	65–75
Advanced (competitive athlete)	80–90 +	75–85 +	75–85 +

7. How often should one train?

Suggested training frequencies are 3–5 times per week. Endurance athletes may train 5–6 days per week, but for health-related aerobic fitness or sports or activities without a great aerobic demand, 3 days per week is adequate.

8. How long should the training sessions be?

The guidelines for aerobic conditioning are 20–60 minutes. About 20 minutes is the minimal duration for maintenance or improvement. Sixty minutes or longer may be required for some long-endurance athletes.

9. What are modes of aerobic exercise?

Aerobic exercises utilize large muscle groups and are continuous and rhythmic in nature. Examples include running, cycling, swimming, stair stepping, aerobic dance, and walking. Exercises that require heavy muscle contractions, such as weight training and sprinting, produce little change in VO_2max.

10. Does it matter which mode of exercise is used?

The answer depends on the intent of training. If a person is exercising for lifetime fitness, the mode does not matter, whereas if someone is training to improve a given sport performance, the mode is important. **Central adaptations** to exercise are relatively nondiscriminatory. Heart rate, stroke volume, and cardiac output changes may occur regardless of the exercise task. In other words, the heart does not know what mode of exercise is used—it simply knows that it must pump more blood. **Peripheral adaptations** to exercise modes are highly task-specific. Neuromuscular recruitment of specific motor units and appropriate blood flow shunts are essential to peripheral physiologic and biochemical adaptations. These changes allow greater tissue utilization of oxygen and improvement of VO_2max.

11. If a runner chose to cycle to improve running performance, which training principle is violated?

Specificity of training. Although a runner may maintain the central component by cycling, the peripheral component is not adequately stimulated because neuromuscular recruitment and blood flow shunts are not the same. Many modes of aerobic exercise may be used interchangeably, however, if health and fitness are the only goals (e.g., health of the heart, lower cholesterol, weight management).

12. How are overload and progression accomplished?

Intensity, frequency, and duration may be manipulated to impose a progressive overload. Intensity of exercise has the greatest influence on improving VO_2max. From the standpoint of progression, frequency should be emphasized first, keeping duration and intensity to a minimum until the desired times per week may be safely achieved. Once the frequency goal has been established, increasing the duration of exercise is emphasized. Intensity is kept low until the desired duration is met. Finally, intensity is manipulated. As fitness levels improve, gradual increases in the intensity of exercise stimulate the improvement of aerobic power. Abrupt increases in frequency, duration, or especially intensity should be avoided because they invite an underpreparation injury.

13. At what point will VO_2max not increase with training?

A genetically determined peak VO_2max may occur in 18–24 months of intense training. Up to 70% of the genetic potential may be achieved in 3 months. Improvements in endurance performances, when VO_2max fails to increase, occur when athletes are able to sustain exercise at a higher percent of VO_2max. Percent utilization of VO_2max is a powerful predictor of endurance exercise performance among individuals with similar aerobic power.

Aerobic Fitness Classifications VO_2max (ml/kg/min)

CATEGORY	MALE AGES		FEMALE AGES	
	13–19	20–29	13–19	20–29
Poor	Below 39	Below 36	Below 30	Below 27
Good	40–50	37–47	31–40	28–37
Excellent	51–59	48–56	41–50	38–47
Highly trained	60–80	57–80	51–65	48–65

14. How much improvement in aerobic power can occur? How long does it take?

The amount of improvement in VO_2max to expect from training is highly individualized and inversely related to the initial level of fitness. An untrained person may experience about a 25% increase in VO_2max in 8–12 weeks. A trained individual may experience a 5% or less improvement in the same time.

15. When should an aerobic training program begin?

When to begin training is dictated by the type of sport and the time at which peak level of conditioning is desired. Athletes in sports such as cross country, track, and swimming may use the season itself as a conditioning period, aiming to peak at the season's end for a championship meet. If a season is 10 weeks long, serious training may start 2–4 weeks before its beginning. Knowing that 8–12 weeks of training are required to obtain significant levels of improvement, an athlete may plan the training period accordingly.

16. How much training is needed?

The amount of training is also dictated by the sport. A football player requires minimal aerobic fitness and may dedicate 3 times per week for 15–20 minutes to aerobic conditioning, whereas a 10-km specialist may train 6 times per week for about 60 minutes, using a variety of high-intensity methods during half of the sessions. The amount of aerobic conditioning is influenced by the aerobic metabolic demand of the sport or event.

17. What is long slow duration training?

The emphasis of long slow duration training is duration rather than intensity. Intensities typically are about 70–80% HRmax, 60–70% of HRRmax, or 60–70% of VO_2max. This approach may be used for lifetime fitness, general conditioning, or as a training mode on days following intense workouts. Long slow duration training should not be used exclusively for the competitive athlete because it lacks the specific neuromuscular and metabolic stress necessary under competitive conditions. An example is a middle-distance runner who runs 6 miles at a 7:30 per mile pace.

18. What is long fast duration training?

Long fast duration training is typified by higher-intensity, moderate-duration forms of exercise. Intensities generally are 90% HRmax, 80–85% of HRRmax, or 80–85% of VO_2max. The athlete maintains a pace just at or below a racing speed. Because the intensity is higher than long slow duration training and the metabolic and neuromuscular components are specific to racing conditions, greater improvements can be made. The physical and psychological demands of long fast duration of training are great; therefore, alternating slow and fast workouts or other training variations is recommended. An example is a middle-distance runner who runs 4 miles at a 5:30 per mile pace.

19. What is interval training?

Interval training may be used to improve aerobic power. By using intervals of intense exercise interspersed with recovery, an athlete may maintain levels of intensity at or above racing conditions for an extended time. Interval training is a high-quality conditioning mode that exemplifies the tenets of exercise specificity. Aerobic training intervals are typically 3–5 minutes in duration performed at or above race paces. Suggested recovery times are from one to one-half the exercise interval time. An example is 3 minutes of exercise with 3 minutes of recovery. Recovery time also may be judged sufficient when the athlete's HR has returned to about 120–130 beats/min. Low-level activity between exercise intervals hastens the removal of lactic acid and thus expedites recovery. The suggested number of intervals is dictated by their length; for example, shorter intervals such as 3 minutes may be repeated 4–8 times, whereas longer intervals such as 5 minutes may be repeated 3–6 times.

20. How should a program be structured?

Most successful programs incorporate all three of the previously described methods. Typically intensive training days or weeks are followed by a corresponding number of easier days or weeks. This approach is necessary physiologically and psychologically. Foss and Keteyian[4] provide an excellent treatment of conditioning programs.

21. What are the special considerations for muscle glycogen depletion and restoration?

Many endurance athletes have chronic glycogen-depletion, which causes their performance to suffer. By and large glycogen depletion is due to overtraining and failure to consume an adequate amount of dietary carbohydrates. It takes approximately 48 hours while eating diets high in carbohydrates for complete restoration from a significantly depleted state. No exhaustive training should take place during this time.

22. Is training two or more times a day better than once a day?

Little scientific evidence indicates that training two or three times per day is better than a single workout. Although more research in this area is necessary, it is generally recommended that the athlete participate in one high-quality training session on scheduled days.

23. Are many long training hours needed for improved performance?

The "more is better" attitude is adopted by many endurance athletes. This attitude invites overtraining injury as well as decreased performance. Athletes who spend 10 or more hours per week in endurance training are probably using the long slow duration method, which is not as productive for providing improvement. Although no equation exists to establish a "perfect" training regimen, the emphasis should be on quality workouts interspersed with adequate low-intensity recovery days.

BIBLIOGRAPHY

1. American College of Sports Medicine: ACSM's Guidelines for Exercise Testing and Prescription. Baltimore, Williams & Wilkins, 1995.
2. American College of Sports Medicine: Position statement on the participation of the female athlete in long distance running. Med Sci Sports 11:ix, 1979.
3. American College of Sports Medicine: Position statement on the recommended quantity and quality of exercise for developing cardiorespiratory and muscular fitness in healthy adults. Med Sci Sports Exerc 22:265–284, 1990.
4. Foss M, Keteyian S: Fox's Physiological Basis for Exercise and Sport. Boston, WBC/McGraw-Hill, 1998.
5. Wilmore J, Costill D: Training for Sport and Activity. Dubuque, IA, William C. Brown, 1988.

15. BUILDING STRENGTH

L. Kay Thigpen, Ph.D.

1. Define strength.

Strength generally refers to a performance characteristic of muscle; for purposes of this chapter, strength is the maximal force a muscle or muscle group can generate.

2. What are strength, weight, and resistance training?

Strength training generally refers to exercises designed to increase the maximal force that a muscle or muscle group can generate voluntarily. Weight training is more specific and refers to the training modality associated with the use of free or machine weights. Resistance training encompasses a wide range of training modalities for strength.

3. What type of exercise is most effective in gaining strength?

Exercises that require voluntary maximal muscular contractions have been shown to be the most effective means of increasing strength. All types of muscular contractions (isometric, isotonic, and isokinetic) produce significant gains in muscular strength.

4. Describe isometric training.

Isometric training refers to the generation of muscular force with no visible joint movement. This type of training occurs when the external resistance is not overcome by internal force generation, as might occur when attempting to push open a locked door.

5. What is isotonic training?

Isotonic training refers to the generation of muscular force with visible joint movement at a variable speed but with a constant external resistance. Isotonic training encompasses free and machine weight training as well as exercises that use therabands or similar devices and exercises that use the body's own weight as resistance (e.g., push-ups, sit-ups).

6. How does isokinetic training differ from isotonic training?

Isokinetic training refers to the generation of muscular force with visible joint movement at a constant speed but with a variable external resistance. Thus, a muscle can generate maximal force throughout its length tension curve.

7. What is variable resistance training?

The terms variable resistance and accommodating resistance refer to specific types of isotonic weight training equipment that attempt to provide a changing external load during the execution of weightlifting exercises through the use of cams or levers.

8. Do variable resistance machines provide an external load that adjusts to the muscle's length tension curve?

Not really. Although equipment manufacturers claim that the external load varies by changing lever lengths during a lift, it is not matched to individual body segment lengths and therefore does not match the muscle's length tension curve.

9. When is isometric training appropriate?

Isometrics are most appropriate when joint motion is not wanted. Isometric training is angle-specific; that is, if the contraction occurs at an elbow angle of 90°, the strength gains occur only at that angle and 20° either side of the training angle. Strength gains are not evident at other joint angles.

10. What is an effective isometric training program?

Maximal isometric contractions are more effective than submaximal contractions. Contractions should be performed daily or several times a day. A small number (3–5) of long-duration contractions (10–30 sec) or a large number (10–30) of short-duration (3–5 sec) contractions provide optimal strength gains.

11. What are the contraindications to isometric training?

Isometrics tend to elevate blood pressure more than the other types of strength training and should be avoided in the elderly and others who are susceptible to hypertension. Another type of training would be more appropriate if a full-body or multiple-joint conditioning program is needed.

12. When is isotonic training indicated?

When strength gains are desired throughout a joint's range of motion.

13. What is an effective program of isotonic training?

Several variables must be considered: number of sets, number of repetitions per set, frequency of training, and intensity. Generally the optimal number of sets is 1–5, with 6–15 repetitions per set. The frequency of training may vary from 1–5 days/week per muscle group, depending on the intensity. Maximal voluntary contractions are essential to increase strength. Research suggests that the more times a muscle is taken to temporary failure, the greater the strength gains. Because of specificity of training, the exact program should reflect the specific goals of the training.

14. When is isokinetic training appropriate?

Isokinetic training is in theory the most effective means of increasing muscle strength, because it allows the muscle to generate maximal force throughout its length-tension curve. However, isokinetic equipment is still extremely expensive, difficult to use properly, and inaccessible to the general public. It is most beneficial during the early stages of rehabilitation. It is also most beneficial when the speed of training needs to resemble the higher speeds of contraction, which would be unsafe to perform with isotonic training.

15. What type of program is most effective in isokinetic training?

The same concerns must be addressed in isokinetic training as in isotonic training with one additional concern—the speed of training. Strength gains are speed-specific. If one wants strength at slow speeds of movement, slow-speed training should be performed. However, intermediate speed training (179°/sec) appears to have the most carryover effect to other speeds. The optimal number of sets and repetitions has not been determined, although most studies have not used fewer than 3 or more than 30. Sets have ranged from 1–10. All combinations have produced significant strength gains.

16. What mechanisms cause increases in strength?

Strength gains may result from neurologic and muscular adaptations.

17. Do neurologic adaptations cause significant gains in strength?

Yes. Research has shown that nearly all strength gains in the first 3–4 weeks of a strength-training program are due to neurologic adaptations. These adaptations come from two primary sources: the body's ability to repress its self-protection reflexes and the body's ability to recruit fully all of the motor units available at appropriate times.

18. What muscular adaptations result in strength gains?

Because the strength of any given muscle fiber is reasonably constant, gains in strength are generally thought to occur when muscle fiber cross-sectional area increases either from hypertrophy or hyperplasia.

19. What is hypertrophy?

Hypertrophy is an increase in muscle fiber size attributed to a greater number of actin and myosin filaments. Resistance training in humans results in increased cross-sectional area of both slow- and fast-twitch muscle fibers, depending on the training protocol. Slow-twitch fibers hypertrophy more with high-volume, low-intensity training and fast-twitch fibers hypertrophy more with low-volume, high-intensity training.

20. What is hyperplasia?

Hyperplasia is defined as the splitting of muscle fibers, which increases cross-sectional area by increasing the number of muscle fibers. Research has demonstrated that hyperplasia occurs in some animals, but evidence suggesting that it occurs in humans is controversial.

21. What is meant by progressive resistance exercises?

To understand this term, one must first understand the principles of overload and adaptation. Overload requires the muscle to exert more force than it would normally encounter, thus ensuring maximal voluntary contractions. The overloaded muscle adapts to this consistently applied overload by physiologic changes that increase strength. Progressive resistance exercise refers to any type of resistance training that adheres to the overload and adaptation principle. One must progressively increase the load to continue the increase in strength.

22. Describe the physiologic adaptations in muscle tissue that result from resistance training.

Cellular adaptations affect aerobic and anaerobic capabilities. These adaptations are listed in the table below.

Adaptations to Resistance Training and Effect of Resistance Training
on Anaerobic and Aerobic Metabolism

SYSTEM/VARIABLE	RESPONSE	METABOLISM	
		ANAEROBIC	AEROBIC
Bone			
Mineral content	Increase		
Cross-sectional area	No change		
Capillary density			
High-volume, low-intensity	No change		
Low-volume, high-intensity	Decrease		Decrease
Connective tissue			
Ligament strength	Increase		
Tendon strength	Increase		
Collagen content	Increase		
Ratio of connective tissue to muscle	No change		
Fuel stores			
Adenosine triphosphatase	Increase	Increase	
Phosphocreatine	Increase	Increase	
Glycogen	Increase	Increase	
Metabolic enzymes			
Creatine phosphokinase			
High-volume, low-load	Increase	Increase	Increase
Low-volume, high-load	Decrease	Decrease	Decrease
Myokinase			
High-volume, low-load	Increase	Increase	Increase
Low-volume, high-load	No change		
Phosphofructokinase			
High-volume, low-load	Increase	Increase	
Low-volume, high-load	No change		
Lactate dehydrogenase			
High-volume, low-load	No change		
Low-volume, high-load	No change		
Carbohydrate metabolism	Increase		Increase
Mitochondrial density	Decrease		Decrease
Muscle			
Size	Increase	Increase	Increase
Number	No change		

23. What changes affect the mitochondria?

Mitochondrial density (the number of mitochondria per volume of muscle tissue) is decreased by a significant increase in muscle mass, even though the number of mitochondria may increase slightly. This change lowers aerobic capacity.

24. How is capillarization affected by resistance training?

A heavy volume of resistance training at moderate-to-high intensity and short rest intervals increase muscle mass and capillarization, resulting in no change in capillary density. However, a low volume of training at a high intensity with long rest periods increases muscle mass but has no effect on capillarization, resulting in a decrease in capillary density and aerobic capacity.

25. Does resistance training affect anaerobic enzymes?

Creatine phosphokinase (CP) and myokinase increase with isokinetic training that resembles circuit training with heavy resistance. In fact, however, CP activity decreases. Phospho-fructokinase and lactate dehydrogenase, both used in glycosis, were found to decrease or show no change due to heavy resistance training.

26. What effect does resistance training have on aerobic enzymes?

The small amount of research on this topic indicates that heavy resistance training does not affect aerobic enzyme activity.

27. Does resistance training affect anaerobic intracellular fuel stores?

Yes. Intramuscular stores of adenosine triphosphate (ATP) and phosphocreatine increase as well as intramuscular glycogen stores. These cellular adaptations enhance the ability of the muscle to generate greater amounts of force for short duration.

28. Does resistance training decrease aerobic capacity?

No. In fact, when resistance training is performed in a circuit, small increases in aerobic capacity have been noted. Some studies have shown a slight decrease in aerobic capacity due to heavy resistance training. This decrease may be easily counteracted by performing a few days of aerobic training.

29. Do increases in muscle mass promote joint injury?

No. Resistance training increases the collagen content of the epimysium, perimysium, and endomysium. Research indicates that the total amount of connective tissue relative to total muscle mass remains relatively constant even in cases of extreme muscular hypertrophy (body-building). Thus joint integrity is not compromised.

30. Is bone affected by strength training?

Bone mineral content is increased by resistance training of high intensity and sufficient duration. However, studies in humans have been unable to confirm changes in bone cross-sectional area due to strength training.

31. What is meant by the terms *concentric* and *eccentric*?

Both terms describe types of muscular contractions that may be isotonic or isokinetic. Concentric contractions occur when the muscle fibers are shortening, as in the lifting phase of a biceps curl. Eccentric contractions occur when the muscle fibers are lengthening, as in the lowering phase of a biceps curl.

32. Is it true that eccentric training is more effective than concentric training?

No. Most studies that have directly compared the two types of training indicate that increases in strength are similar. However, eccentric training tends to generate significantly greater muscular soreness. Training that combines both types is more effective than concentric training alone. During ordinary free and machine weightlifting, every repetition contains a concentric and eccentric phase. To develop maximal benefit from the eccentric portion of the lift, one must lower the weight slowly in a controlled manner.

33. Is athletic performance improved by resistance training?

Although strength training enthusiasts have long promoted improved athletic performance as one of the primary benefits of strength training, research to support this conclusion is sparse.

Studies have shown increases in vertical jump height and decreases in sprint times due to highly specific isotonic and fast-speed isokinetic training protocols.

34. Is there a gender difference in the effects of resistance training?

No. Strength is directly proportional to the cross-sectional area of muscle. Females genetically have less muscle mass and therefore are generally weaker in terms of absolute muscle strength. When relative strength (strength per cross-sectional area) is considered, females are as strong as males. Females tend to exhibit greater percentage increases in strength than males in response to resistance training. Furthermore, resistance training of the upper extremities of females produces greater strength gains than lower extremity training. Both responses can be attributed primarily to the typical muscular training curve.

35. Describe the muscular training curve.

Untrained muscle responds more rapidly to resistance training than trained muscle. The more room for improvement that a muscle has, the more rapid its improvement. Muscles that are near their optimal performance level have less room for improvement and consequently improve less rapidly.

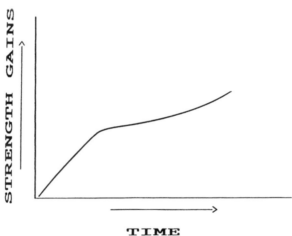

36. Is age a factor in response to resistance training?

No. All ages respond to resistance training. Young and old alike increase strength, although the rate and magnitude of strength gained may vary.

37. Are different programs needed for the extremes of the age continuum?

The same protocols are appropriate, and the safety precautions recommended for young and old are also appropriate for the middle of the continuum. Loads below 6 RM increase the incidence of injury.

38. Do increased levels of testosterone increase muscular hypertrophy in response to resistance training?

Not according to research. There appears to be no correlation between levels of testosterone and muscular response to resistance training.

39. What precautions are needed for resistance training in young adolescents?

Because bone is still developing in adolescents, compression injuries to the epiphyseal plate are a concern. A typical protocol avoids the use of small numbers of repetitions (< 6) with heavy loads (6 RM).

BIBLIOGRAPHY

1. Braith R, Graves J, Leggett S, Pollock M: Effect of training on the relationship between maximal and submaximal strength. Med Sci Sports Exerc 25:132–138, 1993.
2. Castro MJ, McCann DJ, Shaffrath JD, Adams WC: Peak torque per unit cross area differs between strength-trained and untrained young adults. Med Sci Sports Exerc 27:397–403, 1995.
3. Fleck S, Karma W: Designing Resistance Training Programs. Champaign, IL, Human Kinetics Books, 1987.
4. Fleck S, Kraemer W: Resistance training: Physiological responses and adaptations (Part 2 of 4). Phys Sports Med 16(4):109–124, 1988.
5. Fleck S, Schutt R: Types of strength training. Clin Sports Med 4:159–168, 1985.
6. Lillegard WA, Terrio JD: Appropriate strength training. Med Clin North Am 78:457–473, 1994.
7. MacDougall J, Sale D, Alway S, et al: Muscle fiber number in biceps brachii in bodybuilders and control subjects. J Appl Physiol 57:1399–1403, 1984.
8. MacDougall J, Sale D, Elder G, et al: Muscle ultrastructural characteristic of elite powerlifters and body-builders. Eur J Appl Physiol 48:117–126, 1982.
9. Moritani T, DeVries H: Neural factors versus hypertrophy in the time course of muscle strength gain. Am J Phys Med 82:521–524, 1979.
10. Sale D, MacDougall J, Alway S, et al: Voluntary strength and muscle characteristics in untrained men and women and male body builders. J Appl Physiol 62:1786–1793, 1987.
11. Starkey DB, Pollock ML, Ishida Y, et al: Effect of resistance training volume on strength and muscle thickness. Med Sci Sports Exerc 28:1311–1320, 1996.
12. Staff P: The effects of physical activity on joints, cartilage, tendons and ligaments. Scand J Soc Med 29(Suppl):59–63, 1982.
13. Tesch P, Komi P, Hakkinen K; Enzymatic adaptations consequent to long term strength training. J Appl Physiol 46:96–99, 1987.

16. STRENGTH TRAINING IN YOUNG ATHLETES

Stephen G. Rice, M.D., Ph.D., M.P.H., FAAP, FACSM

1. Define strength training.

Strength training (or resistance training) refers to the exertion of muscular force against resistance (such as body weight, machines, barbells, or dumbbells) to improve muscular strength, power, and endurance.

2. Is strength training the same as weightlifting?

Strength training is not to be confused with weightlifting, which is a sport. Strength training generally employs multiple repetitions of submaximal resistance of the purpose of improving muscle strength. In the sport of weightlifting, the object is to lift the maximal weight in a prescribed fashion; such maximal lifts are potentially dangerous to all competitors, especially younger athletes. Two categories of weightlifting are defined. Powerlifting includes the bench press, squat, and dead lift. Olympic lifting consists of the snatch lift and clean and jerk.

3. Who are young athletes?

Young athletes refer to prepubescent (Tanner stages I and II), physically active children. Others, however, include both prepubescent and adolescent athletes.

4. Why do young people strength train?

Primarily, young athletes strength train to enhance physical performances in sports and other physical activities through stronger muscles. Recently, numerous youngsters (early to postpubescent) have turned to strength training to look better or to "buff up." These youngsters are not oriented toward sports; their primary goal is to have attractive physiques.

5. Besides improving muscle strength, what other benefits does strength training provide?

In addition to increasing strength, strength training decreases the severity and rate of common sports injuries, increases power and flexibility (if a program is executed correctly), enhances motor fitness and sports performance, decreases the amount of time needed for rehabilitation of an injury, and improves a young athlete's self-image.

6. Can prepubescent children gain significant strength?

Yes. It has been proved that prepubescent children can improve muscle strength through strength training. In the past 10 years, nearly 20 studies have been done; most scientific evidence strongly suggests that children can significantly increase their strength if the resistance training program is of sufficient duration and intensity. In one study, for example, over a 9-week period, prepubescent children who strength trained improved muscle strength by > 40%, whereas the group that did not train gained < 10%.

7. How do young athletes gain strength?

Unlike adults, who gain strength through muscle hypertrophy (enlarged muscle cells), strength gains in young athletes are more likely due to motor learning (training muscles to respond rapidly and forcefully to the neurologic signals to contract). The mechanism appears to involve (1) increased motor unit activation, (2) changes in motor unit coordination, recruitment, and firing, and (3) possibly intrinsic muscle adaptation, all of which result in increased twitch torque. This also explains how a young man can gain strength without postpubescent levels of androgens (male sex hormones).

8. Can strength training be safe for the young?

Yes. With proper technique and supervision, strength training can be safe for young athletes. The young athlete, however, must be educated to understand that developmentally appropriate goals will be different from the goals of adults and postpubescent adolescents. The presence of an adequate number of alert spotters is also important to a safe experience.

9. What injuries are possible?

Growth plate (epiphyseal and apophyseal) fractures may result from improper execution of certain overhead and leg extension lifts. Stress fractures, musculotendinous strains, osteochondritis dissecans of the knee and elbow, fractured radius and ulna, cervical sprains and fractures, osteolysis of the distal clavicle, spondylolysis, spondylolisthesis, and ruptured lumbar discs in the low back are also possible as a result of improper technique. Some of these injuries may result from trauma (a single event), whereas others are the consequence of overuse (excessive multiple repetitions).

10. How safe is strength training compared with other sports?

According to one study, 7.6% of young athletes reported an injury related to strength training compared with 25.1% reporting a football injury.

11. What safety considerations must be taken during training?

1. A knowledgeable adult with proper training and credentials in conditioning and strength training (C.S.C.S. certification from the National Strength and Conditioning Association) should supervise. The instructor must have specific training and knowledge in dealing with prepubescent young athletes, because techniques used by older adolescents and adults are not appropriate and do not apply to the younger athletes. The ratio of instructors/supervisors to athletes working out must allow adequate supervision and assistance for each young athlete while performing exercises. Sufficient numbers of spotters must be available. A ratio of 10:1 is acceptable; however, additional supervision may be needed during the first few weeks of the program.

2. An athlete must use proper technique with a light enough weight that he or she can do 6–15 slow, controlled repetitions. Young athletes should not try a single-repetition maximum

because injuries may result. A key principle in strength training is to fatigue the muscles (reaching the point of temporary overload or failure) rather than to continue to and beyond the point of pain. By using a weight that requires 6–15 repetitions to achieve muscle fatigue and ensuring proper technique in executing the lifts, a young athlete can safely gain strength with minimal risk of injury.

12. Are blackouts a major concern?

No. Blackouts are easy to prevent; simply exhale as the muscle is contracting and inhale as the muscle is lengthening. The combination of breath-holding (Valsalva maneuver) and isometric contraction of most of the body's other muscles while executing a lift can cause a sudden diversion of cardiac output of blood to the head, resulting in a blackout. By using the proper breathing technique and tightening only the muscles needed to execute a lift, blackouts are easily avoided.

13. Should an athlete with hypertension exercise greater caution?

Yes. The American Academy of Pediatrics recommends that young people with significant cardiovascular problems or persistent hypertension should participate in strength training only after a comprehensive medical examination. Young people with hypertension should inform the instructor so that they receive extra attention during the exercise session. However, young people with only moderate hypertension need not be concerned if they remember to exhale while doing the strenuous part of the lift. Such athletes also should avoid stiffening all of the muscles of the body at once (doing a whole-body isometric contraction). This practice not only increases the pressure of the blood flowing to the head but also is poor technique. The young athlete who partakes of an active physical exercise program, including aerobics and strength training, is likely to improve cardiovascular fitness and muscle strength and to decrease body fat and blood pressure.

14. What lifts need to be avoided?

Young athletes engaged in strength training should avoid complex free weights lifts (generally used in weightlifting), such as the bench press, dead lifts, power cleans, clean and jerk, snatches, and overhead lifts.

15. At what age should young athletes begin a program?

Readiness for sports is the match between a child's level of growth, maturity, and development and the task demands of the sports activity. Growth considers body size, muscle strength, body composition, and aerobic power; maturity examines skeletal age, pubertal age, chronologic age, and level of proficiency of basic motor skills; development speaks to the social, emotional, and cognitive competence of the young athlete.

There is no specific age at which a young athlete should begin. Athletes who start strength training should have the emotional maturity to take directions and understand the limited goals for their age group (learning proper technique, enjoying the workout, and making moderate gains in muscle strength). In addition, young athletes should obtain a physical examination from a doctor knowledgeable in sports medicine to ensure that there are no medical contraindications to initiating the program.

16. Should free weights and machines be used in a program for young athletes?

It depends. Both can increase strength, but each has its advantages and disadvantages. Free weights develop coordinating strength in muscle groups but must be used with a spotter at all times. On the one hand, machines can be good for children because they rarely require a spotter. On the other hand, machines may be oversized and have a minimal weight that is too heavy for the athlete. Determine whether the machines can be adjusted to accommodate the smaller size of young athletes.

17. What kind of strength training program should a young athlete follow?

A young athlete's workout should include a warm-up, lifting session, and cool-down 2 or 3 times per week (with at least 48 hours between sessions). The **warm-up** should consist of about

5–10 minutes of movement exercise (calisthenics) and stretching. The calisthenic or movement exercises are designed to increase cardiovascular circulation slowly and to warm the body to the point of breaking a sweat. Stretches should be done in a static fashion, bringing the muscle to the point where the young athlete begins to feel tension or stress in the muscle (but before he or she experiences pain). Avoid ballistic (bouncing) stretches. Hold each stretch at least 10 seconds (ideally 30 seconds).

The **lifting session** is somewhat self-explanatory. Train large muscle groups first, then smaller muscle groups. Work groups that are antagonistic muscles in pairs (e.g., quadriceps and hamstrings, triceps and biceps). The athlete should concentrate on working a wide variety of muscles (e.g., chest, back, legs, shoulders). One to three sets of 6–15 repetitions with a light weight are recommended. A one-repetition maximum is dangerous and should be avoided.

A 15–20 minute **cool-down** consisting of light calisthenics and stretching should follow each workout.

BIBLIOGRAPHY

1. American Academy of Pediatrics Policy Statement: Strength training, weight and power lifting and bodybuilding by children and adolescents. Pediatrics 86:801–803, 1990.
2. American Academy of Pediatrics, Committee on Sports Medicine and Fitness: Athletic participation by children and adolescents who have systemic hypertension. Pediatrics 99:637–638, 1997.
3. American College of Sports Medicine: The prevention of sports injuries of children and adolescents. Med Sci Sports Exerc 25(Suppl 8):1–7, 1993.
4. American Orthopaedic Society for Sports Medicine: Proceedings of the Conference on Strength Training and the Prepubescent. Chicago, American Orthopaedic Society for Sports Medicine, 1988.
5. Faigenbaum AD: Prepubescent strength training: A guide for teachers and coaches. Natl Strength Condition J 15(5):20–29, 1993.
6. Lillegard WA: Principles of weight training. In Seefeldt V, Brown EW (eds): Program for Athletic Coaches' Education. Carmel, IN, Benchmark Press, 1991, pp 1–19.
7. Lillegard WA: Strength training in children. Sports Med Primary Care 2(8):S5–S8, 1995.
8. Malina RM: Children in the exercise sciences. Res Q Exerc Sport 60:306–317, 1989.
9. Malina RM, Bouchard C: Growth, Maturation and Physical Activity. Champaign, IL, Human Kinetics, 1991.
10. National Strength and Conditioning Association: Youth resistance training: Position statement paper and literature review. Natl Strength Condition J 18(6):62–65, 1996.
11. Ozmun J, Mikesky A, Surburg P: Neuromuscular adaptations following prepubescent strength training. Med Sci Sports Exerc 26:510–514, 1994.
12. Rians CB, Weltman A, Cahill BR, et al: Strength training in prepubescent males: Is it safe? Am J Sports Med 15:483–489, 1987.
13. Risser WL, Risser JMH, Preston D: Weight-training injuries in adolescents. Am J Dis Child 144:1015–1017, 1990.
14. Sewall L, Micheli LJ: Strength training for children. J Pediatr Orthop 6(2):143–146, 1986.
15. Tanner SM: Weighing the risks: Strength training for children and adolescents. Physician Sportsmed 21(6):105–116, 1993.
16. Webb DR: Strength training in children and adolescents. Pediatr Clin North Am 37(5):1187–1210, 1990.

17. FLEXIBILITY

Daniel Blanke, Ph.D.

1. What is flexibility?

Flexibility is the ability to move the joints of the body through the range of motion (ROM) for which they are intended. Each joint of the body is designed to allow a specific amount of motion. An individual lacks flexibility if he or she is unable to produce the amount of motion for which each joint is designed.

2. Range of motion at a joint is limited by what structures?

The type of joint and the shape of the bony structures that make up the joint play a significant role in the ROM possible at the joint. The connective tissue that surrounds the joint and is part of the muscles that cross the joint also is important in limiting the motion at that joint.

3. What is connective tissue?

Connective tissue is one of the most widely varied types of tissue. Although cartilage, bone, blood, and lymph are types of connective tissue, the connective tissue found in tendons, ligaments, intramuscular and extramuscular layers of fascia, and joint capsules is the type of connective tissue that we are concerned about as we discuss joint flexibility. This type of connective tissue is primarily composed of collagenous fibers arranged in a protein-polysaccharide ground substance. It possesses both elastic and plastic properties. This type of connective tissue is referred to as dense or collagenous connective tissue. Dense connective tissue exhibits high tensile strength and therefore is difficult to elongate. Because it is primarily responsible for limiting joint ROM, dense connective tissue is therefore the target of flexibility training. Joint flexibility can be increased through stretching exercises that increase the length of the connective tissue structures. References made to connective tissue in this chapter will be to this dense or collagenous type of connective tissue.

4. How does connective tissue respond to stretch?

When connective tissue is stretched, some of the elongation is elastic and some is plastic. Once the force causing the stretch in the connective tissue is removed, the elastic elements return to their resting length, whereas the plastic components remain elongated. Flexibility training should be designed to produce plastic rather than elastic deformation. Plastic deformation results in a more permanent change in length of the tissue. Low-force loads applied for long periods of time result in a greater incidence of plastic deformation. Stretching connective tissue under conditions of elevated temperature also results in greater plastic deformation. Flexibility training should therefore reflect these force, time, and temperature requirements.

5. What is the range of motion expected at each joint?

The normal ROM for each joint is listed below. It is apparent that there is considerable variation in the ROM expected for each joint.

Average Range of Joint Motion

JOINT	ROM IN DEGREES	JOINT	ROM IN DEGREES
Shoulder		**Hip**	
Flexion	158	Flexion	113
Extension	53	Extension	28
Abduction	170	Abduction	48
Adduction	50	Adduction	31
Horizontal flexion	135	Horizontal flexion	60
Arm at side		Hip in flexion	
Internal rotation	68	Internal rotation	45
External rotation	68	External rotation	45
Arm in 90° abduction		Hip in extension	
Internal rotation	70	Internal rotation	35
External rotation	90	External rotation	48
Elbow		**Knee**	
Flexion	146	Flexion	134
Hyperextension	0	Hyperextension	10
Forearm		**Ankle**	
Pronation	71	Plantar flexion	48
Supination	84	Dorsiflexion	18

(Table continued on following page.)

Average Range of Joint Motion (Continued)

JOINT	ROM IN DEGREES	JOINT	ROM IN DEGREES
Wrist		**Hind foot**	
Extension	71	Inversion	5
Flexion	73	Eversion	5
Ulnar deviation	33	**Fore foot**	
Radial deviation	19	Inversion	33
Thumb		Eversion	18
Abduction	58	**Great toe**	
I-P flexion	81	I-P flexion	60
M-P flexion	53	I-P extension	0
M-C flexion	15	M-P flexion	37
I-P extension	17	M-P extension	63
M-P extension	8	**2nd to 5th toes**	
M-C extension	20	Distal I-P flexion	55
Fingers		Middle I-P flexion	38
Distal I-P flexion	·80	M-P flexion	35
Middle I-P flexion	100	Extension	40
M-P flexion	90	**Cervical spine**	
Distal I-P extension	0	Flexion	38
Middle I-P extension	0	Extension	38
M-P extension	45	Lateral bending	43
		Rotation	45
		Thoracic and lumbar spine	
		Flexion	85
		Extension	30
		Lateral bending	28
		Rotation	38

From the American Academy of Orthopaedic Surgeons: Joint Motion: Method of Measuring and Recording. Chicago, AAOS, 1965.

6. How much flexibility is adequate?

To answer this question it may be best to first ask "flexibility that is adequate for what?" What is considered adequate ROM for a joint can vary somewhat in accordance with the demand placed on the joint. Flexibility is therefore a relative rather than absolute value. If the demand for ROM at a joint is very limited, then the amount of flexibility needed would also be quite limited. On the other hand, if the demand for ROM at the joint is great, then the amount of flexibility required would also be great. Therefore, adequate flexibility would be the ROM at each joint that would allow the individual to carry on the activities of daily living without undue difficulty or injury. If an individual's daily activities do not require much ROM at any joint, then adequate flexibility at each joint would be less than an individual who uses each joint at close to its limit each day.

7. How much flexibility is ideal?

As with adequate flexibility, ideal or optimal flexibility is a relative value. Ideal or optimal flexibility can be described as the required amount of flexibility or ROM at a joint that will allow for maximal performance of a defined activity while protecting the joint from acute or chronic injury. Ideal flexibility of the hip joint of a ballet dancer would be much higher than ideal flexibility of the hip joint of an accountant. Because many jobs require very limited physical activity, the amount of flexibility considered ideal often is determined by an individual's recreational pursuits or exercise behavior. A swimmer requires more shoulder flexibility than a runner. A person interested in sprinting requires more hip flexibility than a person who jogs slowly. This means it is important to consider an individual's daily living activities, job demands, recreational activities, and exercise interests to determine his or her flexibility requirements.

8. Can one have too much flexibility?

Although lack of flexibility can result in poor performance and injury, and ideal flexibility can allow for maximum performance and minimum acute or chronic injury potential, there also is some evidence that excessive flexibility can result in decreased joint stability. There is a trade-off between flexibility and stability. This decrease in joint stability is especially evident when flexibility increases are the result of lengthening the connective tissue structures that stabilize the joint. Deep knee bends may increase the ROM of the knee joint to the point where the knee is more susceptible to chronic or acute instability. An individual's ROM for each joint should be determined by the demands of the individual. Excessive ROM can be associated with decreased stability and a greater potential for injury.

9. What kinds of injuries are common as a result of lack of flexibility?

Individuals with limited flexibility are more susceptible to muscle strains than joint sprains, because the connective tissue surrounding the joint limits the ROM and provides greater support for the joint. Specific limitations in flexibility may contribute to particular problems. Lack of adequate flexibility in the hamstrings is associated with low back pain and pain in the knee and hip in exercisers. Lack of flexibility in the hand and wrist joints may contribute to repetitive motion syndrome or carpal tunnel syndrome.

10. What kinds of injuries are common as a result of too much flexibility?

Individuals with excessive flexibility are more susceptible to joint sprains because the connective tissue surrounding the joint has been elongated, and it therefore does not contribute as effectively to the stability of the joint. Excessive flexibility of a joint may contribute to osteoarthritis or joint pain.

11. How does one increase flexibility?

Several techniques of stretching can be used to increase flexibility safely and effectively. These include static stretching, static stretching with contraction of the antagonist (reciprocal inhibition), static stretching with contraction of the agonist (proprioceptive neuromuscular facilitation, PNF), and static stretching with contraction of the agonist followed by contraction of the antagonist (PNF). Individual exercises for each joint or area of the body should be performed using one or more of these techniques.

12. What is static stretching?

Static stretching is done by slowly moving the joint to the end of the ROM and then holding the position for 5–60 seconds. It is important when moving to the end of the ROM to stop at the point of moderate discomfort and prior to pain. As a result of the slow movement, there is a reduced tendency to elicit the stretch reflex. Static stretch is therefore one of the safest techniques for increasing flexibility.

13. What is static stretching with contraction of the antagonist (reciprocal inhibition)?

Static stretching with contraction of the antagonist is done by slowly moving the joint to the end of the ROM, then isometrically contracting the antagonist muscle group for 5–30 seconds. This is the muscle group directly opposite the muscle being stretched. It is again important to move the joint just to the point of moderate discomfort and no farther. This technique enjoys all the benefits of static stretching with the added benefit of further reducing the tendency to elicit the stretch reflex by actively contracting the antagonist muscle group. By the action of reciprocal inhibition, there is a release of an inhibitory transmitter substance at the spinal cord to reduce the activity of the muscle being stretched.

14. What is static stretching with contraction of the agonist (PNF)?

Static stretching with contraction of the agonist is performed by slowly moving the joint to the end of the ROM and then isometrically contracting the agonist muscle group for 5–30 seconds.

This is a contraction of the muscle group that is being stretched. No movement should occur in the muscle being stretched. The contraction must therefore be isometric. It is theorized that the isometric contraction of the muscle being stretched will relax the muscle, possibly through the action of the Golgi tendon organ, and therefore allow additional ROM at the joint. Minimally, the isometric contraction will put an additional stretch on the connective tissue surrounding the joint and therefore allow greater ROM.

15. What is static stretching with contraction of the agonist followed by contraction of the antagonist (PNF)?

Static stretching with contraction of the agonist followed by contraction of the antagonist is performed by slowly moving the joint to the end of the ROM and then isometrically contracting the agonist muscle group for 5–30 seconds. As with the previous PNF method, this is contraction of the muscle group being stretched. This is followed by relaxing the agonist and contracting the antagonist muscle group, the group opposite the group being stretched, for 5–30 seconds while attempting to stretch the muscle group even more.

16. Are there any types of flexibility exercises that one should avoid?

Although ballistic flexibility exercises will increase an individual's flexibility, this type of flexibility training has been associated with an increase in injury as well. Ballistic flexibility exercises should be avoided.

17. What is ballistic stretching?

Ballistic stretching is performed by quickly moving the joint to the end of the ROM. It often uses bouncing or jerking movements or momentum to force the joint beyond its normal ROM. The movements may be described as pulsing, bobbing, swinging, or kicking movements. Although ballistic stretching has been shown to increase flexibility, it is not recommended as a technique because of the increased potential of injury that is associated with this type of flexibility training. There is a greater tendency for injury as a result of the additional forces created by movement. These forces can lead to muscle or connective tissue tears or bone avulsion.

18. What is the stretch reflex?

The stretch reflex is a protective reflex due to the action of the muscle spindles. When a muscle is stretched rapidly, especially at its greatest length, the muscle spindle sends a stimulus to the central nervous system (CNS), which in turn sends a stimulus back to the muscle. The muscle responds by contracting. The force of contraction is somewhat related to the speed of the stretch. The purpose of this reflex is to protect the muscle and associated joints from injury by limiting the ROM of the muscle. The stretch reflex hampers flexibility training by actively contracting the muscle that is in the process of being elongated. Slow movements that reduce the intensity of the contraction and delay the activity of the stretch reflex until reaching maximum ROM are more desirable than fast movements that elicit the stretch reflex. Flexibility training that uses slow movements therefore reduces the incidence of injury.

19. Which techniques are recommended for a flexibility training program?

In order to improve flexibility, an individual should choose one of the techniques for performing flexibility exercises and then identify specific exercises for each joint. Flexibility exercises should be done daily or more than once per day. Contrary to exercises designed to increase strength, exercises to increase flexibility can be done safely as often as is convenient. Three to five repetitions of each exercise should be performed for best results. It is important that flexibility exercises be done regularly both to increase and maintain the desired joint ROM.

20. What happens if flexibility exercises are stopped?

If you do no flexibility exercises or if you stop doing flexibility exercises, the connective tissue that surrounds the joint and the connective tissue in the muscle will shorten and the ROM of the joint will decrease. This adaptive shortening will continue until the ROM at the joint is maintained by the activities of daily living. The greatest loss of flexibility occurs in the first 2 weeks after termination of flexibility training. After 4 weeks, an individual will continue to lose flexibility but will still be more flexible than prior to starting a flexibility training program. It is therefore important to train for flexibility on a regular basis. If training is not possible because of illness or injury, flexibility will deteriorate, but the increase in joint ROM gained in flexibility training will not be completely eroded even after 4 weeks of inactivity.

21. What effects do habitual movement patterns have on flexibility?

Habitual movement patterns have the greatest effect on flexibility. Moving the joint through a limited ROM will decrease the flexibility of the joint over time owing to adaptive shortening of the muscle and connective tissue. The elastic nature of connective tissue causes it to shorten when no load is applied. To reduce the potential for limited ROM, it is important to exercise the joint through full ROM whenever possible.

22. Is it better to perform the flexibility exercises at a particular time of the day?

Any time of the day is as good as another. An individual may find that he or she is more comfortable performing flexibility exercises at a particular time of the day. Flexibility exercises should be performed when the muscle and connective tissue are warm. It is difficult to elevate tissue temperature deep within large muscles with topical application of heat. In a clinical environment, deep heating methods of diathermy or ultrasound may be beneficial, but in the nonclinical environment, the temperature is best elevated through several minutes of muscle activity. In order to gain maximum benefit of plastic deformation of connective tissue after stretching, the connective tissue should be allowed to cool while the stress is applied. This implies that the most effective flexibility training can be done if the tissue temperature has been elevated and then allowed to cool during the training period. This substantiates the normal practice of training for increased flexibility during the cool-down portion of an exercise bout.

23. Are women more flexible than men?

Girls and women tend to be more flexible than males of the same age. The difference in flexibility between males and females of the same age is partly due to the differences in muscle mass and quantity of connective tissue, but is also is due to the greater tendency for girls and women to participate in activities such as dance, slimnastics, and gymnastics that typically promote flexibility.

24. Are children more flexible than adults?

Flexibility tends to decrease with age. The effects of aging on flexibility can be reduced by consistently participating in a program designed to maintain or enhance flexibility.

BIBLIOGRAPHY

1. Alter M: Science of Flexibility, 2nd ed. Champaign, IL, Human Kinetics, 1996.
2. Alter M: Sport Stretch, 2nd ed. Champaign, IL, Human Kinetics, 1998.
3. American Academy of Orthopaedic Surgeons: Joint Motion: Method of Measuring and Recording. Chicago, American Academy of Orthopaedic Surgeons, 1965.
4. Anderson B: Stretching. Bolinas, CA, Shelter Publications, 1980.
5. Anderson B, Burke E: Scientific, medical, and practical aspects of stretching. Clin Sports Med 10:63–86, 1991.
6. Anderson B, Pearl B, Burke E: Getting in Shape: Workout Programs for Men and Women. Bolinas, CA, Shelter Publications, 1994.
7. Bandy B, Irion J: The effect of time on static stretching on the flexibility of the hamstring muscles. Phys Ther 74:845–850, 1994.
8. Beaulieu J: Stretching for All Sports. Pasadena, CA, Athletic Press, 1980.
9. Beaulieu J: Developing a stretching program. Physician Sportsmed 9(11):59–66, 1981.
10. Donovan G, McNamara J, Gianoli P: Exercise Danger. Dubuque, IA, Kendall/Hunt, 1988.

11. Etnyre B, Lee E: Comments on proprioceptive neuromuscular facilitation stretching techniques. Res Q 58:184–188, 1987.
12. Etnyre B, Lee E: Chronic and acute flexibility of men and women using three different stretching techniques. Res Q 59:222–228, 1988.
13. Knapik J, Bauman C, Jones B, et al: Preseason strength and flexibility imbalances associated with athletic injuries in female collegiate athletes. Am J Sports Med 19:76–80, 1991.
14. Knapik J, Jones B, Bauman C, Harris J: Strength, flexibility and athletic injuries. Sports Med 14:277–278, 1992.
15. Kravitz L, Heyward V: Flexibility training. Fitness Manage 11(2):32–38, 1995.
16. Marieb E: Human Anatomy and Physiology, 3rd ed. Redwood City, CA, Benjamin/Cummings, 1995.
17. McAtee R: Facilitated Stretching: PNF Stretching Made Easy. Champaign, IL, Human Kinetics, 1993.
18. Nelson K, Cornelius W: The relationship between isometric contraction durations and improvement in shoulder joint range of motion. J Sports Med Phys Fitness 31:385–388, 1991.
19. Rasch P: Kinesiology and Applied Anatomy, 7th ed. Philadelphia, Lea & Febiger, 1989.
20. Sapega A, Quedenfeld T, Moyer R, Butler R: Biophysical factors in range-of-motion exercise. Physician Sportsmed 9(12):57–64, 1981.
21. Smith C: The warm-up procedure: To stretch or not to stretch. J Orthop Sports Phys Ther 19:12–17, 1994.
22. Taylor D, Dalton J, Seaber A, Garrett W: Viscoelastic properties of muscle-tendon units. Am J Sports Med 18:300–308, 1990.
23. Thomas T, Zebas C: Scientific Exercise Training. Dubuque, IA, Kendall/Hunt, 1984.

IV. *Environmental Concerns*

18. THERMOREGULATION AND SAFE EXERCISE IN THE HEAT

Mark J. Leski, M.D.

1. Where is the core temperature regulatory center?

The core temperature regulatory center is located in the preoptic area of the anterior hypothalamus.

2. Describe the role of the hypothalamus in regard to heat stress.

When blood bathing the hypothalamus exceeds 37° C (98.6° F), a reflex response (Benzinger reflex) dilates skin blood vessels and causes sympathetic cholinergic stimulation of eccrine sweat glands.

3. What is the hypothalamic set point? How is it affected by exercise?

The hypothalamic set point is a steady state body temperature (generally considered to be 37° C) at which the mechanisms for neither heat elimination nor heat production are active. During exercise, elevation of the set point is followed by an upward shift in core temperature threshold for vasodilation. This may represent an adaptive response that increases the speed of chemical reactions in active tissues.

4. What are the mechanisms of heat dissipation from the body?

The body uses radiation, conduction, convection, and vaporization of water as mechanisms of thermal transfer to the environment. When environmental temperature is well below skin temperature, as much as 70% of heat loss is through radiation, conduction, and convection. The rate of loss through convection depends on the speed of air currents over exposed skin. However, as environmental temperature rises above 68° F, vaporization of water accounts for most heat loss. As ambient temperature approaches body temperature, the body must rely solely on vaporization of water for cooling.

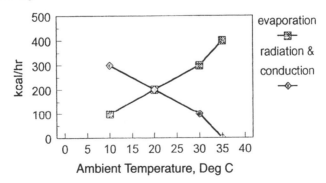

Mechanisms of heat loss related to ambient temperature. (Modified from Gisolfi CV, Wenger CB: Temperature regulation during exercise. Exerc Sport Sci Rev 12:339–372, 1984.)

5. Describe the mechanisms of heat gain in the body.

Heat is gained directly from the reactions of energy metabolism, especially in conversion of biochemical energy into mechanical work. During vigorous exercise, the metabolic rate can increase as much as 20–25 times basal level, producing a theoretical increase in core temperature of $1°$ C every 5 minutes. Heat also may be gained directly from the environment through radiation, conduction, and convection when the ambient temperature is greater than skin temperature. Dark-colored clothing absorbs light and adds to radiant heat gain.

6. How does the circulatory system respond to the demands of exercise in the heat?

In response to exercise in the heat, skin blood vessels dilate and blood is shunted from the visceral organs to working muscles and skin. Total peripheral resistance decreases, and pulse pressure widens. Heart rate and stroke volume increase, improving cardiac output to meet the increased demands on the circulatory system. The physiologic responses to heat stress are summarized by the mnemonic, **Heat Stress Can Speed The Pulse By Skin:**

Heat   = **H**eart rate increases
Stress = **S**troke volume increases
Can   = **C**ardiac output increases
Speed = **S**kin blood vessels dilate
The   = **T**otal peripheral resistance decreases
Pulse = **P**ulse pressure widens
By   = **B**lood is shunted from visceral organs to skin
Skin = **S**weat glands are stimulated

7. What is the latent heat of vaporization?

The latent heat of vaporization is the amount of heat transferred to the environment through vaporization of water. The vaporization of 1 liter of sweat from the body removes approximately 580 kcal of heat (about 0.6 kcal of heat per 1 cc of sweat evaporated).

8. Why is evaporation considered the major physiologic defense against overheating?

As ambient temperature rises, the body must rely more on evaporation for heat loss. A person exercising in the heat may sweat 2–3 L/hr and up to 15 L/day, depending on physical condition. Under conditions that allow rapid evaporation, including cloud cover, steady breezes, and low humidity, daily cooling capacity from sweating is several thousand calories per day.

9. Is sweat a hypo- or hypertonic solution?

Sweat is a hypotonic solution. It promotes conservation of sodium that helps the body retain water in hot conditions.

10. Describe how sweating helps to cool core body temperature.

As sweat in contact with skin evaporates, the heat that was transferred by conduction from the skin to the sweat is now transferred to the environment. This has a cooling effect on the skin. The cooled skin subsequently cools the blood that has been shunted from the interior to the periphery.

11. How much of the cardiac output passes through the skin during heat stress?

In an attempt to transport heated core blood to cooler skin, 15–20% of cardiac output may pass through the skin in severe heat stress.

12. List the factors that influence the rate of total sweat vaporization.

1. The total surface area exposed to the environment
2. The convective air currents (wind velocity)
3. Ambient air temperature
4. Humidity
5. Cloud cover
6. Sweat volume production
7. Clothing able to wick sweat and heat
8. Normal autonomic function

13. Why is relative humidity the most important factor affecting evaporative heat loss?

In high humidity, ambient vapor pressure approximates the vapor pressure of moist skin, which greatly reduces the rate of evaporation and significantly decreases this mechanism of thermal transfer. One continues to sweat, however, resulting in useless water loss that may lead to volume depletion.

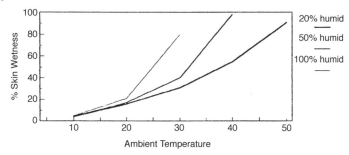

Relationship of ambient temperature and relative humidity to skin wetness at moderate work conditions (3 × basal metabolic rate). (Modified from Schmidt RF, Thews G: Human Physiology. Heidelberg, Springer-Verlag, 1983, p 538.)

14. What is the best indicator of heat stress?

The wet bulb globe temperature index (WBGT) is the best indicator of heat stress and is calculated as follows:

$$WBGT = 0.1 (DBT) + 0.7(WBT) + 0.2(GT)$$

Dry bulb temperature (DBT) is the air temperature recorded with a mercury thermometer. Wet bulb temperature (WBT) takes into account the humidity and is recorded with a similar thermometer surrounded by a wet wick exposed to any air movement (wet bulb thermometer). Globe temperature (GT) is recorded by a thermometer encased in a black globe that absorbs surrounding radiant energy (black globe thermometer). The WBGT is the gold standard; however, the apparatus is expensive. A **sling psychrometer** is also an effective device for measuring heat stress and is about one-tenth the price. In general, exercise should be reduced significantly or not be performed at all if the WBGT is ≥ 85° F (31° C). Charted guidelines for exercise based on WBGT and state of acclimatization are available.[2]

15. Why is an athlete's hydration status important?

The ability of the circulatory and thermoregulatory system to meet the metabolic and thermal stress of exercise is markedly reduced in the volume-depleted state.

16. Describe how volume depletion affects the circulatory system.

As a result of dehydration, blood volume is decreased, and this decrease in turn lowers cardiac filling pressure (left ventricular end diastolic pressure) and stroke volume. A compensatory increase in heart rate results, signaling a general deterioration in circulatory efficiency during exercise. For every liter of water loss, the heart rate elevates about 8 beats/minute, and cardiac output declines one L/min. Volume depletion, represented by a 4% loss in body weight, may reduce blood volume as much as 18%.

17. How does volume depletion reduce the effectiveness of the thermoregulatory system?

A lowered blood volume in the dehydrated state results in decreased blood flow to the skin and hinders heat loss. For every liter of water lost, core temperature rises approximately 0.3° C. A fluid loss as little as 1% of total body weight is associated with a significant elevation in core temperature during exercise. When dehydration becomes extreme, the body stops sweating in an attempt to conserve remaining blood volume. In this state, core temperatures may rise to lethal levels.

Circulatory and Thermoregulatory Effects of Dehydration during Exercise

1. Blood volume decreased	5. Skin blood flow decreased
2. Cardiac filling pressure decreased	6. Sweating may decrease or stop
3. Heart rate increased (compensatory)	7. Core temperature increased
4. Circulatory efficiency deteriorates	

18. What effect does dehydration have on the ability to function during exercise?

In dehydration, delivery of oxygen to working muscles is reduced, resulting in early fatigue. Mild dehydration of 2–3% may reduce work capacity by 15–20%. As dehydration progresses, cognitive function deteriorates and physical capacity becomes seriously compromised. Acute dehydration of 5–6% total body weight may be incompatible with further functioning.

19. What is the best way to monitor hydration status?

Hydration status is best monitored by pre- and postexercise nude, dry body weight. A decrease in body weight after exercise represents fluid loss; a pound of lost weight is equal to 16 oz of water. This fluid should be replaced and weight normalized before the next episode of exercise. Other signs of volume depletion include increased urine specific gravity, decreased urine output, resting tachycardia, and prolonged muscle soreness. **Thirst is not a good indicator of hydration status.**

20. How can one reduce the chance of dehydration while exercising in the heat?

About 400–600 ml (13–20 oz) of cool fluid should be consumed 15–20 minutes prior to exercise. Once exercise begins, consuming a volume of about 150–250 ml (6–8.5 oz) of cool fluid every 15 minutes is recommended. After exercise is completed, the athlete should rehydrate to preexercise body weight. Fluids between 15–22° C (59–72° F) improve palatability and promote fluid replacement.

21. Do electrolyte and carbohydrate solutions slow gastric emptying and rehydration?

High-osmolality solutions slow gastric emptying. However, gastric emptying is influenced primarily by the volume of liquid contained in the stomach. A preexercise fluid bolus combined with ingesting a high volume of liquid during exercise results in greater delivery of fluid to the small intestine. Thus, hydration should not be hindered if the fluid is an isotonic or hypotonic solution with less than 5–6% carbohydrate. In fact, hydration may be improved because people tend to drink more fluid when the fluid is more palatable.

22. Does electrolyte ingestion during exercise improve performance or reduce physiologic strain?

No evidence indicates that electrolyte ingestion during exercise is directly responsible for improving performance. However, solutions that are isotonic and hypotonic have been shown to improve the ability to rehydrate, consequently reducing the physiologic strain of exercising in the heat. The mechanism is three-fold. First, the thirst response is not curtailed by decreasing the osmotic drive when electrolyte solutions are ingested. As a result, athletes tend to drink more. Second, there is a decrease in posthydration diuresis after ingestion of electrolyte solutions. Therefore, athletes retain more water after postexercise rehydration. Finally, electrolyte solutions are generally more palatable, thus improving fluid intake. On the other hand, replacement of electrolytes through fluid intake is not necessary during exercise lasting less than 1–2 hours. Electrolytes may be replaced by eating a well-rounded diet, including fruits and vegetables high in potassium and calcium.

23. When is salt supplementation needed?

With prolonged exercise in the heat, sodium losses can exceed the dietary intake by as much as 8 gm. Sodium supplementation may be accomplished by 1 liter of a 0.1% Na^+ solution (⅓–½ tsp table salt in 1 liter of water). These solutions, however, can be risky. The average American diet contains 9–14 gm of sodium. With ingestion of junk food, the amount quickly increases to 20 gm. In this case, the electrolyte solutions may not be necessary.

24. What is heat acclimatization?

Heat acclimatization is the physiologic changes that improve capacity for exercise in the heat and decrease the discomfort of heat exposure.

25. How can one become acclimatized to the heat?

Four to seven sessions of exercising 1–4 hr per session can acclimatize a person to heat. One should start gradually, alternating 15 minutes of work with 15 minutes of rest, and build up tolerance.[2]

26. List the physiologic effects of acclimatization.

1. Blood volume increased
2. Heart rate lower at a given work load and heat stress
3. Skin vasodilation earlier
4. Sweating initiated earlier
5. Sweating rate increased
6. Sweat sodium concentration decreased
7. Core temperature lower at a given work load and heat stress
8. Perceived intensity of exercise reduced
9. Thermal comfort increases

27. Discuss the role of clothing while exercising in the heat.

Dark colors absorb heat; light colors reflect heat. Therefore, while exercising in the heat, one should wear light-colored clothing to decrease the amount of radiation energy absorbed by the body. Evaporative heat loss occurs only when clothing is wet; therefore, one should not change to dry clothing. Dry clothing retards heat loss from the evaporative route. The down side of wet clothing is that it increases development of chafed skin, tineas, and blisters. Clothing should be loose-fitting to allow good air circulation about the body for evaporative heat loss. Clothing should be washed regularly after exercise because dirt, oil, and salt close the holes in woven cloth, reducing air circulation and wicking of sweat. Heavy clothing or clothing made of polyester or rubber retards evaporation, thereby decreasing heat loss by this method.

28. Why does febrile illness lower the threshold for exercise in the heat?

Febrile illness increases the hypothalamic set point; therefore, heat-dissipating mechanisms do not begin until temperature exceeds that of the new set point. This, along with dehydration, which often accompanies febrile illness because of increased insensible water loss, significantly reduces thermoregulatory capacity and leaves the athlete susceptible to heat injury. Athletes recovering from fever have increased susceptibility to heat illness even after clinical evidence of illness has resolved.

29. Should athletes use sunscreens?

Yes. Besides protecting the skin from aging and skin cancer, sunscreens protect against sunburn. Sunburn reduces the ability of skin to function in the thermoregulatory process.

30. Can medications affect the thermoregulatory system?

Several recreational and prescribed drugs either increase heat production or inhibit heat loss.

Medications Affecting Thermoregulation

DRUG	EFFECT
CNS stimulants (phenylpropanolamine, LSD, cocaine, PCP)	Increase heat production Cause hypothalamic dysfunction
Thyroxine	Increases heat production
Parasympatholytic or anticholinergics	Inhibit sweating

(Table continued on following page.)

Medications Affecting Thermoregulation (Continued)

DRUG	EFFECT
Neuroleptics	Associated with malignant hyperthermia
Beta blockers	Limit cardiac response to heat stress
Diuretics	Possible volume contraction reducing skin perfusion
Opiates	May blunt thirst mechanism
Salicylates	May abet hyperthermia by uncoupling oxidative phosphorylation

CNS, central nervous system; LSD, lysergic acid diethylamide; PCP, phencyclidine.

BIBLIOGRAPHY

1. Allman FL: The effects of heat on the athlete. JAMA 81:307–310, 1992.
2. Bracker MD: Environmental and thermal injury. Clin Sports Med 11(2):419–436, 1992.
3. Gisolfi CV, Wenger CB: Temperature regulation during exercise: Old concepts, new ideas. Exerc Sports Sci Rev 12:339–372, 1984.
4. Gonzales-Alonso J, Heaps CL, Coyle EF: Rehydration after exercise with common beverages and water. Int J Sports Med 13:399–406, 1992.
5. Heat Illness: A Handbook for Medical Officers. US Army Technical Note 91, U.S. Army Research Institute of Environmental Medicine, Natick, MA, 1991.
6. Hubbard RW, Szlyk PC, Armstrong LE: Influence of thirst and fluid palatability on fluid ingestion during exercise. In Gisolfi CV, Lamb DR (eds): Perspectives in Exercise Science and Sports Medicine: Fluid Homeostasis During Exercise. Indianapolis, Benchmark Press, 1990, pp 39–96.
7. Jacobson S: The ill effects of heat. Emerg Med 15:313–324, 1992.
8. Johnson JM: Exercise and the cutaneous circulation. Exerc Sports Sci Rev 20:59–97, 1992.
9. Maughan RJ: Effects of CHO-electrolyte solution on prolonged exercise. In Lamb DR, Williams MH (eds): Perspectives in Exercise Science and Sports Medicine. Carmel, CA, Benchmark Press, 1991, pp 35–89.
10. Maughan RJ, Owens JH, Shirreffs SM, Leiper JP: Post-exercise rehydration in man: Effects of electrolyte addition to ingested fluids. Eur J Appl Physiol 69:209–215, 1994.
11. Maughan RJ, Shirreffs SM, Leiper JB: Rehydration and recovery after exercise. Sport Sci Exerc 9(62):1–5, 1996.
12. McArdle WD, Katch FJ, Katch VL (eds): Exercise Physiology, 2nd ed. Philadelphia, Lea & Febiger, 1986.
13. Mellion MB, Walsh WM, Shelton GL: The Team Physician's Handbook, 2nd ed. Philadelphia, Hanley & Belfus, 1997.
14. Montain SJ, Coyle EF: The influence of graded dehydration on hyperthermia and cardiovascular drift during exercise. J Appl Physiol 73:1340–1350, 1992.
15. Montain SJ, Coyle EF: Influence of the timing of fluid ingestion on temperature regulation during exercise. J Appl Physiol 75:688–695, 1993.
16. Noakes TD, Rehrer NJ, Maugham RJ: The importance of volume in regulating gastric emptying. Med Sci Sports Exerc 23:307–313, 1990.
17. Nose HG, Mack GW, Shi X, Nadel ER: Role of osmolality and plasma volume during rehydration in humans. J Appl Physiol 65:325–331, 1988.
18. Rehrer NJ, Beckets EJ, Brouns F, et al: Effects of dehydration on gastric emptying and gastrointestinal distress while running. Med Sci Sports Exerc 21:540–549, 1989.
19. Rehrer NJ, Brouns F, Beckers E, et al: Gastric emptying with repeated drinking during running and bicycling. Int J Sports Med 11:238–243, 1990.
20. Robertson JW: Preventing heat injury in sports. Phys Sports Med 19(5):31–35, 1991.
21. Schmidt RF, Thews G (eds): Human Physiology. Heidelberg, Springer-Verlag, 1983.
22. Stamford B: How to avoid dehydration. Phys Sports Med 18(7):135–136, 1990.
23. Wilk B, Bar-or O: Effect of drinking flavor and NaCl on voluntary drinking and hydration in boys exercising in the heat. J Appl Physiol 80:1112–1117, 1996.
24. Young AJ: Energy substrate utilization during exercise in extreme environments. Exerc Sports Sci Rev 18:65–119, 1990.

19. HEAT INJURIES

Clark H. Cobb, III, M.D., and John M. Henderson, D.O.

1. What are heat-related illnesses?

Heat-related illnesses or heat injuries are common and challenging disorders of thermoregulation. These disorders lie along a spectrum from mild and self-limited dysfunction to true life-threatening medical emergencies. The underlying pathophysiology reflects heat gain in excess of heat loss.

2. What types of minor heat-related illnesses are commonly seen?

In addition to the more familiar cases of heat stroke and heat exhaustion, heat-related illnesses also include heat edema, heat tetany, miliaria rubra (prickly heat), heat syncope, and heat cramps. Significant sunburn could also be considered a common heat-related injury.

Heat edema—benign, self-limited swelling of the hands and feet that is usually seen in the first few weeks of acclimatization and resolves with cooling, elevation of the affected part, and light compression when necessary (avoid diuretics).

Heat tetany—carpopedal spasm (probably secondary to the normal hyperventilation seen with increased temperature).

Heat syncope—function of decreased vasomotor tone and venous pooling (immediately after stopping exercise) together with elevated body temperature; decreased hydration also contributes.

Miliaria rubra—maculopapular, erythematous rash affecting clothed parts of body when keratin plugs block sweat gland pores; proper hygiene is usually sufficient for treatment.

Heat cramps—cramps of heavily worked muscle groups (lower extremity and abdomen in particular); they appear to wander because the entire muscle is usually not affected; they are usually associated with a whole body salt deficiency. Treatment focuses on sodium replacement (0.1% oral saline solution or IV normal saline).

Weak line rule—Any heat injury in a military unit or among members of an athletic team or work group suggests that others are at risk. Precautions are mandatory.

3. What is the difference between heat exhaustion and heat stroke?

As mentioned, heat-related illnesses lie along a spectrum whose divisions are somewhat arbitrary. Historically, the label **heat exhaustion** has been applied to cases where a patient's temperature did not exceed 102° F and mental status changes were absent. Similarly, **heat stroke** was considered when the temperature was greater than 104° F, mental status was altered, and sweating was absent. We now know that heat exhaustion and heat stroke may be indistinguishable on presentation (the signs and symptoms of multiorgan system dysfunction seen with the latter may not become evident for hours or days). Because heat strokes account for hundreds of deaths in the United States annually, intervention should err on the side of treatment of this more dangerous condition when confusion exists. Any evidence of renal, neurologic, or hepatic injury during the initial 24 hours should lead to the presumptive diagnosis of heat stroke.

4. What is the difference between classic and exertional heat stroke?

Classic heat stroke is often seen during summer heat waves and typically affects poor, elderly, chronically ill, alcoholic, or obese persons. Certain infections and medications increase susceptibility as well. **Exertional heat stroke** also is more common in the summer, but it is not that unusual in the spring and fall. It is frequently seen in athletes, laborers, and military personnel who often sweat profusely. Signs and symptoms are similar in both cases, but the onset may be more rapid in exertional cases.

5. Which endogenous factors predispose to heat injury?

Age (extremes)	Hypokalemia	Sweat gland problems
Dehydration	Alcohol	Drugs (see below)
Obesity	Midday overeating	Past heat injury
Exercise	Heart disease	Sunburn

Drugs that either increase endogenous heat production (e.g., tricyclic antidepressants, amphetamines, lysergic acid diethylamide (LSD), PCP, cocaine) or those that impair heat dissipation (anticholinergics, antihistamines, diuretics, tricyclic antidepressants, beta blockers) place one at increased risk.

6. Which exogenous factors predispose to heat injury?

Increased temperature	No breeze	Inaccurate temperature
Increased humidity	No cloud cover	information

Soldiers deploying to or athletes arriving for competition in a hot environment with little notice will arrive unacclimatized regardless of their physical condition. Acclimatization takes at least a week and often takes 10–14 days of a regimented work–rest cycle program.

7. What are important disorders to consider in the differential diagnosis of heat-related illnesses?

Heat stroke	Malaria	Drug reaction
Meningitis	Influenza	Neuroleptic malignant
Sepsis	Thyroid storm	syndrome
Ethyl alcohol withdrawal	Salicylate overdose	Malignant hyperthermia
Midbrain hemorrhage	Tickborne disease	Atropinism

When a patient has a rectal temperature > 104° F, cooling should begin as early as possible, regardless of the cause, with the intent to cool to a core temperature of 102° F within the first 30–60 minutes.

8. What is important about the early management of heat-related illnesses?

Because the severity of a heat injury is primarily a function of the severity and duration of hyperthermia, the value of prompt recognition, *rapid cooling*, and early transport to a medical facility cannot be overemphasized.

Heat stroke victims may *not* require aggressive intravenous fluids (beware of overshoot hyponatremia as well as pulmonary edema secondary to left ventricular dysfunction).

9. What laboratory abnormalities are expected in significantly heat-injured patients?

Hyperventilation and elevated body temperatures are associated with primary respiratory alkalosis. Metabolic acidosis often follows as a result of increased glycolysis and lactic acid accumulation. Hypoglycemia or hyperglycemia may be seen. Hypokalemia is often seen early and hyperkalemia may develop later (a factor in the EKG abnormalities so often recorded in these cases). Sodium levels vary widely depending to a significant degree on hydration status and type of fluids used in early treatment. Low levels of phosphate, calcium, and magnesium are common. Elevated liver function tests are consistent features and bilirubin may be increased because of both hepatic dysfunction and hemolysis. White blood cell counts may be increased with hemoconcentration and catecholamine circulation, but a drop in platelets is usual (along with falls in coagulation factors V and VIII). Hypoprothrombinemia and hypofibrinogenemia may lead to disseminated intravascular coagulation (DIC). Elevated levels of creatine phosphokinase (CPK) and myoglobin are frequently found in exertional heat stroke patients. The urine is usually concentrated and may contain ketones, protein, or myoglobin.

10. What early treatment options should be employed at the receiving medical facility?

Strict attention to ABC management is obviously the first priority. The second should be **rapid** (0.15° C/min) cooling to 102° F (39° C). The best method for this remains controversial and may be accomplished by immersing the patient in ice or tap water, dousing the patient with water, applying ice packs, or spraying the patient with a cool mist after removing all restrictive clothing. Immersion is probably the most rapid method, but obvious difficulties with cardiovascular monitoring, problems handling a submerged patient who may seize or become incontinent, and the need for a ready supply of ice make it less than ideal. The spray and breeze method is quick and easy and the preferred option in our hands.

Beware of overshoot hypothermia or unmonitored rebound hyperthermia after cooling is complete. (*Remember:* thermoregulation is abnormal for at least several days in cases of severe heat injury).

11. What complications are seen with severe heat injury?

Nearly every organ system may be affected by hyperthermia. Because the brain is extremely sensitive to excess heat, a number of **central nervous system disturbances** are common—e.g., confusion, lethargy, depression, irritability, or delirium. Seizures, cerebellar deficits, and coma may also occur from a decrease in cerebral perfusion or from microinfarcts.

Transient conduction disturbances may be seen on EKG and reflect widespread neuromuscular irritability. Cardiac output is low despite sinus tachycardia (low stroke volume and blood pressure from left ventricular dysfunction). These findings together with heart blocks and tachyarrhythmias are especially prevalent in the cool-down period.

The **pulmonary system** may be affected by increased pulmonary vascular resistance, pulmonary edema, acute respiratory distress syndrome (ARDS), and DIC. Aspiration is not uncommon.

Azotemia may be either renal or prerenal. Acute renal failure may occur in up to 25% of exertional heat stroke patients.

The **liver** is one of the most sensitive organs affected by excess heat. Consistent elevations of liver function tests are seen with heat stroke. Centrilobular necrosis with extensive cholestasis has been observed.

Gastrointestinal dysfunction is common, often manifested by nausea, vomiting, and diarrhea that results from the gastroparesis and ileus frequently observed. Stress ulceration or frank hemorrhage may be seen in severe cases.

Hemostasis is impaired by direct endothelial damage from the heat load, thermal activation of clotting factors, decreased production of clotting factors by an abnormally functioning liver, megakaryocyte damage in the bone marrow, and finally by bone marrow suppression.

12. What treatments are best for the more common complications of heat injury?

Acute renal failure—fluids, furosemide (Lasix), mannitol, dialysis

DIC—fresh frozen plasma, *not* heparin

Seizures or shivering—try diazepam (Valium) (some studies have assessed the benefit of phenytoin [Dilantin] prophylaxis; others have looked at chlorpromazine [Thorazine] as treatment, but Thorazine itself may cause problems with thermoregulation).

Congestive heart failure—use central monitoring and dobutamine if really needed

Dysrhythmias—treat per advanced cardiac life support (ACLS) protocols

There is no sound reason for delayed cooling, narcotics, steroids, antibiotics, dextran, or antipyretics.

13. Why are antipyretics ineffective in managing elevated temperature in heat-related illnesses?

Antipyretics act by lowering the hypothalamic set point that controls body temperature. In infectious disorders, pyrogens are released from granulocytes and affect the supraoptic nucleus to raise the set point. In heat-related illnesses, thermoregulatory cells of the midbrain sustain a direct thermal injury. No pyrogens are released and the set point is not raised. Furthermore, commonly used antipyretics may have detrimental effects on injured hepatic, renal, or gastrointestinal organs.

14. Are children at greater risk for heat-related illnesses?

Children may be at greater risk for heat-related injury for several reasons. Children gain heat more rapidly from the environment, sweat less effectively, produce more metabolic heat for a given work load, and acclimatize slower than adults. Children have a higher mass to surface area ratio and have a lower renal tubular filtration rate. Moreover, children may lack the experience and judgment to perceive early warning signs of impending heat injury.

15. What are the major determinants of prognosis in heat stroke patients?

Rapid reduction of body temperature, proper management of rehydration, control of seizures and other complications, and prompt evacuation to and management in an appropriate medical facility greatly improve survival. Poorer prognostic indicators include an initial temperature > 106° F (the LD_{50} of heat stroke is 108° F), longer duration of hyperthermia, coma lasting > 2 hours (or persisting after temperature has returned to normal), oliguric renal failure, hyperkalemia, and aspartate aminotransferase (AST) levels over 1000 IU.

16. Are most heat stroke patients likely to have a recurrence when heat challenged?

We know that no measured variable consistently predicts recovery or acclimatization, the rate of recovery is unique to each particular case, all heat-injured patients are at higher risk for hyper- and hypothermia, and some victims maintain an elevated CPK for 3 months. However, only about 10% of heat stroke victims will be permanently heat intolerant.

17. What restrictions are prudent after a heat injury?

Mild Cases: No end-organ damage or dysfunction—no running, jumping, prolonged standing or walking, lifting of > 5 lbs, heavy exertion of any type, exposure to adverse environmental conditions for 72 hours. No strenuous activity allowed if body weight drops 5% or more while training. Encourage liberal intake of fluids and food.

Severe Cases: End-organ damage or significant laboratory abnormalities seen—same as above for 72 hours and then exercise at own pace and distance in wet bulb globe temperatures below 86° F for next 90 days. Must have physician reevaluation before resuming usual activities to include a thermoregulatory treadmill stress test to assess the patient's ability to off-load core heat.

BIBLIOGRAPHY

1. Allman FL: The effects of heat on the athlete. J Med Assoc Ga 81:307–310, 1992.
2. Bracker MD: Environmental and thermal injury. Clin Sports Med 11:419–436, 1992.
3. Costrini A: Emergency treatment of exertional heatstroke and comparison of whole body cooling techniques. Med Sci Sports Exerc 22:15–18, 1990.
4. Coyle EF, Montain SJ: Benefits of fluid replacement with carbohydrate during exercise. Med Sci Sports Exerc 24:S324–S330, 1992.
5. Danzl DF: Hyperthermic syndromes. Am Fam Physician 37(6):157–162, 1988.
6. Delaney KA: Heatstroke: Underlying processes and lifesaving management. Postgrad Med 91:379–388, 1992.
7. Epstein Y: Heat intolerance: Predisposing factor or residual injury? Med Sci Sports Exerc 22:29–35, 1990.
8. Heat Illness: A Handbook for Medical Officers. US Army Technical Note 91-3. US Army Research Institute of Environmental Medicine. Natick, MA, June 1991.
9. Hubbard RW, Armstrong LE: Hyperthermia: New thoughts on an old problem. Phys Sportsmed 17(6):97–113, 1989.
10. Jacobson S: The ill effects of heat. Emerg Med, May 15, 1991, pp 313–324.
11. Mellion MB, Walsh WM, Shelton GL: The Team Physician's Handbook. Philadelphia, Hanley & Belfus, 1990.
12. Nash HL: Hyperthermia: Risks greater in children. Phys Sportsmed 15(2):29, 1987.
13. Noakes TD, Berlinski N, Solomon E, Weight L: Collapsed runners: Blood biochemical changes after IV fluid therapy. Phys Sportsmed 19(7):70–81, 1991.
14. Roberts WO: Exercise-associated collapse in endurance events: A classification system. Phys Sportsmed 17(5):49–55, 1989.
15. Robertson JW: Preventing heat injury in sports. Phys Sportsmed 19(5):31–35, 1991.

16. Schwartz M: Recognition and management of heat stroke. Hosp Physician, July 1990, pp 11–20.
17. Scott J: Heat-related illnesses: When are they a true emergency? Postgrad Med 85:154–164, 1989.
18. Shapiro Y, Seidman DS: Field and clinical observations of exertional heat stroke patients. Med Sci Sports Exerc 22:6–14, 1990.
19. Stamford B: How to avoid dehydration. Phys Sportsmed 18(7):135–136, 1990.
20. Tek D, Olshaker JS: Heat illness. Emerg Med Clin North Am 10:299–310, 1992.
21. Young AJ: Energy substrate utilization during exercise in extreme environments. Exerc Sports Sci Rev 18:65–119, 1990.

20. SAFE EXERCISE IN THE COLD AND COLD INJURIES

Brent A. Blue, M.D.

1. What are the most frequent sports injuries associated with cold weather?

Although frostbite and hypothermia are the classic cold weather sports injuries, dehydration, bronchospasm, fatigue, and mechanical injuries occur frequently in the cold environment. These less known cold weather problems occur because of special circumstances associated with low temperatures such as the paresthetic effects of reduced temperature and unfamiliar, as well as the unrecognized, stresses of a cold environment.

2. Are there special precautions for persons who are going to participate in sports in cold environments?

Just like any other sporting activity, the basics are most important. Stretching before exercise is critical for sports such as alpine, Nordic, and back country skiing. These activities involve motions and muscle use that are subject to forces out of the participant's control such as a sudden, unexpected bump in a cross-country track or a dropoff during downhill skiing. Without flexibility, these abrupt motions can tax and injure muscle and ligamentous structures. Because most skiers are weekend or vacation skiers, muscle conditioning is very important. Sudden use of sedentary muscles can precipitate muscle strains and fatigue that may predispose to other more serious injuries.

3. How is fatigue different in the cold?

Many participants report the lack of recognition of fatigue prior to injurious mishaps owing to the subjective lack of the sensation of fatigue in cold weather. The fatigue factor is highlighted by the fact that there are many more serious skiing injuries in the late afternoon than at other times of the day.

4. How is warm-up for activities in the cold different?

Stretching does not produce high levels of thermal energy. However, warm-up should be performed in the cold environment to adjust the thermoregulation of the body progressively. Warm-up should be done with multiple layers of clothing so the body is never shocked by the sudden temperature changes. As the warm-up becomes more aggressive, layers should be shed until full activity is initiated. If the activity is interrupted, such as when a ski racer rests between events, layers should be reapplied.

5. What are the respiratory problems experienced in cold weather?

In cold climates, inspired air must be warmed and humidified by the body as it enters the oral pharynx, trachea, and lungs. When the temperature differential between ambient air and body temperature is large (such as 100° F or more), the air cannot be fully warmed and humidified.

Reactive bronchospasm in normal subjects as well as asthmatics (and those with exercise-induced asthma) is significant. In addition, there is increased mucus production for 12–24 hours after the exposure occurs. Prophylactically inhaled bronchodilators such as albuterol can be very helpful for this unique problem.

6. What common problems are experienced by skiers?

Dehydration and mild hypothermia are the most frequent problems skiers experience. Skiers may become cold from severe or unplanned weather, but even more common, sweating from becoming overheated and/or melting snow on or under clothing results in extensive, evaporative heat loss. The cyclic nature of alpine (downhill) skiing contributes to hypothermia owing to the active metabolic state of actually skiing, alternating with the sedate condition of standing in line and riding the ski lifts. The skier may be unaware of adverse effects of routine medications such as the phenothiazines and anticholinergics.

7. Why is dehydration a factor in the cold?

Dehydration in the cold occurs owing to unperceived loss of fluid with inadequate intake. In very cold weather, humidity approaches zero and large quantities of fluid are lost through exhaled vapor. Cold weather also dulls the thirst response to dehydration. Additionally, the volume of perspiration loss may not be fully appreciated because of voluminous clothing.

8. How is heat lost from the body?

Heat is lost through convection, conduction, evaporation, and radiation in various ways (see below).

Types of Heat Loss

TYPE	METHOD	EXAMPLE
Conduction	Direct contact with cold surfaces	Lying on the snow after injury
Convection	Cold air blowing over skin	Cold air blowing through porous clothing
Evaporation	Evaporation of fluid on the skin	Overheated runner
Radiation	Radiation of heat from the body	Exposed head on skier

9. At what temperature does significant hypothermia occur?

Absolute temperature is less of a factor than preparation for cold. Hypothermia occurs year round. An athlete who knows the weather is extreme is more likely to prepare adequately than one who is facing a more temperate environment. For instance, unexpected immersion in cold water, such as happens to canoeists or white water rafters who go overboard, is a common scenario for hypothermia. Mountain bikers who encounter unexpected storms without proper clothing, unprepared glider pilots at high altitudes, and open water swimmers also are examples of hypothermic victims. Hypothermia also is a frequent finding in injured athletes who are not well protected from the elements while awaiting rescue or evacuation.

10. What is frostbite?

Frostbite is the destruction of the tissue by the freezing of cells. The damage is caused by puncture of the cell wall by ice crystal formation of intra- and extracellular fluid. Frostbite is made worse by the freeze-thaw-freeze cycle. Thus, rewarming should not be attempted until the injured tissue can be kept warm.

11. What temperature is necessary for frostbite?

In order for frostbite, the actual freezing of tissue, to occur, the temperature must be 32° F or lower. Frostbite occurs at exposed areas of the skin such as the ears and nose but also may affect isolated spots such as on the foot where a hole in the stocking is present. Frostbite of the fingers and toes is usually a result of prolonged, unexpected exposure to severe cold without proper protection. Hypothermic and dehydrated patients as well as tobacco users are more susceptible to frostbite.

12. How is frostbite evaluated?

Frostbite is graded by degree similar to burn evaluation. However, frostbite tissue usually recovers more successfully than high-temperature burns, because denaturation of protein associated with heat does not occur with frostbite.

13. How can someone get frostbite without knowing it?

Frostbite can be insidious in onset. For instance, toes in a ski or climbing boot may feel cold and progress to paresthesia without the victim noticing. Once numb, unless intervention occurs, progression to frostbite can go unnoticed by the victim.

14. What are the current treatments for frostbite?

Current therapy centers on gentle, continuous rewarming in 100–104° F water. There is theoretical evidence for the use of calcium channel blockers for peripheral vasodilatation and nonsteroidal antiinflammatory drugs for protection against prostaglandin effect. Tissue should not be rubbed and should be protected from even the lightest trauma. Debridement should **not** be performed unless infection presents. There are many anecdotal reports of dramatic regeneration of severely frostbitten tissue.

15. What is the best rewarming method for hypothermia?

A person with severe hypothermia should be rewarmed in a controlled manner. The patient should be on full cardiac and oximetric monitoring and intravenous access established. A continuous rectal temperature probe is ideal if it does not interfere with rewarming. Adequate staff should be assembled to perform CPR for an extended period of time as well as perform intubation of the patient if he or she is not ventilating. Only then should rewarming begin.

The most effective way to rewarm a severely hypothermic patient is by venous-to-venous hemodialysis. Blood temperature should be raised approximately 1–2° F per hour. If hemodialysis equipment is not available, placement of a nasogastric tube, urinary catheter, peritoneal catheter, and enema tube followed by irrigation with the appropriate warm fluids is a satisfactory but less efficient method. For moderate or mild hypothermia, warming blankets, heated aerosols, and other sources of external heating are usually all that is required.

16. What is the most significant difference between mild and moderate hypothermia?

Although the temperature criteria for moderate hypothermia differ among experts, the most significant clinical differential occurs when the patient becomes so cold that shivering stops. This is crucial because it means the patient will not rewarm intrinsically and requires external heat for recovery. The levels of hypothermia are given below.

Levels of Hypothermia

LEVEL	TEMPERATURE (° F)	MAJOR SYMPTOMS
Mild	> 90	Sense of cold, mild ataxia, shivering, some decrease in cognitive function
Moderate	85–90	Shivering stops, marked cognitive impairment, marked ataxia, somnolence
Severe	< 85	Coma or marked impairment of mental status

17. What is the most frequent complication in rewarming a hypothermic patient?

The most frequent complication is the presence of, or the precipitation of, ventricular fibrillation. Other cardiac arrhythmias may occur during rewarming but require no treatment until core temperature is above 90° F, at which time they should be treated routinely.

18. What is meant by the adage "warm and dead"?

Patients who are severely hypothermic may be comatose and appear to be dead. Severe bradycardia (detectable only by electronic monitoring) or ventricular fibrillation may be present and resuscitatable. Patients should not be declared dead until body temperature has reached 90° F and resuscitation efforts have remained unsuccessful.

19. Should cardiopulmonary resuscitation (CPR) be done on hypothermic patients who are pulseless?

Although controversial, if a patient is severely hypothermic and appears pulseless, CPR should be instituted only if it can easily be sustained until full warming has occurred. When instituted, CPR may be performed at half standard rates. Anecdotal evidence suggests that hypothermic patients are in a state of profound metabolic slowing—a type of suspended animation—and this state should not be disturbed until it can be reversed in a fully controlled environment.

20. Should drugs be used in resuscitation of a hypothermic patient?

Electrolytes and acid-base balance status must be carefully monitored during rewarming but only gentle manipulations of these factors should be attempted. Most cardiac medications will not be pharmacologically active below 88° F and should not be given to prevent a sudden surge or biochemical input as rewarming occurs.

21. What is the cause of death in an avalanche?

The most frequent cause of death in an avalanche is suffocation followed by trauma as a distant second. Hypothermia is rarely a cause.

BIBLIOGRAPHY

1. Biancolini CA, Del Bosco CG, Jorge MA, et al: Active core rewarming in neurologic, hypothermic patients: Effects on oxygen-related variables. Crit Care Med 21:1164–1168, 1993.
2. Bracker MD: Environmental and thermal injury. Clin Sports Med 11:419–436, 1992.
3. Britt LD, Dascombe WH, Rodriguez A: New horizons in management of hypothermia and frostbite injury. Surg Clin North Am 71:345–370, 1991.
4. Darvill FT: Mountaineering Medicine: A Wilderness Medical Guide. Berkeley, CA, Wilderness Press, 1992.
5. Dyment PG (ed): American Academy of Pediatrics, Committee on Sports Medicine: Sports Medicine: Health Care for Young Athletes, 2nd ed. Elk Grove Village, IL, American Academy of Pediatrics, 1991.
6. Edlich RF, Change DE, Birk KA, et al: Cold injuries. Compr Ther 15(9):13–21, 1989.
7. Foray J: Mountain frostbite: Current trends in prognosis and treatment (from results concerning 1261 cases). Int J Sports Med 13(Suppl 1):S193–S196, 1992.
8. Gentilello LM: Advances in the management of hypothermia. Surg Clin North Am 75:243–256, 1995.
9. Gentilello LM, Cobean RA, Offner PJ, et al: Continuous arteriovenous rewarming: Rapid reversal of hypothermia in critically ill patients. J Trauma 32:316–325; discussion, 325–327, 1992.
10. Heller HC, Musacchia KJ, Wang LCH (eds): Living in the Cold: Physiological and Biochemical Adaptations: Proceedings of the Seventh International Symposium on Natural Mammalian Hibernation (10/85). New York, Elsevier, 1986.
11. Kappes B, Mills W, O'Malley J: Psychological and psychophysiological factors in prevention and treatment of cold injuries. Alaska Med 35:131–140, 1993.
12. Kaufman JW, Bagian JP: Insidious hypothermia during raft use. Aviat Space Environ Med 61:569–575, 1990.
13. Lloyd EL: Accidental hypothermia. Resuscitation 32(2):111–124, 1996.
14. Lloyd EL: Hypothermia and Cold Stress. Rockville, MD, Aspen Systems, 1986.
15. Lomax P, Schonbaum E (eds): Thermoregulation: The Pathophysiological Basis of Clinical Disorders. Eighth International Symposium on the Pharmacology of Thermoregulation (8/91). New York, Karger, 1992.
16. Mills WJ: Field care of the hypothermic patient. Int J Sports Med 13(Suppl 1):S199–S202, 1992.
17. Staab DB, Sorensen VJ, Fath JJ, et al: Coagulation defects resulting from ambient temperature-induced hypothermia. J Trauma 36:634–638, 1994.
18. Sutton JR, Coates G, Houston CS (eds): Hypoxia and Mountain Medicine: Proceedings of the Seventh International Hypoxia Symposium. Oxford/New York, Pergamon Press, 1992.
19. Urschel JD: Frostbite: Predisposing factors and predictors of poor outcome. J Trauma 30:340–342, 1990.

20. Vella J, Farrell J, Leavey S, et al: The rapid reversal of profound hypothermia using peritoneal dialysis. Ir J Med Sci 165(2):113–114, 1996.
21. Ward MP, Milledge JS, West JB: High Altitude Medicine and Physiology. Philadelphia, University of Pennsylvania Press, 1989.
22. Wilkerson JA (ed): Hypothermia, Frostbite, and Other Cold Injuries: Prevention, Recognition, and Prehospital Treatment. Seattle, WA, The Mountaineers, 1966.

21. EXERCISE AT HIGH ALTITUDE

Benjamin D. Levine, M.D., and James Stray-Gundersen, M.D.

1. What are the distinguishing physical features of a high-altitude environment?

At high altitude, barometric pressure is reduced, with a parallel decrease in the inspired partial pressure of oxygen (P_IO_2); by 5,500 m (18,000 ft), the atmospheric pressure is reduced to one-half its sea level value and the P_IO_2 is only 75 mmHg. Hypoxia is thus the most prominent physiologic manifestation of high altitude. Temperature also decreases with altitude at a rate of approximately 6.5° C/1,000 m. Other features include dry air (increasing the risk of dehydration), a decrease in air resistance, and an increase in the amount of ultraviolet light (4%/300 m), which increases the risk of sunburn. The range of terrestrial altitudes may be divided into five broad categories, based on increasing physiologic effects:

1. 0–1,000 m	Sea level		4. 3,000–5,000 m	High altitude
2. 1,000–2,000 m	Low altitude		5. 5,000–8,848 m	Extreme altitude
3. 2,000–3,000 m	Moderate altitude			

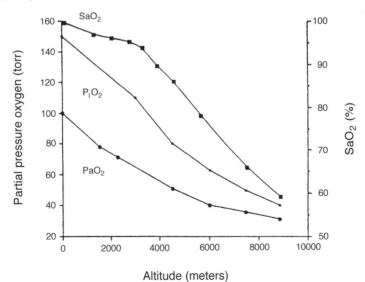

The relationship between altitude, inspired partial pressure of oxygen (P_IO_2), and its associated effect on arterial partial pressure of oxygen (PaO_2) and oxyhemoglobin saturation (SaO_2). Note progressive fall in inspired-arterial gradient for oxygen with increasing altitude, presumably due to hyperventilation and decreases in the atmospheric-alveolar gradient for oxygen. Saturation is well maintained at rest up to 3,000 m, but falls acutely during exercise because of diffusion limitation in the lung (not shown). (Adapted from Hackett PH, Roach RC, Sutton JR: High altitude medicine. In Auerbach PS, Gehr EC (eds): Management of Wilderness and Environmental Emergencies. St. Louis, Mosby, 1989, pp 1–34, with permission.)

2. How does a high-altitude environment affect exercise performance?

Altitude-induced hypoxia reduces the amount of oxygen available to do physical work. Maximal aerobic power (VO_2max) is reduced by approximately 1% for every 100 m above 1500 m in normal individuals. For well-trained athletes, this effect is even greater, and reductions in VO_2max and performance can be identified at altitudes as low as 500 m. Moreover, during exercise at high altitude, ventilation and blood lactate concentration are greater for any given submaximal workrate; an increase in blood lactate concentration increases the sensation of dyspnea and fatigue. However, peak blood lactate concentration is lower in individuals acclimatized to high altitude, a condition that has been termed the *lactate paradox*.

3. Do we know what causes the reduction in maximal aerobic power at altitude or why it appears to be greater in athletes?

The oxygen cascade describes the steps through which oxygen must pass: from the **environment** (determined by altitude achieved), into the **alveoli** (a function of ventilation and therefore the hypoxic ventilatory response), and across the **pulmonary capillary** (limited by diffusion). Oxygen is transported by the **cardiovascular system** (a function of cardiac output and hemoglobin concentration) and eventually diffused into **skeletal muscle** (dependent on muscle capillarity and biochemical state), where it is used by muscle **mitochondria** (influenced by oxidative enzyme activity) for aerobic respiration and production of adenosine triphosphate (ATP). The reduction in VO_2max at altitude probably is due to diffusion limitation in the lung during exercise, which is exacerbated by the high pulmonary blood flow (cardiac output) of endurance athletes. Reduced hypoxic ventilatory drive and pulmonary mechanical limitations also may be present in some highly trained athletes.

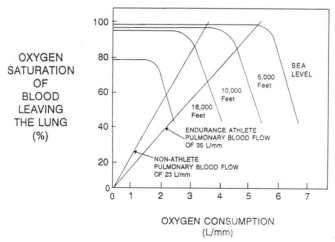

OXYGEN CONSUMPTION
(L/mm)

The effect of oxygen uptake and the requisite pulmonary blood flow (cardiac output) on oxygen saturation of blood leaving the lungs at different altitudes. For an untrained individual with a VO_2max of 3.5 L/min and a peak pulmonary blood flow of 23 L/min, blood is well saturated at sea level and altitudes up to 5,000 ft (1,500 m) at peak exercise. But blood becomes progressively less saturated with exercise at increasing altitude. For an endurance athlete, however, who may have a VO_2max of 5 L/min and a peak pulmonary blood flow of 35 L/min, diffusing capacity is closely matched to oxygen uptake and there is diffusion limitation even at altitudes between sea level and 5,000 ft. This phenomenon likely occurs because the cardiovascular system has a much greater capacity to respond to training than the lung, the diffusing capacity of which is relatively constant. (Adapted from Johnson RL: Pulmonary diffusion as a limiting factor in exercise. Circ Res 20(Suppl 1):S154–S160, 1967.)

4. Can the body adapt to altitude to increase exercise capacity?

Chronic exposure to altitude stimulates the process of acclimatization, which includes a number of physiologic adaptations that improve submaximal work performance at altitude.

Increases in alveolar ventilation and reductions in mixed venous oxygen content are primarily responsible for maximizing exercise capacity at altitude. Probably the most important adaptation that may improve sea level performance is an increase in hemoglobin and hematocrit, which increases the oxygen-carrying capacity of the blood and improves aerobic power. Moreover, peripheral uptake of oxygen by skeletal muscle may be facilitated by increased capillary density, mitochrondrial number, and tissue myoglobin concentration as well as by increased concentrations of 2,3-diphosphoglycerate. Buffer capacity of skeletal muscle is also increased, which may improve anaerobic capacity and endurance. Moreover, substrate utilization is enhanced by increasing mobilization of free fatty acids and increasing dependence on blood glucose, thus sparing muscle glycogen. The result is decreased accumulation of metabolites such as lactate or ammonia during submaximal exercise. Together these adaptations may be sufficient to restore exercise capacity to near-sea-level values at low or moderate altitudes of < 2,500 m. At higher altitudes, acclimatization is not sufficient to restore VO_2max to normal, and even acute erythrocyte infusion is not beneficial.

With higher altitudes (> 2,500 m) and rapid ascent rates (> 300 m sleeping altitude/day above 3,000 m), a maladaptive state may develop called acute mountain sickness (AMS). AMS is characterized by headache, nausea, anorexia, fatigue, and difficulty with sleeping. Fortunately, this process is usually mild and self-limited; in such cases, rest and mild analgesics are sufficient treatment. In some individuals, however, AMS may progress to more severe and life-threatening high-altitude pulmonary or cerebral edema, in which case immediate descent is mandatory.

5. How long does acclimatization take to develop?

The ventilatory changes begin immediately on exposure to the hypoxic environment and continue to increase over the first few days at altitude. This hyperventilation causes respiratory alkalosis, which stimulates renal excretion of bicarbonate over the first week to normalize acid-base balance. The sympathetic nervous system is activated acutely with increases in sympathetic nerve activity and arterial concentrations of epinephrine. The result is an increase in heart rate and cardiac output so that tissue oxygen delivery remains nearly constant with sea-level values. By 2–3 weeks, systemic and regional blood flow have returned toward sea-level values as oxygenation improves.

Hematocrit and hemoglobin concentration increases within 24–48 hours because of a reduction in plasma volume rather than an increase in red cell mass. Erythropoietin begins to increase within the first few hours of hypoxia and peaks by approximately 48 hours. Erythropoietin levels remain elevated only for 1–2 weeks at altitude despite continued exposure, and red cell mass increases slowly in a time-dependent fashion. It may take as long as 1–2 years of continued altitude exposure for sea-level natives to acquire the same red blood cell mass as high-altitude natives at the same altitude. Most of the metabolic changes appear to be complete by 3–4 weeks of altitude exposure. The ultrastructural changes in capillary density, mitochondrial number and muscle fiber size probably take weeks to months to become complete.

6. Does exercise at altitude provide any advantages above and beyond the development of acclimatization?

Whether hypoxic exercise provides an enhancement of the training effect during altitude training is controversial and probably depends on both mode and intensity of training. When a small enough muscle mass is used (i.e., one leg) so that the same absolute workrates can be performed under hypoxic and normoxic conditions, hypobaric hypoxic exercise results in greater increases in endurance, accompanied by greater increases in oxidative enzyme capacity than normoxic exercise training. Although one study of swimming rats suggested that the same synergistic effect can be observed in whole-body exercise, this theory has been difficult to prove in humans. In general, controlled studies of trained athletes have not been able to confirm a benefit of hypoxic exercise without concomitant acclimatization.

7. Do the physiologic consequences of altitude affect the way an athlete will train?

Definitely. Athletes train faster and at greater aerobic power at sea level than at altitude. During high-intensity, interval-type workouts, running speed, oxygen uptake, heart rate, and lactate are lower at altitude, suggesting that interval workouts are best performed as close to sea level as possible. During base training, running speed and oxygen uptake are lower at altitude, but heart rate is the same as at sea level, and submaximal lactate is slightly higher. **The net balance between acclimatization and reduction in training intensity by hypoxia is the ultimate determinant of the outcome of altitude training in endurance athletes.**

8. How should an athlete prepare for competition at altitude?

If possible, adequate time for acclimatization should be allowed to maximize performance at altitude. Most of the short-term benefits of acclimatization are obtained after 2–3 weeks. For competition at altitude, this period should allow maximal acclimatization while at the same time minimizing the detraining that may occur during training at altitude. Some athletes and coaches believe that if adequate time for acclimatization is not possible, competing immediately on arrival at altitude may be best. However, this hypothesis has not been rigorously tested.

9. Does altitude affect all athletes similarly?

No. Altitude affects endurance athletes and sprinters in different ways. For endurance events lasting longer than about 2 minutes, performance is significantly impaired at altitude because of the hypoxia-induced reduction in aerobic power. However for short, sprint events (400 m or less), most of the ATP required for muscular contraction of fast-twitch fibers comes from glycolytic metabolism, which is not dependent on oxygen availability. The reduced air resistance at altitude thus actually improves sprint performance. For this reason, all times in events shorter than 400 m were very fast in the Mexico City Olympics (altitude 2,100 m) in 1968, and many world records were set. However, times for all events longer than 1,500 m were substantially slower than at sea level.

10. How about recreational athletes who hike, climb, or mountain bike but are not interested in athletic competition?

Of course, recreational athletes also are affected by the hypoxia of altitude. However, for non–endurance-trained individuals who plan to perform exercise at altitude, exercise training at sea level provides important advantages. In fact, after a training program at sea level, endurance and maximal aerobic power improve to the same extent at altitude and at sea level in untrained subjects.

11. Does exercise training at altitude improve sea-level performance?

Many scientists, athletes, and coaches have been intrigued by the similarities between altitude acclimatization and endurance training. Numerous anecdotal reports since the 1940s have suggested that endurance athletes may achieve some benefit from altitude training for sea-level performance. The ultimate result has depended on the type of athlete studied, the altitude achieved, and the methods of testing and training. Runners improve more than swimmers, and athletes training at lower altitudes improve more than athletes training at higher altitudes (over 4,000 m). Rarely considered in these studies, however, is the effect of supervised training per se. A training camp has the advantage of carefully supervising training and nutrition, treating injuries quickly and appropriately, and removing the stresses of every-day life that may distract from training. This factor may be important to the improvement seen in uncontrolled studies. When appropriate control groups have been included, living and training at altitude have not proved to be superior to similar training at sea level.

12. Are there any alternative strategies to take advantage of the benefits of acclimatization yet minimize the detrimental effects of detraining?

The authors recently demonstrated that living at moderate altitude (2,500 m) but training at low altitude (1,250 m) (living high–training low) results in acclimatization without detraining, thereby improving sea-level performance. Athletes who perform this type of training develop an increase in red blood cell mass volume, a proportional increase in maximal aerobic power, an increase in the VO_2 at maximal steady state (ventilatory threshold), and an improvement in race time over 5,000 meters. Such an improvement in race time was not seen in control groups that lived and trained at moderate altitude or lived and trained in a similar mountainous training camp environment but at sea level.

13. How high should an athlete live to achieve the optimal result?

Acclimatization to altitude depends on oxygen delivery to peripheral tissues, which decreases linearly with oxyhemoglobin saturation. Thus red cell mass does not appear to increase until PaO_2 decreases below approximately 65 mmHg, when saturation begins to fall. For most individuals, this threshold altitude is approximately 2,200–2,500 m, although some small changes have been reported in endurance athletes at altitudes as low as 1,250 m. Above 2,500 m such adaptations are likely to be greater with increasing altitude unless acute mountain sickness intervenes or marked hypoxia (above 4,000 m) results in a catabolic state characterized by weight loss with reduction in muscle mass. An altitude of 2,500–2,800 m thus appears to maximize acclimatization and minimize complications.

14. How high should an athlete train?

High-intensity, interval workouts should be conducted as close to sea level as possible, preferably below 1,500 m, to maximize running speed and training intensity. The appropriate altitude at which to conduct base training is less definitive. Base training at low altitude allows relatively normal training intensity and may prevent the loss of heat acclimatization that often accompanies living in the mountains. In contrast, base training at altitude may facilitate an increase in mitochondrial aerobic enzyme activities and maximize peripheral oxygen utilization. Recent data from the authors suggest that maximal aerobic power and 5,000 m time may show similar improvement with the "high-low" approach and by living at moderate altitude, performing base training at moderate altitude, and interval training at low altitude ("high-high-low"). The "high-high-low" approach minimizes the logistical difficulties inherent in twice daily travel to a low-altitude environment and thereby opens up more training sites. It is important to emphasize, however, that if base training is performed too hard (i.e., at too high an intensity at altitude) the overtraining syndrome may result. Moreover, altitude training is not a substitute for a focused, well-designed training program with appropriate rest and nutrition.

15. How soon after returning from altitude should an athlete plan to compete?

Most athletes and coaches believe that the best performances are delivered 2–3 weeks after returning from altitude. This observation may be related to rapid alterations in skeletal muscle acid-base balance after return from altitude. Alternatively, a period of normoxic training may be necessary to maximize neuromotor coordination, particularly if all interval workouts have been performed under the slower training conditions of moderate altitude. Recently, the authors demonstrated that at least when the "high-low" strategy is employed, fast racing times are obtained immediately on return from altitude and persist for at least 3 weeks at sea level.

16. What special considerations need to be addressed before training at altitude?

Nutritional factors, particularly iron stores, play a critical role in the ability to respond to altitude training. In a series of studies involving more than 100 competitive distance runners training at altitude, 40% (60% of women and 25% of men) were found to have reduced iron stores based on a low serum ferritin level. The athletes with low ferritin levels prior to altitude exposure (male and female) were unable to increase the volume of red cell mass (blood volume minus plasma volume) and did not increase VO_2max or improve running performance. Because iron is a critical moiety in myoglobin as well as mitochondrial cytochromes, iron deficiency may not only compromise oxygen-carrying capacity but also inhibit oxygen extraction (a-v O_2 difference) and reduce VO_2max and performance, even in nonanemic athletes. Thus iron stores must be normalized before undertaking a period of altitude training. Normalization may require high doses of oral iron (up to 500 mg elemental iron/day in divided doses), which are usually best tolerated in liquid, pediatric preparation (Feosol, 5–20 ml, 1–3 times/day, taken with vitamin C, 30 minutes before or 60 minutes after a meal).

BIBLIOGRAPHY

1. Adams WC, Bernauer EM, Dill DB, Bomar JB: Effects of equivalent sea-level and altitude training on VO₂max and running performance. J Appl Physiol 39:262–265, 1975.
2. Hackett PH, Roach RC, Sutton JR: High altitude medicine. In Auerbach PS, Gehr EC (eds): Management of Wilderness and Environmental Emergencies. St. Louis, Mosby, 1989, pp 1–34.
3. Hansen JR, Vogel JA, Stelter GP, Consolazio CF: Oxygen uptake in man during exhaustive work at sea level and high altitude. J Appl Physiol 26:511–522, 1967.
4. Levine BD, Stray-Gundersen J: A practical approach to altitude training: Where to live and train for optimal performance enhancement. Int J Sports Med 13(Suppl 1):S209–S212, 1992.
5. Levine BD, Stray-Gundersen J: "Living high-training low": Effect of moderate-altitude acclimatization with low-altitude training on performance. J Appl Physiol 82:102–112, 1997.
6. Maher JT, Jones LG, Hartley LH: Effects of high altitude exposure on submaximal endurance capacity of men. J Appl Physiol 37:895–898, 1974.
7. Mizuno M, Juel C, Bro-Rasmussen T, et al: Limb skeletal muscle adaptation in athletes after training at altitude. J Appl Physiol 68:496–502, 1990.
8. Reeves JT, Wolfel EE, Green HJ, et al: Oxygen transport during exercise at altitude and the lactate paradox: Lessons from Operation Everest II and Pikes Peak. Exerc Sports Sci Rev 20:275–296, 1992.
9. Sutton JR, Reeves JT, Wagner PD, et al: Operation Everest II: Oxygen transport during exercise at extreme simulated altitude. J Appl Physiol 64:1309–1321, 1988.
10. Terrados N, Jansson E, Sylven C, Kaijser L: Is hypoxia a stimulus for synthesis of oxidative enzymes and myoglobin? J Appl Physiol 68:2369–2372, 1990.

22. SCUBA AND DIVING MEDICINE

Joseph L. Torres, M.D.

An increased interest in the underwater environment has been demonstrated by an ever-growing number of scuba divers. In the United States alone, there are over 5 million certified scuba divers. Because diving is not restricted to coastal areas and is being done in lakes and quarries, and classes are usually taught in pools, physicians must be made aware of the problems an individual may encounter during and after a dive.

1. What does scuba mean?
It is an acronym for self-contained underwater breathing apparatus.

2. What laws of physics should a diver always keep in mind?
Boyle's law: The volume of a gas varies inversely with pressure.
Henry's law: The amount of a given gas that is dissolved in a liquid at a given temperature is directly proportional to the partial pressure of that gas.

3. What is an atmosphere?
The measure of barometric pressure at sea level is equal to 1 atmosphere, 760 mmHg (millimeters of mercury) or 14.7 psi (pounds per square inch). This is a pressure exerted on a human body from its environment at sea level. As a diver descends past 33 feet, the atmospheric pressure doubles.

4. What are the bends?
This is a condition in which Henry's law applies. As ambient pressure increases, a greater amount of nitrogen and oxygen is dissolved in the blood and distributed throughout the body tissues. As divers ascend and ambient pressure decreases, nitrogen diffuses out of tissues and supersaturation in the blood stream occurs. With a rapid ascension, the nitrogen dissolved in the tissues

is released too quickly and forms bubbles in the blood stream that may block blood flow to vital areas of the body and cause pain in the limbs and abdomen. This is also known as decompression sickness.

5. What types of decompression sickness exist?

Type I is mild and generally presents as pruritus, an urticarial rash, and joint pain that usually subsides within 30 minutes and at times without treatment. Type II is severe and usually appears within 30 minutes after a diver surfaces. It requires immediate transport of a diver to a recompression chamber. Symptoms include weakness, sensory deficit, blurred vision, headaches, "staggers" with disturbances to the labyrinth and vestibular function, and "chokes" from nitrogen bubbles in the pulmonary vasculature.

6. How is decompression sickness treated?

The diver is brought back to simulated depth in a recompression chamber in order to dissolve the nitrogen bubbles. Oxygen is administered at the highest concentration possible, and hydration is maintained.

7. Can decompression sickness be avoided?

Yes. It can be avoided by controlling the rate of ascent and pausing at several depths during the ascent as directed by decompression tables.

8. What is a decompression table?

The U.S. Navy and the Royal Navy have developed tables that demonstrate the depths and lengths of time a diver should stop during ascent in order to equilibrate the body's oxygen and nitrogen content and prevent decompression sickness.

9. Is there a safe depth that does not require a stop in order to equalize the nitrogen oxygen content of the body?

Yes. Short dives as deep as 35 feet may not require a stop; but even at this shallow depth, Boyle's law and Henry's law still apply. So a diver should not risk ascending too quickly on any dive. Because the oxygen and nitrogen dissolved in the body expand and come out of solution as the diver ascends, it is important that the diver exhale this stream of gas continuously and avoid breathholding. When ascending, the diver should follow the smallest exhaled air bubbles toward the surface.

10. What is the PADI wheel?

The Professional Association of Diving Instructors (PADI) simplified the diving table into a small plastic wheel, which makes it easier for the diver to determine at what depths it is necessary to stop during ascent (see figure, top of next page).

11. What is barotrauma?

It is tissue injury that occurs when there is failure of a gas-filled body space to equalize its internal pressure with its external pressure. Boyle's law applies to this event; gas expands as the diver ascends. Barotrauma of the middle ear during descent is probably the most common disorder in divers.

12. Can barotrauma occur in any tissue space?

Yes. The organ at greatest risk is the lung, where pneumothorax may occur and be life threatening.

13. What is the most dangerous sequela of pulmonary barotrauma?

Air embolism. A nitrogen bubble in an artery travels to the brain and causes focal neurologic deficits or strokelike syndromes. A diver with air embolism should be transferred to the nearest hyperbaric oxygen facility immediately.

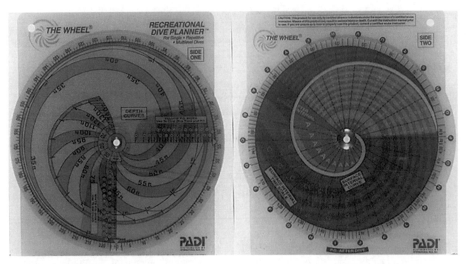

Source: Recreational Dive Planner-Wheel™, by Diving Science and Technology Corp., 1989. Reprinted with permission from International PADI, Inc.

14. What does hyperbaric oxygen do in treating barotrauma?

It increases the oxygenation of hypoxic brain tissue, decreases postembolic brain edema, and helps dissolve any persistent nitrogen bubbles in the blood stream.

15. What other types of barotrauma exist?

Paranasal sinus barotrauma is the second most common form. When the inner ear is affected, alternobaric vertigo may occur.

16. What is "rapture of the depth"?

This phenomenon occurs when the partial pressure of nitrogen in the central nervous system increases and causes a pleasant drowsiness that gradually develops into narcosis. The greater the ambient pressure, the greater the partial pressure and, consequently, the greater the narcosis.

17. How is nitrogen narcosis in a diver recognized?

Symptoms are similar to those encountered with alcohol intoxication.

18. What factors may make nitrogen narcosis more probable?

Alcohol, fatigue, cold water, and increased carbon dioxide tension.

19. What can be done for nitrogen narcosis?

The diver should ascend to a depth of less than 100 feet.

20. What is mixed gas diving?

Mixed air diving is use of different mixtures of oxygen, helium, and nitrogen. These mixtures help to increase bottom time and depth while decreasing the chances of CNS toxicity from oxygen and nitrogen narcosis. Two different agencies, American NITROX Divers Institute (ANDI) and the International Association of NITROX Diving (IAND), have introduced NITROX to sports diving. The National Oceanographic and Aeronautical Administration (NOAA) has established standards for mixed gas diving.

21. When doing a physical examination on a diver, which conditions are absolute contraindications to diving?

In general, any condition that may put the diver or anyone in his or her group at risk is considered to be a contraindication to diving. Absolute contraindications of greater importance include a history of spontaneous pneumothorax, chronic obstructive pulmonary disease (COPD), pulmonary blebs, and asthma requiring medication. Relative contraindications are conditions that may alter consciousness; for example, insulin-dependent diabetes mellitus or claustrophobia.

22. Is pregnancy a contraindication for scuba diving?

Yes. Pregnancy is a contraindication because of the changes in barometric pressures that occur while diving.

23. Can wheelchair-bound patients scuba dive?

If they do not have any absolute contraindication for diving, they may do so with proper supervision.

24. How soon can a person fly in a commercial airliner after diving?

A safe rule of thumb is to wait a minimum of 12 hours before flying.

25. Where can information be obtained in case of an emergency or for location of the nearest hyperbaric oxygen chamber?

In the United States, the Diver Alert Network provides 24-hour information. It is based out of Duke University in Durham, NC; the telephone number is 919-685-8111.

BIBLIOGRAPHY

1. Dreifuss FE: Epileptics and scuba diving. JAMA 253:1877, 1985.
2. Eile S: Importance of dive tables in scuba diving. West J Med 146:750, 1987.
3. Madorsky JG, Madorsky AG: Scuba diving: Taking the wheelchair out of wheelchair sports. Arch Phys Med Rehabil 69(3 Pt 1):215, 1988.
4. Melamed Y, Shupak A, Bitterman H: Medical problems associated with underwater diving. N Engl J Med 1:30, 1992.
5. Michalodimitrakis E, Patsalis A: Nitrogen narcosis and alcohol consumption—A scuba diving fatality. J Forens Sci 32:1095, 1987.
6. Millington JT: Scuba diving and pregnancy. Am Fam Physician 40:61, 1989.
7. Millington JT: Physical standards for scuba divers. J Am Board Fam Pract 1:194, 1988.
8. Mount T, Gilliam B: Mixed Gas Diving: The Ultimate Change for Technical Diving. San Diego, CA, Watersport Publishing, 1993.
9. Orlowski JP: Adolescent drownings: Swimming, boating, diving and scuba accidents. Pediatr Ann 17:125–128, 131–132, 1988.
10. Parell GJ: Conservative management of inner ear barotrauma resulting from scuba diving. Otolaryngol Head Neck Surg 93:393, 1985.
11. Replogle WH, Sanders SD, Keeton JE, Phillips DM: Scuba diving injuries. Am Fam Physician 37:135, 1988.
12. Wedman G: Diabetes and scuba diving. Diabetes Educ 13:267, 1987.

V. Protective Equipment

---

23. PROTECTIVE EQUIPMENT: FOOTBALL

Cindy J. Chang, M.D., and Kristine L. Burke, M.D.

---

1. What types of football helmets are being used today?

Helmets currently fall into two major categories: (1) padded and (2) air and fluid filled, with combinations of both types. The shell is made of a hard, resilient plastic (polycarbonate or acrylonitrile butadiene styrene, ABS), and the inner bladder or liner can be pads made of energy-absorbing foams, air chambers that can be inflated or deflated for optimal fitting, or glycerin filled to help further lessen helmet impacts.

An older type of helmet being phased out of use is the suspension helmet. Bishop compared 6- to 8-year-old helmets and found suspension helmets to be markedly inferior under impact conditions to the padded and padded-suspension helmets.[6] This is thought to be due to the stretching of the webbing materials used in the suspension helmets, which reduces the distance between the head and shell, permitting the head to contact the shell on impact.

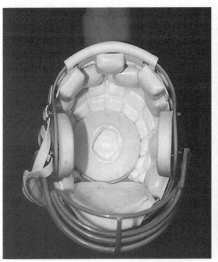 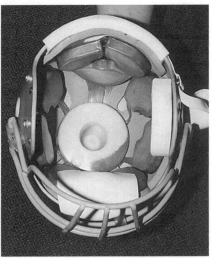

Different types of football helmets. *Left,* padded and air-filled cells. *Right,* fluid-filled cells.

2. How should a football helmet be properly fit?

General preparation. Try to fit the helmet when the hair is at normal hair length and at the length it will remain throughout the season. For example, if longer hair is cut later, the helmet will fit too loosely. It may also be important to fit the helmet when the hair is dry or wet, depending on the time of the season and amount of sweating during play. Observe any noticeable head-shape variations in the players, which may require a special fit and even a custom-made helmet.

1. **Proper entering of the helmet.** Spread the ear flaps by placing the thumbs or fingers in the ear holes of the helmet. Put the helmet directly over the head, then tilt it backward and rotate it to the front while pulling it down into position. The helmet should fit snugly around all parts of the player's head (front, sides, and crown), with no gaps between the pads and the head or face. It should also cover the base of the skull but should not impinge on the cervical spine when the neck is extended.

2. **Crown adjustment.** The helmet should sit approximately 1 to 2 fingerbreadths (approximately 0.75 to 1.0 inch) above the eyebrows. Press straight down on the top of the helmet and exert firm pressure. The helmet should not come down over the eyes.

3. **Side-to-side check.** Ask the player to hold his or her head straight forward and attempt to turn the helmet on the head. It should turn only slightly if properly fit. However, if the head is long and oval-shaped, there may be excessive room on the sides, which spacers or extra pads can correct.

4. **Jaw pad fit.** Check to see if the pads fit the jaw area snugly to prevent lateral rocking of the helmet.

5. **Chin-strap fit.** The four-point chin strap (some NFL players still use a two-point chin strap) provides added protection by restricting forward and backward movements of the helmet, preventing lacerations over the bridge of the nose. It should be comfortably snug, with equal tension on both sides. Rocking the helmet back and forth should produce no movement.

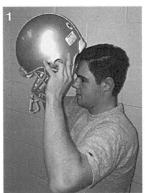
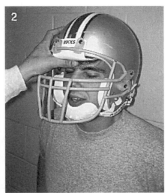

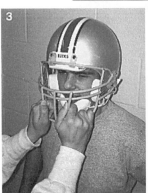
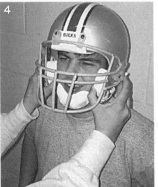
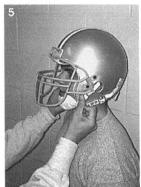

Fitting a football helmet.

Final check. Enter the player's name or number in the helmet to ensure that each player always wears his or her own helmet. Last, remember that the helmet must be routinely checked for proper fit. If air-bladder helmets are used by a team traveling to a different altitude and air pressure, the fit must be rechecked.

3. Do football helmets have to pass any safety standards?

Yes. A major influence on football helmet standardization in the United States is the National Operating Committee on Standards for Athletic Equipment (NOCSAE). This organization was established in 1969 for the purpose of making competitive sports as free from injury as possible through protective equipment standards; it identified as its highest priority the issues of head injuries in football. Since 1978 for colleges and 1980 for high schools, all new football helmets must have a NOCSAE certification.

To be NOCSAE approved, a helmet must be able to tolerate forces applied to it in many different areas and withstand repeated blows of high mass and low velocity (e.g., running into a goalpost or hitting the ground with the head). However, this does not mean that the helmet is completely fail-safe. To make each player and his or her family members aware of the inherent risks involved in playing football, each helmet must have a visible exterior warning label.

Testing new helmets to ensure their safety also does not guarantee that they will remain safe. If alterations are made in the helmet later that do not comply with NOCSAE standards (e.g., improper mounting of the face mask), the helmet's NOCSAE certification becomes invalid. Also, a random selection of helmets from a high school football team revealed that 75% of those that were 3 years old failed the NOCSAE test.[3] There are currently no rules requiring routine reconditioning of the helmets, although NOCSAE standard recertification is done yearly by some larger colleges for liability reasons. Riddell, a manufacturer of sports equipment, carried a 5-year shell warranty on the majority of its helmets.

WARNING:

Do not strike an opponent with any part of this helmet or face mask. This is a violation of football rules and may cause you to suffer severe brain or neck injury, including paralysis or death. Severe brain or neck injury may also occur accidentally while playing football.

NO HELMET CAN PREVENT ALL SUCH INJURIES.
YOU USE THIS HELMET AT YOUR OWN RISK.

Warning label found on football helmets.

4. Why are there so many different types of face masks?

Face masks are selected depending on the position played and the protection needed. Linemen usually wear a full cage with a middle bar to prevent accidental injuries to the eyes, nose, and face from opposing linemen's fingers. For the quarterback, running backs, and wide

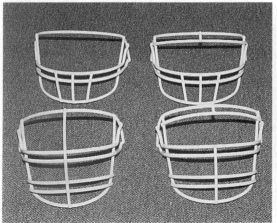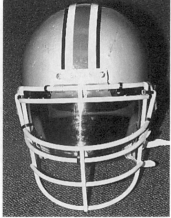

Left, The wide variety of face masks used in football. *Right,* A face mask with an eye shield.

receivers who need an unobstructed view, an intermediate style is used that will provide adequate facial protection yet enable visualization of a wider view of the playing field. Rarely, punters and placekickers in the NFL are still seen wearing a single-bar face mask, which offers protection only from large objects directed horizontally. Ideally, no face protection should have less than two bars. For players who have fractured the mandible in the past or who simply desire more protection in that area, a posterior inferior bar can be added bilaterally or unilaterally to the cage face mask. Despite the protection of the face mask, eye injuries with permanent visual loss can still occur from inadvertent finger penetration. Because of this, some authorities are advocating the use of a Plexiglas eye shield; these shields can be clear or tinted.

5. Are mouth guards mandatory?

Yes, except in the NFL. In 1962, major agencies, including the National Federation of High Schools and National Intercollegiate Athletic Association, mandated that football players must wear mouth guards; in 1973, the NCAA also adopted mandatory mouth guard requirements. Since the adoption of face masks and mouth guards for use in football, mouth injuries have been reduced more than 50%.[21] Besides protecting the teeth and soft tissue, the intraoral mouth guard absorbs and dissipates the shock of chin blows, which reduces the incidence of fractured jaws and helps to prevent cerebral concussions and neck injuries.

To enforce compliance, the NCAA enacted a ruling starting in the 1990 football season that football players must wear colored intraoral mouth guards to increase their visibility. Although the NFL still does not require its professional football players to wear mouth guards, many players are doing so voluntarily.

6. What types of mouth guards are available?

Three types of mouth guards are used in football: (1) ready-made, which is the least expensive but most uncomfortable; it interferes with breathing because it is held in position by clenching the teeth together; (2) mouth-formed, fit by submerging in boiling water and then molding directly to the teeth in the maxillary arch; best if done by a dentist; and (3) custom-made, formed over an impression of the maxillary arch; this must also be constructed by a dentist and is the most expensive. All three types of mouth guards are retained on the upper jaw.

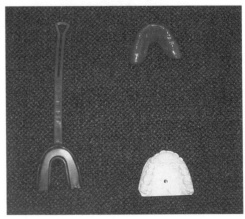

Ready-made (*left*) and custom-made (*right*) mouth guards.

7. What are the differences in types of shoulder pads? How should they be fitted?

There are two general types of pads, flat and cantilevered. The cantilevered type is bulkier and offers greater protection to the shoulder muscle complex; therefore, it is used by those players who block and tackle. The cantilever strap, which disperses impact forces over a wider area, can be found on the inside or outside of the pads. The flat type, which offers less protection but a greater range of motion about the shoulder, is used by the quarterback and wide receiver.

In fitting shoulder pads, the following rules are applied:

1. To initially estimate the size of the pad needed, a measurement is made from one acromioclavicular joint to the other. Do not estimate the fit of the pads based on weight, as no two players' musculature are the same.

2. The tip of the inside shoulder pad should fit just to the lateral aspect of the shoulder.

3. The shoulder pads should cover the sternum and clavicles. The neck opening should provide adequate space for the player to extend the arms overhead without impingement of the neck, but must not be so large as to allow excessive sliding.

4. The elastic axilla straps are tightened as comfortably as possible, so that an impact of a blow will be distributed evenly.

5. The flaps, or epaulets, should be large enough to cover the deltoid area.

6. The shoulder pads must be constantly inspected for cracks, frayed strings or straps, or broken rivets.

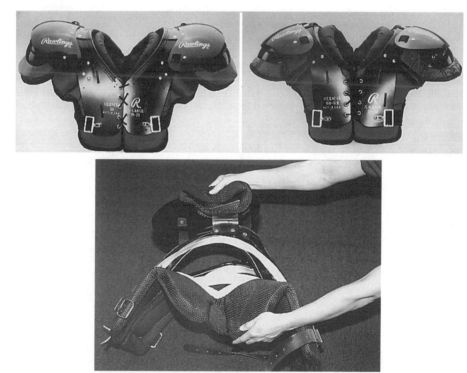

Above, Shoulder pads for a lineman (*left*) and a quarterback or wide receiver (*right*). (Photographs courtesy of Rawlings Sporting Goods Company, St. Louis, MO). *Below,* A view of the cantilevered shoulder pad.

8. What other types of protective devices can be used for the shoulder?

If necessary, additional protection can be provided to the shoulder complex with larger anterior and posterior pads to cover the deltoid, teres major, and latissimus muscle areas. An injured acromioclavicular (AC) joint also can be further protected with a custom-fitted donut pad taped to the shoulder or with a "spider" AC pad, which is worn underneath the shoulder pads to elevate them off of the AC joint.

Different types of shoulder restraint braces also are used for those players with chronically dislocating shoulders. All are designed to limit abduction and external rotation and thereby reduce the incidence of anterior subluxation or dislocation. However, because of this limitation in range of motion, the player's capabilities may also be reduced.

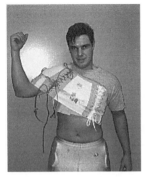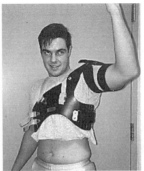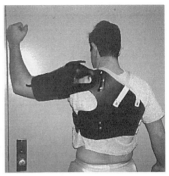

Types of shoulder restraints. *Left,* West Point shoulder harness. *Center* and *right,* Shoulder subluxation inhibitor (SSI). (Marketed by Physical Support Systems, Wyndham, NH).

9. Under what conditions should neck rolls or collars be worn?

The use of neck rolls has been advocated in those players who have suffered "stingers" or brachial plexus injuries previously and are returning to participation. They also have been used for players with neck problems without associated stingers and for the *prevention* of these injuries. However, most of the neck rolls used for these purposes have had limited success, primarily because of improper fit; therefore, they are not able to prevent neck motion, especially neck extension. This is more of a problem in the high school athlete, where the neck roll is thermoformed and comes in three standard sizes. At the collegiate and professional levels, the neck rolls are designed to attach securely to the shoulder pads; one design is part of a plastic frame that then bolts onto the pads.

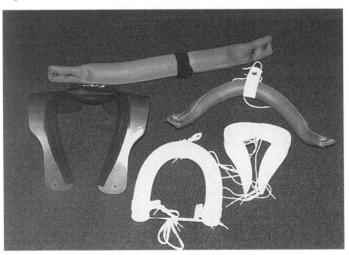

Different types of neck rolls.

10. What other types of protective devices are used for the thorax and limbs?

Other areas of the body that need protection are the arms, chest, ribs, thighs, hips, buttocks, knees, and groin. Biceps pads are worn by offensive linemen to prevent myositis ossificans. Sternum and back plates that attach to the pads offer greater protection to those regions. There are several types of rib pads; the most common are wrap-around rib protectors that attach to the shoulder pads or are suspended over the shoulders.

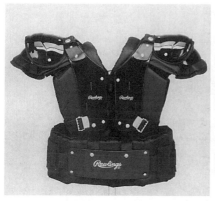 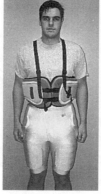 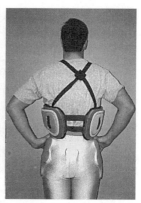

Types of rib pads (*Left,* photograph courtesy of Rawlings Sporting Goods Company, St. Louis, MO.)

Hip pads designed to protect the iliac crest, greater trochanter, and coccyx come in three basic types: snap-in, wrap-around, and girdle. The most commonly used are the girdle type; along with the thigh and knee pads, these fit into specially designed pockets in the girdle shells and football pants. A basic error in wearing these pads is to let them slide down over the iliac crest, thus offering no protection and increasing risk of a painful hip pointer injury.

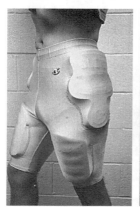 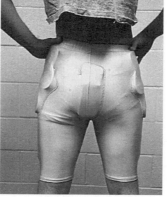

Types of hip pads.

Gloves for defensive linemen have protective metacarpophalangeal and finger padding; gloves for offensive linemen have extra padding on the entire dorsum and along the heels of the hands.

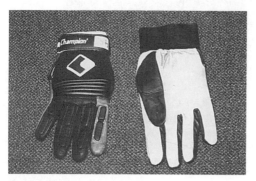

Examples of padded gloves.

11. How can the playing surfaces affect the choices of protective equipment used?

Artificial playing surfaces for football have been implicated as causing an increase in certain types of injuries. Both new artificial turf and 5-year-old artificial turf have less ability to absorb impact force than sod. Prepatellar and olecranon bursitis are far more common on artificial surfaces.[13] Prevention and reduction of severity can be accomplished with additional knee protection and the use of elbow pads.

Soft tissue injuries of the great toe, commonly referred to as "turf toe," also have increased in incidence with the advent of artificial turf. Turf toe is a sprain of the plantar capsule ligament complex of the metatarsophalangeal (MTP) joint of the great toe. Because the most common mechanism of injury is hyperextension of the MTP joint, shoe wear and the hardness of the artificial playing field are thought to be contributory to the problem. If playing on artificial turf, a metal plate built into the front sole of the shoe or contained within an insole may help to prevent this type of hyperextension.

Regardless of the type of playing surface, a large number of knee and ankle injuries occur in a noncontact situation. Therefore, the type of shoe worn and the type and condition of the playing surface have been implicated as causative factors. One study found that the resurfacing of playing fields and the wearing of shorter cleats reduced the rates of injury of the lower extremities by 42%.[10]

The two basic types of shoes worn by the football player are those with detachable cleats and those with a molded rubber-cleated sole. The former, with the five-in-front and two-in-back arrangement, is commonly worn on natural turf and should conform to a 0.5-inch cleat length as dictated by the National High School Federation and the NCAA. The latter, with the multi-short-cleated sole, is more commonly used on artificial turf. Although this type of shoe has seemed to produce fewer injuries to the knee and ankle, when conditions are wet, it can accumulate more dirt and mud and thus provide less traction.

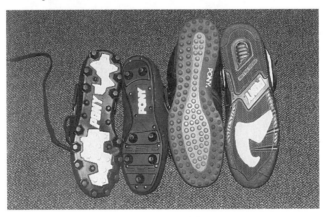

Variations in football shoes.

CONTROVERSIES

12. What is the role of prophylactic knee bracing in football?

There are three types of knee braces: (1) prophylactic, designed to prevent or reduce the severity of knee injury; (2) rehabilitative, designed to allow protected motion of an injured knee treated operatively or nonoperatively; and (3) functional, designed to provide stability for an unstable knee. Because the knee is the most frequently injured joint in football and the medial collateral ligament is the most frequently injured ligament, much attention has focused on attempts to decrease the number of knee injuries and, specifically, medial knee injuries. Players most at risk are offensive and defensive linemen, linebackers, and tight ends. One method to protect the medial knee is to provide additional external support with lateral stabilizing bars. Such prophylactic knee braces are widely used by players at all levels of skill, although conclusions in the literature about their value have been divergent. Requa and Garrick's review of nine studies evaluating the efficacy of knee braces demonstrated lack of agreement.[19] Some studies actually found a higher incidence of injury in players who were wearing braces than in players who were not. More recent research has begun to clarify the confounding variables. Both the West Point[23] and Big Ten[1] investigations showed a consistent trend toward reduction in MCL injuries in collegiate football athletes wearing knee braces when the variables of position, string (starters, substitutes, and nonplayers), and session (game or practice) were controlled. All players experienced decreased injury rates except athletes in the skill positions during games. Although consistent, the absolute values of these trends did not reach statistical significance with one exception. Athletes in the nonplayers group, whose only contact experience occurred during practice (i.e., third string), had a significantly higher injury rate with brace wear than without, regardless of position played.

Many organizations, including the American Academy of Pediatrics[2] and the American Academy of Orthopedic Surgeons, have recommended against the use of prophylactic knee bracing as standard football equipment because of lack of substantial proof of efficacy. **The current evidence supporting prophylactic knee bracing suggests benefit for certain player groups, but it is not compelling and, therefore, does not mandate compulsory or routine use.** The decision to wear a brace should be left to the player. No claim should be made to the player, coach, or parent that the brace is effective in prevention of injury.

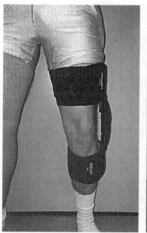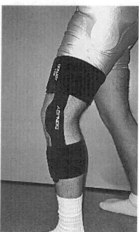

A prophylactic knee brace.

13. Is the helmet to blame for the increased incidence of neck injuries?

No. Faulty techniques are the most common cause of neck injury. A contributing factor also can be the improper fit of the helmet.

When the sport of American football evolved in the mid-1800s, protective football equipment did not exist; 23 fatalities occurred in 1905. By the 1920s, research was focused on the development of protective equipment such as pads and helmets. The first helmet was made of various layers of sturdy leather. However, it was not until 1939 that helmets became required equipment in college football and not until 1943 for the National Football League. In the 1950s, the development of plastics brought about the creation of plastic rigid helmets, which offered more protection, had higher impact strength, and were more resistant to damage. A chin guard to secure the helmet in place and protect the chin from lacerations was also added; later face masks were placed to further protect the mouth and other facial structures.

Unfortunately, athletes began feeling so secure wearing these helmets that they began to use them as weapons against their opponents by spear tackling them and causing new types of injuries. Data collected between 1959 and 1963 compared with data from 1971 to 1975 demonstrated that although both intracranial hemorrhages and intracranial deaths had decreased (by 66% and 42%, respectively), there was a large increase in the number of fractures and dislocations and permanent cervical quadriplegia (204% and 116%, respectively).[25] The improved protective capabilities of the helmets accounted for the decrease in head injuries, but also led to the development of playing techniques that used the top of the helmet as the initial point of contact, which placed the cervical spine at risk for serious injury.

As a result of these findings, in 1976 rule changes were implemented by the NCAA and National Federation of High School Athletic Associations (NFHSAA) that prohibited the use of the top of the helmet as the initial point of contact in striking an opponent during a tackle or block. Since then, there has been a decrease in both the total number of cervical spine injuries and those resulting in quadriplegia at both the high school and college levels.

14. Which is more effective at preventing ankle injuries—taping or commercial ankle supports?

Proper proprioceptive and strength training of the ankle may be the most effective method of prevention.[4] But it is becoming clearer that commercial prophylactic ankle stabilizers may be an effective alternative to the costly and time-consuming practice of ankle taping for each athletic episode. Both softshell (lace-up type) and semirigid (e.g., Aircast Sport Stirrup) stabilizers have been found to decrease the frequency of ankle injury.[24] Some studies have shown a lower risk of ankle injury with ankle taping as well. But taping also has been shown to lose up to 40% of its initial support after only 10 minutes of exercise[20] and to be ineffective at resisting inversion under body-weight load after 40 minutes of vigorous exercise.[16] Concerns about functional impairment with stabilizing braces have been disputed by two recent investigations demonstrating no difference in selected performance tasks among braced and unbraced participants.[9,15] Other factors should be considered in the selection of prophylactic ankle support. Ankle taping requires not only materials such as underwrap and tape but also someone skilled in its application. Cost estimates for ankle taping per team of collegiate football players range from $16,000–$40,000 per season. On the other hand, after they have been properly fitted, commercial braces are self-applied and reusable and may be less expensive over the course of a season.

15. What is "spatting"? Is it effective for decreasing injuries?

Spatting is the prophylactic application of tape to the ankle and heel over the shoe to provide additional stability to the ankle. Although many professional football players and some college level players use this method of taping, it has not been well studied. Only one investigation addressed this technique, and it focused on how spatting affected the interaction of the shoe and playing surface.[11] Because half of the sole of the shoe is covered when spatted, it is not surprising, as the authors note, that shoe-surface interface friction for both anterior translation and rotational torque was reduced significantly. Such laboratory models have been designed to address the underlying causes of noncontact anterior cruciate ligament injuries in particular, but the effect of this reduction in friction on injury rates in vivo is unknown. With so little information available to evaluate the usefulness of spatting, its current widespread use may be more a matter of individual style than science.

ACKNOWLEDGMENT

Special thanks to Richard Strauss, M.D., Dan Swain, and Rob Sloan for their assistance with the photos.

BIBLIOGRAPHY

1. Albright JP, Powell JW, Smith W, et al: Medial collateral ligament knee sprains in college football: Effectiveness of preventive braces. Am J Sports Med 22(1):12–18, 1994.
2. American Academy of Pediatrics Committee on Sports Medicine: Knee brace use by athletes. Pediatrics 85:228, 1990.

3. Arnheim DD: Modern Principles of Athletic Training. St. Louis, Times Mirror/Mosby College, 1989.
4. Ashton-Miller JA, Ottaviani RA, Hutchinson C, Wojtys EM: What best protects the inverted weightbearing ankle against further inversion? Evertor muscle strength compares favorably with shoe-height, athletic tape, and three orthoses. Am J Sports Med 24:800–809, 1996.
5. Baker BE: The effect of bracing on the collateral ligaments of the knee. Clin Sports Med 9:843–851, 1990.
6. Bishop PJ, Norman RW, Kozey JW: An evaluation of football helmets under impact conditions. Am J Sports Med 12:233–236, 1984.
7. Deppen RJ, Landfried MJ: Efficacy of prophylactic knee bracing in high school football players. J Orthop Sports Phys Ther 20(5):243–246, 1994.
8. Gieck J, McCue FC: Fitting of protective football equipment. Am J Sports Med 8:192–196, 1980.
9. Gross MT, Clemence LM, Cox BD, et al: Effect of ankle orthoses on functional performance for individuals with recurrent lateral ankle sprains. J Orthop Sports Phys Ther 25(4):245–252, 1997.
10. Halpern B, Thompson N, Curl WW, et al: High school football injuries: Identifying the risk factors. Am J Sports Med 15:S113–S117, 1987.
11. Heidt RS, Dormer SG, Cawley PW, et al: Differences in friction and torsional resistance in athletic shoe-turf surface interfaces. Am J Sports Med 24:834–842, 1996.
12. Hodgson VR: National Operating Committee on Standards for Athletic Equipment football helmet certification program. Med Sci Sports 7:225–232, 1975.
13. Larson RL, Osternig LR: Traumatic bursitis and artificial turf. J Sports Med 2:183–188, 1974.
14. Levy M, Skovron ML, Agel J: Living with artificial grass: A knowledge update. Am J Sports Med 18:406–412, 1990.
15. Macpherson K, Sitler M, Kimura I, Horodyski M: Effects of a semirigid and softshell prophylactic ankle stabilizer on selected performance tests among high school football players. J Orthop Sport Phys Ther 21(3):147–152, 1995.
16. Manfroy PP, Ashton-Miller JA, Wojtys EM: The effect of exercise, prewrap, and athletic tape on the maximal active and passive ankle resistance to ankle inversion. Am J Sports Med 25:156–163, 1997.
17. Mellion MB, Walsh WM, Shelton GL (eds): The Team Physician's Handbook, 2nd ed. Philadelphia, Hanley & Belfus, 1997.
18. Ranalli DN: Prevention of craniofacial injuries in football. Dent Clin North Am 35:627–645, 1991.
19. Requa RK, Garrick JG: Clinical significance and evaluation of prophylactic knee brace studies in football. Clin Sports Med 9:853–869, 1990.
20. Rovere GD, Clarke TJ, Yates CS, Burley K: Retrospective comparison of taping and ankle stabilizers in preventing ankle injuries. Am J Sports Med 16:228–233, 1988.
21. Roy S, Irvin R: Sports Medicine: Prevention, Evaluation, Management, and Rehabilitation. Englewood Cliffs, NJ, Prentice-Hall, 1983.
22. Saal JA: Common American football injuries. Sports Med 12:132–147, 1991.
23. Sitler M, Ryan J, Hopkinson WJ, et al: The efficacy of a prophylactic knee brace to reduce knee injuries in football: A prospective randomized study at West Point. Am J Sports Med 18:310–315, 1990.
24. Sitler M, Ryan J, Wheeler B, et al: The efficacy of a semirigid ankle stabilizer to reduce acute ankle injuries in basketball: A randomized clinical study at West Point. Am J Sports Med 22:454–461, 1994.
25. Torg JS: Epidemiology, pathomechanics, and prevention of football-induced cervical spinal cord trauma. Exerc Sport Sci Rev 20:321–338, 1992.

24. PROTECTIVE EQUIPMENT: BASEBALL, SOFTBALL, HOCKEY, WRESTLING, AND LACROSSE

Scott Naftulin, D.O., and Douglas B. McKeag, M.D., M.S.

GENERAL CONSIDERATIONS

1. What general characteristics should protective equipment possess?

Protective equipment should prevent injury and protect injured areas from further injury. Ideally, the equipment should not interfere with functional performance or be harmful to other athletic participants. In addition, the equipment should be easily maintained, durable, reliable, affordable, and, if possible, custom fit.

2. Is the use of protective equipment mandatory in sports?
The National Collegiate Athletic Association (NCAA) has established rules governing the use of protective equipment in many college sports including wrestling, baseball, men's lacrosse, and ice hockey.

NCAA Mandated Use of Protective Equipment

SPORT	EQUIPMENT
Baseball	Double-ear flap helmet while running or batting Throat guard on catcher's mask
Ice hockey	Helmets with fastened chin straps Face masks Internal mouthpiece
Men's lacrosse	Helmet with face mask, chin pad, and strap Chest and throat protector for goaltender Upper intraoral mouthpiece Protective gloves
Wrestling	Protective ear guards

3. How does one know if the equipment is of sufficient quality?
Certification standards have been established for certain protective equipment through the National Operating Committee on Standards for Athletic Equipment (NOCSAE; pronounced "noxey"). The Sports Equipment and Facilities Committee of the American Society for Testing and Materials (ASTM) is also involved in establishing equipment standards. The seal "Meets NOCSAE Standard" (see below) is permanently stamped on the outside rear portion of each helmet meeting the quality standards. A list of these helmet models can be obtained from the Executive Director of NOCSAE (Ben W. Ashley, c/o Wallace, Saunders, Austin, Brown and Enochs, 10111 West 87th Street, Overland Park, KS 66282-2290).

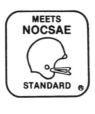
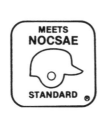
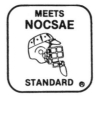

4. What protection does the mouthpiece (mouth guard) provide?
The use of a properly fitted mouthpiece unequivocally reduces the number and severity of dental injuries. Several studies have also demonstrated intraoral mouth guards to be effective in the reduction of concussive forces to the head.

5. List the criteria of an "ideal" mouth guard.
The ideal mouth guard should (1) fit comfortably between the upper and lower teeth without interfering with respiration, (2) remain in a stable, accurate position without external force, (3) be resilient and resistant to deformation from chewing, (4) have an external attaching point for easy removal, and (5) cover all of the teeth except the last two molars of players over 14 years of age.

6. What are the different types of mouth guards available?

Essentially, there are three types of mouth guards: (1) custom-fitted, (2) mouth-formed (boil and bite), and (3) stock, or off-the-shelf (ready-to-wear) (see below). It is generally agreed that the custom-fitted mouth guard most readily meets the criteria for the ideal mouthpiece. However, the cost for outfitting a team with the custom-fitted type may be prohibitive.

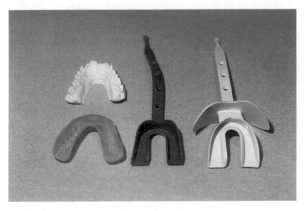

Custom, mouth-formed, and stock mouth guards (*left to right*).

7. What is the risk of eye injury in these sports?

Sports can be classified as low risk, high risk, and extremely high risk for eye injury. Low-risk sports do not involve a thrown or hit ball, a bat or a stick, or close aggressive play with body contact. High-risk sports involve a high-speed ball or puck, the use of a bat or stick, close aggressive play with intentional or unintentional body contact and collision, or a combination of these factors. Examples include hockey, lacrosse, racquetball, baseball, and softball. Eye protection devices are available for these sports. In contrast, extremely high-risk sports for eye injury are the combative sports such as boxing and wrestling, for which effective eye protection devices are not available.

8. What are the current guidelines for eye protection in sports?

In 1989, the International Federation of Sports Medicine (FIMS) issued a position statement on "Eye Injuries and Eye Protection in Sports." Recommendations for eye protection were based on the sports' risk of eye injury (see question 7 above) and the presence or absence of eye disease. Eye examination and counseling were also recommended as an integral part of the preparticipation physical examination.

9. Do normal "streetwear" eyeglass frames with 2-mm polycarbonate lenses provide sufficient protection against eye injury?

These types of glasses give adequate, cosmetically acceptable protection for routine use by active people. Such glasses are recommended for daily wear by the visually impaired or functionally one-eyed athlete. They are also satisfactory for athletes in competition who wear eyeglasses and participate in low-risk sports. However, glass lenses, ordinary plastic lenses, and open (lenseless) eye guards do not provide adequate protection for persons involved in active sports. In fact, their use can increase the risk and severity of eye injury.

10. Which eye protective equipment is recommended?

Molded polycarbonate frames and lenses are suggested for contact lens wearers and athletes who ordinarily do not wear glasses but participate in moderate-risk to high-risk, noncontact sports such as baseball and softball (see figure, next page). A face mask or helmet with face protection is required for use in high-risk contact or collision sports such as ice hockey or baseball (catcher). The molded polycarbonate protective eyewear may be used in combination with the helmet and/or face mask for additional protection. The face mask should consist of metal wire, coated wire, or a transparent polycarbonate shield.

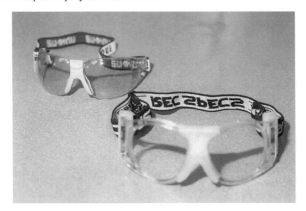

Polycarbonate protective eyewear.

11. What protection is available for male genitalia?
Protective cups are available as stock items that fit into a jockstrap or athletic supporter. These protective devices should be used in sports involving high-velocity projectiles, especially in such positions as baseball catcher or hockey goaltender.

12. What types of knee braces are available?
Three types of knee braces are generally used: (1) functional, (2) prophylactic, and (3) rehabilitative. Functional knee braces are used during athletic activities to provide functional support to unstable knees. Frequently functional braces are also prescribed after reconstructive surgery. Prophylactic knee braces are designed to prevent injury, but their use remains controversial. The rehabilitative braces are used postoperatively or after acute injuries during the rehabilitation process. Knee sleeves or compression bands are frequently used to provide additional comfort to the athlete with disorders such as patellofemoral pain. However, these sleeves or bands do not provide any significant support or stability to the knee.

BASEBALL AND SOFTBALL

13. How are baseball and softball batting helmets tested?
After mounting a helmet on a synthetic head model, an air cannon is used to fire a baseball at the helmet at specific speeds, angles, and locations. Shock measurements are taken and the Severity Index is calculated and compared with the NOCSAE Standard to determine if the helmet meets the standard.

14. Is there a real risk of eye injury in baseball?
In 1988, baseball remained the leading cause of sports-related eye injuries seen in emergency departments. Baseball injuries have been reported to account for approximately one-third of the total number of eye injuries incurred while children were participating in sports.

15. What can be done to prevent baseball-related eye injuries?
In a study in children, over one-third of the injuries occurred while the child was batting.[9] Therefore batting helmets equipped with a clear protective shield covering the eyes should be provided. In fact, the Sports Eye Safety Committee of the National Society to Prevent Blindness

recommended in 1984 that baseball batters of ages 4–14 years should wear helmets with face protectors. These protectors also protect facial bones from injury.

16. What are breakaway bases?

The regular bases used in baseball and softball are anchored by 5-inch metal rods. In contrast, the breakaway base uses suction cups to adhere to a baseplate installed in the field.

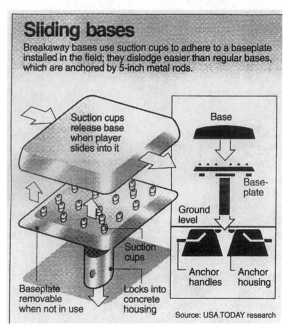

Breakaway baseball/softball bases. (Copyright 1993, USA Today. Reprinted with permission.)

17. Are breakaway bases effective in injury prevention?

The most common injuries in softball are related to sliding. Sliding-related injuries are decreased by approximately 98% with the use of breakaway bases. The Centers for Disease Control estimates breakaway bases would prevent 1.7 million injuries annually, saving 2 billion dollars per annum in acute medical care costs nationally. A recent study also suggests the bases would be effective in college and minor league baseball without interfering with plays or umpires' calls.

18. What other protective equipment is available for baseball and softball?

Although sliding-related injuries are the most common in these sports, collisions and falls also result in injury. Padded backstops, deformable walls, and field maintenance would prevent the majority of injuries in collisions and falls.

HOCKEY

19. Has the use of helmets and face masks in ice hockey been effective in injury prevention?

Eye injuries in ice hockey were common in Canada and the United States until helmets and face masks were required. A significant decrease in these injuries was found following the implementation of rules requiring face masks. Estimates project an annual prevention rate of 70,000 eye and facial injuries in 1,200,000 protected players at a savings of over 10 million dollars in medical expenses. In addition, facial injuries including the traumatic loss of teeth usually caused by the hockey stick of opponents is reduced by the use of the face masks and mouth guards.

20. List the protective equipment usually worn by ice hockey players.

In addition to the helmet, face mask, and mouthpiece mandated by the NCAA, players wear (1) shoulder pads, (2) elbow pads, (3) protective gloves, (4) padded pants, and (5) shin guards.

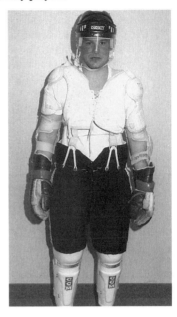

21. What protective equipment do field hockey players wear?

The players wear shin guards, and mouth guards are commonly used. The goaltender also wears a helmet, face mask, gloves, and chest protector.

LACROSSE

22. List the protective equipment usually worn by men's lacrosse players.

In addition to the protective equipment mandated by the NCAA, players wear shoulder pads and elbow pads. Some players also wear rib protectors.

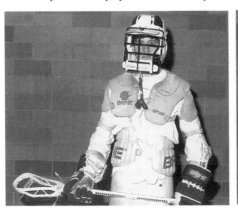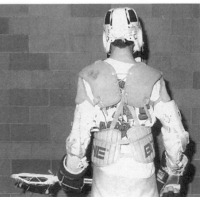

23. What protective equipment do the women's lacrosse players wear?

Some players wear mouth guards. No other protective equipment is usually worn, except by goaltenders.

WRESTLING

24. What function do the ear guards or wrestling headgear serve?

The ear guards are useful in protecting against the formation of auricular hematomas, which cause the cosmetic deformity known as "cauliflower ear." The headgear may also reduce concussive forces to the head.

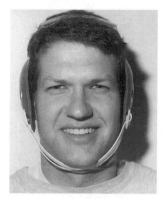 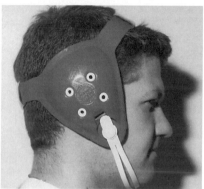

BIBLIOGRAPHY

1. Arnheim DD: Modern Principles of Athletic Training. St. Louis, Times Mirror/Mosby College Publishing, 1989.
2. Hickey JC: The relation of mouth protectors to cranial pressure and deformation. JADA 74:735–740, 1967.
3. International Federation of Sports Medicine: Eye injuries and eye protection in sports. Br J Sports Med 23:59–60, 1989.
4. Janda DH, Wild DE, Hensinger RN: Softball injuries: Aetiology and prevention. Sports Med 13:285–291, 1992.
5. Janda DH, Wojtys EM, Hanklin FM, et al: A three-phase analysis of the prevention of recreational softball injuries. Am J Sports Med 18:632–635, 1990.
6. Landry GL: Sports injuries in childhood. Pediatr Ann 21:165–635, 1992.
7. McKeag DB, Hough DO: Primary Care Sports Medicine. Carmel, IN, Brown & Benchmark, 1993.
8. Moore M: Corrective mouth guards: Performance aids or expensive placebos? Phys Sportsmed 9(4):127–132, 1981.
9. Nelson LB, Wilson TW, Jeffers JB: Eye injuries in childhood: Demography, etiology, and prevention. Pediatrics 84:438–441, 1989.
10. Pashby TJ: Eye injuries in Canadian amateur hockey. Am J Sports Med 7:254–257, 1979.
11. Podesta L, Sherman MF: Knee bracing. Orthop Clin North Am 19:737–745, 1988.
12. Reid DC: Sport Injury Assessment and Rehabilitation. New York, Churchill Livingstone, 1992.
13. Sims FH, Simonet WT, Melton LJ III, Lehn TA: Ice hockey injuries. Am J Sports Med 16(Suppl 1):586–596, 1988.
14. Torg JS: Cervical spine injuries. Med Sci Sports Exerc 17:295–303, 1985.
15. Vinger P: Sports eye injuries: A preventable disease. Ophthalmology 88:108–113, 1981.
16. National Operating Committee on Standards for Athletic Equipment Manual. Kansas City, MO, NOCSAE/National Federation, 1993.

VI. Sports Nutrition

25. ERGOGENIC ASPECTS OF SPORTS NUTRITION

Ann C. Grandjean, Ed.D., and Jaime S. Ruud, M.S., R.D.

1. What is an ergogenic aid?

An ergogenic aid is any substance that helps to increase work output. The term is used to describe drugs and dietary regimens believed by some to (1) increase strength and endurance, (2) increase concentration, (3) decrease pain, and (4) delay the onset of fatigue.

2. Name the different types of ergogenic aids.

Ergogenic aids can be classified into five categories: mechanical (e.g., equipment), psychologic (e.g., hypnosis), physiologic (e.g., sodium bicarbonate), pharmacologic (e.g., caffeine), and nutritional (e.g., carbohydrate loading).

3. Give some examples of nutritional ergogenic aids.

Dietary regimens used to alter glycogen levels and supplements, both nutritive and non-nutritive, are examples of nutritional aids. Water also can be considered a nutritional aid; compared with dehydration, maintaining a hydrated state will reduce body core temperature and improve performance time when exercising in the heat.

4. How do nutritional aids increase performance?

Nutritional aids are hypothesized to increase performance by (1) increasing energy stores in the body, (2) facilitating the biochemical reactions that produce energy, and (3) modifying the biochemical changes contributing to fatigue.

5. What exactly is carbohydrate loading?

Carbohydrate loading is the process of manipulating the diet and amount of exercise in an effort to increase glycogen stores in the muscles. There are several variations of the carbohydrate loading technique.

6. Which regimen is the best?

The regimen that is most effective with the fewest side effects is to reduce activity gradually during the week before competition, with complete rest the day before the event. The diet should provide adequate calories and 10 gm of carbohydrate per kilogram of body weight.

7. Is carbohydrate loading recommended for all athletes?

This regimen is beneficial for endurance athletes: for example, distance runners, cross-country skiers, road cyclists, and some swimmers. It is not recommended for athletes participating in events such as sprints and sports such as football, basketball, and wrestling.

8. Are there any harmful side effects to carbohydrate loading?

Carbohydrate loading can cause increased water retention and subsequent weight gain. Other side effects that have been reported are stiffness and a feeling of heaviness. Additionally, some athletes may experience gastric discomfort (flatulence and diarrhea) on very high-carbohydrate diets.

9. What other types of nutritional aids do athletes use?

Vitamins (both oral and injectable), minerals, pseudovitamins, and non-nutritive supplements comprise a large portion of the nutritive ergogenic aids used by athletes. Surveys show that C, E, and B-complex vitamins are the most popular vitamins used by athletes. Pseudovitamins and non-nutritive supplements include such compounds as vitamin B15 (calcium pangamate), inosine, and coenzyme Q10.

10. What is creatine?

Creatine is a compound made by the liver, kidney, and pancreas. It is found in meat and fish in quantities of approximately 4 gm/kg (2.2 lb). Creatine is stored mainly in skeletal muscle as free creatine or bound to a phosphate molecule. The phosphate molecule serves as an immediate source of energy for muscle contraction. Theoretically, supplementation with creatine should benefit the adenosine triphosphate-phosphocreatine (ATP-PCr) energy system.

11. How is creatine used?

Creatine is used by athletes from a wide range of sports, including power sports such as weightlifting and wrestling, team sports such as football and volleyball, and sports requiring short, explosive action such as the 100-meter dash and discus throw. Recommended doses and regimens vary. The standard loading dose is 20–30 gm/day for 5–7 days followed by a maintenance dose of 2 gm/day. Common recommendations are to take creatine with a carbohydrate (glucose) drink or to combine it with other amino acids.

12. Does taking creatine improve performance or increase muscle gain?

Preliminary studies show that creatine supplementation may increase intramuscular concentrations of PCr, enhance anaerobic power, speed recovery from intermittent high-intensity exercise, enhance muscular strength, and increase lean body mass. However, there are gaps in the research, and not all studies have reported significant changes. Furthermore, creatine has not been tested in athletes younger than 18, a group easily influenced by advertising and testimonials from professional athletes.

13. What are the potential side effects or risks associated with creatine use?

Muscle cramping, diarrhea, and weight gain have been reported by athletes using creatine. The potential may exist for elevated uric acid levels, which may result in gout-like symptoms in some athletes. The long-term effects of supplemental creatine have yet to be established.

14. Does strenuous exercise increase nutrient requirements that cannot be met by food alone?

Exercise does not increase the need for minerals or most vitamins. It is often thought that athletes may need higher amounts of vitamins involved in energy metabolism. This is true for thiamine. The recommended dietary allowance for thiamine is 0.5 mg for every 1000 calories of food and no less than 1.0 mg per day for people consuming 2000 calories or less per day. So, yes, in fact, the requirement for thiamine increases as activity increases, but the intake of this vitamin will increase as the athlete eats more food to meet energy needs.

15. Can taking a vitamin-mineral supplement help?

If the athlete is consuming enough calories to maintain body weight and those calories are provided by a wide variety of foods, the athlete probably will not benefit from supplements.

On the other hand, if the athlete is restricting food intake to lose weight or omits entire food groups from the diet (e.g., meat, milk) a vitamin-mineral supplement providing the nutrients most likely to be deficient may be beneficial. For example, if an adolescent gymnast does not include milk or red meat in the diet, he or she may be at increased risk for low intakes of calcium, iron, and zinc. Likewise, athletes may find that their intake of fruits and vegetables drops dramatically when they are on the road. In these cases, a multivitamin supplement may be indicated.

Although supplements can prevent inadequate intakes of a few nutrients, they cannot make up for a diet that is inadequate overall.

16. What about amino acid supplements? Can they help?

Promotions of amino acid supplements have included statements claiming that they will increase muscle mass during weight training and prevent protein catabolism during prolonged endurance exercise. Amino acids are sold individually or in various combinations. Arginine and ornithine are frequently promoted as a "natural steroid," and arginine and lysine are claimed to promote weight loss. However, research on protein and amino acid supplements shows no beneficial effects on strength, power, hypertrophy of muscle, or physiologic work capacity.

17. What are the risks associated with taking amino acid supplements?

Athletes consuming adequate dietary protein are consuming adequate amounts of essential amino acids. Dietary excesses can interfere with optimal physiologic efficiency, which in turn may lead to decreases in performance and health risks. A survey of popular strength and fitness magazines reported that the doses for amino acids ranged from 350 mg for some single amino acids to 40,000 mg for unspecified amino acids.

18. Is caffeine a proven ergogenic aid?

Research findings do not agree 100%, but several studies show that caffeine (9–15 mg/kg) may raise serum free fatty acids during exercise, thus sparing glycogen and prolonging endurance performance. Another possible ergogenic benefit of caffeine is the psychologic stimulant effect. Caffeine has not been shown to enhance speed or power in nonendurance athletes. Although athletic governing bodies allow levels of caffeine that represent normal use, a urinary level exceeding 12 μg/ml is grounds for disqualification. To reach this limit, an athlete must drink 6–8 cups of coffee in one sitting and be tested within 2–3 hours.

19. Do herbal products enhance athletic performance?

Although many herbs are promoted as performance enhancing, no scientific data exist to support these claims. Furthermore, athletes need to be aware that using herbs can be dangerous. Ginseng, an herbal root sold whole or in capsule form as an extract, powder, or tea, is promoted as an "energizer"; however, at doses as low as 3 gm a day, high blood pressure and symptoms such as insomnia, nervousness, confusion, depression, and edema have been reported. Many herbal teas contain high levels of caffeine. For athletes with a low tolerance to caffeine, these products can negatively affect the nervous system. Additionally, some herbal compounds contain ephedrinelike compounds that can result in a positive drug test for banned substances.

20. How do you evaluate nutritional ergogenic aids?

There are three important steps to evaluating new products on the market. Ask the following questions:
1. Does the claim make sense?
2. Does scientific research from accredited journals back it up?
3. What are the health consequences to the athlete?
4. What issues of liability and legality are involved?
5. Does the substance have the potential of being harmful?
6. Is the substance on the ban lists of the United States Olympic Committee or the National Collegiate Athlete Association?

21. What about the psychological effects of using ergogenic aids?

A major consideration when evaluating the effectiveness of any ergogenic aid or nutritional supplement is the "placebo effect." The placebo effect is a physiologic improvement brought about by a psychological mechanism. Studies show that placebos are effective about one-third of the time.

BIBLIOGRAPHY

1. Butterfield G: Ergogenic aids: Evaluating sport nutrition products. Int J Sport Nutr 6:191–197, 1996.
2. Greenhaff PL: Creatine and its application as an ergogenic aid. Int J Sport Nutr 5:S100–S110, 1995.
3. Hultman E, Greenhaff P: Creatine ingestion and exercise performance in humans. Strength Condition 17:14–15, 1995.
4. Philen RM, Ortiz DI, Auerbach SB, Falk H: Survey of advertising for nutritional supplements in health and bodybuilding magazines. JAMA 268:1008–1011, 1992.
5. Rosenbloom C, Millard-Stafford M, Lathrop J: Contemporary ergogenic aids used by strength/power athletes. J Am Diet Assoc 92:1264–1266, 1992.
6. Sherman WM, Wimer GS: Insufficient dietary carbohydrate during training: Does it impair athletic performance? Int J Sport Nutr 1:28–44, 1991.
7. Tarnopolinsky MA: Protein, caffeine and sports. Phys Sportsmed 21:137–149, 1993.
8. Williams MH: Ergogenic and ergolytic substances. Med Sci Sports Exerc 24:S344–S348, 1992.

26. A HEALTHY DIET FOR ATHLETES

Ann C. Grandjean, Ed.D., and Jaime S. Ruud, M.S., R.D.

1. What is the best diet for an athlete?

The best diet for the athlete is one that considers physiologic, sociologic, and psychologic factors. Many different dietary patterns will provide good nutrition, but a wide variety of foods is the basis of an optimal diet.

2. Are there certain dietary guidelines an athlete should follow?

The Dietary Guidelines for Americans are seven basic principles developed by the government to serve as the foundation of a healthy diet.

Dietary Guidelines for Americans

1. Eat a variety of foods.
2. Balance the food you eat with physical activity. Maintain or improve your weight.
3. Choose a diet with plenty of grain products, vegetables, and fruits.
4. Choose a diet low in fat, saturated fat, and cholesterol.
5. Choose a diet moderate in sugar.
6. Choose a diet moderate in salt and sodium.
7. If you drink alcoholic beverages, do so in moderation.

3. But the guidelines do not indicate specific foods or how much to eat. Is there a food guide that is more specific?

The food pyramid is an outline of what to eat each day based on the Dietary Guidelines for Americans. It recommends a certain number of servings from each of six food groups as shown in the figure on the following page. Each of these food groups provides some, but not all, of the nutrients that an athlete needs; thus, no one food group is more important than another. All athletes should have at least the lowest number of servings for each group. However, because of their body size and level of training, athletes may need more than even the larger number of recommended servings.

4. How many calories does an athlete need to maintain weight?

Calorie requirements vary from person to person and depend on body size, age, level of physical training, and climate. To determine average calorie intake, multiply body weight in pounds by one of the numbers in the following table. Example: a 170-pound male whose activity

Food Guide Pyramid

A Guide to Daily Food Choices

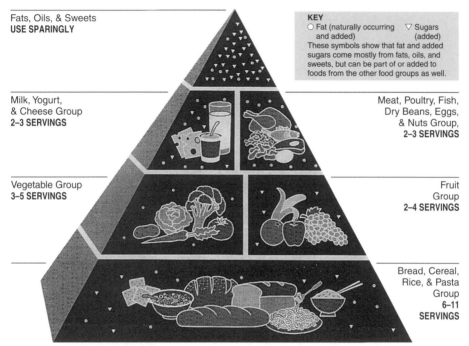

Fats, Oils, & Sweets
USE SPARINGLY

KEY
○ Fat (naturally occurring   ▽ Sugars
and added)   (added)
These symbols show that fat and added
sugars come mostly from fats, oils, and
sweets, but can be part of or added to
foods from the other food groups as well.

Milk, Yogurt,
& Cheese Group
2–3 SERVINGS

Meat, Poultry, Fish,
Dry Beans, Eggs,
& Nuts Group,
2–3 SERVINGS

Vegetable Group
3–5 SERVINGS

Fruit
Group
2–4 SERVINGS

Bread, Cereal,
Rice, & Pasta
Group
**6–11
SERVINGS**

SOURCE: U.S. Department of Agriculture/U.S. Department of Health and Human Services

Use the Food Guide Pyramid to help you eat better every day . . . the Dietary Guidelines way. Start with plenty of Breads, Cereals, Rice, and Pasta; Vegetables; and Fruits. Add two to three servings from the Milk group and two to three servings from the Meat group.

Each of these food groups provides some, but not all, of the nutrients you need. No one food group is more important than another—for good health you need them all. Go easy on fats, oils, and sweets, the foods in the small tip of the Pyramid.

is moderate needs about 3230 calories a day (170×19). These numbers represent averages. Some athletes need fewer calories, whereas others need more.

Factors* for Estimating Daily Energy Allowances at Various Levels of Physical Activity for Men and Women Ages 19 to 50

ACTIVITY LEVEL	MEN	WOMEN
Light	17	16
Moderate	19	17
Heavy	23	20

Adapted from National Research Council, 1989.[6]
* Kilocalories per pound of body weight per day.

5. How do athletes know they are getting enough calories?

Athletes who maintain their weight are eating as many calories as they expend. The table above can serve as a rough estimate, but the exact number of calories needed varies greatly among athletes. The best guide for calorie intake is body weight.

6. What should an athlete eat before competition?

An athlete's performance depends more on long-term dietary practices than on the last meal prior to an event. The primary goal of the precompetition meal is to provide fluid and energy for the athlete during performance. Physiologically, the most significant consideration is that the meal not interfere with the stresses associated with athletic performance. It should consist of foods the athlete likes, foods that are well tolerated (do not cause gastrointestinal upset), and foods the athlete usually eats.

7. I have heard that water is very important for athletes.

Water is the most important nutrient for the athlete. Without adequate water, performance can suffer in less than an hour. Water is necessary for the body's cooling system. It also transports nutrients throughout the body and maintains adequate blood volume.

8. How much water should an athlete drink?

Water needs are determined by water loss. If fluid loss by sweat and urine exceeds fluid intake, the athlete becomes dehydrated. Therefore, adequate fluid intake before, during, and after workouts and competition is important. The American College of Sports Medicine (ASCM) recommends 500 ml (17 oz) of fluid 2 hours before exercise followed by another 500 ml (17 oz) 15–20 minutes before exercise. During exercise, athletes should start drinking early and at regular intervals at a rate sufficient to replace fluids lost through sweating.

9. Why are athletes advised to increase the amount of carbohydrate in their diet?

Carbohydrate is the primary fuel used during exercise. The body converts dietary carbohydrate to muscle glycogen—one of the sources of energy for the working muscle. Carbohydrate stores in the body are limited; when depleted, the athlete may experience fatigue or feeling of "staleness."

10. How much carbohydrate do athletes need?

Like calories, carbohydrate needs vary depending on body size and the intensity of the sport. Nonendurance athletes need about 5 gm of carbohydrate per kilogram of body weight per day. Athletes participating in endurance events such as road cycling, distance running, and distance swimming need between 8 and 10 gm/kg/day. To determine how many grams of carbohydrate an athlete needs, divide body weight in pounds by 2.2 to get weight in kilograms. Then multiply the number of kilograms by 5 or 8 depending on the sport and training demands.

11. Do athletes need more dietary protein than nonathletes?

Research shows that changes occur in protein metabolism with exercise. The RDA for sedentary individuals is 0.8 gm/kg bw/day. Endurance athletes require 1.2–1.4 gm/kg bw/day, and strength athletes require 1.4–1.8 gm/kg bw/day.

12. Are there certain groups of athletes in which protein intake is a concern?

Although many athletes eat more protein than they need, female athletes, and amenorrheic athletes in particular, may not get enough protein. Studies show that amenorrheic athletes have lower protein, fat, and energy intakes than regularly menstruating athletes. This may be due in part to vegetarian or other restricted eating patterns. Wrestlers who are "cutting weight" to compete in a lower weight class may also have low protein intakes.

13. Can a vegetarian athlete get the proper nutrients for health and performance?

The key to a healthful vegetarian diet is to eat a variety of foods and enough calories to support the athlete's training schedule. Diets that exclude all animal foods may be low in calories, protein, vitamin B12, iron, zinc, and calcium. Thus, vegetarian athletes need to be aware of the plant foods that are good sources of these nutrients. Maintaining ideal competitive weight is the best determination of adequate calorie intake.

14. Does exercise increase the need for vitamins and minerals?

The need for some vitamins and minerals may increase during strenuous exercise, but this increase is small and can be accomplished by eating a balanced diet and consuming adequate calories. In situations where an athlete is restricting food intake, a vitamin-mineral supplement may be warranted.

15. Will taking supplements help boost energy and improve performance?

If dietary intake is adequate, vitamin and mineral supplements will not improve performance. However, female athletes often do not get enough iron and calcium in their diets. Low calcium intake may reduce peak bone mass in young women and increase risk of stress fractures. True iron deficiency can affect energy levels and decrease performance. Most cases of iron deficiency can be reversed by increasing dietary iron and/or the use of an iron supplement.

BIBLIOGRAPHY

1. American College of Sports Medicine: Position stand on exercise and fluid replacement. Med Sci Sports Exerc 28:i–vii, 1996.
2. Greenleaf JE: Problem: Thirst, drinking behavior, and involuntary dehydration. Med Sci Sports Exerc 24:645, 1992.
3. Haymes EM: Vitamin and mineral supplementation to athletes. Int J Sport Nutr 1:146, 1991.
4. Kaiserauer S, Snyder AC, Sleeper M, Zierath J: Nutritional, physiological, and menstrual status of distance runners. Med Sci Sports Exerc 21:120, 1989.
5. National Research Council: Recommended Dietary Allowances, 10th ed. Washington, DC, National Academy Press, 1989.
6. Reimers KJ, Ruud JS, Grandjean AC: Sport Nutrition. In Mellion MB (ed): Office Sports Medicine, 2nd ed. Philadelphia, Hanley & Belfus, 1996, pp 22–34.
7. U.S. Department of Agriculture and U.S. Department of Health, Education and Welfare: Nutrition and Your Health: Dietary Guidelines for Americans, 3rd ed. Home and Garden Bulletin No. 232. Washington, DC, U.S. Department of Agriculture, 1990.
8. U.S. Department of Agriculture: The Food Pyramid. Washington, DC, U.S. Government Printing Office, 1992.

27. FLUIDS AND ELECTROLYTES

Jaime S. Ruud, M.S., R.D., and Ann C. Grandjean, Ed.D.

1. Why is water the athlete's most important nutrient?

Water must be consumed regularly and in sufficient amounts to ensure normal functioning of the body and thermal regulation. Failure to replace water loss results in dehydration, which can cause decrements in performance.

2. What are the effects of exercise on water balance?

Under conditions of thermal and metabolic stress, sweating is the primary method of thermoregulation. The greater the intensity and duration of the sport, the greater the heat production and sweat loss.

3. Which athletes will heat and humidity affect?

All athletes need to be aware of the harmful effects of heat, humidity, and dehydration. However, in addition to high activity levels, athletes such as soccer players, road cyclists, and marathoners may also be exposed to high temperature, high humidity, and sunlight. For these athletes, fluid losses can be sizable, and core body temperature can climb to dangerous levels if hydration is not maintained.

4. How much fluid can an athlete lose?

During intense prolonged exercise, some athletes can lose up to 6–8 lb (2.7–3.6 kg) of sweat per hour.

5. What is the best way to determine water loss?

Keeping track of the athlete's body weight on a daily basis is the most accurate method for determining water loss. If the athlete experiences a weight loss of 1–3% from the previous day's activity, rehydration is essential. For every pound lost, the athlete should drink 2 cups (16 oz) of fluid.

6. What if the athlete does not have access to a scale?

Fluid loss can also be assessed by the volume and color of urine. An adult's urine volume is about 1.2 qt every 24 hours. Therefore, infrequent urination can be an indication. If urine volume is less than 1 qt a day, the athlete needs to drink more fluid. Urine that is dark in color or strong in odor also indicates that the athlete may be dehydrated.

7. How much fluid should an athlete consume?

Everyone should consume at least eight 8-ounce glasses of fluid per day. Most athletes need more. The American College of Sports Medicine (ACSM) recommends that athletes drink 500 ml (17 oz) of fluid 2 hours before exercise followed by another 500 ml (17 oz) 15–20 minutes before exercise to replace water lost through sweat. During a work-out or competition, athletes should start drinking early and at regular intervals at a rate sufficient to replace fluid loss.

8. What are the effects of dehydration on performance?

The most serious effect of dehydration resulting from failure to replace lost fluid is impaired heat dissipation, which may increase body core temperature to extremely high levels > 40° C (104° F). Fluid loss at 1% of body weight impairs thermoregulation; at 3–5%, the body's ability to utilize oxygen efficiently is impaired; and at 7% loss, collapse is likely.

Adverse Effects of Dehydration

Percent of Body Weight Loss		
0	–	
1	–	Thirst threshold, and threshold for impaired exercise thermoregulation leading to decrement in physical work capacity
2	–	Stronger thirst, vague discomfort and sense of oppression, loss of appetite
3	–	Dry mouth, increasing hemoconcentration, reduction in urinary output
4	–	Decrement of 20–30% in physical work capacity
5	–	Difficulty in concentrating, headache, impatience, sleepiness
6	–	Severe impairment in exercise temperature regulation, increased respiratory rate leading to tingling and numbness of extremities
7	–	Likely collapse if combined with heat and exercise

Adapted from Greenleaf JE, Harrison MH: Water and electrolytes. In Layman DK (ed): Nutrition and Aerobic Exercise. Washington, DC, American Chemical Society, 1986, pp 107–124.

9. What are the warning signs of heat illness?

When the body temperature rises excessively, heat illness can occur. Warning signs of heat illness include dizziness, nausea, confusion, headache, flushing, rapid pulse, and fainting.

10. How can you prevent heat illness?

Encourage athletes to drink fluids before, during, and after practice sessions and competition. Schedule rest and water breaks. Wear light, loose clothing that allows free circulation of air. Remove outer clothing when it gets wet—wet clothing reduces the skin's ability to cool.

11. Are there any other factors that increase the risk of heat illness?

Disease, lack of sleep, depletion of glycogen or glucose, some medications, and a sudden increase in the athlete's training activity can contribute to heat illness.

12. Does the athlete need to replace electrolytes, such as sodium and potassium, that may be lost through sweat?

Sodium is the mineral most affected by physical exercise. Under extreme conditions, athletes who sweat profusely, who are not acclimated to the heat, or who have low sodium intakes may experience heat cramps or exhaustion due to sodium imbalance. In most cases, however, the athlete's typical diet provides ample sodium, potassium, and other electrolytes to replace sweat losses. During events lasting longer than 1 hr, the ACSM recommends 0.5–0.7 gm of sodium per liter of water to promote fluid retention and enhance palatability.

13. Should the athlete consume an electrolyte solution?

Sport drinks are not high in sodium. The best way to meet sodium needs is by eating a variety of foods. Sodium is found naturally in many foods and beverages that athletes eat and drink. But some athletes may need to increase their intake of foods higher in sodium (e.g., pizza, ham, salted snack foods) or to salt foods during meals.

14. What is the best fluid replacement beverage?

For most athletes who are exercising for 1 hour or less in moderate temperature, plain water or sports drinks meet the athlete's needs. During endurance exercise (events lasting longer than 90 minutes of continuous effort), the best fluid replacement beverage is one that tastes good, does not cause gastric upset, and provides a source of carbohydrate for energy.

15. Is one sport drink better than another?

Studies show that commercial sport beverages containing 4–8% carbohydrate in the form of glucose, glucose polymers, or sucrose are all absorbed quickly and help maintain blood glucose levels during exercise. Beverages containing fructose leave the stomach more slowly and, if levels are high enough, may cause cramps, diarrhea, and nausea in some athletes.

16. What is the major benefit of a sport drink?

Generally, sport drinks taste good and thus stimulate voluntary fluid intake. A major benefit of consuming sport drinks is to supply carbohydrate to help maintain blood glucose levels and to delay fatigue during events lasting longer than 1 hr.

BIBLIOGRAPHY

1. American College of Sports Medicine: Position stand on exercise and fluid replacement. Med Sci Sport Exerc 28:i–vii, 1996.
2. Greenleaf JE: Problem: Thirst, drinking behavior, and involuntary dehydration. Med Sci Sports Exerc 24:645–656, 1992.
3. Mellion MB, Shelton GL: Thermoregulation, heat illness, and safe exercise in the heat. In Mellion MB (ed): Office Sports Medicine, 2nd ed. Philadelphia, Hanley & Belfus, 1996, pp 45–57.
4. Ruud JS, Reimers KR, Grandjean AC: Fluids and electrolytes for exercise in the heat. In Mellion MB (ed): Office Sports Medicine, 2nd ed. Philadelphia, Hanley & Belfus, 1996, pp 58–64.
5. Sawka MN: Physiological consequences of hypohydration: Exercise performance and thermoregulation. Med Sci Sports Exerc 24:657–670, 1992.

VII. Behavioral and Psychological Problems

28. DRUGS AND DOPING: ANABOLIC STEROIDS AND GROWTH HORMONE

Robert W. Heck, M.D., and John A. Lombardo, M.D.

1. What are anabolic steroids?

Anabolic steroids, or more appropriately anabolic-androgenic steroids (AAS), are synthetic hormones that are analogues of testosterone. Like testosterone, these hormones are synthesized from the parent compound cholesterol, and various modifications made to the cholesterol compound yield AAS with differing properties. For example, the efficacy of orally administered AAS can be greatly improved by alkylation at the 17α position. This change slows the first-pass metabolism by the liver and thus increases its potency. The efficacy of the parenterally active AAS is enhanced by esterification of the 17β-hydroxyl group. This modification yields a more lipid-soluble compound with extended activity.

2. What are the effects of testosterone on the human body?

Testosterone affects nearly every system and tissue in the human body. There are two main actions of testosterone on the human body:

Androgenic (masculinizing): deepens the voice and stimulates growth of facial hair and development of sexual organs, for example.

Anabolic (tissue building): stimulates the development of muscle mass and enhances long bone growth.

3. Is it possible to separate the anabolic from the androgenic effects of AAS?

No. AAS are synthesized to minimize the androgenic effects, but to date all commercially available AAS preparations have some androgenic properties.

4. Why isn't "natural," unaltered testosterone used by athletes instead of AAS?

Natural, unaltered testosterone is rapidly cleared by the liver when taken orally and has a short half-life when given intramuscularly; therefore, it is ineffective and inconvenient to use clinically. However, simple changes to the hormone structure or the delivery vehicle have yielded AAS that are more potent and longer acting than testosterone.

Additionally, testosterone is a relatively potent androgen but a less potent anabolic drug. By comparison, animal studies show an anabolic to androgenic potency ratio of 0.07 for testosterone, whereas the ratio for stanozolol is 4.3 and for Wy3475 (another AAS) the ratio is 20.

Nevertheless, because of the increased amount of drug testing to which athletes are subjected, natural testosterone has become more popular. Although the androgenic effects are increased, the risk of detection is reduced (but not eliminated). There have been reports of athletes using scrotal patches to deliver a relatively consistent amount of testosterone.

5. How are AAS administered?

Orally, intramuscularly, or transdermally. Athletes may use numerous drugs with varying routes of administration simultaneously (stacking) or may alternate routes of administration over time. Some athletes think that stacking enhances the anabolic effects of the drugs.

6. What is the typical AAS regimen used?

Many regimens have been reported varying from athlete to athlete, gym to gym, and sport to sport. Dosages have been reported to range from 5 to 100 times physiologic dose. The serious user typically starts with an oral AAS, becomes impressed with the gains, and raises the dose or adds another drug. Eventually, the experienced user switches to parenteral preparations and adds other drugs, such as antiestrogens and human chorionic gonadotropin (hCG) to inhibit the adverse effects, such as gynecomastia due to aromatization of the androgens and testicular atrophy, respectively.

Whereas the daily production of testosterone in an adult male is about 7 mg, steroid users commonly take 50 mg a day, and doses of 100–200 mg are not unusual. The "orals" with shorter half-lives are typically taken daily (up to three times a day), and the "parenterals" can be injected on a weekly or biweekly basis.

The annual use pattern varies with the sport and the likelihood of being tested. The unrestricted user typically "cycles" on and off several times per year for several years in concert with competition dates. Cycles refer to periods "on" the drugs, and normally the cycle length is 6–12 weeks, alternating with 6–12 weeks drug free or low dose to maintain physiologic testosterone levels. A typical 12-week cycle incorporates two to four drugs in escalating doses that peak either in mid cycle ("pyramid") or at the end of the cycle.

If event drug testing is expected, the regimen is adjusted to current knowledge of detection times. Following a cycle of high-dose nandrolone decanoate, metabolites can be detected in the urine for months; short-acting, water-based injectables and oral AAS may only be detectable for days or weeks. Experienced users are knowledgeable about these drugs and detection methods, and if event testing is the only testing, the athletes can generally beat the system.

7. What benefit is reaped by cycling?

Three main reasons for cycling have been suggested.

1. Cycling allows the body to return to normal function between cycles. Endogenous testosterone levels, sperm production, and the entire hypothalamic-pituitary-gonadal axis are affected by AAS use. The "off" cycle is believed to return these functions to normal.

2. History suggests that cycling may decrease the incidence of harmful side effects associated with anabolic steroid use.

3. There seem to be diminishing anabolic effects with prolonged drug use, that is, tachyphylaxis. Cycling eliminates the need for increasing drug dosages to attain desired effects.

8. Do endogenous testosterone levels return to normal after cessation of AAS use?

Yes. But the time required for the hypothalamic-pituitary-testicular axis to return to normal after steroid withdrawal varies and is related to the amount of drug used and the cycle length.

9. What are the effects of AAS use on sperm production?

Numerous investigators report oligospermia (small number of sperm in semen), azoospermia (lack of sperm in semen), and decreased testicular tissue on biopsy associated with AAS use. These changes have been shown to resolve after discontinuation of the drugs, but the number and morphology of the sperm may remain abnormal for 12–24 months. Treatment of these individuals as hypogonadal with testosterone can further prolong the natural recovery.

10. Are there any other potential adverse effects of AAS?

Many other systems are affected adversely by AAS use:

Endocrine with a decrease in the secretion of the gonadotropins, follicle-stimulating hormone (FSH) and luteinizing hormone (LH), irregular menses in women, and often irreversible gynecomastia in men.

Gastrointestinal with cholestasis and jaundice when used to treat refractory anemia in humans, steroid-induced tumors in the livers of rats and mice, and benign hepatomas, peliosis hepatitis, as well as hepatocellular carcinoma reported in patients using oral antibiotic steroids for various medical conditions and athletes using drugs for performance enhancement.

Cardiovascular with hypertension, changes in lipid profiles (decrease in high-density lipoprotein cholesterol and increase in total cholesterol), and cardiac muscle changes such as hypertrophy and cardiomyopathy in animal studies and human case reports.

Musculoskeletal with weakening of connective tissue reported in animal studies.

Dermatologic with excessive acne, alopecia, and temporal hair recession.

Psychiatric with aggressive behavior, depression, dependency, irritability, frequent mood swings, and libido changes.

Immunologic with reported lowering of immunoglobulins (IgA, IgM) and enhanced natural killer cell activity.

Hematologic with increased hematocrits and hypercoagulability.

11. Have there been any life-threatening processes associated with AAS use?

Case reports exist associating AAS use with the following:

Peliosis hepatitis and hepatocellular carcinoma	Pulmonary embolisms
Cardiomyopathy and ultimately congestive heart failure	Brain tumors
Thrombosis of coronary arteries and myocardial infarction	Wilms' tumors
Cerebrovascular accidents	

Although the evidence for these links is inconclusive, the case load of these complications among athletes is growing despite the extremely low incidence.

12. Are there any special risks for prepubescent users and women?

Youths may experience accelerated maturation and premature closure of growth plates with AAS use. Women users can experience irreversible masculinization (e.g., hirsutism, clitoral enlargement, and deepening of the voice).

13. Can an athlete become dependent on AAS?

The physiologic addictiveness of AAS is not known but has been suggested by anecdotal reports of withdrawal symptoms, such as depression, low levels of energy, and headaches. A few cases of apparent dependency in multidrug AAS abusers have been reported in the literature that are strikingly similar to dependencies observed with other substances. Further support for physiologic dependence on these drugs resides in the numerous reports demonstrating the role of opiate peptides in the mediation of sex steroid effects on the central nervous system.

Psychologic dependency with a major behavioral component appears likely with AAS. Data from a large national high school survey indicate that approximately one-quarter of AAS users report behaviors, perceptions, and opinions that are consistent with psychological dependence; for example, their unwillingness to stop use, their perceptions of risks and benefits of use, and their rationalization of use.

Both expectations from the drugs and the user's needs have a powerful effect on behavior following administration. ASS can leave the athlete feeling good about himself or herself because of increase self-esteem and positive peer admiration that may be precipitated by improved appearance and performance. Clearly, such outcomes encourage continued AAS use, as do the altered mood states that have often been reported with higher levels of AAS use; for example, increased self-confidence, feelings of euphoria and of well-being, sometimes to the point of true grandiosity with hypomania or frank mania.

When the athlete discontinues these drugs, he or she may note a decrease in energy and drive, a decrease in strength and size, and a let-down from the euphoria of the drugs. Some athletes feel "weak" or "small" when off the drugs, whereas others feel they cannot be competitive in their sport without the help of steroids. These feelings of inadequacy certainly can lead to prolonged uninterrupted AAS use.

14. I understand there is some controversy as to the efficacy of AAS as ergogenic aids. Is there any scientific support for their use?

Aerobic capacity: Conflicting data exist and are inconclusive. There may be a slight increase in red blood cell production with AAS use, which would enhance endurance by increasing

O_2 delivery. Alternatively, AAS may improve endurance event performance by increasing the user's ability to perform high-intensity work.

Body composition: Evidence exists that AAS administration results in a positive effect on lean body mass with exercise,[14] and there is a dose response to these drugs regardless of exercise.[8]

Strength: Contradictory reports exist in the literature. However, based on the results of available scientific data and overwhelming anecdotal reports by athletes, it can be surmised that there can be gains in strength with AAS use.

15. What is the mechanism by which AAS affect ergogenicity in athletes?

A number of mechanisms have been proposed for the actions of androgens on muscular strength and lean body mass:

Increase in protein synthesis

Inhibition of the catabolic effect of glucocorticoids

Effects on central nervous system and neuromuscular junction

Placebo effect

16. Do the ergogenic benefits of AAS persist after cessation of use?

It is not really known how much if any of the gains remain after the drugs are stopped.

17. Can a physician legally prescribe AAS for performance enhancement in athletes?

No. Anabolic steroids are Schedule III federally controlled substances with restricted use in the United States. Some state laws also prohibit the prescription of AAS for performance enhancement.

18. Is it true that only high-level and professional athletes use AAS?

Absolutely not. Some estimates of AAS use in high school males are as high as 5–11%. Some of these are participants in competitive sports, whereas others are not. In collegiate athletes, the incidence ranges from 2–20%, and in elite athletes up to 44%.

19. How can AAS users be identified?

Random and event urine testing is done on national, international, collegiate, and professional athletes. There is minimal testing in the high school system. One should be suspicious of steroid use in the athlete who shows excessive gains in size or strength over a short period of time, excessive acne, especially on the shoulders, personality change, or facial feature changes (frontal bossing, increased mandible size). However, one must also realize that many of the aforementioned changes may also occur naturally in athletes of all ages and maturity levels.

20. What is growth hormone?

Human growth hormone is a 191–amino acid polypeptide secreted by the somatotrope cells of the anterior pituitary. Prior to 1985, the only source was human cadavers; however, with the success of recombinant DNA techniques, a synthetic form identical to endogenous human growth hormone has become available. Consequently, the supply has increased, and the misuse of growth hormone is on the rise.

21. Why is growth hormone being used by athletes?

There are three actions of growth hormone that the athlete perceives as beneficially ergogenic: (1) stimulation of protein and nucleic acid synthesis in skeletal muscle, (2) increase in lipolysis and overall decrease in body fat, and (3) enhancement of healing after musculoskeletal injuries. Growth hormone has the additional appeal to the athlete in that it is not detectable by present urine drug testing techniques.

22. Is there any scientific support for using growth hormone as an anabolic aid?

Some studies have shown beneficial effects of growth hormone on lean body mass and strength gains. However, most studies support such findings in individuals who are growth hormone-deficient. Few studies have addressed the effects of growth hormone on lean body mass and strength in normal individuals who are not growth hormone-deficient.

23. What is the mechanism of action of growth hormone?

It is not fully understood how growth hormone works, but its effects are at least partly mediated through insulinlike growth factors (IGF)—formerly known as somatomedins—which are produced in the liver, kidneys, and peripheral target tissues. Growth hormone has a relatively short half-life. When administered intravenously, the concentration of circulating growth hormone peaks in 1 hour and returns to baseline in 3 hours. IGF levels, however, increase at 3 hours and remain elevated for 9–24 hours.

The growth-promoting actions of human GH (hGH) on skeletal tissues are insulinlike in stimulating amino acid uptake and protein synthesis. Paradoxically, although this insulinlike effect opposes that of cortisol, the action of hGH on carbohydrate and fat metabolism opposes that of insulin, being synergistic with cortisol in exerting lipolytic and diabetogenic effects.

24. Does growth hormone have an effect on healing of injuries?

There is insufficient evidence to reach any conclusion on this question at this time.

25. What are the potential adverse effects of growth hormone?

Excess of endogenous growth hormone causes gigantism in prepubertal individuals and acromegaly in adults. Because there is no good screening test for hGH, identification of adverse effects in users is only anecdotal. Only a few cases of athletes with early symptoms of acromegaly have been reported.[3] Acromegaly is characterized by bony overgrowth, being particularly noticeable in the mandible and the supraorbital ridges, and the enlargement of the hands and feet. Other symptoms include the manifestation of muscular weakness, arthritis, impotence, hyperlipidemia, diabetes, and cardiomyopathy.

26. Are there other anabolic agents being used by athletes?

Certain food products are being promoted as having anabolic properties. These include amino acids, plant steroids and extracts, and chromium picolinate. Certain amino acids have been shown to increase levels of endogenous growth hormone in athletes. Some plant steroids (sterols) such as yohimbine bark extract are being used as anabolic agents, but it is unlikely that the human body can convert the plant sterol into a usable human AAS. Chromium picolinate is claimed by some to increase lean body mass, probably via its effect on insulin-induced protein metabolism; however, further studies are necessary before any valid conclusions can be made.

Two other types of drugs are being used by athletes as ergogenic acids, hCG and beta agonists, such as clenbuterol. Human chorionic gonadotropin (hCG), the hormone of pregnancy, given intravenously or intramuscularly, has been shown to increase both endogenous testosterone and epitestosterone levels in users, and it is being used by athletes alone and in combination with AAS to elevate endogenous testosterone levels and to minimize testicular atrophy. The mechanism of anabolic action of beta agonists is still unknown.

Creatine monohydrate is used with increasing frequency by athletes. Creatine is part of an energy molecule used by the body during repetitive bouts of short-burst, high-intensity activity. Some scientific data and many anecdotal reports support the effectiveness of creatine at increasing lean body mass and strength with high-intensity workouts. There have been anecdotal reports of increases in muscle strains in athletes using creatine.

The precursors of testosterone are presently marketed by supplement producers. The most popular is DHEA. Another is androstenedione. These precursors may be metabolized in the body to testosterone. The amounts that are absorbed and the efficacy have not been shown. Positive drug tests due to these substances have been reported. There seems to be some contradiction in the fact that testosterone is a controlled substance whereas precursors that are one and two steps from testosterone are produced with no controls.

27. What would you suggest to the athlete who wants to increase lean body mass and strength?

Most importantly, the athlete should be instructed on proper exercise, adequate nutrition, and rest. Occasionally, an athlete will seek to accelerate his or her gains through the use of anabolic agents. Most of these anabolic agents have no scientific basis for their use and have not undergone sufficient scientific review for validation.

From an ethical standpoint, one should emphasize that using anabolic agents is "cheating." How would you feel being in an athletic competition knowing that one of your opponents was using ergogenic aids? Would you feel cheated, or worse yet, would you feel coerced into using the drugs yourself? This is the main problem with these substances.

BIBLIOGRAPHY

1. Ariel G, Saville W: Anabolic steroids: The physiological effects of placebos. Med Sci Sports 4:124–126, 1972.
2. Catlin DH, Hatton CK: Use and abuse of anabolic and other drugs for athletic enhancement. Adv Intern Med 36:399–425, 1991.
3. Cowart VS: Human growth hormone: The latest ergogenic aid? Phys Sportsmed 16:175–185, 1988.
4. Crist DM, Peake GT, Egan PA, Waters DL: Body composition response to exogenous GH during training in highly conditioned adults. J Appl Physiol 65:579–584, 1988.
5. de Boer D, DeJong EG, van Rossum JM, Maes AA: Doping control of testosterone and human chorionic gonadotropin: A case study. Int J Sports Med 12:46–51, 1991.
6. Ferenchick GS, Kirlin P, Potts R: Steroids and cardiomyopathy: How strong a connection? Phys Sportsmed 19:107–110, 1991.
7. Ferenchick GS: Anabolic/androgenic steroid abuse and thrombosis: Is there a connection? Med Hypotheses 35:27–31, 1990.
8. Forbes GB, Porta CR, Herr BE, Griggs RC: Sequence of changes in body composition induced by testosterone and reversal of changes after drug is stopped. JAMA 267:397–399, 1992.
9. Hasten DL, Rome EP, Franks BD, Hegsted M: Effects of chromium picolinate on beginning weight training students. Int J Sport Nutr 2:343–350, 1992.
10. Johnson MD: Anabolic steroid use in adolescent athletes. Pediatr Clin North Am 37:1111–1123, 1990.
11. Kicman AT, Cowan DA: Peptide hormones and sport: Misuse and detection. Br Med Bull 48(3):496–517, 1992.
12. Kochakian CD: History of anabolic-androgenic steroids. NIDA Research Monograph: Anabolic Steroid Abuse 102:29–59, 1990.
13. Lombardo JA: Anabolic-androgenic steroids. NIDA Research Monograph: Anabolic steroid abuse 102:69–73, 1990.
14. Lombardo JA, Hickson RC, Lamb DR: Anabolic/androgenic steroids and growth hormone. In Lamb DR, Williams MH (eds): Ergogenics: Enhancement and Performance and Exercise in Sport. Carmel, IN, Brown & Benchmark, 1991, pp 249–284.
15. Maltin CA, Delday MI, Hay SM, et al: The effect of the anabolic agent, clenbuterol, on overloaded rat skeletal muscle. Biosci Rep 7(2):143–149, 1987.
16. Martikainen H, Alen M, Rahkila P, Vihko R: Testicular responsiveness to human chorionic gonadotropin during transient hypogonadotropic hypogonadism induced by androgenic-anabolic steroids in power athletes. J Steroid Biochem 25(1):109–112, 1986.
17. Martineau L, Horan MA, Rothwell NJ, Little RA: Salbutamol, a β_2-adrenoceptor agonist, increases skeletal muscle strength in young men. Clin Sci 83:615–621, 1992.
18. Uzych L: Anabolic-androgenic steroids and psychiatric-related effects: A review. Can J Psychiatry 37:23–27, 1992.
19. Wagner JC: Enhancement of athletic performance with drugs: An overview. Sports Med 12(4):250–265, 1991.
20. Yesalis CE, Vicary JR, Buckley WE, et al: Indications of psychological dependence among anabolic-androgenic steroid abusers. NIDA Research Monograph: Anabolic Steroid Abuse 102:29–59, 1990.

29. DRUGS AND DOPING: BLOOD DOPING AND RECOMBINANT HUMAN ERYTHROPOIETIN

Robert C. Gambrell, M.D., FACSM, and John A. Lombardo, M.D.

1. What is blood doping?

Blood doping is the infusion of blood into an individual with a normal level of red blood cells (RBCs) to induce erythrocythemia. The intent of this induced erythrocythemia is to increase the oxygen-carrying capacity of the blood and thus increase the endurance performance of that individual. Blood can be transfused from a matched donor (homologous transfusion) or reinfused from the same individual after removal and a period of storage (autologous transfusion).

2. How is blood doping done?

An athlete would typically have 1 or 2 units of blood removed 4 to 8 weeks before an antici-pated athletic event and have the RBCs preserved via glycerol freezing. The athlete continues to train allowing the hemoglobin level to return to normal. One to 7 days before the athletic event, the RBCs are then thawed, reconstituted with saline, and reinfused over 1 to 2 hours. This process obviously requires a great deal of technical support not only in the removal and reinfusion of the blood but also in the separation of the RBCs from the plasma, freezing the RBCs, and their sub-sequent thawing and reconstitution.

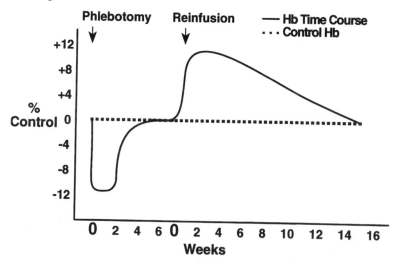

Time course of hematologic changes following the removal and reinfusion of approximately 900 ml of autol-ogous freeze-preserved blood. (From Gledhill N: Blood doping and related issues: A brief review. Med Sci Sports Exerc 14:183–189, 1982, with permission.)

3. Does blood doping really work?

Although early studies of blood doping reported variable results, recent studies have shown that maximal aerobic capacity and endurance exercise capacity can be improved by infusing at least 900 ml of blood. Faster endurance racing times also have been observed after blood doping.[2,14] Major reasons for the contradictory findings of earlier studies were the use of inade-quate reinfusion volumes, premature reinfusion of the blood following withdrawal, and storage of blood by refrigeration rather than by freezing.

4. What kind of athlete would use blood doping?

Blood doping increases endurance performance and has reportedly been used by endurance athletes such as cross country skiers, marathoners, triathletes, and cyclists in an attempt to gain a competitive advantage. Although reports of blood doping occurred during the 1970s, it was not until the 1984 Olympics when seven members of the U.S. Olympic cycling team (four medalists) admitted to receiving blood transfusions that its use was substantiated. Elite athletes at national and international levels of competition may have many reasons to resort to blood doping if they think that it may give them an advantage. The intense pressure and high expectations that they may be subjected to by coaches and trainers, the athletes' own high aspirations, and the prospect of lucrative endorsement contracts that may follow championships or medals are only a few reasons that blood doping may be used.

5. What are the risks associated with blood doping?

Blood transfusions from matched donors (homologous transfusions) carry the risk of hepatitis, AIDS, and transfusion reactions. Induced erythrocythemia has all the potential risks that have been described with polycythemia, including hypertension, congestive heart failure, and stroke. Recent controlled studies of blood doping, using autologous transfusions of 900–1350 ml to avoid risks of blood-borne disease and transfusion reactions, have not been shown to produce significant problems. Blood doping under these tightly controlled conditions appears relatively safe.

6. What is rEPO?

Erythropoietin is a hormone produced primarily by the kidneys that stimulates erythropoiesis. It induces RBC production by stimulating the proliferation, differentiation, and maturation of erythroid precursor. Recombinant human erythropoietin (rEPO) is a genetically engineered substance that has been produced from the successful cloning and expression of the human erythropoietin gene. rEPO has been successfully used to treat the anemia of chronic end-stage renal disease and shows tremendous promise in the treatment of other forms of anemia.

7. Why would an athlete use rEPO?

A great deal of concern exists about the possible use of rEPO by athletes to stimulate erythropoiesis and induce erythrocythemia in an attempt to gain a competitive advantage. The use of rEPO could be seen as an easier method of blood doping by the athlete because it does not require the support of a blood bank, and the injection of rEPO could be done in the privacy of the athlete's home, providing much more confidentiality. Additionally, autologous transfusions require the athlete to go through a 4–6 week period of relative anemia that may impair his or her performance during a critical period in the season, which does not occur with rEPO use.

8. Does rEPO improve athletic performance?

A study by Ekblom and Berglund[6] showed an increase in VO_2max and hemoglobin concentrations for 15 healthy male subjects given rEPO over 6 weeks to be similar to increases after the acute infusion of autologous blood. This suggests that rEPO use would impart a competitive advantage to the athlete, but the precise relationship of increasing the VO_2max and improvement in athletic performance is still unproven.

9. How is rEPO administered?

Most of the clinical experience with rEPO has been with intravenous administration in patients on hemodialysis, but it also can be given subcutaneously, achieving similar results.

10. What are the adverse effects of rEPO?

rEPO use in hemodialysis patients has been associated with arterial hypertension, thrombosis of vascular access (e.g., arteriovenous shunt), and a so-called flulike syndrome. The flulike syndrome may be accompanied by light headache and muscle pain usually occurring some hours after the last injection of rEPO.

11. Are there any risks associated with rEPO use?

Extreme concern exists about the potential problems that rEPO may pose to the competitive athlete. The vast majority of experience with rEPO comes from patients with end-stage renal disease and is difficult to extrapolate to athletes, but the limited evidence that exists is disturbing. A suspicious increase in the number of deaths among competitive cyclists in Europe may be attributed to the use of rEPO.

The most ominous problem with rEPO comes from the belief by many athletes that if a little is good, then a lot must be better. If the athlete is left to monitor his or her own administration of rEPO, there is a great potential to increase the hematocrit to dangerous levels. The resulting polycythemia may be further aggravated by the dehydration that occurs with endurance events. In Ekblom's study of athletes given rEPO over a 6-week period, it was noted that they developed a significant increase in systolic blood pressure in response to submaximal exercise.[5] An exaggerated elevation of blood pressure and polycythemia with exercise present an ideal setting for stroke, myocardial infarction, or other catastrophic events to occur.

12. Is blood doping legal?

Blood doping, defined as the administration of blood or related blood products, including erythropoietin, to an athlete other than for legitimate medical treatment is banned by the International Olympic Committee (IOC), United States Olympic Committee (USOC), and National Collegiate Athletic Association (NCAA). The USOC and IOC take the position that any evidence confirming that blood doping was used will result in suspension for a maximum of 3 months with the first offense, 2 years for the second, and a lifelong ban for the third from events sanctioned by their organizations.

13. Are there any tests to detect blood doping or rEPO use?

Blood doping was not specifically forbidden by the IOC until after the 1984 Olympics when U.S. cyclists admitted to receiving blood transfusions. This prohibition went into effect in spite of the fact that there was no test that could unequivocally detect blood doping. In spite of considerable work that has been done in this area, present tests can detect only about 50% of blood-doped athletes who have used refrigerated blood. No reliable analytical technique is available to detect rEPO use as an ergogenic agent.[6] Serum erythropoietin levels can be measured and determined to be high but the ergogenic effect may last for weeks after discontinuing its use. Difficulty arises in the fact that blood doping and rEPO are naturally occurring substances and simply detecting their presence does not indicate inappropriate use. A further challenge in detection is the fact that all testing being investigated requires a blood sample, which is currently not allowed by the IOC or NCAA.

BIBLIOGRAPHY

1. Berglund B: Development of techniques for the detection of blood doping in sports. Sports Med 5:127–135, 1988.
2. Brien AJ, Simon TL: The effects of red blood cell reinfusion on 10 km race time. JAMA 257:2761–2765, 1987.
3. Eichner ER: Sports anemia, iron supplementation, and blood doping. Med Sci Sports Exerc 24(suppl): S315–S318, 1992.
4. Ekblom B: Blood doping, oxygen breathing, and altitude training. In Strauss RH (ed): Drugs and Performance in Sports. Philadelphia, W.B. Saunders, 1987.
5. Ekblom B, Berglund B: Effect of erythropoietin administration on maximal aerobic power. Scan J Sci Sports 1:88–93, 1991.
6. Gareau R, Audran M, Baynes RD, et al: Erythropoietin abuse in athletes [letter]. Nature 380(6570):113, 1996.
7. Gledhill N: Blood doping and related issues: A brief review. Med Sci Sports Exerc 14:183–189, 1982.
8. Kicman AT, Cowan DA: Peptide hormones and sport: Misuse and detection. Br Med Bull 48:496–517, 1992.
9. Leith W: Cyclists don't die like this. In Sunday Review, Independent on Sunday. London, Newspaper Publishing, July 14, 1991, pp 3–4.
10. Nielson OJ: Recombinant human erythropoietin: Experimental and clinical applications. Med Bull 38:355–370, 1991.

11. Sawka M, Young A, Muza S, et al: Erythrocyte reinfusion and maximal aerobic power. JAMA 257: 1496–1499, 1987.
12. Simon TL: Induced erythrocythemia and athletic performance. Semin Hematol 31(2):128–133, 1994.
13. Wagner JC: Enhancement of athletic performance with drugs. Sports Med 12(4):250–265, 1991.
14. Williams MH, Wesseldine S, Somma T, Schuster R: The effect of induced erythrocythemia upon 50-mile treadmill run time. Med Sci Sports Exerc 13:169–175, 1981.
15. Zanjani ED, Ascensao JL: Erythropoietin. Transfusion 29:46–57, 1989.

30. DRUGS AND DOPING: AMPHETAMINES AND OTHER AGENTS

R. Trent Sickles, M.D., and Edward P. Dominguez

1. What are stimulants?

Stimulants are agents that increase organic activity primarily through their effects on the central nervous system (CNS) and peripheral nervous system. The effects of these agents vary widely with regard to their effects on the CNS, skeletal muscle, and smooth muscle. Each of these properties has the potential to affect performance either beneficially or adversely in an individual athlete. In some instances, stimulants have been shown to increase muscle contractility and speed reaction time.

2. Why are stimulants used by athletes?

Perceived performance-enhancing agents are utilized by athletes to gain an edge on the competition. The desire to win is driven in part by the competitive nature of athletics and to a large degree by the value that society places on winning. Stimulants are used by athletes for two primary purposes: for their effects in combating fatigue and speeding reaction time or for their appetite-suppressing effects to lose weight.

3. How common is amphetamine use by athletes?

The replication of the national study of the substance use and abuse habits of college student-athletes in 1989 reported that athletes' self-reported use of amphetamines was 3%.[1] This is significantly less than the 8% self-reported use in the original survey in 1985.

4. Do amphetamines have any performance-enhancing effects?

Amphetamines are potent sympathomimetic agents. Their effects on peripheral tissues are thought to be due to release of norepinephrine from adrenergic nerve endings and from direct action on alpha- and beta-adrenergic receptors. CNS effects are primarily in the cerebral cortex, where they cause an increase in motor activity, increase alertness, and diminish the sense of fatigue. No conclusive evidence exists that amphetamines improve performance. When performance has been reduced by fatigue, improvement has been seen with the performance of certain tasks. This may be related to an improved attitude toward performing the task.

5. Are there any adverse effects of amphetamines on performance?

Side effects of amphetamines may decrease performance in individual athletes. These include anxiety during their use or depression following their withdrawal, tremor, hyperthermia, vasoconstriction, variable gastrointestinal effects, cardiac arrhythmias, and sudden death. Agitation and acute psychosis can be seen and would obviously adversely affect performance.

6. What other stimulants are commonly used by athletes?

Both over-the-counter and prescription drugs that have stimulant properties and that are commonly used by athletes both for therapeutic and for possible performance-enhancing effects are listed below.

Over-the-counter medications:
  Caffeine
  Decongestants
    Ephedrine
    Pseudoephedrine
    Phenylpropanolamine
  Antiasthmatic medications
    Epinephrine
  Nicotine

Prescription medications:
  Theophylline
  Beta-agonists
    Salbutamol (albuterol)
    Metaproterenol
    Terbutaline
    Isoproterenol
    Bitolterol
    Clenbuterol (outside U.S.A.)
  Amphetamines
  Decongestants
    Most over-the-counter medications are
    available in prescription strength

7. Describe the potential performance-enhancing properties of caffeine.

Caffeine, like theophylline and theobromine, is a xanthine derivative. Caffeine stimulates the CNS, producing decreased fatigue and possibly improving psychomotor coordination. Caffeine stimulates voluntary skeletal muscle and has been shown to decrease muscle fatigue and thereby increase performance in endurance events. The improvement in performance during endurance events may be due to caffeine's effects on glycogen. Caffeine promotes the release of free fatty acids into the blood stream and thereby preserves glycogen stores as a ready source of energy. Conflicting evidence exists regarding increased muscle contractility and increased explosiveness.

8. How much caffeine must be consumed to achieve performance-enhancing levels?

The effects vary widely from one individual to another. No evidence exists that a threshold exists over which performance is likely to be improved. However, doses of 250–350 mg have been shown to enhance performance in endurance athletes. To achieve banned levels of caffeine in the body, most athletes would need to consume five or six cups of regular coffee within 2 hours of competition.

9. What are the adverse effects of high-dose caffeine consumption?

Agitation, irritability, and tremulousness are the most common side effects of acute ingestion of caffeine. Supraventricular arrhythmias, although less common, also can occur in susceptible individuals. Addiction, dependency, and withdrawal can occur in long-term users. Finally, caffeine acts as a moderate diuretic and may accelerate dehydration.

10. What effect does nicotine have on athletic performance?

Athletes use nicotine for a variety of reasons, including its stimulant properties and its mood-altering effects, which may provide a calming sensation in some individuals and a stimulating effect in others. Nicotine also has mild appetite-suppressive properties that are perceived as beneficial by some athletes. No evidence exists that nicotine enhances performance. Given the well-known adverse effects of tobacco use (both smoking and smokeless), the use of nicotine-containing products should be strongly discouraged.

11. Do decongestants like pseudoephedrine and phenylpropanolamine have any performance-enhancing properties?

These agents and other sympathomimetic amines act by stimulating both alpha- and beta-adrenergic receptors to produce their primary effects on the upper respiratory mucosa. They may also have mild CNS stimulatory effects in some susceptible individuals and thereby decrease the sensation of fatigue. Phenylpropanolamine also has been shown to have mild appetite-suppressing properties that are perceived as beneficial by some athletes. No scientific evidence exists concerning efficacy in enhancing competitiveness following acute ingestion.

12. Do herbs such as ginseng with stimulant properties have performance-enhancing effects?

Ginseng is derived from the roots of several species of *Panax*, a Chinese plant. Its chemical structure is similar to pseudoephedrine. No evidence exists that ginseng or other herbs with stimulating effects enhance performance.

13. Are there any prescription medications with stimulant properties that affect performance?

Beta-agonists, frequently used in the management of reactive airway disease, may have ergogenic benefits, although sound evidence regarding their performance-enhancing effects is lacking. Evidence exists that clenbuterol, a beta-agonist available in Europe and other countries outside the U.S., may have anabolic effects. Contradictory evidence exists regarding salbutamol. Theophylline also has been shown to enhance performance in endurance events in some individuals, although its side effects, especially diuresis and gastrointestinal intolerability with acute dosing, limit its use in most athletes. For obvious ethical reasons, physicians should never prescribe these medications for their possible performance-enhancing effects but only for approved indications.

14. Which stimulants are "banned substances"?

Most athletic governing bodies ban stimulants during competitive events. However, appropriate use of medication is acceptable in all but the highest levels of competition. Inhaled beta-agonists are generally not banned. Theophylline for the management of chronic asthma also is usually acceptable. Decongestants are allowed when prescribed by a physician by the NCAA but are banned by the USOC and IOC. Caffeine below threshold levels as determined by each governing body also is allowed. The NCAA and the IOC have drug hotlines that can be contacted whenever there is any question regarding "legal" use of stimulants by competitive athletes.

15. If there are no proven performance-enhancing effects associated with stimulants, why are they banned?

Many of these drugs have perceived ergogenic properties by athletes. When they are used by athletes to gain an edge on the competition and the perception of athletes is that there is a benefit, then other athletes are coerced into taking them to remain competitive. Contradiction exists in the scientific literature regarding the potential performance-enhancing effects of various stimulants. As long as a question remains regarding their effects on performance, most governing bodies will tend to err on the side of restricting their use. The spirit of fair and ethical competition is against the use of drugs for performance enhancement.

16. What clinical evidence exists for an athlete's usage of carnitine during training or competition?

Carnitine, specifically the physiologically active L-carnitine, is found mostly in skeletal and heart muscle. This vitamin-like carboxylic acid is often used by athletes to enhance aerobic endurance. The basis for this practice is in vitro studies that show carnitine's role in transport of long-chain fatty acids into mitochondria for oxidation—a major source of energy during prolonged exercise—and its stimulant activity of pyruvate dehydrogenase, which enhances glucose utilization and prevents lactic acid build-up. Recent clinical studies of athletes have shown little support for these theories and no improvement in athletic performance.

17. Why has the beta-agonist clenbuterol become a popular performance-enhancing agent?

Clenbuterol is used medically in the inhaled form to treat bronchial constriction. However, in animal models it has been shown to lead to skeletal muscle hypertrophy, to prevent protein breakdown, and to reduce subcutaneous fat. Its long half-life and exceptional potency have made it popular as a possible performance-enhancing drug even without substantial evidence in human trials. It is reportedly ingested in capsule or tablet form in dosages twice that for treating bronchial spasms. Although categorized as a stimulant-doping substance and prohibited by the

United States Olympic Committee and other regulatory agencies, it can still be obtained illegally by athletes at some "health food" stores, by illegal mail order, or by other means. More research is necessary to determine the direct effects of clenbuterol on humans and the potential performance-enhancing benefits, if any.

18. What should the athlete know about the creatine supplements available in "health food" stores?

Creatine exists in muscle as creatine phosphate. Creatine supplementation has been shown to increase stored creatine phosphate loads, resulting in greater capacity for immediate energy production and additional buffer of lactic acid. Creatine supplementation also has been shown to enhance short-term strenuous exercise performance in some recent clinical studies using dosages of 20–30 gm/day for 5–6 days. No benefits to endurance exercise have been found. Supplementation also has led to weight increase, but further investigation is necessary to find out whether this gain is lean mass or water retention. Supplementation dosages of 0.3 gm/kg of body mass for 6 days are commonly used by athletes. Creatine has no known adverse side effects and is not prohibited by any sports governing bodies. More studies are needed before any definite benefits of creatine can be shown. Other studies have shown no significant benefits.

19. Should the insulinomimetic agent, vanadyl sulfate, be recommended to athletes interested in improving strength?

Vanadyl sulfate is best known for its insulinlike effects and potential role in diabetes mellitus treatment. It is currently marketed as a strength-enhancing compound that promotes increased muscle quality and better performance. At present no clinical evidence supports these claims.

20. How can sodium bicarbonate enhance an athlete's performance? When should it be used?

Oral supplementation of sodium bicarbonate has been shown to delay the onset of fatigue during high-intensity anaerobic activity in some studies. It is hypothesized that this effect is due to the buffering of lactic acid in the blood and muscles by bicarbonate. The decreased muscle acidosis and reduced feeling of fatigue may improve performance in high-intensity anaerobic activity as well as recovery time between repeated activities in some athletes. Along with the buffering activity of bicarbonate, the involvement of sodium in intravascular volume enhancement also may be a factor in improved performance.

Sodium bicarbonate ingestion is often used in association with competitive activities lasting for 1–7 minutes. Sodium bicarbonate ingestion has not been shown to enhance performance in activities of shorter duration. The dosage that has shown performance enhancement in some athletes is 300 mg/kg of body weight 1–2 hours before competition. This dosage is medically safe but may produce gastrointestinal disturbances in some individuals.

BIBLIOGRAPHY

1. Anderson W, McKeag D: Replication of the national study of substance use and abuse habits of college student athletes. Technical report. Mission, KS, National Collegiate Athletic Association, 1989.
2. Bird SR, Wiles J, Robbins J: The effect of sodium bicarbonate on 1500-m racing time. J Sports Sci 13:339–403, 1995.
3. Clarkson PM: Nutrition for improved sports performance. Sports Med 21:393–401, 1996.
4. Fawcett JP, Farquhar SJ, Walker RJ, et al: The effect of oral vanadyl sulfate on body composition and performance in weight-training athletes. Int J Sports Nutr 6:382–390, 1996.
5. Heinonen OJ: Carnitine and physical exercise. Sports Med 22:109–132, 1996.
6. Hultman EK, Soderlund K, Timmons JA, et al: Muscle creatine loading in men. Appl J Physiol 81:232–237, 1996.
7. Jonas AP, Sickles RT, Lombardo JA: Substance abuse. Clin Sports Med April 1992.
8. Prather ID, Brown DE, North P, Wilson JR: Clenbuterol: A substitute for anabolic steroids? Med Sci Sports Exerc 27:1118–1121, 1995.
9. Reider B (ed): Sports Medicine: The School Age Athlete. Philadelphia, W.B. Saunders, 1991.

10. Spann C, Winter ME: Effect of clenbuterol on athletic performance. Ann Pharmacother 29:75–77, 1995.
11. Strauss RH (ed): Drugs and Performance in Sports. Philadelphia, W.B. Saunders, 1987.
12. Williams MH: Nutritional ergogenics in athletics. J Sports Sci 13:563–574, 1995.

31. EATING DISORDERS

Deborah L. Squire, M.D.

1. The term "eating disorder" includes what specific diagnoses?

The primary diagnoses categorized as eating disorders include anorexia nervosa (AN), bulimia nervosa (BN), and eating disorder not otherwise specified (NOS). An eating disorder NOS is one that does not meet the DSM IIIR criteria for either AN or BN.

2. What is the incidence of eating disorders in the general population?

The most vulnerable population is female high school and college students from middle to upper socioeconomic class. Between 0.2 and 1.0% of that population develop AN; about 4% of that population develop BN.

3. How common are anorexic or bulimic symptoms (not necessarily the full-blown disease) in the female high school population?

Anorexic and Bulimic Symptoms in Adolescent Girls

ATTITUDE OR BEHAVIOR	% OF POPULATION
Concerns about weight and eating	
Desire weight loss	81
Perceive self overweight	42
Fear weight gain	16
Fear look fat	27
Worry about overeating	35
Weight control behaviors	
Dieted in last year/serious dieting	63/12
Fasted in last year/serious fasting	20/5
Vomited in last year/serious vomiting	8/1
Laxative use in last year/serious laxative use	2/0.4
Diuretic use in last year/serious diuretic use	0.9/0.3
Used diet pills in last year/serious diet pill use	17/4
> 2 behaviors last year	27
> 2 serious behaviors last year	5
Binge eating	
Large binge	7
Recurrent binges	6
Solitary binge	93
Binge discomfort	81
Binge distress	11

From Whitaker AH: Pediatr Ann 21:752, 1992,[12] with permission.

4. Are athletes more likely than nonathletes to use pathogenic weight control (PWC) techniques (fasting, vomiting, laxatives/diuretics, severe caloric restriction, excessive exercise, diet pills)?

While there is inconclusive evidence that athletes use PWC behaviors or are obsessed with weight *more* than nonathletes, there is evidence that they are affected *at least* as often.

Percentage of 182 Female Athletes Using at Least One PWC Behavior

SPORT	%
Field hockey	50
Gymnastics	74
Softball	23
Tennis	24
Volleyball	21
Track & field	26
Distance track	47

From Rosen LW, et al: Phys Sportsmed 14(1):79, 1986,[7] with permission.

5. Does the use of PWC behaviors predispose the athlete to develop an eating disorder?

The answer to this question remains unknown. Use of PWC behaviors, *by itself*, may not have any long-term consequences for the athlete. If, however, the athlete also has the psychological risk factors for AN/BN, then familiarity with PWC behaviors *may* facilitate development of an eating disorder. More research needs to be done to determine whether, as athletes find themselves in more competitive situations, those athletes who have Eating Disorder Inventory (EDI) scores similar to patients with AN or BN go on to develop a full-blown eating disorder.

6. Is the incidence of eating disorders higher in athletes than in nonathletes?

There is inconclusive evidence to support the suggestion that athletes are more prone to eating disorders than nonathletes. Clearly, athletes are *at least* as likely to have an eating disorder as a nonathlete. Studies of athletes in sports that emphasize leanness (gymnastics, track and field, diving, cross country, volleyball, ballet) have found the highest incidence of eating disorders.

7. How common are eating disorders among males?

Between 5% and 10% of those diagnosed with an eating disorder are males.

8. According to the American Psychiatric Association (DSM-IV), what are the diagnostic criteria for AN?
  1. Disturbance of body image
  2. Intense fear of becoming obese
  3. Absence of more than 3 consecutive menses
  4. Weight loss of at least 15% of original body weight
  5. Refusal to maintain body weight over a minimum normal weight for age and height

9. How would you describe the athlete most likely to develop an eating disorder?

The athlete who develops an eating disorder is commonly the "perfect" offspring, student, and athlete. She is a high-achieving, perfectionistic individual with low self-esteem; although she usually excels in academics and athletics, she is rarely satisfied with her performance. In fact, the very characteristics that may predispose to the development of AN are the characteristics viewed as desirable by many coaches. The multiple time constraints placed on this driven athlete result in a regimentation in day-to-day living that limits her opportunities to develop into an independent, mature, and responsible young adult. Although she can control little else in her life, the one thing she learns to control is her weight.

10. What is the average age of presentation with the diagnosis of AN?

The average age of presentation with AN is 15 years, although the curve of age at presentation has two peaks. The first is at 13 years, when pubertal changes cause the adolescent to focus on body image. The second is at age 17–18 years, when stresses associated with separating from home become prominent. The collegiate athlete often develops symptoms between the freshman and sophomore years.

11. What are common symptoms of AN?
- Compulsive exercising
- Tearful, uptight, overly sensitive
- Intense fear of becoming fat
- Amenorrhea
- Wears baggy clothing and layers of clothing
- High intake of caffeine-containing beverages
- Anxiety at mealtime
- Isolation from family and friends
- Cuts food into small pieces
- Extreme sensitivity to cold
- Sleep disturbance
- High consumption of sugar-free gum

12. What are common signs of AN?
- Significant weight loss
- Hyperactivity
- Distorted body image
- Rough, dry skin
- Vellous hair on back and extremities
- Atrophy of breast tissue
- Bradycardia
- Hypothermia
- Low blood pressure
- Thinning of scalp hair
- Carotenemia
- Atrophy of vaginal mucosa

13. What is the earliest symptom of AN?

Amenorrhea precedes other symptoms of AN in 16% of cases and is coincident with the onset of AN or early weight loss in 55% of cases. The diagnosis of AN should be included in the differential diagnosis for any athlete presenting with amenorrhea.

14. What other historical clues should lead you to consider the possibility that an athlete has AN?

Many athletes with AN assiduously limit the fat in their diets; they are proud of the fact that they are "eating better than they ever have." Not uncommonly, their percent calories contributed by fat is less than 10%. To accomplish this, the athlete essentially eliminates dairy products and meat and high-protein foods from the diet. The patient may claim to have a lactose-intolerance or announce the philosophical decision to become a vegetarian. There is a resistance to use of lactose-containing dairy products and a reluctance to eat the variety and amount of food necessary for balanced nutrition for a vegetarian.

Ultimately, the athlete with AN will show a decrease in performance; not only does the athlete have a marked loss of muscle mass and strength, she often also is hypoglycemic. This affects her mental as well as physical abilities on the playing field. A significant tip-off to the presence of an eating disorder may be the response to injury; athletes with AN become very anxious when injury prevents them from engaging in the excessive exercise regimen that helps them control weight gain. Furthermore, amenorrhea and nutritional deficiencies predispose the athlete with AN to stress fractures; indeed, the sports medicine community has recently identified the "female athlete triad": amenorrhea, eating disorders, and osteoporosis.

15. What is the differential diagnosis of AN?

The differential diagnosis should include any illness that may present with weight loss and amenorrhea. Most are easily eliminated at the initial evaluation; others, such as hypothalamic tumors, may require more extensive evaluation.
- Pregnancy
- Hyperthyroidism
- Diabetes mellitus
- Addison's disease
- Overtraining
- Depression
- Malignancy
- Inflammatory bowel disease
- Hypothalamic tumor

16. According to the American Psychiatric Association (DSM-IV), what are the diagnostic criteria for BN?
1. Recurrent episodes of binge eating—twice a week for 3 months
2. Overly concerned about body weight and shape
3. Fear of not being able to stop eating voluntarily
4. Depressed mood and self-deprecating thoughts following binges
5. At least one of the following:
    - Inconspicuous eating during a binge
    - Termination of binge by abdominal pain, sleep, social interruption, self-induced vomiting
    - Repeated attempts at weight loss through self-induced vomiting, severely restrictive diets, cathartics or diuretics, or excessive exercise
    - Repeated weight fluctuations > 10 lbs
6. Bulimic episodes not due to anorexia nervosa or other physical disorder

17. What are common symptoms of BN?
- Frequent vomiting
- Inconspicuous binge eating
- Difficulty swallowing and retaining food
- Petty stealing of money (to pay for binges)
- Secretive behavior
- Trips to bathroom after meals
- Weakness, headaches, dizziness
- Overconcern with personal appearance

18. What are the common signs of BN?
- Lymphadenopathy
- Puffiness around face (below cheeks)
- Frequent weight fluctuations
- Abrasions on backs of knuckles (from inducing vomiting)
- Loss of tooth enamel
- Damage to throat and halitosis
- Subconjunctival hemorrhages

19. Why is it so difficult to diagnose a patient with bulimia?
Bulimics, by their very nature, are secretive and vehemently deny their problem. The physical signs described above occur late in the course of illness or may never develop. Because weight is often in the normal range, it is difficult to obtain objective evidence of the illness. Studies have shown that less than one-third of normal-weight bulimics had ever discussed their problem with a professional.

20. What are the medical complications of restricted caloric intake resulting in low weight?
- Amenorrhea
- Osteoporosis
- Bradycardia
- Hypothermia
- Decreased peripheral circulation
- Depression/suicidal ideation
- Xerosis of skin/coarse hair
- Decreased renal function
- Kidney stones
- Growth retardation
- Peripheral edema
- Congestive heart failure
- Dizziness/syncope

21. What are the medical complications of binge eating?
- Obesity
- Acute stomach dilatation
- Depression
- Peripheral edema
- Gastric rupture
- Suicidal ideation

22. In addition to the signs and symptoms described above, what are the medical complications of self-induced vomiting?
- Hypokalemia
- Dehydration
- Arrhythmias
- Hematemesis
- Metabolic alkalosis
- Muscle weakness
- Chronic nasal congestion
- Esophageal rupture

23. What medical complications are seen with the chronic use or abuse of diuretics?
- Hypokalemia
- Arrhythmias
- Dehydration
- Muscle weakness

24. What medical complications are associated with the chronic use of diet pills?
- Hypertension
- Myocardial infarction
- Anxiety
- Cardiovascular stroke
- Seizures
- Hyperactivity

25. What are the complications of chronic laxative use?
- Dehydration
- Electrolyte abnormalities
- Muscle weakness
- Constipation (laxative dependency)
- Dizziness and syncope
- Arrhythmias
- Rectal bleeding
- Peripheral edema

26. Does chronic laxative use help in weight control?
No.

27. What should be included in the laboratory evaluation of a suspected eating disorder?
There is no set work-up for eating disorders; laboratory tests should be tailored to the individual's presenting signs and symptoms. The following tests should be considered:

Laboratory Tests for Eating Disorders

TEST	PRESENTING SIGN OR FUNCTION TESTED
CBC, reticulocytes, ferritin	Anemia
Electrolytes	Na, Cl, K, CO_2
U/A, BUN, Creatine	Renal function
EKG	Arrhythmias, U waves, QT prolongation
Stool guaiac	Occult blood
Serum amylase	Occult vomiting
Beta HCG	Pregnancy
LH, FSH, prolactin	Hypothalamic/pituitary function

28. What are the essential components in the treatment of an athlete with an eating disorder?
Early identification of the problem and prompt institution of interventional therapy are associated with the best prognosis. The athlete is followed by a team, including the medical physician, nutritionist, and psychotherapist. The key member of this group is the therapist; until the athlete is able to develop healthy coping skills, she depends on the pathologic control of her weight as a way of handling the stresses she encounters. At various points in her treatment, the athlete may benefit from individual, family and/or group therapy. Management must be individualized; as the athlete responds to counseling, ongoing dietary counseling allows her to gradually improve her nutritional status. Continued participation in her sport must be dependent upon compliance with the treatment program.

29. How can eating disorders be prevented?
The prevalence of PWC behaviors and obsession with weight among high school females makes the area of nutrition and body image an extremely important focus for discussion during routine health maintenance exams. For many high school athletes, their only contact with the health care system is for a presports physical. Consideration should be given to screening for PWC behaviors/eating disorders as part of this exam. The athlete should be asked what she thinks about her current weight and what she feels her ideal weight should be. Positive nutritional

counseling regarding safe and appropriate weight loss should be provided to both the athletes and coaching staff.

BIBLIOGRAPHY

1. Borgen JS, Corbin CB: Eating disorders among female athletes. Phys Sportsmed 15(2):89, 1987.
2. Brooks-Gunn J, Burrow C, Warren MP: Attitudes toward eating and body weight in different groups of female adolescent athletes. Int J Eating Disorders 6:749, 1988.
3. Clark K, Parr R, Castelli (eds): Evaluation and Management of Eating Disorders: Anorexia, Bulimia, and Obesity. Champaign, IL, Life Enhancement Publications, 1988.
4. Dick RW: Eating disorders in NCAA athletic programs. Athletic Training 26:136, 1991.
5. Dummer GM, Rosen LW, Heusner WW, et al: Pathogenic weight-control behaviors of young competitive swimmers. Phys Sportsmed 15(5):75, 1987.
6. Rosen LW, Hough DO: Pathogenic weight-control behaviors of female college gymnasts. Phys Sports med 16(9):141, 1988.
7. Rosen LW, McKeag DB, Hough D, et al: Pathogenic weight control behavior in female athletes. Phys Sportsmed 14(1):79, 1986.
8. Selby R, Weinstein HM, Bird TS: The health of university athletes: Attitudes, behaviors, and stressors. Journal of American College Health 39:11, 1990.
9. Taub DE, Blinde EM: Eating disorders among adolescent female athletes: Influence of athletic participation and sport team membership. Adolescence 27:833, 1992.
10. Thompson RA, Sherman RT: Helping Athletes with Eating Disorders. Champaign, IL, Human Kinetics, 1993.
11. Warren BJ, Stanton AL, Blessing DL: Disordered eating patterns in competitive female athletes. Int J Eating Disorders 9:565, 1990.
12. Whitaker AH: An epidemiological study of anorectic and bulimic symptoms in adolescent girls: Implications for pediatricians. Pediatr Ann 21:752, 1992.
13. Whitaker A, Davies M, Shaffer D, et al: The struggle to be thin: A survey of anorexic and bulimic symptoms in a non-referred adolescent population. Psychol Med 19:143, 1989.

32. EXERCISE ADDICTION

James R. Barrett, M.D., C.A.Q.

1. What is exercise addiction?

In its most general definition, exercise addiction is an unhealthy reliance on exercise for daily functioning, often becoming the sole coping mechanism to deal with daily stresses. More specifically, exercise addiction, like other addictions, has three characteristics: dependence, tolerance, and withdrawal.

Dependence is the feeling that exercise is necessary in order to feel good, often to the exclusion of commitments to marriage, job, and friends.

Tolerance indicates that more and more exercise is needed to achieve the same level of "feeling good." Some sources feel tolerance is difficult to apply to exercise addiction and do not use it in their definition.

Withdrawal symptoms are a key feature of exercise addiction. Some sources believe that they are critical in determining the existence and degree of addiction. These symptoms are generally described as feeling tired or weak 24–36 hours after a regularly scheduled exercise session is missed. Symptoms such as depression, anxiousness, irritability, relationship problems, and restlessness also are common.

An inherent difficulty in defining exercise addiction and identifying addicts is that this addiction is looked on in a positive light as opposed to alcohol or other drug addictions. People with exercise addiction tend to look good and feel good about themselves. This leads to positive reinforcement of the addiction. It is not until significant injury such as a stress fracture or family/work problems develop that the negative effects of the addiction are manifested.

2. What other names are used to connote exercise addiction?

Many names have been used to describe exercise addiction. Some of the more commonly used are fitness fanaticism, obligatory running, exercise dependence, exercise commitment, exercise abuse, running anorexia, and morbid exercising.

3. What causes exercise addiction?

The cause of exercise addiction is not known. A relationship between this addiction and the release of endorphins may eventually explain the cause, but this has not been well studied at this time. Researchers have found it very difficult to do clinical studies to determine the cause of exercise addiction. For example, one researcher could not get a subset of his subjects to stop exercising no matter how much he offered to pay them.

4. How many people have exercise addiction?

Although the exact prevalence is unknown, it is a small subset of people who regularly exercise.

5. Can we predict who is at risk for becoming addicted to exercise?

Although there seem to be some similarities between anorexic patients and exercise addicts, no factors have been found that predispose a person to exercise addiction.

6. What is the most common presentation of exercise addiction?

Exercise addicts most commonly do not present to physicians. When they do, it is usually for a persistent overuse injury. Injuries such as stress fractures, strains, sprains, and bursitis are all common presenting problems. These problems tend to be resistant to treatment because exercise addicts are reluctant to follow treatment regimens that may include stopping exercise or even decreasing it.

7. What types of questions can be asked to screen for exercise addiction?

Although several research questionnaires have been developed to screen for exercise addiction, currently there is no standardized questionnaire used in screening. To determine if an exercise addiction exists, the physician might ask questions about the motivation for exercise; whether exercise interferes with family, friends, or job; how much and how often they exercise; whether they keep a log of exercising; whether they have any withdrawal symptoms when they are not able to exercise; and whether they have a history of recurrent overuse injuries.

8. Is exercise addiction more common in any particular sport?

Running is the most common sport associated with exercise addiction, but other aerobic sports such as cycling, aerobic dancing, rowing, speed skating, and swimming also can be associated with exercise addiction. Even sports such as basketball, tennis, wrestling, volleyball, and racquetball have exercise addicts.

9. Is exercise addiction associated with other addictions or psychological problems?

Exercise addicts tend not to become addicted to substances such as alcohol or other drugs. They tend to stay away from any substances that might negatively affect exercise. Some researchers have found similarities between exercise addiction and anorexia. Both groups tend to be preoccupied with food and exercise. The reasons for using exercise are different in the two groups—anorexics use exercise for weight control, whereas exercise addicts use it as a coping mechanism.

10. Is there a distinction between overtraining, staleness, burnout, and exercise addiction?

There is a considerable amount of confusion surrounding these terms. Most sources tend to make a distinction between them even though there is some overlap of the terms. The European literature uses the term overtraining generically to include staleness.

In American literature, **overtraining** is the process by which staleness occurs. Overtraining is a method used by athletes to achieve a higher level of performance. It involves "overloading the system without adequate recovery."[6] An example of this is a distance swimmer who trains at increased distances with an increased intensity every day without allowing rest days or easy days during training.

Staleness is characterized by a lack of improvement in performance or even a deterioration during training or in competition. Frequently, symptoms such as fatigue, myalgias, insomnia, weight loss, decreased libido, and mood disturbances such as depression and anxiety occur.

Burnout describes the mental fatigue that can occur during intense training. It is likened to the burnout that can occur in an occupational setting.

Exercise addiction is the unhealthy reliance on exercise for daily functioning. Overtraining, staleness, burnout, and exercise addiction can occur in combination or as separate conditions.

11. What is the best way to manage patients with exercise addiction?

Exercise addicts are difficult to treat. There are no standard protocols for treatment. In most cases, exercise is a symptom of an underlying problem; therefore, treatment is best accomplished by identifying and remedying this underlying cause such as job or family stressors. Treatment of the overuse injuries associated with exercise addiction is described in Section IX of this book. The principles of relative rest and cross-training are often helpful in treating many of these injuries. Some exercise addicts are not able to change their exercise patterns and only stop exercising when the injury causes severe enough disability to preclude exercise.

12. What are the consequences of continued exercise addiction?

Overuse injuries (many of which become intractable), marital difficulties, social/career problems, and eating disorders can all be consequences of continued exercise addiction.

BIBLIOGRAPHY

1. Anthony J: Psychologic aspects of exercise. Clin Sports Med 10:171–180, 1991.
2. Baekeland F: Exercise deprivation: Sleep and psychological reaction. Arch Gen Psychiatry 22:365–369, 1970.
3. Chalmers J, Catalan J, Day A: Anorexia nervosa presenting as morbid exercising. Lancet 1:286–287, 1985.
4. de Coverley Veale D: Exercise dependence. Br J Addict 82:735–740, 1987.
5. Ellickson K: Psychological aspects of exercise and sport. In Strauss R (ed): Sports Medicine, 2nd ed. Philadelphia, W.B. Saunders, 1991, pp 299–306.
6. Kuipers H, Keizer H: Overtraining in elite athletes: Review and directions for the future. Sports Med 6:79–92, 1988.
7. Morgan W: Negative addiction in runners. Phys Sportsmed 7:57–70, 1979.
8. Morgan W, Brown D, Raglin J, et al: Psychological monitoring of overtraining and staleness. Br J Sports Med 21:107–114, 1987.
9. Morgan W, Costill D, Flynn M, et al: Mood disturbance following increased training in swimmers. Med Sci Sports Exerc 20(4):408–414, 1988.
10. Raglin J: Exercise and mental health: Beneficial and detrimental effects. Sports Med 9:323–329, 1990.
11. Sachs M, Pargman D: Running addiction. In Running as Therapy: An Integrated Approach. Lincoln, NE, University of Nebraska Press, 1984, pp 231–252.
12. Szabo A: The impact of exercise deprivation on well-being of habitual exercisers. Aust J Sci Med Sport 27(3):68–75, 1995.
13. Veal DM: Psychological aspects of staleness and dependence on exercise. Int J Sports Med 12:S19–S22, 1991.
14. Wichmann S, Martin DR: Exercise excess: Treating patients addicted to fitness. Phys Sportsmed 20:193–200, 1992.
15. Yates A, Leehey K, Shisslak C: Running—An analogue of anorexia? N Engl J Med 308:251–255, 1983.

33. PSYCHOLOGICAL PROBLEMS OF THE ATHLETE

Todd P. Hendrickson, M.D.

GENERAL CONSIDERATIONS

1. Are athletes more at risk than nonathletes for developing mental health problems?

No. Most athletes suffer the same types of mental health problems that are seen in nonathletes, including depression, anxiety, and substance abuse. One difference in athletes may be the lower incidence of chronic mental health problems such as schizophrenia and dementia.

2. What type of clinicians work with athletes on their mental health problems?

M.D.s (psychiatrists)   Ed.D.s (doctors of education)
Ph.D.s (clinical psychologists)   M.S.W.s (social workers)

When selecting a counselor for working with athletes, it is important to check licensure and other qualifications and to inquire about the clinician's education and training.

3. Generally, what is the focus of the sports psychiatrist or psychologist in working with athletes?

- Clinical problems, with the emphasis on diagnosis and treatment
- Issues of performance enhancement, usually through psychological skills training
- Health and wellness, through the use of education models
- Social issues, including interpersonal relationships and teamwork (group therapy)

4. What types of treatment modalities are commonly used by the sports therapist?

Psychotherapy (both individual and group)
Pharmacotherapy (use of medications)

5. How does the sports psychiatrist or psychologist interact with other members of the sports medicine team?

The ideal situation is for the therapist to work within the sports medicine group, consulting with the sports medicine physicians, physical therapists, athletic trainers, and coaches.

6. How are referrals generated?

Most referrals come from the sports medicine team, coaches, parents, and other people concerned with the athlete's progress or problem areas.

7. How is the issue of confidentiality treated?

Confidentiality is mandatory when dealing with problem issues that the athlete discusses. The athlete must give permission for the sports therapist to communicate information about diagnosis or treatment. The only exception to this rule is issues that may endanger either the athlete or someone else. The protected relationship between clinician and patient includes issues of chemical dependency as well as the potential diagnosis of a mental health problem.

EVALUATION AND ASSESSMENT

8. How is the mental status examination used in working with athletes?

The mental health status examination is a diagnostic tool that generates both signs and symptoms, which are then clustered together to arrive at a specific psychiatric diagnosis.

9. What are the components of the mental status examination?

The mental status examination, which is a measure of psychological fitness, contains the following features:

1. Commentary on the general attitude and behavior of the patient
2. A description of the patient's affect (emotional responsiveness) and mood (subjective feelings of the patient)
3. Thought content (what the patient thinks about)
4. Though processing (includes cognitive or intellectual functioning)
5. Insight and judgment into self and problems

10. How often is psychological testing required in working with the athlete?

Psychological testing may be helpful in organizing the overall picture of the athlete's health. It can be extremely beneficial when diagnostic issues are confusing or when treatment plans meet with resistance.

11. Is there one psychological test that seems to work best with athletes?

No. Several psychological tests assess different portions of the patient's mental status:

1. Personality can be assessed by the Minnesota Multiphasic Personality Inventory (MMPI).
2. Mood can be assessed by the Hamilton Depression Rating Scale.
3. Anxiety can be assessed by the Sport Competition Anxiety Test (SCAT).
4. Thought disorders (i.e., psychosis) can be assessed by the Symptom Checklist-90 (SCL/90).

PSYCHIATRIC DISORDERS AND SYNDROMES

12. How is depression diagnosed in the athlete?

Use of the mnemonic IN SAD CAGES can be helpful.

In	loss of **int**erest in pleasurable activities
S	**s**uicidal ideation
A	**a**ctivity (usually decreased)
D	**d**ysthymia (depressed feeling)
C	**c**oncentration (usually decreased)
A	**a**ppetite (usually involves weight loss)
G	**g**uilt feelings
E	**e**nergy (usually decreased)
S	**s**leep (usually decreased)

The presence of six or more of these criteria at any one time is highly indicative of major depression.

13. Do all depressive illnesses require treatment with medications?

No. Major depression as described above is best treated with a combination of both medication (antidepressants) and psychotherapy. Adjustment disorders occur when athletes have a depressed mood in reaction to specific psychosocial stressor(s). Such reactive depressions are probably best treated by dealing with the stressor at hand and may not require the use of medications except for patients who have significant difficulty with anxiety or sleep disturbance. Organic depression (depression caused by either medications or medical illness) is best managed by treating the underlying medical condition (e.g., steroid withdrawal, hypothyroidism).

14. What is the most common anxiety disorder seen in athletes?

Social phobia is common among athletes. In most situations, it is seen by the clinician primarily as performance anxiety. The athlete may feel embarrassed, humiliated, or excessively scrutinized. The key to the diagnosis is that the anxiety increases as the performance approaches.

15. Can injuries precipitate psychiatric illness?
Yes. Two psychiatric conditions commonly seen after injury are adjustment disorder with depressed mood (depression as an emotional reaction to the stress of injury) and posttraumatic stress disorder (symptoms of extreme anxiety and depression, and reexperience of the original stressor through either flashbacks or nightmares). It should be noted, however, that most athletes do not suffer psychiatric illness after physical injury.

16. What is the treatment choice for obsessive-compulsive disorder in athletes?
Obsessive-compulsive disorder, which is characterized by intrusive, obsessive thoughts and compulsive rituals, is best treated with clomipramine (Anafranil), usually at a dose of 100–250 mg/day.

17. What are pathogenic weight control behaviors?
Commonly seen in patients with eating disorders, these behaviors include the following:
Body dissatisfaction (i.e., body image distortion)
Frequent use of the bathroom after meals (i.e., purging behavior)
Preoccupation with food and food preparation
Ongoing loss of weight despite the emergence of physical problems
Secretive behavior with regard to meals and eating
Compulsive drive to be thin
Hoarding of food
Excessive exercise to burn off calories

18. What are the most common substances of abuse among athletes?
Number one is still alcohol. Other substances abused by athletes are psychostimulants (e.g., cocaine and amphetamines), anabolic steroids, and central nervous system depressants (e.g., benzodiazepines and opiate-narcotic analgesics).

19. What are some of the psychiatric symptoms seen in abuse of anabolic steroids?
Mania (elevated mood with heightened sense of self-importance and exaggerated grandiosity)
Depression (often seen when athletes are withdrawing or weaning from anabolic steroids)
Anxiety (organic; typically expressed as irritability and agitation; often seen when stacking multiple steroids at the same time)
Psychosis (paranoid feelings, self-persecution)

20. What is a personality disorder?
Personality disorders become evident when the patient's personality traits become inflexible and maladaptive, causing either impairment in social or occupational functioning or subjective distress. Often this maladaptive behavior occurs in the sports context (defiance, narcissism, self-injurious behavior, exaggeration of behavior, passive-aggressive behavior).

21. How does the clinician recognize passive-aggressive behavior in the athlete?
The passive-aggressive athlete typically procrastinates, resists demands, finds excuses for delays, and usually finds fault with others. Lack of assertiveness and indirectness are common features. As with most personality disorders in athletes, these personality traits typically bring out strong feelings of discomfort in the clinician working with the athlete.

22. Can psychiatric disorders be seen in young athletes (i.e., children and adolescents)?
Yes. One of the most common illnesses in young athletes is depression, usually manifested by behavioral changes and/or somatic complaints with limited physical pathology. Other illnesses not infrequently seen in children include:
Attention deficit hyperactivity disorder (ADHD)
Oppositional defiant disorder
Conduct disorder (antisocial behavior)

TREATMENT

23. How does the clinician decide which antidepressant to use for treatment of the depressed athlete?

The following flow sheet may be helpful:
1. Patient's previous response to the medication
2. Family history of response to the medication
3. Target symptoms (e.g., use of a more sedative antidepressant for people with insomnia)
4. Side-effect profile (e.g., especially important in athletes, who typically desire few side effects)
5. Clinician's personal preference and previous experience

24. Is there an ideal medication for treatment of depression?

Not necessarily. However, antidepressants with limited side effects (fluoxetine/Prozac, paroxetine/Paxil, nortriptyline/Pamelor, sertraline/Zoloft) may be especially useful in athletes who do not desire excessive fatigue or strong anticholinergic side effects.

25. What are the best understood neurotransmitters involved in depressive illness?

Norepinephrine, epinephrine, and serotonin are the neurotransmitters that seem to be involved in depressive illness.

26. What is the most untoward side effect of Prozac (fluoxetine) in the treatment of depression?

Akathisia is an extrapyramidal type of symptom that can be extremely bothersome to the athlete. It is evidenced by extreme restlessness and inability to sit still and requires immediate attention. Akathisia can be alleviated by an anticholinergic medication such as diphenhydramine hydrochloride (25–50 mg intramuscularly or orally) or benztropine mesylate (0.5–1.0 mg intramuscularly or orally) and may necessitate discontinuation of the antidepressant medication.

27. How long does it take most antidepressants to work?

For reasons not yet elucidated, antidepressant response typically occurs within 2–6 weeks after initiation of therapy. This long-term approach requires an adequate trial to determine therapeutic level.

28. What are the most common findings in antidepressant toxicity?

Anticholinergic toxicity (tachycardia, hypertension, and delirium)
Arrhythmias (AV conduction abnormalities)
Seizures
Orthostatic hypotension

29. What is the treatment of choice for panic attacks?

If the panic attacks are persistent and pervasive and indicate the possibility of panic disorder (i.e., syndrome), then alprazolam (Xanax) is usually effective at a dosage of 1–3 mg/day. The dosage can also be divided—i.e., 0.5–1.0 mg every 4–6 hours.

30. Are there any contraindications for use of benzodiazepines (anxiolytics) in athletes?

1. Care must be taken in prescribing benzodiazepines for patients with chemical dependency problems, especially central nervous system depressants such as alcohol and sleeping pills.
2. Benzodiazepines are additive in effect with the concurrent use of alcohol.
3. Long-term use may foster both dependence on and tolerance of the same medication.

Benzodiazepines are typically underutilized by mental health professionals because of the fear of dependence. They should be used in combination with nonmedication treatments (e.g., relaxation training, stress management) in the management of most anxiety symptoms and disorders.

31. What is psychotherapy?

Psychotherapy is the process through which the patient forms a therapeutic alliance with the therapist with the goal of resolving symptoms and problems. Many different types of psychotherapy can be extremely useful in helping the athlete. Most psychotherapy done by nonpsychiatric professionals is supportive.

32. Is psychotherapy as effective as medication in the treatment of depression?

Both are effective. However, research suggests that the combined use of medication and psychotherapy may provide the quickest results—especially in major depression and dysthymia (chronic depression for more than 2 years).

BIBLIOGRAPHY

1. Ashe AR: A Hard Road to Glory. New York, Warner Books, 1988.
2. Cassem NH, Hackett TP: Handbook of General Hospital Psychiatry, 2nd ed. PSG Publishing, 1987.
3. Kaplan HI, Sadock BJ: Synopsis of Psychiatry, 6th ed. Baltimore, Williams & Wilkins, 1991.
4. Marks IM: Fears, Phobias and Rituals. Oxford, Oxford University Press, 1987.
5. Silva JM, Weinberg RS: Psychological Foundations of Sport. Champaign, IL, Human Kinetic Publishers, 1984.

34. PSYCHOLOGICAL TECHNIQUES TO ENHANCE PERFORMANCE

Todd P. Hendrickson, M.D.

1. What is performance enhancement?

For the sports psychiatrist or psychologist, performance enhancement includes strategies, both cognitive and behavioral, that assist the athlete in improving performance. These strategies include behavioral methods (such as relaxation training) and cognitive strategies (such as goal-setting and positive self-talk) that help to develop certain skills that can be applied to the sport environment.

2. What is the "flow" experience?

Athletes typically describe flow experience as an activity or performance that was done without tremendous effort or thought and induced a subjective feeling of "being in the groove" (often a sense of euphoria). These experiences are not typically described as commonplace.

3. List some of the psychological characteristics of peak performance.

Peak performance can be categorized in three different areas of skill development:
1. Physical skills development
   Adequate technical and physical preparation: repetition of skills
2. Emotional skills development
   Regulation of anxiety and arousal
   Subjective feelings of self-confidence
   Feeling passionately about the performance
3. Cognitive skills development
   Clearly defined goals
   Use of visual imagery on a regular basis
   Concentration on the here and now (i.e., focus on the task at hand)
   Ability to control distractions and sense of commitment and determination (i.e., assertiveness)
   Positive expectation of successful outcome

4. Can the clinician use the same strategies for performance enhancement in all athletes?

Despite the many different types of intervention strategies, care must be taken to individualize each program to maximize effectiveness and to give the athlete as active a part as possible. Different athletes may require different strategies; for example, some athletes may not need to work as much as others on relaxation or goal-setting strategies.

5. List some of the techniques that are used to decrease performance anxiety.

It is crucial that the athlete learn through practice the skill of relaxation. Some of the following techniques can be helpful:

Deep diaphragmatic breathing	Autogenic training	Meditation
Progressive muscle relaxation	(self-suggestions	Massage therapy
Mental (visual) imagery	or self-statements)	Exercise itself
Biofeedback	Yoga	

All of the above techniques can be used either individually or in combination to provide the skills necessary to achieve relaxation.

6. What is visual (mental) imagery?

Mental imagery is a practice in which the athlete creates certain mental images of the self, a particular idea, or a desired or experienced emotional response. It can be used to produce mechanical and technical images of performance (past, present or future) or kinesthetic images of control, comfort, and relaxation.

7. For what purposes do athletes use mental imagery?

Often athletes use mental imagery to correct mistakes in past performances, to visualize future performances, and to create a relaxed environment in which they can solve problems more clearly. The use of imagery to produce relaxation is extremely helpful in multiple clinical situations, including technical instruction, injury rehabilitation, and problem-solving.

8. Does mental imagery work?

At this time it is difficult to determine whether the images created in the mind directly correlate with athletic performance because most of the data come from self-reports. However, a growing number of athletes at all levels personally attest to its effectiveness in their own training programs. It is clear that imagery used as a relaxation tool can increase the ability to concentrate and decrease the effect of distracting thoughts.

9. How can an athlete "bust out" of performance decrements (slumps)?

A typical slump-busting program includes the following:

1. Identification of the problem through self-evaluation and feedback from others
2. Repetition of past experiences of breaking through performance plateaus (i.e., if it has been dealt with before, it can be dealt with again in the same fashion)
3. Open communication with other athletes and coaches about their experiences dealing with the same problems
4. Ability to evaluate one's own performance (i.e., the detection of technical, emotional, or cognitive flaws that may disrupt performance)
5. Sense of commitment to making a change
6. Development of a strategy or plan to change the nature of the performance
7. Self-monitoring of the plan itself (the ability to give oneself feedback or to get it from others)

It is important to discuss performance plateaus as a normal part of athletic development. The key issue seems to be the time it takes to return to a more desirable level of performance.

10. What is the best way to set goals?

First, one must identify areas of strength and weakness in the sports performance. Areas of weakness are fertile ground for the development of specific strategies for improvement. Once this self-evaluation is done, it is much easier to establish both short- and long-term goals to achieve the desired outcome. It is important to get feedback from others, and a buddy system is also extremely helpful.

11. What are the key components to a typical training program for psychological skills?
  1. Psychological skills assessment
     Development of self-awareness (self-monitoring of performance)
     Development of techniques to control anxiety
     Establishment of self-esteem (understanding the self and the ability to change)
     Stress management
     Communication and interpersonal skills
     Motivational strategies (i.e., concepts of goal-setting)
     Development of leadership style
     Concentrational focus
  2. Methods of development
     Practice
     Educational model (i.e., the athlete learns about concepts and techniques)
     Specific intervention strategies (e.g., imagery, relaxation)

Note: Care must be taken to apply the methods and techniques to the sport setting. This is best done with the supervision of a sports specialist who is trained in these areas.

Adapted from Vealey RS: Future directions in psychological skills training. Sport Psychol 2:318–330, 1988.

12. What is desensitization training?
   Desensitization training is the gradual ability to tolerate or to become insensitive to negative disturbances and situations that may create significant anxiety or discomfort. In the context of sports, it is useful when athletes are apprehensive about some aspect of their performance.

13. How can desensitization be achieved in the sports context?
   The key issue is exposure therapy. Theoretically, gradual exposure to the situation that produces anxiety or discomfort helps to condition the athlete in tolerance. Therapy should begin with exposure to situations that are easier to tolerate rather than to the most difficult situation that the athlete has to face.

14. What are some of the uses of exposure to desensitization therapy?
   This type of training can be especially helpful for situational anxiety (e.g., free-throws in basketball) and certain phobias (e.g., fear of being judged harshly, fear of failure in a given situation). It parallels the role of repetitive practice in the development of athletic skills (i.e., increased exposure correlates with decreased anxiety as skills are developed).

15. List the key elements for a successful sports team.
   Open communications between athletes and coaching staff
   Development of team pride and tradition
   Community involvement in the sport experience (i.e., public relations)
   Common goals and expectations
   Support for the value of unique personal contribution (i.e., avoidance of excessive cohesiveness)
   Periodic team meetings and individual meetings with athletes and coaching staff (attempt to avoid communication only in crisis situations)
   Use of leaders within the team (i.e., team captains with a sense of responsibility can be a liaison between the coach and players)
   Focus and commitment to skill development
   Development of team depth (i.e., skill development for all players)
   Competition within the practice environment

16. What are the characteristics of effective communication?

Honesty, clarity, consistency, and sincerity. Sarcasm and ridicule should be avoided.

17. What are some of the key features seen in athletes with leadership ability?

Ability to communicate openly with teammates as well as coaches and other athletic staff

Ability to make decisions in a firm but democratic manner

Respect from others

Role-modeling (the leader sets the example for others)

Sense of humor

Proficiency in the sport (credibility)

Ability to solve problems in a rational way

18. How can an athlete build self-confidence?

Typically the athlete's confidence is based on his or her thoughts, beliefs, and experiences. Therefore, development of confidence includes the following:

Fitness, conditioning and repetition (i.e., development of physical skills)

Exposure to competitive stress

Ability to take time out (i.e., the ability to make adjustments and to change)

Effort (enthusiasm and intensity of activity)

Concentration on task (i.e., the activity at hand) rather than outcome (winning vs. losing)

Note that confidence can also be facilitated by the development of skills in nonathletic areas such as academics, interpersonal relationships, and spirituality.

19. How can the athlete improve his or her concentration abilities?

Ideally, concentration should keep all thoughts directed toward the athlete's next opportunity. This requires the following:

Concentration on the here and now (i.e., the task at hand)

Relaxation (increases the effectiveness of concentration)

Thinking forward, not backward

Trying to avoid thinking about what's wrong (i.e., focus on successful performance)

Thinking about tasks rather than outcomes

20. When working with the athlete, how can one create a motivational environment?

Development of mutual trust

Variety in training (avoiding boredom through challenge and stimulation)

Organization (i.e., practices)

Openness and clarity of communication

Positive talking and reinforcement

Instructional feedback when correcting mistakes

Incorporating the athlete into the sports plan and program

Allowing for social development (e.g., fun, travel, and humor)

BIBLIOGRAPHY

1. Ashe AR: A Hard Road to Glory. New York, Warner Books, 1988.
2. Cassem NH, Hackett TP: Handbook of General Hospital Psychiatry, 2nd ed. PSG Publishing, 1987.
3. Kaplan HI, Sadock BJ: Synopsis of Psychiatry, 6th ed. Baltimore, Williams & Wilkins, 1991.
4. Marks IM: Fears, Phobias and Rituals. Oxford, Oxford University Press, 1987.
5. McGuane T: The Best American Sports Writing. New York, Houghton Mifflin Company, 1992.
6. Mellion MB, Walsh WM, Shelton GL (eds): The Team Physician's Handbook, 2nd ed. Philadelphia, Hanley & Belfus, 1997.
7. Nideffer RM: Athlete's Guide to Mental Training. Champaign, IL, Human Kinetic Publishers, 1984.
8. Silva JM, Weinberg RS: Psychological Foundations of Sport. Champaign, IL, Human Kinetic Publishers, 1984.
9. Wiese DM, Weiss MR: Psychological rehabilitation and physical injury: Implications for the sportsmedicine team. Sport Psychol 1:318–330, 1987.

10. Williams JM: Applied Sport Psychology—Personal Growth to Peak Performance, 2nd ed. Mayfield Publishing, 1993.
11. Vealey RS: Future directions in psychological skills training. Sport Psychol 2:318–330, 1988.

35. OVERTRAINING

Thomas R. Sachtleben, M.D.

1. How does overtraining relate to general training principles?

Training principles are incorporated into athletic training programs to maximize physical performance. Both endurance and strength training use incremental increases in training loads to stimulate physiologic stress and subsequent adaptation. A well-designed training program includes overload training within exercise tolerance levels, along with adequate recovery periods that optimize training improvements. This approach—called periodization of training—aids in the timing of an athlete's peak performance. Overtraining occurs when excessive exercise stress transcends the body's ability to adapt and leads to reductions in athletic performance. Homeostasis is not restored, and thus biochemical, physiologic, and immunological systems become altered.

2. How are the different types of overtraining categorized?

Overload training is the process of stressing athletes at higher levels than those to which they are accustomed. thus providing stimulus for physiologic adaptation.

Training fatigue is the normal response that athletes experience after several days of heavy training

Overreaching describes reduced maximal performance capacity as a result of short-term high-intensity training. This form of overtraining carries a favorable prognosis, and recovery usually takes from several days to 2 weeks. It is often a component of a specific training regimen intended to stimulate physiologic adaptation.

The **parasympathetic form** of overtraining includes decreased sympathetic activity at rest. Primary symptoms include inhibition with an impassive temperament, long periods of sleep, and depression. Decreased performance due to parasympathetic overtraining results primarily from excessive aerobic activity.

The **sympathetic form** of overtraining includes increased sympathetic activity at rest. Common symptoms include an increased resting heart rate, decreased appetite, restlessness, and excitability. Impaired performance results primarily from anaerobic exercise.

3. What is overtraining syndrome?

The overtraining syndrome consists of various symptoms in an athlete who has engaged in a training program that has exceeded the body's physiologic and/or psychological limitations. The athlete's physical performance declines, and the ability to maintain a desired intensity level of training lessens. This multisystem disorder results from an imbalance between exercise and adequate recovery. The overtraining syndrome, also referred to as staleness, is a state of chronically depressed performance accompanied by various physiologic and psychological symptoms.

4. What is the difference between overtraining and exercise-related fatigue?

Exercise-related fatigue is the anticipated response to an overload training stimulus. The functional capacity of the athlete is only temporarily impaired, and the recovery process ensures the renewal of energy sources and may even supercompensate to above baseline levels. As opposed to exercise-related fatigue, which may last from several days up to 2 weeks and carries a favorable prognosis, overtraining may take several weeks to months for complete recovery. Further impairment of physical performance and alterations of mood state characterize the overtraining syndrome.

5. What is the clinical picture of overtraining syndrome?

Athletes often present with a cluster of symptoms, the most common of which are fatigue, depression, and heavy muscles. Additional symptoms include decreased appetite, weight loss, excessive sweating, and an increased resting heart rate. Further questioning may reveal poor sleep, decreased libido, decreased competitive drive, and emotional lability. Alternatively, the athlete's only symptom may be impaired performance.

Common Symptoms Associated with Overtraining

Increased resting heart rate	Decreased performance
Weight loss	Irritability
Poor healing	Restlessness
Insomnia	Diffuse myalgias and arthralgias
Loss of appetite	Reduced concentration
Frequent upper respiratory infection	Depression
Sore throat, lymphadenopathy	Emotional lability
Heavy feeling in legs	Increased evening fluid intake

6. What is delayed-onset muscle soreness (DOMS)?

DOMS is an overuse syndrome manifested by aching, sore muscles following unaccustomed exercise or rigorous activity. Athletes often complain of weak, stiff muscles that are extremely tender and swollen. Eccentric exercise, the usual antecedent for DOMS, is associated with muscle and other soft tissue disruption. A subsequent inflammatory response ensues, and creatine kinase levels rise dramatically, peaking 48–72 hours after the initial exercise. Symptoms usually abate over the next several days, although sometimes they may last up to 5–7 days. Severe DOMS affects performance by reducing strength, impairing glycogen repletion, and decreasing the economy of movement.

7. What psychologic components contribute to overtraining syndrome?

Disturbance of an athlete's mood is one of the key components of the overtraining syndrome, and may be associated with increases in training volume and/or intensity. Symptoms related to decreased performance include fatigue, difficulty in concentrating, depression, and irritability. An athlete's rating of perceived exertion (RPE) is increased at a given workload. The Profile of Mood States (POMS) is frequently used to measure alterations in psychopathologic parameters. This scale can be used to monitor an athlete's mood during times of increased stress as a means of detecting overtraining.

Endurance athletes also need to be monitored for detrimental training regimens that lead to physical and psychological breakdown. Multisport athletes and marathoners often exhibit obsessive-compulsive behavior in their attempt to log immense yardage or mileage in their training schemes. These obsessive-compulsive tendencies are difficult to detect but may be exposed by a thorough history.

8. What are the immunologic aspects of overtraining?

Athletes appear to be more susceptible to infections during periods of high intensity training. Specifically, a high frequency of upper respiratory tract infections (URTI) in elite endurance athletes has been linked to the overtraining syndrome. A higher incidence of URTI has been associated with increased training volumes in distance runners.[7] Secretory immunoglobulin A (IgA) concentrations were lowered after intense daily exercise in both runners and swimmers.[13] Levels of plasma glutamine, an essential nutrient for cells of the immune system, and natural killer cell activity are also depressed in overtrained athletes.

9. How does overtraining affect the cardiovascular system?

The hallmark alteration is an increased basal heart rate as opposed to the expected brady-cardia found in highly trained athletes. Increases of 5–10 beats per minute are suggestive, and increases greater than 10 beats per minute are often considered diagnostic. Maximal heart rate and maximal oxygen uptake are also reduced, correlating with decreased peak performance. One of the pathophysiologic mechanisms implicated in the overtraining syndrome is a relative drop in plasma volume secondary to dehydration and chronic fluid deficiency. In addition, impaired left ventricular contractility and decreased stroke volume have been observed in ultra-endurance athletes.

10. What endocrinologic changes occur with overtraining?

Decreased levels of free testosterone and increased cortisol levels have been observed in overtrained athletes. Both hormones play a significant role in protein and carbohydrate metabo-lism; thus, the testosterone/cortisol ratio is often used to reflect the anabolic/catabolic balance in athletes. Although endocrine parameters used to monitor training remain experimental, it has been recommended that a 30% decline in the testosterone/cortisol ratio in athletes suggests over-training. This ratio may aid in the early diagnosis of overtrained athletes.

Hypothalamic dysfunction also appears to be a component of the overtraining syndrome. Studies of overtrained endurance athletes have demonstrated reduced cortisol, adrenocorti-cotropic hormone, growth hormone, and prolactin release after insulin-induced hypoglycemia. Gonadotropin-releasing hormone (GnRH) and luteinizing hormone secretion are also impaired in some overtrained athletes.

Catecholamine levels are also influenced by overtraining and may be involved in its patho-genesis. Disturbed autonomic regulation and impaired utilization of anaerobic lactate reserves may lead to decreased maximal serum lactate levels and decreased maximal performance. Although nocturnal release appears to be suppressed in overtrained athletes, exercise-related re-lease of catecholamines is increased.

11. How does overtraining syndrome occur?

Overtraining syndrome results from an imbalance between training and recovery. Limited rest and training overload beyond an athlete's ability to recover and adapt lead to an overtrained state. A combination of endogenous and exogenous factors induce overtraining. Each athlete has an individual and variable recovery potential and exercise capacity, as well as a multitude of non-training stress factors. In addition, many incidents of overtraining are secondary to training errors and/or rapid increases in training intensity.

12. Which athletes are at greatest risk of overtraining?

Endurance athletes are at higher risk of overtraining because of their prolonged periods of exercise training. Young athletes are also at risk, because often they are pushed too hard or too fast by overzealous coaches and parents. For example, young track athletes are often entered in 3 or 4 events during a single track meet.

Adult runners often compete in too many road races per season and do not allow enough rest between competitions. Competitive swimmers also use high training volumes and commonly train several times per day. Multisport athletes (e.g., triathletes, pentathletes, decathletes) fre-quently struggle to balance appropriate rest while simultaneously training for multiple sports. Female athletes, particularly those in sports with extra emphasis placed on performance and physical appearance, may overtrain in pursuit of thinness.

13. What is in the differential diagnosis of overtraining syndrome?

Viral infection	Subclinical myocarditis
Anemia	Iron deficiency
Hypothyroidism	Chronic fatigue syndrome
Infectious mononucleosis	Psychological illness

14. What means are available to aid in the detection of overtraining?

Decreased performance is often the first sign of an overtrained athlete. Although there are no widely accepted diagnostic criteria for the overtraining syndrome, performance decrements associated with other recognized indicators of overtraining may be sufficient to make the diagnosis. Additional markers for overtraining include an increased resting heart rate, weight loss, frequent illness, sleep disturbances, and increased thirst and evening fluid intake.

Recently, glutamine has emerged as a possible indicator of exercise stress and has shown promise as a means of detecting overtraining. Glutamine homeostasis is altered during various types of catabolic states. Plasma glutamine responds to both endurance and short-term, high-intensity exercise, and overload training has been shown to result in depressed levels that require prolonged recovery.[17]

Impaired immune function has been linked to depressed levels of glutamine secondary to overtraining. Glutamine functions as a fuel source in both lymphocytes and macrophages. Depressed levels of glutamine in overtrained athletes may be responsible for compromised ability to respond to immunologic challenge and increase the overtrained athlete's susceptibility to infection. Further research is needed to clarify glutamine's role in exercise stress and overtrained athletes.

15. How can overtraining syndrome be prevented?

Prevention is paramount because of the risk of injury, illness, premature retirement, and sustained decrements in performance. Unfortunately, no universally accepted laboratory test can be used to monitor overtraining. Periodization of training separates the various phases of training, such as endurance work, speed work, skill training, and tapering into limited periods for maximal performance. The principle of periodization allows athletes adequate rest between training sessions and can prevent breakdown during periods of hard training. Coaches need to be aware of unique differences in each athlete's tolerance to stress and appropriately balance and individualize training sessions. Proper attention to specific training practices can prevent training errors, which are the most common cause of running injuries. High-intensity training without rest days and sudden increases in mileage or intensity must be avoided. Daily mood monitoring with a Profile of Mood State (POMS) questionnaire has been used with success to reduce overtraining. Training should be appropriately decreased when deteriorating moods are detected and increased when mood is improved.

16. What treatments can be offered to athletes who have overtrained?

There is no specific treatment protocol for overtraining syndrome. Thus, the focus must be on early recognition and appropriate prevention. A reduction in training volume and/or intensity may be adequate for recovery. Athletes need reassurance and proper counseling about the importance of rest and relaxation techniques. Massage and hydrotherapy are often used as regeneration strategies. An open communication line with coaching personnel is crucial, and field tests for physical conditioning help coaches to guide gradual increments in training. Attention to proper nutrition and fluid supplementation is recommended. Cross-training and reduction in competitions also aid in the recovery process.

17. Can the stressors of rigorous training be monitored?

The Profile of Mood States (POMS) can be used to monitor an athlete's mood during a specific training period. Studies using POMS have successfully identified athletes suffering from the stress of overtraining. Elevated catecholamine levels at rest and reduced blood lactate levels after maximal exercise also have been used as objective markers of overtraining. Measurement of other physiologic parameters also have been investigated, but results have been inconsistent and their value for monitoring overtrained athletes remains unproven: Morning heart rate, heart rate recovery, and exercise performance during standardized submaximal exercise can be useful monitoring tools. In addition, self-monitoring with daily training logs and self-reported ratings of well-being are valuable means for monitoring overtraining.

BIBLIOGRAPHY

1. Barron JL, Noakes TD, Levy W, et al: Hypothalamic dysfunction in overtrained athletes. J Clin Endocrinol Metab 60:803–806, 1985.
2. Budgett R: The overtraining syndrome. BMJ 309:465–468, 1994.
3. Dressendorfer RH, Wade C, Scaff JH: Increased morning heart rate in runners: A valid sign of overtraining? Physician Sportsmed 13:77–86, 1985.
4. Fields KB: Running. In Sallis RE, Massimino F (eds): ACSM's Essentials of Sports Medicine. St. Louis, Mosby, 1997, pp 579–591.
5. Fry RW, Grove JR, Morton AR, et al: Psychological and immunological correlates of acute overtraining. Br J Sports Med 28:241–246, 1994.
6. Fry RW, Morton AR, Keast D: Periodisation and the prevention of overtraining. Can J Sports Sci 17:241–248, 1992.
7. Heath GW, Ford ES, Craven TE, et al: Exercise and the incidence of upper respiratory tract infections. Med Sci Sports Exerc 23:152–157, 1991.
8. Hooper SL, Mackinnon LT: Monitoring overtraining in athletes. Sports Med 20:321–327, 1995.
9. Hooper SL, Mackinnon LT, Howard A, et al: Markers for monitoring overtraining and recovery. Med Sci Sports Exerc 27:106–112, 1995.
10. Ketner JB: Overtraining. In Mellion MB, Walsh WM, Shelton GL (eds): The Team Physician's Handbook, 2nd ed. Philadelphia, Hanley & Belfus, 1997, pp 243–247.
11. Ketner JB, Mellion MB: The overtraining syndrome: A review of presentation, pathophysiology, and treatment. Med Exerc Nutr Health 4:138–147, 1995.
12. Lehmann M, Foster C, Keul J: Overtraining in endurance athletes: A brief review. Med Sci Sports Exerc 25:854–862, 1993.
13. Mackinnon LT, Hooper S: Mucosal (secretory) immune system response to exercise of varying intensity and during overtraining. Int J Sports Med 15:S179–S183, 1994.
14. McKenzie DC: Overtraining. In Torg JS, Shephard RJ (eds): Current Therapy in Sports Medicine. St. Louis, Mosby, 1995, pp 526–530.
15. Parry-Billings M, Budgett R, Koutedakis Y, et al: Plasma amino acid concentrations in the overtraining syndrome: Possible effects on the immune system. Med Sci Sports Exerc 24:1353–1358, 1992.
16. Rowbottom DG, Keast D, Goodman C, Morton AR: The haematological, biochemical and immunological profile of athletes suffering from the overtraining syndrome. Eur J Appl Physiol 70:502–509, 1995.
17. Rowbottom DG, Keast D, Morton AR: The emerging role of glutamine as an indicator of exercise stress and overtraining. Sports Med 21:80–97, 1996.
18. Smith LL: Causes of delayed onset muscle soreness and the impact on athletic performance: A review. J Appl Sport Sci Res 6:135–141, 1992.

36. ABUSE AND ADDICTION: ALCOHOL AND STREET DRUGS

Gary A. Green, M.D., FACP, and Aurelia Nattiv, M.D.

1. What is the most common drug abused by intercollegiate athletes?

Alcohol is the most frequently abused drug by athletes. Despite increased awareness of alcohol and drug use among athletes and the increased number of drug education and drug-testing programs for college athletes, alcohol use continues to be a significant problem for athletes as well as nonathletes. In the 1991 study by Anderson et al., 89% of college athletes reported using alcohol within the preceding 12 months.

2. Are athletes at higher risk for using alcohol and other drugs than the general population?

Most studies comparing the frequency of alcohol and drug use among athletes and nonathletes report similar or slightly less use among athletes. However, a multicenter study of lifestyles and health risks of collegiate athletes found that collegiate athletes were at higher risk than nonathletes for both quantity and frequency of alcohol consumption. A higher prevalence of abuse is reported among athletes for two drugs: smokeless tobacco among baseball and football players, and anabolic steroids among high school and collegiate athletes, especially those involved in football, wrestling, and track and field.

3. Can alcohol use affect athletic performance?

Yes. Alcohol is a depressant, not a stimulant, and can diminish athletic skills, negatively affecting ability and performance. Strength, power, speed, and muscular and cardiovascular endurance may decrease with acute ingestion. With increased ingestion of alcohol, psychomotor skills are impaired, including reaction time, speech, balance, and coordination. Metabolic and physiologic functions, such as energy metabolism, maximum oxygen consumption (VO_2max), heart rate, stroke volume, cardiac output, muscle blood flow, respiratory dynamics, and arteriovenous oxygen difference, are not substantially influenced.

4. How can the recreational drinker be distinguished from someone who has a problem with alcohol?

Differentiation is difficult. Although alcohol use is ubiquitous, the percentage of patients that suffer debilitating effects is relatively small. In addition, many of the physical and social effects of alcoholism require 10–20 years of alcohol abuse. The clinician caring for adolescent and young adult athletes sees only the beginning of the problem.

Because of patient denial, the traditional physician screening questions such as "How much do you drink?" and "How often?" are relatively meaningless. To assist physicians, two short questionnaires have been developed. The first is the Michigan Alcoholism Screening Test (MAST), a 25-question screening tool that later was shortened to the 13-question Short Michigan Alcoholism Screening Test (SMAST).

An even briefer tool that has gained widespread popularity because of its simplicity is the CAGE questionnaire. It is a four-question survey that has been validated by a number of studies and can easily be included in a routine patient history. The CAGE questionnaire does not confirm the diagnosis of alcoholism but suggests to the physician that further investigation is warranted.

CAGE Questionnaire

1. Have you ever felt you ought to cut down on your drinking?
2. Have people annoyed you by criticizing your drinking?
3. Have you ever felt bad or guilty about your drinking?
4. Have you ever had a drink first thing in the morning
(eye opener) to steady your nerves or get rid of a hangover?

Two or more positive answers indicates the probability of alcoholism. A single positive answer deserves further evaluation.

5. What other lifestyle behaviors involving alcohol and/or drugs may place athletes at higher risk for health problems or injury?

Motor vehicle accidents represent the number one cause of morbidity and mortality in adolescents and young adults. Approximately 50% of accidents involve drivers under the influence of alcohol or drugs. Recent studies have concluded that collegiate athletes may be at higher risk for driving under the influence of alcohol or drugs, riding with an intoxicated driver, and using seatbelts and helmets less often. Similar studies in high school athletes found that they exceeded the speed limit more often than nonathletes and were less likely to wear helmets when driving a moped, motorcycle, or bicycle. Collegiate athletes were also at higher risk for less contraceptive use, greater number of sexually transmitted diseases, and increased numbers of sexual partners.

High risk-taking behaviors have been found to be more frequent in male vs. female athletes and to be more common in athletes participating in contact vs. noncontact sports. Athletes with one risk-taking behavior have been found to be at higher risk for multiple risk-taking behaviors. Future research is needed to focus on interventions that promote positive lifestyle behaviors in high-risk groups.

6. When do athletes start using alcohol and drugs?

According to the 1997 NCAA Study of Substance Abuse and Abuse Habits of College Student-Athletes, the majority of collegiate athletes reported that their experience with alcohol and drugs begins in junior high and high school. Fifty-two percent of anabolic steroid users began in junior high or high school. These data are consistent with other studies demonstrating that 38% of high school students (athletes and nonathletes) who had used steroids reported initial use at 15 years of age or younger. The NCAA found that 77% of athletes began alcohol use before entering college. Effective primary drug education and intervention programs need to be targeted to students at the elementary and junior high levels, in addition to high school and college levels, to prevent future problems with drug and alcohol abuse.

7. Why is smokeless tobacco use so prevalent in sports? What are the risks?

The use of smokeless tobacco is quite common among athletes of all ethnic and racial groups. The 1997 NCAA Survey reported that 21% of all athletes had used smokeless tobacco. The prevalence is much higher in male athletes and athletes involved in baseball and football. The recent NCAA study found that 45% of baseball players and 30% of football players use smokeless tobacco. The use of smokeless tobacco has continued despite efforts to control its consumption. Efforts include the prohibition of radio and television advertising, warning labels on the product, and laws to ban sales to people under the age of 18. In addition, the NCAA banned smokeless tobacco use in all NCAA sanctioned events; the penalty for use is expulsion from the contest. After much protest, baseball has also banned the use of smokeless tobacco from minor league games, although it is still allowed at the major league level.

The use of smokeless tobacco greatly increases the risk of oral cancers. Users are exposed to high concentrations of nicotine and nitrosamines as well as other known carcinogens, such as polycyclic aromatic hydrocarbons and radiation-emitting polonium. The mean survival rate for persons with oral cancer is 50% at 5 years.

8. Can cocaine cause problems in athletes?

Yes. The well-publicized deaths of basketball star Len Bias and football player Don Rogers in 1986 alerted the public to the potential dangers of cocaine abuse in athletes, including ventricular arrhythmias and coronary artery vasospasm. Vasospasm may cause coronary thrombus formation, even in the presence of normal arteries, that may result in acute myocardial infarction or sudden death. In addition, cerebrovascular accidents and seizure activity may result from central nervous system stimulation. Hyperthermia is another potentially serious complication of cocaine abuse, especially in athletes who exercise in hot and humid environments.

Cocaine may cause feelings of euphoria, decreased fatigue, and grandiosity of thought, often distorting the athlete's perception of his or her performance. Although reflex speed may be increased, movements are often uncoordinated and unsynchronized.

Cocaine, in the form of crack or powder, is an addictive drug with many potential deleterious effects. Professional help is indicated for athletes who abuse cocaine. Despite efforts to publicize the effects of cocaine, it seems that not all athletes are listening: 1.5% of NCAA athletes surveyed in 1997 admitted to using cocaine during the previous year.

9. Can an athlete have marijuana in his or her system and not be disqualified after drug testing?

Yes. Certain cutoff levels are used in urine drug testing as indicators of drug abuse. For marijuana, the NCAA cutoff is 15 ng/ml of tetrahydrocannabinol (THC) as detected by gas chromatography. Each athletic organization determines its banned list of substances and appropriate cutoff levels. The International Olympic Committee (IOC), which is primarily concerned with ergogenic aids, does not include marijuana on its banned list.

Various factors can affect the detection of such drug levels, including frequency, quantity of ingestion, and elimination time of drugs in the urine. For marijuana, the elimination time can be

3–5 weeks or more, depending on a number of variables, including percent body fat and method of ingestion.

10. How do athletes circumvent drug testing and avoid detection?

The increasing use of drugs by athletes has led to the growth of drug testing to ensure that an athlete is "clean." Unfortunately, there are many loopholes in drug testing that athletes attempt to exploit. The most common method is to know the half-life of the drug. This knowledge is the main limitation to announced testing at events such as the Olympic Games or NCAA championship events. An athlete merely needs to know the date of an event and how long a drug persists in the system to calculate when to stop its use. To counteract this strategy, the NCAA and many other organizations now test randomly throughout the year.

Athletes also frequently go to great lengths to substitute someone else's (clean) urine for their own. Male athletes have been known to catheterize themselves and pour clean urine into their bladder before a test. This practice can result in disastrous urinary tract infections. Female athletes have released small bags of clean urine, hidden internally, to simulate urination. Such ploys remind those in charge of drug testing programs to be aware of the lengths to which athletes will go to avoid detection. The increasing amount of money available to athletes provides a great temptation to circumvent rules against use of banned substances.

11. Is clenbuterol a type of anabolic steroid?

When four power athletes tested positive for clenbuterol at the 1992 Summer Olympics, the immediate assumption was that clenbuterol represented a new anabolic steroid. In actuality, clenbuterol is a beta-agonist that has been available in Europe since 1977 and is used as a bronchodilator, much like albuterol in the United States.

12. Why do athletes who are trying to improve strength turn to a bronchodilator used to treat asthma?

In animal studies clenbuterol has been found to enhance contractile tension in muscle and to induce true muscular hypertrophy. The mechanism may be that catecholamines can reduce amino acid release from muscle; however, why clenbuterol is more effective than other beta-agonists remains to be determined. Extrapolating from animal data, it seems that the anabolic dose for clenbuterol is much higher than the therapeutic dose used to treat asthma and may exceed safety limits.

13. Can other asthma medications improve performance?

The data are somewhat conflicting with regard to the ergogenic effect of other bronchodilators, including albuterol. Signorile et al. concluded that acute administration of albuterol (180 μg) can have an ergogenic effect on short-term power output. Bedi et al. found an increase in forced expiratory flow (FEF) parameters and improvement in sprint time. Others found no ergogenic effect of the beta-2 agonist salbutamol. At present, beta-2 agonists are legitimate drugs for the treatment of asthma, including exercise-induced asthma, which affects a significant number of athletes (11% of athletes in the 1984 Olympics). IOC requires a note from a physician if the athlete is using beta-2 agonists. More research needs to be performed before these drugs are banned.

14. How do nonsteroidal antiinflammatory drugs (NSAIDs) work? Are they used as ergogenic aids?

NSAIDs are widely used by athletes for their antiinflammatory and analgesic properties. The exact mechanisms of action of NSAIDs are not completely known. The antiinflammatory action is believed to be primarily through interference with the metabolism of arachidonic acid by inhibition of cyclooxygenase and synthesis of prostaglandins. It has been generally assumed that the analgesic effect of NSAIDs results from the same mechanism, thereby relieving pain secondary to inflammation. Considerable data now support a centrally mediated mechanism of action that, at least for some NSAIDs, affects nociceptive pathways independent of prostaglandin synthesis. From the available data, three NSAIDs have been demonstrated unequivocally to provide additional analgesic benefit to concomitant physical therapy—azapropazone, ketoprofen, and naproxen. All three have been demonstrated to have analgesic efficacy comparable with high-efficacy opioids. The extent and site of the central action are unknown; the extent to which the analgesic efficacy includes a peripheral component is also unclear.

15. What is the "best" NSAID?

In the United States, over 30 different types of NSAIDs are available in prescription and over-the-counter formulations. It is the most prescribed class of drugs in the U.S. with over 30 billion tablets consumed annually. NSAIDs are a broad class of compounds that to some degree possess analgesic and antiinflammatory properties. Although each NSAID has similar characteristics, they vary in terms of the relative degree of both beneficial and adverse effects. Because of this wide variability, the "best" NSAID depends on the particular indication, the desired effect, and the side-effect profile of each drug. For example, in a patient with gastrointestinal sensitivity who requires an NSAID, nabumetone or etodolac is a good choice because of the reduced risk of GI upset. Because of this variability, there is no one "best" NSAID therapy; it must be individualized according to the predicted interaction of drug and patient.

16. Can gamma hydroxybutyrate (GHB) increase strength? Is it safe?

GHB is also known as sodium oxybate, sodium oxybutyrate, gamma hydroxybutyrate sodium, Gamm-OH, 4-hydroxy butyrate, gamma hydrate, and Somatomax PM. In the United States it has been advertised as facilitating sleep and weight control and as having euphoric effects. It has been particularly targeted for body builders because of the claim that it produces growth hormone release. This claim is derived from the fact that GHB has many of the properties of a neurotransmitter and can cross the blood-brain barrier. It has been shown that GHB facilitates slow-wave sleep in the laboratory. Slow-wave sleep is associated with growth hormone release—thus the use of GHB by body builders.

The actual effects of this theoretical process on muscle mass are not known. However, at least 57 cases of GHB poisoning were reported during a 5-month period in 1990 across nine states. No deaths were reported, but 11 patients needed hospitalization and 9 required ventilatory support for depressed respiration. In addition, GHB has been reported as a "date rape" drug; women who were unknowingly given GHB have been raped after they fell asleep from its effects.

In November of 1990, the Food and Drug Administration issued an advisory that GHB should be used only under experimental protocols for narcolepsy and is otherwise unsafe. Despite these warnings, GHB continues to be used by athletes.

17. Can ephedrine be an ergogenic aid?

Ephedrine, a sympathomimetic amine, is found in many over-the-counter preparations, especially diet aids. It has become increasingly common as an ergogenic aid because of its stimulant properties. The 1997 NCAA Study of Substance Abuse revealed that 51% of ephedrine users stated that the main reason for use was to improve athletic performance. To address this problem, the NCAA added ephedrine to its banned drug list in 1997; there is a 1-year suspension for a positive test.

BIBLIOGRAPHY

1. Amadio P Jr, Cummings DM, Amadio PB: NSAIDs revisited: Selection, monitoring, and safe use. Postgrad Med 101:257–271, 1997.
2. American College of Sports Medicine Position Statement: The use of alcohol in sports. Med Sci Sports Exerc 14(6):ix-x, 1982.
3. Anderson WA, Albrecht RR, McKeag DB, et al: A national survey of alcohol and drug use by collegiate athletes. Phys Sportsmed 19(2):91–104, 1991.
4. Anderson WA, McKeag DB: Replication of the National Study of the Substance Use and Abuse Habits of College Student-Athletes. Mission, KS, The National Collegiate Athletic Association, 1989.
5. Baumert P, Henderson J, Thompson N: Health risk behaviors of adolescent participants in organized sports [abstract]. In Proceedings of the Second Annual Meeting of the American Medical Society of Sports Medicine. Sun Valley, ID, July 16–20, 1993.

6. Bedi JF, Gong H Jr, Horvath SM: Enhancement of exercise performance with inhaled albuterol. Can J Sport Sci 13:144–148, 1988.
7. Buckley WE, Yesalis CE III, Friedl KE, et al: Estimated prevalence of anabolic steroid use among male high school seniors. JAMA 260:3441–3445, 1988.
8. Buchsbaum DG, Buchanan RG, Centor RM, et al: Screening for alcohol abuse using CAGE scores and likelihood ratios [see comments]. Ann Intern Med 115:774–777, 1991.
9. Cantwell JD, Rose FD: Cocaine and cardiovascular events. Phys Sportsmed 24(11):77–82, 1986.
10. Centers for Disease Control: Leads from the MMWR. Multistate outbreak of poisonings associated with illicit use of gamma hydroxy butyrate. JAMA 265:447–448, 1991.
11. Chin MY, Kreutzer RA, Dyer JE: Acute poisoning from gamma-hydroxybutyrate in California. West J Med 156:380–384, 1992.
12. Connolly GN, Orleans CT, Kogan M: Use of smokeless tobacco in major-league baseball players. N Engl J Med 318:1281–1285, 1988.
13. DeMeersman R, Schaeffer D, Martelli M: The effects of a sympathomimetic drug on maximal aerobic capacity. J Sports Med 26:251–257, 1986.
14. Ewing JA: Detecting alcoholism. The CAGE questionnaire. JAMA 252:1905–1907, 1984.
15. Goodwin JS: Mechanism of action of nonsteroidal anti-inflammatory agents. Am J Med 77(1A):57–64, 1984.
16. Green GA, Puffer JC: Drugs and doping in athletes. In Mellion MB, Walsh WM, Shelton GL (eds): The Team Physician's Handbook, 2nd ed. Philadelphia, Hanley & Belfus, 1997, pp 212–238.
17. Hasson SM, Daniels JC, Divine JG, et al: Effect of ibuprofen use on muscle soreness, damage, and performance: A preliminary investigation. Med Sci Sports Exerc 25(1):9–17, 1993.
18. Haupt HA: Ergogenic aids. In Reider B (ed): Sports Medicine: The School Age Athlete. Philadelphia, W.B. Saunders, 1991, pp 52–66.
19. Lombardo JA: Stimulants and athletic performance. II: Cocaine and nicotine. Phys Sportsmed 14(12): 85–89, 1986.
20. Marwick C: Increasing use of chewing tobacco, especially among younger persons, alarms Surgeon General [news]. JAMA 269:195, 1993.
21. McCormack KM, Brune K: Toward defining the analgesic role of nonsteroidal anti-inflammatory drugs in the management of acute soft tissue injuries. Clin J Sports Med 3:106–117, 1993.
22. McKenzie DC, Rhodes EC, Stirling DR, et al: Salbutamol and treadmill performance in elite non-atopic athletes. Med Sci Sports Exerc 15:520–522, 1983.
23. Meeuwisse WH, Hopkins SR, McKenzie DC, McGavan A: The effect of salbutamol on performance in elite nonasthmatic athletes. Med Sci Sports Exerc 23:S134, 1991.
24. Meeuwisse WH, McKenzie DC, Hopkins SR, Road JD: The effect of salbutanol on performance in elite nonasthmatic athletes. Med Sci Sports Exerc 24:1161–1166, 1992.
25. Milhorn HT Jr: The diagnosis of alcoholism [see comments]. Am Fam Physician 37(6):175–183, 1988.
26. Morton AR, Papalia SM, Fitch KD: Changes in anaerobic power and strength performance after inhalation of salbutamol in nonasthmatic athletes. Clin J Sports Med 3:14–19, 1993.
27. Muscling in on clenbuterol [editorial]. Lancet 340:403, 1992.
28. National Collegiate Athletic Association: Study of substance abuse and abuse habits of college athletes, 1997 [unpublished].
29. Nattiv A, Puffer JC: Lifestyle and health risks of collegiate athletes. J Fam Pract 33:585–590, 1991.
30. Nattiv A, Puffer JC, Green GA: Lifestyles and health risks of collegiate athletes—A multicenter study. Clin J Sports Med 7(4):262–272, 1997.
31. Signorile JF, Kaplan TA, Applegate B, Perry AC: Effects of acute inhalation of the bronchodilator, albuterol, on power outlet. Med Sci Sports Exerc 24:638–462, 1992.
32. Survey shows steroid use on decline. National Collegiate Athletic News 34(32):1, 1997.
33. Tambylm R, Berkson L, Dauphinee WE, et al: Unnecessary prescribing of NSAIDs and the management of NSAID-related gastropathy in medical practice. Ann Intern Med 127:429–438, 1997.
34. Tennant FS Jr: Dealing with cocaine use by athletes. Sports Med Dig 6(11):1–3, 1984.
35. Toohey JV, Corder BW: Intercollegiate sports participation and nonmedical drug use. Bull Narc 33(3):23-27, 1981.
36. Voy RO: The U.S. Olympic Committee experience with exercise-induced bronchospasm, 1984. Med Sci Sports Exerc 18:328–330, 1986.
37. Wolfe MM: NSAIDs and the gastrointestinal mucosa. Hosp Pract 31(12):37–48, 1996.
38. Zeman RJ, Hirschman A, Hirschman ML, et al: Clenbuterol, a beta 2-receptor agonist, reduces net bone loss in denervated hindlimbs. Am Physiol 261 (2 Pt 1):E285–E289, 1991.

VIII. General Medical Problems

37. INFECTIONS IN ATHLETES

Paul R. Stricker, M.D., and Gary A. Green, M.D.

1. What effect does exercise have on the immune system?

The immune system appears to be influenced by the physical and psychological stress of exercise, and the immunology of exercise is an active area of research. The relationship between exercise and infection has been investigated in part by examining changes that occur among many components of the immune system. Results have been limited by inconsistencies in exercise protocols and duration/intensity of the exercise. Because of these difficulties, results reported in the literature are often conflicting.

Clinical research has focused on the influence of exercise on the development of infection. Immune parameters have been investigated and show fairly consistent changes under acute and chronic exercise conditions. Acute exercise has often used exercise treadmill tests or cycle/arm ergometry, whereas chronic exercise refers to long-term high-intensity activity such as marathon running, cross-country skiing, competitive cycling, and swimming.

Although the clinical significance of many of the immune system changes is yet to be determined, some trends can be observed. The chart below summarizes some of the frequently measured parameters of the immune system in relation to acute and chronic exercise; namely, total white blood cell (WBC) count, lymphocyte count, neutrophil activity, natural killer cell activity, serum immunoglobulin (Ig), complement (C) activity, and salivary IgA.

	WBCs	Lymphocytes	Neutrophil Activity	NK Cell Activity	Serum Ig	C3, C4	Salivary IgA
Acute	↑↑	↑*	↑	↑	NC	NC	↓ or NC
Chronic	↑†	↓	↓	↑	NC	↓	↓↓‡

NC, no significant change.

* Rapid initial rise in response to epinephrine, then decrease as epinephrine diminishes and longer-acting cortisol is still present.

† Although chronic exercise induces increased WBC count with each bout as with acute exercise, the rise is to a lesser degree than in nonchronic exercisers, and the actual resting WBC in chronic exercisers is often decreased.

‡ Not only does salivary IgA decrease more with chronic exercise, but baseline levels also appear to decrease.

2. Are athletes more susceptible to infections?

Although exercise can affect certain immune parameters, the actual clinical relevance remains unclear. Whether athletes are more susceptible to acquiring infections also is controversial, but increasing evidence supports that elite athletes may be at greater risk than people who exercise at a more moderate level. Multiple studies have shown that marathoners and runners have increasing risk of upper respiratory infections (URIs) with higher training mileage and during the early 1–2 week postrace period. Another concept is that people who exercise may not have fewer infections, but the duration of illness may be shorter than in nonexercisers. However, the opposite results also have been found in similar investigations. In addition, these studies cannot take into account changes in immunity that result from neuroendocrine changes due to the psychologic stress of training and competition.

Although limitations apply to some of the available studies (e.g., survey studies, lack of control groups), more of the recent studies are correcting these problems. Growing evidence indicates that moderate exercise may decrease the risk of URIs, whereas heavy chronic exercise may increase that risk. An important point is not to discourage people from exercising because of the possible effects from overexertion, but to encourage them because of the possible benefits of moderate levels of exercise.

3. Should a person exercise with a cold or a fever?

Most studies of URIs and exercise have been either inconclusive or have resulted in conflicting findings. Some case reports indicate that exercise during the incubation period of some illnesses may worsen the disease, particularly enteroviral infections. Two sports-related sudden deaths due to myocarditis may have been reported during athletic activity. This suggests that exercise during a viral infection may lead to myocarditis if the virus has the propensity to cause myocarditis.

Even though there are no clear-cut guidelines with regard to training during an illness, common sense is a good place to start. If the athlete feels too ill to participate, then he or she should not participate. However, there are studies that demonstrate detrimental effects of febrile illnesses on muscle strength and endurance, so even elite athletes should avoid training during these types of illnesses. It is probably safe for most athletes to continue to participate with minor cold symptoms that improve with or do not interfere with their training. If, however, signs of systemic illness appear (e.g., significant fever, myalgias, loss of appetite, extreme fatigue, swollen painful lymph glands), it is in the athlete's best interest not to train or compete for 10–14 days to avoid a prolonged decrease in performance and/or severe complications such as cardiomyopathy.

Heat production during exercise can lead to heat exhaustion when coupled with a malfunctioning thermoregulatory system that occurs with a fever. Sweating after a fever "breaks" could aggravate dehydration, especially if combined with diarrhea or vomiting.

4. What effects do anabolic steroids have on the immune system?

Physical changes of the body and enhanced performance induced by androgenic/anabolic steroids (AAS) are well known. Harmful effects on the cardiovascular system, liver, and reproductive system are also common knowledge.

However, the effects of AAS on the immune system has been minimally investigated. Immunoglobulins have been found to be significantly lower in AAS users when compared with controls, and lymphocyte proliferation in vitro tends to be higher in AAS users. These changes are of unknown clinical significance.

5. What is "walking pneumonia"?

Correctly referred to as a lung infection due to *Mycoplasma pneumoniae*, this condition involves a 10- to 14-day incubation period and destruction of ciliated respiratory mucosal cells. Initial symptoms are similar to influenza and include sore throat, malaise, and possible fever. The disease progresses gradually with productive sputum and occasional coughing paroxysms. Physical examination tends to be relatively benign compared with the patient's symptoms. The disease is generally mild when compared with the more severe types of pneumonia; hence the old term "walking pneumonia." Spontaneous recovery is usually the rule following the 1- to 2-week illness, but reactive airways can develop during the recovery period. Erythromycin or any of the newer macrolides, such as clarithromycin or azithromycin, are the antibiotics of choice.

An important fact for athletes and team physicians is that *M. pneumoniae* is the most common lung infection pathogen in the 5- to 35-year-old age group and seems to appear in areas of close contact, such as school, the military, dormitories, families, and athletic teams.

6. Will antibiotics affect performance?

Athletes often refuse antibiotics because they think the medication will adversely impact their performance. This topic is unfortunately an area of research that has been relatively untouched.

In a double-blind crossover study using amoxicillin in physically active healthy subjects, there was no statistical evidence to suggest any negative effect of the antibiotic on aerobic work capacity and leg extension strength. In a more recent randomized, double-blind, placebo-controlled study, similar conclusions were found using three different antibiotics (ampicillin, tetracycline, and trimethoprim/sulfamethoxazole) with no deleterious effect on aerobic capacity or muscle strength.

Obviously, medication should not be withheld in athletes with infections that would respond to appropriate antibiotics. Although only a small number of antibiotics have been studied, they represent antibiotics that may be prescribed to athletes for problems such as acne and not for actual illness. Most significantly ill athletes may not feel like training or competing, but healthy athletes who are prescribed an antibiotic for some other reason should know that apparently antibiotics in and of themselves are not detrimental to performance.

7. Why are water athletes more predisposed to "swimmer's ear"?

Otitis externa, or swimmer's ear, is initiated by epithelial breakdown of the external auditory canal. This breakdown can occur from trauma but also by any condition that causes the loss of the protective waxlike acidic cerumen and lipid epithelial coating. Constant immersion during water sports produces a moist environment that helps strip away the protective substances and raises the pH of the ear canal allowing pathogens to invade the tissues of the canal. The various organisms include *Pseudomonas, Proteus,* and other gram-negative bacteria; fungi such as *Aspergillus* and *Mycoplasma*; or viruses. The athlete should refrain from water activity until the infection has cleared. This restriction does not occur as much from a contagious standpoint but to allow the use of medicated ear drops as the canal heals and regains some protection.

8. What are the implications of infectious mononucleosis in an athlete?

Infectious mononucleosis is an acute, usually self-limited viral lymphoproliferative disease caused by communicable transmission of the Epstein-Barr virus. Implications for athletes are twofold: (1) issues of transmission and (2) interference with and return to training.

The attack rate is highest from ages 15 to 25. The virus is excreted in saliva, which is the usual route of transmission whether it be through direct contact, airborne droplets, or sharing utensils. With a 30- to 50-day incubation period, the disease can be spread unknowingly.

Owing to the symptoms of malaise, headache, fever, sore throat, loss of appetite, and significant fatigue, athletes are usually unable to train. A simultaneous streptococcal pharyngitis can occur and should be treated with penicillin or erythromycin (ampicillin causes a severe rash). Mild hepatitis is often seen, and a mild thrombocytopenia also can occur. Other complications are more serious and are incompatible with athletic activity (and sometimes incompatible with life), such as severe airway obstruction due to enlarged tonsils and adenoids, Guillain-Barré syndrome, and splenic rupture.

9. How long should an athlete with mononucleosis be restricted?

The main reason for restriction involves splenic enlargement and its potential for rupture, which can be lethal. Splenic rupture is infrequent, occurring in about 0.1–0.2% of all cases, and can happen during contact trauma as well as with a mild Valsalva maneuver during defecation. Unfortunately, many enlarged spleens are not palpable, so athletes with infectious mononucleosis should be restricted from athletic activity for a certain period of time regardless of how quickly symptoms of the illness resolve. Most splenic ruptures occur between days 4 and 21 of the illness, and rupture after 4 weeks is rare.

Application of this information leads to the general guideline that easy athletic activity can be resumed approximately 3 weeks after the onset of illness if the spleen is not enlarged or tender, the patient is afebrile, liver enzymes are normal, and any complications are resolved. A month after the onset of the illness, contact sports may be resumed if splenomegaly is absent. Because physical examination for an enlarged spleen is notoriously unreliable, ultrasonographic measurements (normal length < 14 cm) should be considered if there is any suspicion of splenomegaly.

10. Which contagious diseases are significant for athletes?

With increased perspiration, heat, friction, and specific gear, certain contagious skin infections can be easily transmitted among athletes. In addition, contact with infected aerosol droplets also can easily occur in many close contact sports.

There have been at least 33 reports of infectious disease outbreaks associated with sports activities, most of which have involved person-to-person contact, such as herpes gladiatorum among wrestlers. Other modes of spread have included common-source transmission (i.e., drinking water) of enteroviral infections among football and soccer players, as well as airborne spread of measles associated with basketball and gymnastics competitions.

11. What measures can be taken to reduce spread of infections among athletes?

Team physicians and trainers can help prevent transmission by emphasizing good hygiene practices, screening examinations for certain sport-specific risks (such as herpes in wrestlers), ensuring up-to-date immunization status, and temporary suspension of an infectious athlete from participation.

It also has been reported that certain clothing materials may make a difference in the spread of herpes among wrestlers. It was found that during seasons with cotton jerseys, there were fewer instances of herpes gladiatorum than when the team wore heavier more abrasive polyester-cotton gear.

BIBLIOGRAPHY

1. ACSM: Stand on the Use of Anabolic-Androgenic Steroids in Sports. Indianapolis, IN, 1984.
2. Berkow R, Fletcher A (eds): Merck Manual, 15th ed. Rahway, NJ, Merck & Co., 1987.
3. Burstein R, Hourvitz A, Epstein Y, et al: The relationship between short-term antibiotic treatments and fatigue in healthy individuals. Eur J Appl Physiol 66:372–375, 1993.
4. Calabrese LH, Kleiner SM, Lombardo JA: The effect of anabolic steroids on the immune response in male body builders (abstract). Med Sci Sports Exerc 19:S52, 1987.
5. Dershewitz R (ed): Ambulatory Pediatrics. Philadelphia, J.B. Lippincott, 1988.
6. Edwards AJ, Bacon TH, Elms CA, et al: Changes in the populations of lymphoid cells in human peripheral blood following physical exercise. Clin Exp Immunol 58:420–427, 1984.
7. Eichner ER: Infection, immunity, and exercise. Phys Sportsmed 21:125–135, 1993.
8. Eichner ER: Infectious mononucleosis: Recognition and management in athletes. Phys Sportsmed 15:61–71, 1987.
9. Goodman RA, Solomon SL, Osterholm MT, et al: Epidemiology of infectious diseases in sports. Presentation for the annual meeting of the American Medical Society for Sports Medicine, San Diego, July 9, 1992.
10. Haines JD Jr: When to resume sports after infectious mononucleosis: How soon is safe? Postgrad Med 81:331–333, 1987.
11. Hanson PG, Flaherty DK: Immunological responses to training in conditioned runners. Clin Sci 60:225–228, 1981.
12. Kuipers H, Verstappen FT, Reneman RS: Influence of therapeutic doses of amoxicillin on aerobic work capacity and some strength characteristics. Am J Sports Med 8:274–279, 1980.
13. Mackinnon LT, Hooper S: Mucosal (secretory) immune system responses to exercise of varying intensity and during overtraining. Int J Sports Med 15:179–183, 1994.
14. Mackinnon LT, Tomasi TB: Immunology of exercise. Ann Sports Med 3:1–4, 1986.
15. McCarthy DA, Dale MM: The leukocytosis of exercise. Sports Med 6:333–363, 1988.
16. Nieman DC: Exercise, upper respiratory tract infection, and the immune system. Med Sports Sci Exerc 26:128–139, 1994.
17. Peters EM, Bateman ED: Ultramarathon running and upper respiratory tract infections: An epidemiological survey. S Afr Med J 64:582–584, 1983.
18. Russell WR: Paralytic poliomyelitis. Br Med J 1:465–471, 1949.
19. Sitorious MA, Mellion MB: General medical problems in athletes. In Mellion MB, Walsh WM, Shelton GL (eds): The Team Physician's Handbook, 2nd ed. Philadelphia, Hanley & Belfus, 1997.
20. Smith JA, Telford RD, Mason IB, et al: Exercise, training, and neutrophil microbicidal activity. Int J Sports Med 11:179–187, 1990.
21. Stamford B: Exercise and the common cold. Phys Sportsmed 15:197, 1987.
22. Strauss RH (ed): Sports Medicine. Philadelphia, W.B. Saunders, 1984.
23. Strauss RH, Leizman DJ, Lanese RR, et al: Abrasive shirts may contribute to herpes gladiatorum among wrestlers. N Engl J Med 320:598–599, 1989.

24. Tharp GD, Barnes MW: Reduction of saliva immunoglobulin levels by swim training. Eur J Appl Physiol 60:61–64, 1990.
25. Thompson SP, McMahon LJ, Nugent CA: Endogenous cortisol: A regulator of the number of lymphocytes in peripheral blood. Clin Immunol Immunopathol 17:506–514, 1980.

38. HIV/AIDS IN ATHLETES

Christopher A. McGrew, M.D.

1. What is the risk of human immunodeficiency virus (HIV) transmission in sports and athletics?

At present, there are no epidemiologic studies assessing the transmission rate of HIV (or other bloodborne pathogens such as the viruses causing hepatitis B or C) during athletic activities. Given the high prevalence of these infections in the general population (not just athletes),[10] it is reassuring that there are no well-documented examples of such transmission in sports. The one reported case of possible transmission of HIV in sports by contact of bloody wound to bloody wound[21] is considered unconfirmed and invalidated.[5,11] Experience gathered from occupational exposure in the health care setting and extrapolated to the sports arena shows that any risk of sports-related transmission is unlikely. The risk of transmission for parenteral exposures is likely influenced by a variety of factors, including the size of the inoculant and the route of entry. Most parenteral exposure has been associated with deep intramuscular penetrations with hollow-bore needles. These conditions are unlikely to be duplicated in the sports setting. In the health care setting, mucocutaneous transmission has been reported retrospectively; each one of these rare cases involved large quantities of blood and prolonged exposure along with a portal of entry such as nonintact skin.[10] Prospective analysis of HIV-infected blood exposure to mucous membranes or nonintact skin has revealed no cases of such transmission. Over 1,000 cases have been studied.[12] Despite such negative data, when significant blood exposures do occur, there is a theoretical, although extremely low (incalculable), chance of transmission. The estimated *potential risk* of transmission of HIV has been calculated in a few circumstances involving football. For example, Brown et al. reported the estimated risk for transmission in the National Football League at less than 1 per 85 million game contacts.[13] Even this infinitesimal estimate of the risk of transmission is probably exaggerated, given that the calculations in this particular study assumed the transmission risk associated with a deep, hollow-bore needle stick. This is not typical of what could happen in sports. Potential sports transmission estimates probably should use the data associated with mucocutaneous exposure, which would result in an even smaller risk estimate. In general, participants in sports are subject to the same risk of HIV infection as any other individual in the general population by the usual routes of sexual activity and intravenous (IV) drug abuse. (However, their potential for risky behaviors may be increased.[17]) In addition, traveling athletes should be aware that they may be exposed to a population with a higher prevalence of the virus than seen in the United States. They could, for example, be offered medical treatment, unscreened blood transfusion, or injections with a contaminated needle that may put them at increased risk for acquiring the HIV virus.

2. Should athletes be tested for HIV?

Mandatory testing or widespread HIV screening is not justified for medical reasons as a condition for athletic participation/competition.[1,2,5,6,11,16,18] HIV testing of an athlete should be based on personal behavior risk factors. Any consideration of an HIV testing program in the athletic setting must be mindful of the practical, medical, scientific, legal, and ethical problems that it poses. No testing program, despite how widespread, is justifiable because it would probably fail to further diminish the extremely low (theoretical) risk of HIV transmission in sports.

3. Should participation restrictions be placed on an HIV-infected individual in any sport?

Athletes should not be restricted from participating in any sport merely because they are infected with the HIV virus. The decision to advise continued athletic competition should be individualized and involve the athlete and the athlete's personal physician. Variables that must be considered include the athlete's current state of health and the status of the HIV infection, the nature and intensity of his or her training, and the potential contribution of stress from athletic competition. There is no evidence that exercise and training of moderate intensity is damaging to the health of HIV-infected individuals. High-level training and competition *may* be deleterious to the overall state of medical and physical health and should be considered.[5,12,16,20]

4. What is the role of medical personnel on the sideline?

The role of the medical personnel on the sideline should be defined by common sense and adherence to basic principles of hygiene. Universal precautions should be followed by all health care providers. Preventive measures should focus on the recognition and immediate treatment of bleeding wounds. Pre-event preparation includes proper care for existing wounds. Abrasions, cuts, or weeping wounds that may serve as a source of bleeding or as a port of entry should be covered with an occlusive dressing that will withstand the demands of competition. Necessary equipment and supplies important for compliance with universal precautions should be available to the caregivers. These supplies include appropriate gloves, disinfectant and bleach solutions, antiseptic, designated receptacles for soiled equipment or uniforms, bandages or dressings, and a container for appropriate disposal of sharps. Occasionally, protective eyewear will be necessary (e.g., when drilling a subungual hematoma, blood may spurt out and protective eyewear is necessary). Early recognition of uncontrolled bleeding during an event is the responsibility of officials, athletes, and medical personnel. Participants with active bleeding should be removed from the event as soon as practical. Bleeding must be controlled and the wound must be covered in such a way to withstand the activity's demands.

In terms of uniforms, any participant whose uniform is saturated with blood must have that uniform changed before returning to competition. Small amounts of blood stain on a uniform that are rapidly dried do not require removal of the participant or uniform change. Minor cuts and abrasions that are not bleeding should be cleaned and covered during scheduled breaks in play. Any equipment or area such as a wrestling mat soiled with blood should be wiped up immediately with disposable paper towels or cloths. The contaminated area should be disinfected with a solution of one part household bleach and nine parts water, which should be prepared fresh daily. After the event, all blood-soaked uniforms or towels are collected for washing in hot water and detergent.

Many athletic contests and practices, especially at the community or scholastic level, occur without medical personnel attendance. Coaches and officials who may be involved in primary first aid should adhere to the same precautions as above. All personnel involved with sports should be trained in basic first aid and infection control.[1,2,6,14–18,20,21]

5. What are other blood-borne pathogens to be concerned with?

Hepatitis B and hepatitis C also should be of concern. Hepatitis B and C viruses are more easily transmitted than HIV. Both are transmitted through parenteral exposure, mucous membrane and nonintact skin exposure, and even potentially by household contact with a chronic hepatitis B virus carrier with whom one is not involved in sexual activity or IV needle sharing. Although incalculable, transmission of hepatitis B on the playing field has a relatively higher theoretical risk than transmission of HIV; therefore, even if HIV was not an issue, universal precautions and general hygienic practices would be indicated in the athletic arena.[7,14]

6. What is the influence of exercise on HIV infection?

In general, exercise is a safe and beneficial activity for the HIV-infected person. HIV-infected individuals should begin to exercise while healthy and adopt strategies to help them maintain an exercise program throughout the course of the disease. The use of exercise can play an important role in the management of HIV disease while improving the quality of life.[5]

7. What are some general recommendations for exercise activity for the HIV-infected person?

Before initiating any type of exercise training, all HIV-infected individuals regardless of age or stage of disease should have a complete physical examination, discuss exercise plans with their physician, and comply with American College of Sports Medicine (ACSM) testing and prescription guidelines. If the athlete is healthy, asymptomatic, and HIV seropositive, unrestricted exercise activity may continue along with continued competition. Special attention must be paid to avoid overtraining. When the CD_4 counts have dropped below 500, the athlete may continue exercise training; however, terminating competition may be recommended, and some authors have suggested that the athlete should avoid exhaustive exercise. Viral load—quantitative measurement of HIV RNA—gives an indication of the amount of current viral activity and has been shown to correlate with disease progression. Research is needed to determine the usefulness of this lab test in evaluating the effects of exercise on the HIV-infected person. Once diagnosed with AIDS, the athlete should be encouraged to remain physically active, continue exercise training on a symptom-limited basis, avoid strenuous exercise, and reduce or curtail exercises during acute illness.[5,13,20]

BIBLIOGRAPHY

1. American Academy of Pediatrics Committee on Sports Medicine and Fitness: Human immunodeficiency virus (acquired immunodeficiency syndromes [AIDS] virus) in the athletic setting. Pediatrics 88:640–641, 1991.
2. American Medical Society for Sports Medicine and American Orthopedic Society for Sports Medicine Position Statement on HIV and other bloodborne pathogens in sports. Clin J Sports Med 5:199–204, 1995.
3. Brown L, Drotman P, Chu A, et al: Bleeding injuries in professional football: Estimates of the risk for HIV transmission. Ann Intern Med 122:271–275, 1995.
4. Calabrese L, Kelley D: AIDS and the athlete. Phys Sportsmed 17(1):127–132, 1989.
5. Calabrese L, LaPerriere A: Human immunodeficiency virus infections, exercise, and athletics. Sports Med 15:1–7, 1993.
6. Canadian Academy of Sports Medicine Task Force on Infectious Disease in Sports: HIV as it relates to sport. Clin J Sports Med 3:63–65, 1993.
7. Federal Register: Blood Borne Pathogens. Federal Register Rules and Regulations, 56(235):64175–64182, 1991.
8. Friedland G, Klein R: Transmission of the human immunodeficiency virus. N Engl J Med 317:1125–1134, 1987.
9. Gayle HD, Kelling RP, Garcia-Gunon M, et al: Prevalence of the human immunodeficiency virus among university students. N Engl J Med 323:1538–1541, 1990.
10. Gershom R, Vlakov D, Nelson K: The risk of transmission of HIV through non-percutaneous, non-sexual modes—A review. AIDS 4:645–650, 1990.
11. Goldsmith MF: When sports and HIV share the bill, smart money goes on common sense. JAMA 267:1311–1314, 1992.
12. Henderson D, Fahey B, Schmidt J, et al: Risk for occupational transmission of human immunodeficiency virus type I (HIV-1) associated clinical exposures: A prospective evaluation. Ann Intern Med 113:740–746, 1990.
13. Henry K: HIV and sports: Should infected patients stay in the game? Your Patient and Fitness 6:5–10, 1992.
14. IDEM. Update: Universal precautions for prevention of transmission of human immunodeficiency virus, hepatitis B virus and other bloodborne pathogens in health care settings. MMWR 37:377–382, 387–388, 1989.
15. Landry G: Aids in Sport. American Coaching Effectiveness Program. Champaign, IL, Human Kinetics, 1989.
16. McGrew C, Dick R, Schniedwind K, Gikas P: Survey of NCAA institutions concerning HIV/AIDS policies and universal precautions. Med Sci Sport Exerc 25:917–921, 1993.
17. Nattiv A, Puffer J: Lifestyles and health risks of collegiate athletes. J Fam Pract 33:585–590, 1991.
18. NCAA Sports Medicine Handbook, 1996–97 Guideline 2H: Blood-Borne Pathogens and Intercollegiate Athletics. Overland Park, KS, National Collegiate Athletic Association, 1996, pp 24–28.
19. OSHA Instructions CPL 2-2, 44C March 6, 1992. OSHA Office of Public Affairs, 200 Constitution Avenue, N.W., Washington, DC 20210.
20. Seltzer D: Educating athletes on HIV disease and AIDS: The team physician's role. Phys Sportsmed 21(1):109–115, 1993.

21. Torre D, Sanpietro C, Ferraro G, et al: Transmission of HIV-1 infection via sports injury. Lancet 335:1105, 1990.
22. Webster DL, Kaiser DA: An infection control policy for the athletic training setting. Athletic Training 26:72–74, 1991.
23. Welch MJ, Sitper MR, Horodyski M: Should athletic trainers be concerned about HIV? Guidelines for athletic trainers. Athletic Training 24:27–28, 1989.

39. DIABETES MELLITUS

Morris B. Mellion, M.D., and Kris E. Berg, Ed.D.

1. Should diabetics exercise?

Lifelong physical activity is an important component of diabetes mellitus treatment. A recent study (Helmrich et al.) demonstrated that the development of non–insulin-dependent diabetes mellitus, especially in individuals at high risk for the disease, was inversely proportional to the amount of leisure time physical activity in their lives.

2. What are the benefits of exercise to the diabetic?

Exercise increases insulin sensitivity by enhancing receptor site binding. The exercising diabetic may experience increased glucose uptake at a given insulin concentration. The effect persists for several hours and may last as long as 24 hours in some individuals. Consequently, the exercising diabetic may be able to reduce doses of insulin or oral hypoglycemic medications. Occasionally, non–insulin-dependent diabetics may even discontinue medication.

Exercise is a valuable component of weight management. Weight loss in the obese, non–insulin-dependent diabetic enhances blood glucose control and thereby reduces complications.

Many diabetics find that as they begin an exercise program they pay closer attention to their diet and monitor their blood glucose more frequently. Because blood glucose management is the key to reducing complications of diabetes and all of the above factors contribute to that management, the incidence and severity of retinopathy, microangiopathy, and neuropathy may be reduced in well-controlled exercising diabetics. The importance of blood glucose control was recently observed in a 10-year multicenter study with more than 14,000 people with type I diabetes. The incidence and severity of diabetic sequelae were reduced about 50–70% for patients monitoring blood glucose four or more times daily and taking insulin via pump or injections four or more times daily. There may even be some improvement in these conditions with prolonged, tightly controlled blood glucose levels.

Exercise plays a major role in the reduction of other cardiovascular risk factors, which may combine with diabetes to produce arteriosclerotic heart disease. Exercise improves serum lipids (reduces LDL cholesterol and triglycerides and increases HDL cholesterol), reduces blood pressure, increases fibrinolysis, and decreases stress. Furthermore, the American Heart Association recently recognized sedentary living to be a fourth primary risk factor.

Finally, exercise has a major psychological benefit. The exercising athlete who becomes more active in the control of his or her blood sugar and metabolic function feels a new sense of control that extends to many areas of personal behavior. A higher level of self-confidence often results.

3. Are there contraindications to exercise for the diabetic?

The major contraindications for exercise in the diabetic relate to complications of the disease. Diabetics with peripheral neuropathy or microangiopathy must avoid exercise that may traumatize the feet. The pounding effect of running and jumping exercises may be damaging, particularly if sensory nerve function is reduced. Swimming and bicycling may be good alternatives.

These diabetics should pay special attention to their feet by examining them daily, keeping them well lubricated, wearing properly fitting shoes and socks to avoid blisters, corns and calluses, and treating any foot injuries immediately. Diabetic athletes should exhibit special care when trimming their nails and should use a pumice stone to control callus development.

Diabetics with proliferative retinopathy should avoid strenuous activity that might raise their systolic blood pressure above 180 mmHg. Particular concerns include weightlifting and isometric exercises, which may cause dramatic increases in blood pressure. Exercise in an inverted position should also be avoided because it may increase intraocular pressure and threaten retinal damage. Scuba diving should be avoided because of the effect of increased water pressure on the retina. Additionally, pounding or jarring activities such as running, jumping, collision sports, and gymnastics should all be avoided.

The final contraindication to exercise in the diabetic is that it may not be safe to exercise if blood glucose is not well controlled.

4. How does the blood glucose level affect conditioning and performance?

When the blood glucose level is tightly controlled, the athlete's body performs better physiologically. Consequently, the ability to train and compete is improved. At optimal blood glucose levels, the body uses both glucose and fat as fuel sources in a more normal manner. As a result, there is less protein degradation and an opportunity to build increased muscle mass. Muscle and glycogen stores are replenished more completely, and more water is stored in the cells, giving the athlete increased exercise and heat tolerance.

5. Is it safe to exercise with high or low blood glucose levels?

Both situations may be dangerous. Although exercise generally causes a drop in blood glucose, if the blood glucose level exceeds 250–300 mg/dl at the initiation of exercise, blood glucose may rise rather than fall during exercise. If ketosis has begun before exercise, ketone production will continue to rise, sometimes dangerously. This phenomenon may be due to a low insulin level or low insulin sensitivity, as well as to the release of counter-regulatory hormones such as catecholamines and cortisol.

On the other hand, a low blood glucose level at the onset of exercise predisposes to hypoglycemia. In both cases, it is wise to get the blood sugar back into normal range before beginning exercise. Preventing and dealing with these states require assessment of blood glucose about 30 minutes before exercise.

6. What are the other important issues in blood glucose regulation for the exercising diabetic?

The initial bodily response to an exercise demand is the breakdown of muscle glycogen to provide adenosine triphosphate (ATP). As exercise continues, the muscles begin to use blood glucose. Early in exercise insulin blocks hepatic glycogenolysis as well as lipolysis. If the insulin level is adequate, glucose from the blood stream is taken up by the muscle cells and used as fuel. As the blood glucose level declines in response to uptake by the cells, glucagon and catecholamines are released and stimulate first hepatic glycogenolysis and later gluconeogenesis. It is important not to exercise with excess insulin in the blood, which may inhibit the production of glucose by the liver. To prevent hypoglycemia during exercise, the blood insulin level must be reduced. Reducing pre-meal insulin and exercising about 30–60 minutes after a meal works well. The exact amounts of food consumed and insulin used must be balanced with the energy expended during exercise. Measuring blood glucose before and after exercise allows modifications to be made that provide a safe and effective blood glucose response.

In exercise exceeding 45 minutes, carbohydrates (about 1–2 exchanges) should be consumed with fluid every 30–40 minutes. Blood glucose monitoring is also helpful in avoiding problems. Glucose and fat metabolism are complex and multifactorial. Consequently, whenever long-duration and novel exercise is performed, additional blood glucose testing is essential. Diabetic athletes have successfully completed marathons, mountain climbing, and even the Hawaiian Iron Man Triathlon using this approach.

7. Is there a best time of day to exercise?

Hypoglycemia is least likely to occur when exercising in the morning and most likely to occur when exercising in the evening because of a diurnal variation in growth hormone level. Diabetics exercising in the evening should anticipate reduced need for any insulin that peaks after the evening meal and consider consuming more food before and possibly after exercise. If the diabetic athlete is to compete in the evening, it is important to experiment with altered insulin and food intake several times in advance with situations that mimic the actual conditions of competition. Because of the prolonged effect of exercise on insulin sensitivity, blood glucose should be measured 3–4 hours after exercise and, depending on the intensity and duration of the exercise, even in the middle of the night.

8. Does exercise affect insulin absorption? Are there special considerations for injection site?

Exercise performed within 1 hour of injecting regular insulin speeds its absorption and time to peak effect. Similarly, exercise performed within $2\frac{1}{2}$ hours after injecting intermediate insulin speeds absorption and reduces the interval until peak effect. There is some controversy as to whether the choice of injection site adds to the basic effect of exercise in accelerating the peak effect. Until all doubt is removed, there is enough evidence in the literature to warrant selecting the injection site according to the type of exercise performed. Diabetics using insulin should not use the thigh as an injection site before predominantly running and jumping sports. Similarly, the arm and shoulder should not be used before activities involving intensive use of the upper extremities. The most consistent absorption rates of insulin occur when injected in the abdomen.

Consistency is also important for the exercising diabetic. Preferably, the diabetic should exercise about an hour after a meal. But whatever the relation of exercise to meals and injection site, the diabetic will do better if he or she uses the same exercise pattern routinely.

9. When should blood glucose be measured in relationship to exercise?

Blood glucose should be measured before and after exercise. During prolonged and/or high intensity exercise, a special effort may be made to measure the blood glucose during exercise. More frequent measurements are warranted during and after exercise on hard days of training and during tournaments. To prevent hyperglycemia, frequent measurements should be made during reduced training the day of and before a competition.

10. What is post-exercise delayed-onset hypoglycemia? Can it be prevented?

Post-exercise delayed-onset hypoglycemia is a condition that may occur several hours to a full day after intense or prolonged exercise. It generally results from two synergistic phenomena. A prolonged intense bout of exercise will increase insulin sensitivity for several hours, and up to 24 hours. The same exercise may deplete muscle and liver glycogen stores. If the insulin level is adequate, these stores will be replenished at the expense of circulating blood glucose. The result of the increased cellular uptake and glycogen storage may be a precipitous drop in blood glucose, resulting in hypoglycemia. It can be prevented by reducing pre-exercise insulin, increasing pre-exercise, intra-exercise, and post-exercise carbohydrate intake, and monitoring post-exercise blood glucose level frequently. Hypoglycemic reactions are common at night following vigorous daytime activity. Some diabetics must awaken in the middle of the night to assess blood glucose and eat if needed.

11. What are additional guidelines to prevent hypoglycemia during exercise?

Measure blood glucose before exercise. If the blood glucose is less than the 130 mg/dl, the diabetic should consume two carbohydrate exchanges for each 30–45 minutes of light-to-moderate exercise (less than 60% of VO$_2$max) and three exchanges before heavy exercise (at greater than 70% of VO$_2$max). If the blood glucose is 130–180 mg/dl, the athlete should consume one carbohydrate exchange for 30–45 minutes of light-to-moderate exercise and two exchanges for 30–45 minutes of heavy exercise. If the blood glucose is 180–240 mg/dl, no food supplement is warranted before light-to-moderate or up to 30 minutes of heavy exercise. If performing greater than 30 minutes of heavy exercise, perform a second blood glucose reading during exercise and use the above criteria for further supplementation. If the blood sugar is 250 mg/dl or higher, exercise should be deferred because the presence of counterregulatory hormones may cause the blood sugar and ketone levels to rise during exercise.

When exercise lasts for several hours (e.g., marathons, bicycle touring, mountaineering, triathlons, tournament play) **the athlete's insulin dose should be reduced by 20–50%**. For some athletes the reduction applies only to insulin peaking during exercise; but for others it must include the total daily insulin. **Food supplementation** (approximately one carbohydrate exchange or 60 kcal) should be consumed every 30–45 minutes. **Blood glucose monitoring** during the event is extremely helpful. **Simulation of the event** prior to the competitive situation is definitely useful in determining the individual's response to exercise stress.

A common finding in active diabetics, particularly athletes, is a rise in blood glucose after exercise. This occurs because catecholamine secretion increases as exercise intensity rises. Consequently, if the liver's release of glucose exceeds the rate of utilization by muscle, the blood glucose rises. It is paradoxical and surprises many diabetic athletes. Some veteran diabetic athletes anticipate this effect and eat a bit less food before vigorous exercise. This can be done only if a person is willing to do added blood glucose testing (immediately before and after exercise).

12. Should diabetics gain or lose weight?

Insulin-dependent diabetes mellitus (type I diabetes) is characterized by reduced capacity for insulin secretion due to a beta-cell defect. Type I diabetics are characteristically lean. The combination of exercise and good blood glucose control may enable them to increase weight by building muscle mass.

Non–insulin-dependent diabetes mellitus (type II diabetes), on the other hand, may result from a relative decrease in insulin secretion and/or impaired tissue sensitivity to insulin. Type II diabetics are often obese and may have hyperlipidemia. For type II diabetics, exercise may be useful in an effort to lose weight, raise HDL cholesterol, and reduce levels of LDL cholesterol and triglycerides.

13. What special aspects of preparticipation physical evaluation are indicated for diabetics?

First, good blood glucose control should be evaluated. A record of routine preprandial and bedtime blood glucose monitoring should be reviewed and glycosylated hemoglobin should be obtained.

Careful physical examination should be performed to look for microangiopathy and peripheral neuropathy. The retinas should be evaluated by ophthalmoscopic examination. Urinalysis, BUN, and creatinine may be used to screen for nephropathy. If these levels are borderline or abnormal, a 24-hour urine specimen should be analyzed for creatinine clearance.

An exercise electrocardiogram should be performed if the athlete is over 40 years old, has had diabetes for over 25 years, or has one or more primary risk factors for arteriosclerotic cardiovascular disease.

14. What precautions are necessary for treatment of early or impending hypoglycemia?

In spite of the best efforts at good management, hypoglycemia may occur during or after exercise. Most athletes have some warning signs of hypoglycemia, which tend to be the same for that individual. However, after many years, signs and symptoms typically become less dramatic and obvious. Tightly controlled diabetics in particular find this a problem. Glucose gel or tablets should be readily accessible to them in case of sudden severe hypoglycemia. In severe hypoglycemia, treatment with 1 mg of glucagon subcutaneously or intramuscularly may be warranted. The glucagon causes rapid release of hepatic glycogen.

Mild hypoglycemia should be treated with easily absorbed simple sugars (i.e., candy, juice, dextrose) followed by complex carbohydrates for a more prolonged response. The diabetic should keep a candy or sugar source available at all times. It is a good policy to have a supplemental feeding readily available as well.

15. What are the long-term effects of exercise on insulin requirements?

The need for both insulin and oral hypoglycemics is reduced in the early months of an exercise training program and remains low as long as the diabetic continues exercising at the same level. Mature exercising diabetic athletes usually require 0.5–0.6 units of insulin per kilogram of body weight or less, whereas sedentary diabetics require 0.5–1.0 units per kilogram. Some type II diabetics may eventually be able to discontinue insulin or oral hypoglycemic medication due to the effect of exercise on insulin sensitivity and weight loss resulting from the exercise program.

BIBLIOGRAPHY

1. Allen DB, MacDonald MJ: Preventing post-exercise late-onset hypoglycemia. Practical Diabetology 8(1):1–6.
2. American College of Sports Medicine and American Diabetes Association. Joint position statement: Diabetes mellitus and exercise. Med Sci Sports Exerc 29:i–iv, 1997.
3. American Diabetes Association: Exercise and NIDDM. Diabetes Care 13:785–789, 1990.
4. Berg K: Blood glucose regulation in an insulin-dependent diabetic backpacker. Phys Sportsmed 11(12):101–104, 1983.
5. Berg K: Metabolic disease: Diabetes mellitus. In Seefeldt V (ed): Physical Activity and Human Well Being. Reston, VA, American Alliance of Health, Physical Education, Recreation and Dance, 1986.
6. Berg K: Diabetic's Guide to Health and Fitness. Champaign, IL, Human Kinetics, 1986.
7. Berg KE: The diabetic athlete. In Mellion MB, Walsh WM, Shelton GL (eds): The Team Physician's Handbook, 2nd ed. Philadelphia, Hanley & Belfus, 1997, pp 189–193.
8. Berg KE: Guidelines for physically active diabetics. In Mellion MB (ed): Office Management of Sports Injuries and Athletic Problems. Philadelphia, Hanley & Belfus, 1988, pp 110–116.
9. Berg K: Weight training for persons with diabetes mellitus. Strength Conditioning 17:42–45, 1995.
10. Bergman M, Auerhahn C: Exercise and diabetes. Am Fam Physician 32(4):105–111, 1985.
11. Costill DL, Cleary P, Fink WJ, et al: Training adaptations in skeletal muscle of juvenile diabetics. Diabetes 28:812–822, 1979.
12. Ekoe JM: Overview of diabetes mellitus and exercise. Med Sci Sports Exerc 21:353–355, 1989.
13. Fahey PJ, Stallkamp ET, Kwatra S: The athlete with type I diabetes: Managing insulin, diet and exercise. Am Fam Physician 53:1611–1617, 1996.
14. Helmrich SP, Ragland DR, Leung RW, Paffenbarger RS Jr: Physical activity and reduced occurrence of non-insulin dependent diabetes mellitus. N Engl J Med 325:147–152, 1991.
15. Jensen MD, Miles JM: The roles of diet and exercise in the management of patients with insulin-dependent diabetes mellitus. Mayo Clin Proc 61:813–819, 1986.
16. Larsson Y, Persson B, Sterky G, Thoren C: Functional adaptation to vigorous training and exercise in diabetic and nondiabetic adolescents. J Appl Physiol 19:629–635, 1964.
17. Mayer-Davis EJ, D'Agostino R Jr, Karter AJ, et al: Intensity and amount of physical activity in relation to insulin sensitivity: The insulin resistance atherosclerosis study. JAMA 279:669–674, 1998.
18. McCarren M: DCCT: Why do it? And why'd it take so long? Diabetes Forecast 6:42–62, 1993.
19. Robbins DC: Managing the diabetic athlete. Phys Sportsmed 17(12):45–54, 1989.
20. Wallace MB, Mills BD, Browning CL: Effects of cross-training on markers of insulin resistance/hyperinsulinemia. Med Sci Sports Exerc 29:1170–1175, 1997.
21. Wallberg-Henriksson H: Acute exercise: Fuel homeostasis and glucose transport in insulin-dependent diabetes mellitus. Med Sci Sports Exerc 21:356–361, 1989.

40. HYPERTENSION AND EXERCISE

Jeffrey L. Tanji, M.D.

1. Is exercise useful as a therapeutic modality for the control of hypertension?

According to the report of The Fifth Joint National Committee on Detection, Evaluation and Treatment of High Blood Pressure, published in 1992, nonpharmacologic therapy, including moderate exercise, is the first-step recommendation for the management of mild hypertension. Mild hypertension in this report is defined as a diastolic blood pressure between 90 and 100 mmHg.

Currently, more than 30 human and 20 animal longitudinal studies have demonstrated the benefit of an ongoing exercise regimen for the control of high blood pressure. Each of the studies uniformly presents the following common issues for such training. The exercise is described as aerobic in nature, of moderate intensity, and must be performed three to five times per week.

2. What are the proposed mechanisms that explain the benefit of exercise in the treatment of high blood pressure?

Most often cited are mechanisms involving the reduction of sympathetic nervous tone for the control of mild hypertension with exercise. In most studies, plasma catecholamine concentrations have been used as an index of sympathetic nervous system activity. A decrease in absolute weight has been shown in the Trials of Hypertension Prevention Study to be associated with decreased blood pressure, whereas decreased percentage of body fat has been shown to be associated with the drop in blood pressure in other studies. One of the more intriguing mechanisms for an explanation for the reduction of blood pressure with exercise is the insulin hypothesis. Described as both "syndrome X" by Reaven[15] or the "deadly quartet" by Kaplan,[11] the insulin hypothesis states that hypertension, type II diabetes mellitus, hyperlipidemia, and obesity are four related factors that exist in the same metabolic milieu of elevated serum insulin levels, elevated adrenergic tone, and increased insulin resistance.

3. What is the practical significance of the insulin hypothesis?

Given that a common metabolic milieu exists that results in the combination of hypertension, type II diabetes mellitus, hyperlipidemia, and obesity, management of one condition such as control of high blood pressure with the use of a diuretic may actually worsen other parameters. Hyperlipidemia, hyperglycemia, and hyperuricemia are all described as side effects with the use of diuretic medications. The use then of one agent that may improve the parameters of an isolated cardiovascular risk factor may in fact then worsen parameters of other cardiovascular risk factors. What is particularly appealing about exercise for the management of high blood pressure is the fact that exercise can simultaneously address multiple risk factors and, therefore, alleviate this problem.

4. Specifically how much exercise is advisable for the control of mild hypertension?

The American College of Sports Medicine in 1990 recommended for aerobic exercise that it be 20–60 minutes in duration, three to five times per week at 60–90% of one's maximal heart rate. The predicted maximal heart rate (PMHR) can be determined using the equation PMHR = 220 minus the person's age. Therefore, anywhere between 1 and 5 hours per week of aerobic exercise done at moderate intensity, defined as between 60 and 70% of one's predicted maximal heart rate, is probably the optimal range for blood pressure control.

5. Is weightlifting contraindicated for patients with high blood pressure?

The answer is both yes and no. High-weight, low-repetition resistance training has been associated with marked elevations in both systolic and diastolic blood pressure in a study by MacDougall et al.,[13] even in normotensive subjects. However, another study, by Harris and Holly,[7] demonstrates that low-weight, high-repetition resistance training has been associated with an antihypertensive effect as opposed to an effect resulting in marked elevation of blood pressure.

6. What is the meaning of a markedly exaggerated blood pressure response to exercise, such as might be encountered during an exercise treadmill stress test?

The hypertensive response to exercise, defined as an elevation in systolic blood pressure in excess of 200–225 mmHg, has been associated in normotensive individuals with a greater predisposition to develop hypertension at a later date. Numerous studies, both prospective and retrospective, have demonstrated that this correlation exists. More work needs to be done, however, before general screening of the population can be recommended for the purposes of screening for hypertension.

7. What are the effects of exercise with commonly used antihypertensive agents?

Diuretics, a popular first-line agent for the treatment of hypertensives may not be the optimal agent for the exercising athlete. In particular, hypokalemia may be exacerbated during acute bouts of exercise, when relatively high levels of catecholamines are released. Dehydration, a side effect during chronic exercise training, may also be exacerbated by diuretics.

Beta-blockers also are often used as first-line agents. All beta-blockers can potentially reduce exercise tolerance and the level of perceived exertion associated with each level of exercise. In particular, nonselective beta-blockers are absolutely contraindicated for exercising adults. During exercise, beta-blockers may increase serum potassium through a mechanism that is not well understood. Thus serum potassium should be closely monitored in these patients. Heat dissipation may be impaired by beta-blockers either by reduction of blood flow to the skin or by direct reflex vasoconstriction; therefore, patients who are prescribed beta-blockers should be well aware of signs and symptoms of hyperthermia. Selective beta-blockers generally should not be contraindicated in exercising adults because they have fewer side effects than nonselective agents.

Angiotensin-converting enzyme inhibitors and calcium channel blockers have a low side effect profile in exercising adults. Prazosin and doxazosin also are associated with very few side effects in exercising individuals.

In the most recent Fifth Joint National Committee on Evaluation, Detection and Treatment of High Blood Pressure, diuretics and beta-blockers are listed as first-line therapeutic agents for the pharmacologic management of high blood pressure. Although these agents are quite cost effective, the potential for side effects in exercising adults is much higher with these agents.

BIBLIOGRAPHY

1. American College of Sports Medicine: Guidelines for Graded Exercise Testing and Exercise Prescription. Philadelphia, Lea & Febiger, 1990.
2. Davidoff R, Schamroth CL, Goldman AP, et al: Post-exercise blood pressure as a predictor of hypertension. Aviat Space Environ Med 53:591–594, 1982.
3. Dlin RA, Hanne N, Silverberg DS, et al: Follow-up of normotensive men with exaggerated blood pressure response to exercise. Am Heart J 106:316–320, 1983.
4. Duncan JJ, Farr JE, Upton SJ, et al: The effects of aerobic exercise on plasma catecholamines and blood pressure in patients with mild essential hypertension. JAMA 254:2609–2613, 1985.
5. Esler M, Jennings G, Korner P, et al: Assessment of human sympathetic nervous system from measurements of norepinephrine turnover. Hypertension 11:3–20, 1988.
6. Ferrannini E, Buzzigoli G, Bonadonna R, et al: Insulin resistance in essential hypertension. N Engl J Med 317:350–357, 1987.
7. Harris KA, Holly RG: Physiological response to circuit weight training in borderline hypertensive subjects. Med Sci Sports Exerc 19:246–252, 1987.
8. Hill JF, Bulpitt CJ, Fletcher AE: Angiotensin-converting enzyme inhibitors and the quality of life: The European trial. J Hypertens 3(Suppl):S91–S94, 1985.
9. Jette M, Landry F, Sidney K, et al: Exaggerated blood pressure response to exercise in the detection of hypertension. J Cardiopulmo Rehabil 8:171–177, 1988.
10. Joint National Committee on Detection, Evaluation and Treatment of High Blood Pressure: The Fifth Report of the JNC. Bethesda, MD, NHLBI, NIH, Oct 30, 1992.
11. Kaplan NM: The deadly quartet: Upper-body obesity, glucose intolerance, hypertriglyceridemia, and hypertension. Arch Intern Med 149:1514–1520, 1989.
12. Kiyonaga A, Arakawa K, Tanaka H, et al: Blood pressure and hormonal response to aerobic exercise. Hypertension 7:125–131, 1985.
13. MacDougall JD, Tuxen D, Sale DG, et al: Arterial blood pressure response to heavy resistance exercise. J Appl Physiol 58:785–790, 1985.
14. Modan M, Halkin H, Almog S, et al: Hyperinsulinemia: A link between hypertension, obesity and glucose intolerance. J Clin Invest 75:809–817, 1985.
15. Reaven GM: Insulin resistance, hyperinsulinemia and hypertriglyceridemia in the etiology and clinical course of hypertension. Am J Med 90(suppl 2A):7S–12S, 1991.
16. Tanji JL: Exercise and the hypertensive athlete. Clin Sports Med 11:291–302, 1992.
17. Tanji JL, Champlin JJ, Wong GY, et al: Blood pressure recovery curves after submaximal exercise: A predictor of hypertension at ten-year follow-up. Am J Hypertens 2:135–138, 1989.
18. Tipton CM: Exercise, training and hypertension: An update. Exerc Sports Sci Rev 19:447–505, 1991.
19. Tipton CM, Matthes RD, Marcus KD, et al: Influence of exercise intensity, age and medication on resting systolic blood pressure of SHR populations. J Appl Physiol 55:1304–1310, 1983.

41. EXERCISE-INDUCED ASTHMA

Morris B. Mellion, M.D., and Roger H. Kobayashi, M.D.

1. What is exercise-induced asthma?

Exercise-induced asthma (EIA) is a respiratory problem in which shortness of breath occurs with vigorous exercise in affected individuals. Intensive exercise for 5–10 minutes or longer causes a decrease of 15% or greater in breathing capacity as measured by forced expiratory volume in one second (FEV_1) or peak expiratory flow rate (PEFR). This decrease may occur either during or after the exercise period. Normal individuals commonly have a 10% fall in FEV_1 after exercise; however, in EIA the fall is greater. A decrease of 20% or less is considered mild EIA, a 20–40% decrease is considered moderately severe, and a 40% or greater decrease is severe.

2. Is this a common problem?

EIA is quite common and occurs in 10% of all athletes, 40–50% of those with allergic rhinitis, and 80–90% of asthmatics. Of 597 U.S. athletes competing in the Summer Olympics of 1984, 67 had asthma or EIA; 41 of these 67 athletes won medals—a greater proportion than nonasthmatic Olympians.

3. Is EIA easy to diagnose?

Although the symptoms of bronchospasm during or immediately after exercise are usually straightforward, in many patients the diagnosis is difficult. The patient may be unaware of the bronchospasm and may experience only vague chest discomfort or complain of "being out of shape." In children, cough and lack of endurance are common symptoms. Often children with EIA avoid vigorous play and their parents are unaware that there is a problem. Clinical clues to the diagnosis of EIA are listed below.

Clinical Clues to Exercise-induced Asthma

Obvious clinical clues	Subtle clinical clues
Wheezing	Cough
Dyspnea on exertion	Chest congestion
Chest tightness	Chest discomfort or pain
	Shortness of breath
	Increased susceptibility in cold air
	Patient feels "out of shape"
	Lack of energy (especially in children)
	Frequent colds
	Problems occur while running but not while swimming
	Patient is unable to run 5 minutes without stopping

From Mellion MB, Kobayashi RH: Exercise-induced asthma. Am Fam Physician 45:2671–2677, 1992.

4. What factors influence the onset and severity of EIA?

(1) The type of exercise, (2) the intensity of exercise, (3) the duration of exercise, and (4) the conditions under which the exercise occurs are principal factors. Sports that require continuous activity at a relatively high percentage of aerobic capacity are more likely to cause EIA. The more intense the activity, the greater the incidence and severity of attacks. Duration of exercise is also important. Up to a point, the severity of EIA varies proportionately with the duration of exercise. However, some athletes find that if they run a longer distance, even after becoming symptomatic, they can actually "run through" their bronchospasm.

5. How does the environment affect EIA?

Exercise in cold, dry air makes EIA worse; exercise in warm, moist air generally reduces the incidence and severity. Moreover, a variety of stimulants may have an additive effect until their sum exceeds a threshold. The components of the stimulus, such as cold air, allergens, irritants, air pollutants, and viral infections, may vary from season to season.

Stimuli that Contribute to Attacks of Exercise-induced Asthma

Exercise	Pollutants
Cold	Allergens
Low humidity	Dust
Respiratory infections	Irritants
Fatigue	Automobile exhaust and commercial
Emotional stress	pollutants, especially SO_2, NO_2, O_3
Athletic overtraining	

From Kobayashi RH, Mellion MB: Exercise-induced asthma, anaphylaxis, and urticaria. Primary Care 18:809–831, 1991.

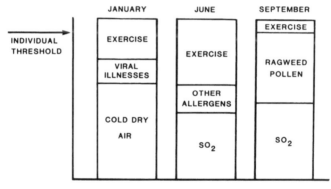

Relative contribution to exercise-induced bronchospasm in an individual who has EIA and ragweed hay fever. (From Kobayashi RH, Mellion MB: Exercise-induced asthma and related problems. In Mellion MB (ed): Office Management of Sports Injuries and Athletic Problems. Philadelphia, Hanley & Belfus, 1988.)

6. What are the etiologic factors in exercise-induced asthma?

(1) Exercise-induced mediator release from mast cells and granulocytes, (2) respiratory heat loss causing bronchial vascular bed dilation, (3) respiratory water loss causing increased pulmonary tissue osmolarity, (4) sympathetic mediation through vagus nerve innervation. The net result of these factors is airway narrowing.

7. What is the "late-phase response"?

In some patients with EIA a second episode of bronchospasm may occur 4–8 hours after exercise. This late-phase response results from the activity of inflammatory mediators such as eosinophil chemotactic factor of anaphylaxis, platelet-activating factor, and the leukotrienes (LTC_4, LTD_4, LTE_4).

8. How is the diagnosis of EIA confirmed?

Often it is not necessary to confirm a classic presentation characterized by repeated episodes. When the diagnosis is obvious, empirical treatment is reasonable. When the diagnosis is unclear, either informal or formal testing may be carried out.

9. How is formal exercise testing for EIA conducted?

Formal testing consists of measuring pulmonary function before and after 5–8 minutes of vigorous exercise on a treadmill at 90% of predicted maximum heart rate. Pulmonary function parameters are measured before exercise, after exercise, and every 5 minutes thereafter for 20–30 minutes. A decrease of 15% or greater in FEV_1 or PEFR is considered a positive test.

10. How sensitive is formal testing for EIA?

It is not as sensitive as exercising outdoors. Air temperature and humidity are different from the field setting, and the air may be cleaner.

11. How is informal exercise testing for EIA conducted?

Informal testing may be accomplished adjacent to a physician's office. First, the patient's pulmonary function is measured. The patient then exercises outdoors at the intensity that usually brings on an attack, completing the exercise at the physician's office, where pulmonary function is measured once again. Running up and down stairs is also sufficiently strenuous to precipitate bronchospasm. Another option is to measure the athlete's PEFR before and after a normal workout using a peak flowmeter.

12. If these tests are negative and suspicion is high, is there another type of test that will help diagnose EIA?

Methacholine challenge, which is a more sensitive but less specific test for bronchial hyperreactivity, may be used.

13. What is the initial treatment for mild to moderate EIA?

The treatment of choice is an inhaled beta$_2$ agonist from a metered-dose inhaler taken 10–60 minutes before exercise. A second line of treatment is the use of inhaled cromolyn sodium or nedrocromil sodium by metered-dose inhaler 15–30 minutes before exercise. If neither is successful alone, the two medications should be used together. If the combination fails to prevent EIA, it is reasonable to evaluate the patient further and decide whether the patient has an ongoing problem that needs more comprehensive treatment. Ipratropium bromide inhaled 1–2 hours before exercise may be helpful in some patients. Theophylline also may be helpful but should be used continuously rather than just before exercise. Citirizine, astemizole, loratadine and other newer antihistamines, and some calcium antagonists are less effective.

Beta Agonists Used to Treat Exercise-induced Asthma

DRUG	TRADE NAME	DOSE (10–60 MIN BEFORE EXERCISE)	APPROVED FOR NCAA USE	APPROVED FOR OLYMPIC USE
Albuterol	Proventil Ventolin	2–4 puffs	Yes	Yes
Bitolterol	Tornalate	1–2 puffs	Yes	No
Metaproterenol	Alupent Metaprel	2–4 puffs	Yes	No
Pirbuterol	Maxair	2 puffs	Yes	No
Terbutaline	Brethine	2–4 puffs	Yes	Yes

Adapted from Mellion MB, Kobayashi RH: Exercise-induced asthma. Am Fam Physician 45:2671–2677, 1992.

14. Are there newer agents which may be available soon?

Salmeterol, a longer acting beta$_2$-antagonist and nedocromil sodium, a new drug similar to cromolyn sodium, have been shown to be effective in EIA. Leukotriene inhibitors, platelet activating factor inhibitors, and other chemokine inhibitors are being evaluated.

15. Does standard treatment prevent the late-phase response?

Currently available beta$_2$-agonists are not effective in preventing the late-phase response, but cromolyn sodium, nedocromil sodium, and both oral and inhaled corticosteroids are. Longer-acting beta$_2$-agonists, such as salmeterol, may also be effective.

16. Does exercise conditioning affect EIA?

Exercise conditioning reduces the incidence and severity of the EIA attack. The well-conditioned athlete can perform the same workload with less increase in minute ventilation and, consequently, less respiratory heat and water loss than the poorly conditioned athlete. Thus, the well-conditioned athlete is less likely to have an attack of EIA.

17. What is the refractory period?

Generally, an attack of EIA begins to resolve within 20 minutes. For a period of 1–3 hours thereafter, the patient may be "refractory" to an additional attack in spite of a repeated exercise stimulus. Some athletes use short bursts of repeated physical activity to induce a refractory period as a training technique, thereby avoiding a significant attack. It is likely that the refractory period is caused by endogenous release of epinephrine and/or norepinephrine in response to exercise.

18. What special advice may be given to athletes with EIA to help prevent attacks?

Athletes with EIA might choose activities with recurrent short bursts of exercise rather than long, vigorous bursts. In winter in more northerly climates, athletes with EIA tend to do better in indoor sports where temperature and humidity are higher. Athletes should breathe through the nose as much as possible and use a slow, deep, and rhythmic pattern to provide more efficient airflow and relaxation. Obviously, this approach can be used only in lower intensity exercise. Those with allergic rhinitis should control their symptoms. If it is necessary to exercise outdoors in a cold, dry, or polluted climate, a surgical face mask may warm, humidify, and purify the inspired air and reduce the incidence of EIA. Use of approved medications *before* exercise is highly useful.

19. Should athletes with EIA be discouraged from participating in sports?

No. They can enjoy a broad range of vigorous physical activities if they develop proper athletic conditioning and use warm-up and repetitive and short exercise bursts to induce the refractory period. If these maneuvers do not succeed, then pharmacologic treatment is appropriate. Proper patient education and treatment can result in successful athletic participation in a wide range of sports and climates.

BIBLIOGRAPHY

 1. Anderson SD: Current concepts of exercise-induced asthma. Allergy 38:289–302, 1983.
 2. Barnes PJ, Holgate ST, Laitenen LA, et al: Asthma mechanisms, determinants of severity and treatment: The role of nedocromil sodium. Clin Exp Allergy 25:771–787, 1995.
 3. Bierman CW, Spiro SG, Petheram I: Characterization of the late response in exercise-induced asthma. J Allergy Clin Immunol 74:701–706, 1984.
 4. Eggleston PA: Methods of exercise challenge. J Allergy Clin Immunol 73(5 Pt 2):666–669, 1984.
 5. Konig P, Hordvik NL, Kreutz C: The preventive effect and duration of action of nedocromil sodium and cromolyn sodium on exercise-induced asthma (EIA) in adults. J Allergy Clin Immunol 79:64–68, 1987.
 6. Kobayashi RH, Mellion MB: Exercise-induced asthma, anaphylaxis, and urticaria. Sports Med Primary Care 18:809–831, 1991.
 7. Kyle JM, Walker RB, Hanshaw SL, et al: Exercise-induced bronchospasm in the young athlete: Guidelines for routing, screening and initial management. Med Sci Sports Exerc 24:856, 1992.
 8. Mellion MB, Kobayashi RH: Exercise-induced asthma. Am Fam Physician 45:2671–2676, 1992.
 9. National Asthma Education Program: Expert Panel Report. Guidelines for the diagnosis and management of asthma. J Allergy Clin Immunol 88(3 Pt 2):425–534, 1991.
10. Nelson HS: β-adrenergic bronchodilators. N Engl J Med 333:499–506, 1995.
11. Noviski N, Bar-Yishay E, Gur I, Godfrey S: Exercise intensity determines and climactic conditions modify the severity of exercise-induced asthma. Am Rev Respir Dis 136:592–594, 1987.
12. O'Byrne PM, Dolovich J, Hargreave FE: Late asthmatic responses. Am Rev Respir Dis 136:740–751, 1987.
13. Pierson WE, Covert DS, Koenig JQ: Air pollutants, bronchial hyperactivity, and exercise. J Allergy Clin Immunol 73(5 Pt 2):717–721, 1984.
14. Spector SL: Leukotriene inhibitors and antagonists in asthma. Ann Allergy Asthma & Immunol 75:463–470, 1995.

15. Stearns DR, McFadden ER Jr, Breslin FJ, Ingram RH Jr: Reanalysis of the refractory period in exertional asthma. J Appl Physiol 50:503–508, 1981.
16. Svenonius E, Arborelius M Jr, Wiberg R, Ekberg P: Prevention of exercise-induced asthma by drugs inhaled from metered aerosols. Allergy 43:252–257, 1988.
17. Virant FS: Exercise-induced bronchospasm: Epidemiology, pathophysiology, and therapy. Med Sci Sports Exerc 24:851–855, 1992.
18. Voy RO: The U.S. Olympic Committee experience with exercise-induced bronchospasm, 1984. Med Sci Sports Exerc 18:328–330, 1986.
19. Woolley M, Anderson SD, Quigley BM: Duration of protective effect of terbutaline sulfate and cromolyn sodium alone and in combination on exercise-induced asthma. Chest 97:39–45, 1990.

42. EXERCISE-INDUCED URTICARIA AND ANAPHYLAXIS

Gregory L. Landry, M.D.

1. What is the difference between urticaria and angioedema?

Urticaria represents localized nonpitting edema of the superficial dermis. Angioedema is well-demarcated edema involving deeper layers of the skin and subcutaneous tissues.

2. What is anaphylaxis?

Anaphylaxis is a life-threatening condition that involves upper airway distress or hypotension. Urticaria or angioedema may or may not occur with anaphylaxis.

3. If an athlete develops hives while exercising, is there a risk of anaphylaxis?

Maybe. It depends on whether the athlete has exercise-induced urticaria (EIU) or cholinergic urticaria (CU). CU is associated with small punctate lesions, 2–4 mm in diameter, which may coalesce. These small hives develop in response to the increase in body temperature produced by exercise that stimulates histamine release. If the athlete has CU, he or she may have noticed that "hives" occurred previously with passive warming, such as in a hot shower or sauna. CU may be associated with bronchospasm, but progression to anaphylaxis is rare. EIU involves larger lesions that measure 1.0–2.5 cm in diameter. There may be progression to angioedema and anaphylaxis.

4. It sounds like differentiation of these entities may be important. Are there any tests available to distinguish CU from EIU?

The diagnosis of EIU or CU is usually made on the basis of the history. Provocative testing is unnecessary in the majority of cases. If the diagnosis is unclear, two tests can be performed that are specific for CU, but they are not very sensitive. **Passive heat challenge** elevates serum histamine levels and produces urticaria in individuals with CU. This can be achieved by warming the patient with a heating blanket or by immersing an extremity in hot water (40–42°C) to raise the body core temperature 0.5–1.5°C. A **methacholine stimulation test** (intradermal injection of acetyl methylcholine chloride) will usually produce 2- to 4-mm urticaria in patients with CU but not in those with EIU. A negative test does not exclude a diagnosis of CU.

5. How is CU treated?

Antihistamines such as hydroxyzine and diphenhydramine are helpful, but at least a third of patients find the symptoms mild enough that they do not desire treatment. It is important to ask about associated symptoms related to anaphylaxis. Athletes with EIU are clearly at risk for anaphylaxis unless one can be sure they have CU.

6. What other symptoms does an athlete with EIU report that should make one think of exercise-induced anaphylaxis (EIAna)?

Classic EIAna produces a range of symptoms that include cutaneous warmth and flushing, pruritus and urticaria, and angioedema that may often progress to laryngeal edema, bronchospasm, and hypotension. It is difficult to make a definite diagnosis of EIAna unless there is upper airway distress or hypotension.

Just to make things more confusing, there also is a variant form of EIAna that is associated with smaller lesions without pulmonary symptoms and is capable of progression to hypotension. To help distinguish these entities, these anaphylactic diseases have been divided into three patterns, as shown in the table below. It has also been suggested that these patterns may represent a continuum rather than three distinct entities.

Patterns of Exercise-induced Anaphylaxis or Urticaria

DISEASE	SIZE OF SKIN LESIONS	RESPIRATORY SYMPTOMS	SHOCK	PRECIPITATORS
Cholinergic urticaria	2–4 mm	Yes	Rare	Exercise, passive warming
Classic EIAna	1.0–2.5 cm	No	Frequent	Only exercise
Variant EIAna	2–4 mm	No	Frequent	Only exercise

Modified from Nichols AW: Exercise-induced anaphylaxis and urticaria. Clin Sports Med 11:303, 1992.

7. Why is exercise-induced anaphylaxis abbreviated EIAna instead of EIA?

Because EIA is often used for exercise-induced asthma. EIAna makes it more clear that anaphylaxis is being discussed.

8. Why does exercise trigger anaphylaxis?

The mechanism of exercise in triggering EIAna is not well understood. It appears that food ingestion plays an important role as a coprecipitator in over half of the patients with this disorder.

9. Describe an attack of EIAna.

The classic symptoms of EIAna often occur approximately 5 minutes into a bout of exercise, but the symptoms can occur at any time during exercise. In a survey of patients with EIAna, Wade et al.[5] found that pruritus was the most common symptom associated with EIAna, occurring in 92% of individuals. Urticaria was reported in 83%, angioedema in 78%, and respiratory symptoms in 59%. The athlete who reports that sometimes exercise produces a warm feeling with some itching and an associated feeling of "impending doom" does not need to see a psychiatrist. He likely has EIAna!

10. How can one differentiate asthma from anaphylaxis?

It is not always easy to differentiate these two entities, but exercise-induced asthma usually only produces respiratory symptoms such as dyspnea, cough, wheezing, and chest tightness. It is usually not associated with other symptoms.

11. What foods are associated with anaphylaxis?

Virtually any food can coprecipitate an episode of EIAna. Surprisingly, the most common food associated with EIAna is raw celery. Any meal has been reported to increase the risk of an episode in some individuals, and among the reports of coprecipitating foods are shellfish, peaches, grapes, wheat, cabbage, and alcohol. Medications have also been reported to be factors and they include aspirin, nonsteroidal anti-inflammatory drugs (NSAIDs), antibiotics, and over-the-counter (OTC) cold remedies.

12. What kinds of exercise will most likely produce anaphylaxis?

The more intense the exercise, the more likely symptoms of EIAna will occur. Therefore, running is the most frequently reported activity associated with EIAna, but EIAna has been reported with a variety of exercise activities.

13. Does the environment make a difference?

In 64% of individuals, a warm environment increased the chances of an attack, whereas 23% reported that cold weather was more of a problem. High humidity predisposed to an attack in 32%.

14. Does EIAna cause death?

Despite the increased recognition of this entity and reports of over 1000 cases, EIAna has not been reported to be a cause of death.

15. Is EIAna hereditary?

Not usually, but it has been reported in one family.

16. How is EIAna treated?

The only medication known consistently to reverse the progression of an anaphylactic attack is epinephrine. Vascular support and airway maintenance may be necessary if the reaction is severe. Antihistamines also are frequently used.

17. Can EIAna be prevented?

Avoidance of exercise during environmental conditions that are risky helps some individuals with recurrent episodes. Pretreatment with antihistamines usually produces significant improvement. Hydroxyzine hydrochloride and diphenhydramine hydrochloride are the most effective agents, but sedation is a significant side effect of these drugs for a significant number of patients. The dose must be titrated upward slowly depending on clinical response and sedation. It must be remembered that many patients will develop a tolerance to the sedating effect and should be encouraged to stick with hydroxyzine or diphenhydramine for several weeks before switching to a different antihistamine. In addition, some individuals have taken up to 150 mg of hydroxyzine to prevent symptoms.

Other antihistamines have been used and have been reported to be helpful. The H_2 antagonist cimetidine has been helpful in some cases.

Avoidance of coprecipitating foods or medications is very important in the prevention of recurrences. Avoidance of food for at least 4 hours before exercise has been strongly recommended. Some individuals avoid symptoms of EIAna by exercising exclusively in the morning after an overnight fast. For individuals who get recurrent symptoms, an exercise and food diary is imperative to identify potential coprecipitants.

Individuals with EIAna should not exercise alone and must carry epinephrine with them during exercise at all times.

BIBLIOGRAPHY

1. Briner WW, Bruno PJ: Case report: 30-yr-old female with exercise induced anaphylaxis. Med Sci Sports Exerc 23:991, 1991.
2. Nichols AW: Exercise-induced anaphylaxis and urticaria. Clin Sports Med 11:303, 1992.
3. Sheffer AL, Austen KF: Exercise-induced anaphylaxis. J Allergy Clin Immunol 73:699, 1984.
4. Sheffer AL, Tong AKF, Murphy GF, Lewis RA, et al: Exercise-induced anaphylaxis: A serious form of physical allergy associated with mast cell degranulation. J Allergy Clin Immunol 75:479, 1985.
5. Wade JP, Liang MH, Sheffer AL: Exercise-induced anaphylaxis: Epidemiologic observations. In Biochemistry of the Acute Allergic Reactions: Fifth International Symposium. New York, Alan R. Liss, 1989, pp 175–182.

43. THE ATHLETE WITH EPILEPSY

Donald R. Bennett, M.D., and Barry D. Jordan, M.D., M.P.H.

1. Are epileptics at increased risk for having seizures during physical exercise?

No. "Epilepsy prefers to attack when the person is off guard, sleeping, resting, idling."[9] Since ancient times, the rarity of exercise-precipitated seizures has been documented. These writings also suggest that a regular physical exercise program may be helpful in improving seizure control. The reasons for this remain speculative. Changes in acid-base balance, the release of β-endorphins, in brain tissue (β-endorphins tend to inhibit seizures), sensory inhibition, and increased vigilance and attention have been suggested.

2. Do you believe that epileptics attending high schools and colleges are well represented on various athletic teams?

They are underrepresented. In a high school district with a total enrollment of 5792 students, not 1 of the 17 epileptics identified by the school nurse participated in team sports. Only 1 of approximately 3000 student athletes participated in sports (gymnastics) in a Division 1 National College Athletic Association (NCAA) conference.

3. Does a regular physical exercise program adversely affect the pharmacokinetics of antiepileptic drugs?

Theoretically, exercise may reduce serum levels of the anticonvulsant drugs because of its hepatic enzyme-inducing effect, and postexercise ketosis may increase serum levels. However, limited studies in adults taking phenytoin and valproic acid have shown that physical training does not significantly alter serum anticonvulsant levels. More recent evidence suggests that gabapentin levels may be reduced during exercise as the result of increased creatinine clearance associated with increased cardiac output and increased renal blood flow. The pharmacokinetics of antiepileptic drugs also may be altered by significant changes in weight or body composition.

4. Is the injury rate for epileptics who participate in sports the same as for their peers?

Yes. There is no evidence that seizure-related injuries are increased in epileptics participating in sports. The same injury rate (3%) has been reported for epileptics as well as nonepileptics regardless of whether they were participating in sports. Only 9 of 274 (3.3%) consecutive immersion accidents were associated with seizures. All patients survived without neurologic deficits.

5. Do repeated blows to the head during collision or contact sports increase the seizure frequency in epileptics?

Probably not, although the data supporting this are limited. Based on their 34-year experience in caring for over 15,000 epileptic children, two neurologists could not recall a single instance of seizure recurrence after head trauma in any of their epileptic athletes.

6. What is the most frequent cause of accidental death during a seizure?

Drowning. Accidents are responsible for 7% of epileptic deaths; however, only 5% of these are related to injuries incurred during a seizure. Bath tub drownings—not drowning in the sea or swimming pool—account for most of the immersion deaths. The risk of drowning secondary to a seizure during swimming may be reduced by using the buddy system or swimming in the presence of a lifeguard.

7. What is the prognosis for epilepsy?

Contrary to popular belief, epilepsy is not a lifelong condition. Studies in children have shown the remission rate for epileptics who have been seizure free on medication for 2–4 years is approximately 65% to 75% after the antiepileptic drugs are withdrawn. Many of these remissions are permanent. Most relapses will occur during the first few months to 1 year after withdrawing the medication.

8. Should epileptics whose seizures are under excellent control (no seizures in the past year) be allowed to participate in collision or contact sports?

Yes. The results from a survey of 6 neurologists on whether epileptics whose seizures are under excellent control can participate in collision or contact sports are tabulated below. Of the 22 sports, the only activities contraindicated were auto racing, boxing, motorcycling, rodeo, and ski jumping. With less optimal control, the number of these sports as well as other athletic activities recommended for participation will naturally decrease.

Recommendations for Participating in Collision and Contact Sports for Epileptics Whose Seizures Are Under Excellent Control

SPORT	P Q C	SPORT	P Q C	SPORT	P Q C	SPORT	P Q C
Auto racing	–	Field hockey	+	Motorcycling	–	Soccer	+
Bob sledding	±	Football	+	Polo	±	Water polo	±
Boxing	–	Gymnastics	+	Rodeo	–	Water skiing	±
Cycling	+	Ice hockey	+	Rugby	+	Wrestling	±
Diving	±	Karate/Judo	+	Downhill skiing	+		
Equestrian	+	Lacrosse	+	Ski jumping	–		

P, Recommend participation; Q, questionable participation; C, contraindicated.

9. How would you evaluate an epileptic in previous excellent seizure control who suffered a breakthrough seizure during practice or competition?

The first step is to establish whether the seizure was provoked by a head injury, hyperthermia, metabolic or electrolyte abnormalities, excessive fatigue, sleep deprivation, or subtherapeutic anticonvulsant serum levels. The history, physical examination, and the results of the blood studies should provide the answers. In addition, a computed tomographic (CT) scan of the head should be obtained if you suspect a head injury, the neurologic examination is abnormal, particularly if focal deficits such as a hemiparesis are present, or if the postictal period is prolonged.

10. Suppose the serum anticonvulsant levels were subtherapeutic in the epileptic discussed in question 9. When should he or she be allowed to resume practice?

The most common cause for a breakthrough seizure is noncompliance in taking anticonvulsant drugs. If the level is subtherapeutic, and previous serum anticonvulsant serum levels had been therapeutic, resume the same dose and recheck the level. The time when this should be done is dependent on the half-life of the anticonvulsant (5 × the drug half-life). For example, the average half-life of phenytoin is 24 hours. Therefore, the serum level should be checked 5 days later when a steady state should have been achieved. Once the level is therapeutic, the athlete can resume playing the sport.

If the anticonvulsant level is therapeutic, the athlete should not be allowed to compete, particularly in contact or collision sports, unless cleared to do so by a neurologist.

11. What side effects from anticonvulsant medications may interfere with athletic performance?

A variety of side effects, including fatigue, somnolence, dizziness, diplopia, decreased concentration, ataxia, and impaired coordination, may result from anticonvulsant use. Accordingly, potential side effects that may influence an athlete's performance or ability to compete safely should be recognized.

12. Can seizures result from exercise?

Yes, but rarely. Exercise-induced seizures may occur during prolonged exercise such as marathons or triathlons. Such seizures may be associated with underlying metabolic disturbances such as hyponatremia, hypomagnesemia, and hypoglycemia.

BIBLIOGRAPHY

1. A Randomized Study of Antiepileptic Drug Withdrawal in Patients in Remission. The Medical Research Council Antiepileptic Drug Withdrawal Study Group. Lancet 337:1175–1180, 1991.
2. Bennett DR: Sports and epilepsy: To play or not to play. Semin Neurol 1:345–357, 1981.
3. Bennett DR: Unpublished data.
4. Borgà O, Juhlin-Dannfeldt A, Dahlquist R: Plasma levels and protein binding of phenytoin during exercise in man: The effect of elevating free fatty acids. Pharmacology 16:37–43, 1978.
5. Fischer A, Daute KH: The risk of an accident in sport and at games in epileptic children. Med Sport (Berlin) 28:93–95, 1988.
6. Gates JR, Spiegel RH: Epilepsy, sports and exercise. Sports Med 15:1–5, 1993.
7. Hauser WA, Annegars JF, Elveback LR: Mortality in patients with epilepsy. Epilepsia 21:399–412, 1980.
8. Jordan BD: Epilepsy in the athlete. In Mellion MB, Walsh WM, Shelton GL (eds): The Team Physician's Handbook, 2nd ed. Philadelphia, Hanley & Belfus, 1997, pp 325–331.
9. Lennox WG, Lennox MA: Epilepsy and Related Disorders, Vol. 2. Boston, Little, Brown, 1960, pp 823–824.
10. Livingston S, Berman W: Participation of epileptic patients in sport. JAMA 224:236–238, 1973.
11. Livingston S, Pauli LL, Pruce I: Epilepsy and drowning in children. Br Med J 2:515–516, 1977.
12. Marsh TD, Garnett WR, Poyner WJ, Pellock JM: Effects of exercise on valproic acid pharmacokinetics. Clin Pharmacol 2:62–64, 1983.
13. Pearn J, Bart R, Yamaoka R: Drowning risks to the epileptic: A study from Hawaii. Br Med J 2:1284–1285, 1978.
14. Tettenborn B, Kramer G: Total patient care in epilepsy. Epilepsia 33(Suppl 1):528–532, 1992.
15. van Linschoten R, Backx FJG, Mulder OGM, Meinardi H: Epilepsy and sports. Sports Med 10:9–19, 1990.
16. Zielinski JJ: Epilepsy and mortality rate and cause of death. Epilepsia 15:191–201, 1974.

44. EXERCISE-INDUCED HEADACHE

Mark S. Williams, D.O., Kenneth B. Batts, D.O., and John M. Henderson, D.O.

1. Describe the characteristics of exertional or exercise-induced headaches.

Athletes may encounter sports-related headaches during or after competition. Usually the headaches are benign and can be described by specific characteristics inherent to participation in the event. The typical headache is abrupt in onset, and throbbing; location varies. The headache may persist as a dull ache after the event, but usually resolves within a few hours and is not associated with neurologic defects. In each activity, intrathoracic pressure may be increased by coughing, bending over, sexual orgasm, or Valsalva maneuver, resulting in increased intracranial pressure and decreased cerebral blood flow, which lead to headache. Treatment should focus on the precipitating cause.

2. What is the most common type of exercise-induced headache?

Tension headaches occur as commonly in athletes as in the general population. The pain is described as a dull, constant, bandlike pressure originating in the occipitocervical region and radiating to the temporofrontal area of the head. The headaches may be daily or seasonal and vary in intensity, location, and duration. Although the actual mechanism is thought to be constant contraction of scalp muscles, additional psychologic factors such as fatigue, anxiety, emotional stress, and depression may play a role in headache attacks.

3. How should you evaluate an athlete who presents with a headache?

First and foremost, a thorough history of headache characteristics, duration, and relation to the athletic endeavor should be obtained. For athletes with recurrent headaches and no neurologic sequela, a headache diary describing diet, medication usage, psychosocial stressors, and pre-headache activities can be helpful in determining a pattern to the headaches and devising strategies for therapy. Ominous signs and symptoms may need further neurologic evaluation and hospitalization. Treatment needs to be individualized so that the athlete can compete without limiting his or her performance.

4. Describe an effort headache.

Effort headaches occur in various sporting events such as marathons and triathlons, in which the participants are exposed to extremes of heat, humidity, altitude, and inadequate nutrition. The headaches usually occur at the end of exercise, last for at least 1 hour, and have migrainous qualities such as unilateral location, visual aura, and vomiting. Treatment consists of maintaining hydration during the event, along with proper conditioning and warm-up periods to adapt the sympathetic nervous system gradually, thereby preventing the vascular imbalance of a migraine headache.

5. Name the five forms of posttraumatic headaches.

Posttraumatic Headaches

FORM	EXAMPLE
Chronic muscle contraction	Resembles muscle contraction headache
Migraine-like	Footballer's migraine, indistinguishable from migraine headache
Mixed	Mixture of above, muscle contraction headache with super-imposed migraine
Dysautonomic	Injury to sympathetic fibers near carotid artery may result in Horner's syndrome
Second-impact	Caused by multiple minor blows to the head

6. What is footballer's migraine?

Footballer's migraine was first described in British athletes participating in club soccer games as a classic migraine occurring immediately after a player headed the ball. Associated symptoms include visual field deficits, nausea, and vomiting. The migraine is thought to result from distortion and spasm of the basal cerebral blood vessels from an improper "header." Skilled soccer players hit the ball with the frontal region of the head rather than the parietal portion of the skull, which requires contraction of the lateral neck muscles to direct the ball to a teammate. This same headache pattern has been reported in American football, rugby, boxing, and wrestling.

7. What is second-impact catastrophic headache?

Second-impact headache develops after repeated contact to the head, producing diffuse brain swelling and loss of vasomotor tone. Increased intracranial pressure results in midbrain and temporal lobe compression, cranial nerve palsies, and diminished function of the reticular-activating center. Posttraumatic headaches may lead to coma or a postconcussive syndrome with sequelae of persistent headaches, inability to concentrate, and irritability that last several months after the event.

8. What are the characteristics of weightlifter's headache?

Weightlifter's headache occurs during power lifting as the athlete performs a Valsalva maneuver that increases the intrathoracic and intracranial pressures. The headache is usually located in the occipital or upper cervical region and has been described as an abrupt, burning pain gradually persisting as a dull, steady ache that incapacitates the athlete. In certain cases, the headache may be induced by strain of the cervical ligaments and persist for weeks. Cervical spine radiographs should be performed to identify vertebral instability from spondylolysis and spondylolisthesis as well as vertebral body or disc compression.

9. What is the pathophysiology of an altitude headache during acute mountain sickness?

During the ascent to elevations above 3000 meters, mountain climbers hyperventilate to maintain minute volume in the hypoxic environment, thus producing cerebral vasoconstriction and an aura. The effort of climbing also increases blood pressure, resulting in extracranial vasodilation and the pain of a migrainous headache. Hyperventilation syndrome leads to reduction in carbon dioxide (decreased PCO_2) and respiratory alkalosis. To compensate, the kidneys increase excretion of bicarbonate (decreased HCO_3), producing metabolic acidosis. Altitude headaches can be prevented by acclimatization, gradual ascent to higher elevations, and prophylaxis with acetazolamide. Treatment in the acute situation with neurologic symptoms of cerebral edema includes rapid descent, oxygen, and corticosteroids.

10. What types of headaches are associated with diving?

Divers experience vascular headaches due to carbon dioxide accumulation from "skip breathing." They also experience muscle contraction headaches from contracting the orofacial muscles tightly around the mouthpiece. Goggle headaches result from pressure on the cutaneous supraorbital and infraorbital facial nerves from tight-fitting masks.

11. Describe how athletic equipment may contribute to headaches.

One cause of headaches is external compression of the skull produced by helmets or headgear used for protection in many modern sports. Football, lacrosse, hockey, cycling, and skydiving require helmet use for participation. Other sports, such as wrestling, boxing, and scuba diving, require forms of head or face protection that may produce compression-type headache. Simple repairs and adjustments to faulty or tight headgear may resolve and prevent significant discomfort for the athlete. Many helmets require pneumatic devices for a proper fit. Mouthguards used to protect the dentition of athletes must be properly fitted but may initiate headaches by causing abnormal closure of the temporomandibular joint.

12. What drug regimens are available for treating headaches in athletes?

Each treatment regimen should be individualized so as not to affect the athlete's performance adversely and to provide maximal relief of symptoms and not hide a serious intracranial problem. The most common medications used for relief of certain headaches in athletes and their adverse effects are listed in the tables below.

Common Drug Therapy for Headaches in Athletes

HEADACHE TYPE	DRUG THERAPY
Benign exertional headache	Acetaminophen, nonsteroidal antiinflammatory drugs (NSAIDs)
Tension headache (muscle contraction)	NSAIDs, muscle relaxants
Migraine (common, classic)	Abortive: ergotamine tartrate, naproxen sodium, Midrin, sumatriptan Prophylactic: beta-blockers, calcium channel blockers, NSAIDs, tricyclic antidepressants
Footballer's migraine	Prophylactic ergotamine
Weightlifter's headache	NSAIDs
Altitude headache	Prophylactic acetazolamide, corticosteroids

Major Adverse Effects of Specific Medications for Exercise-induced Headaches

MEDICATION	ADVERSE EFFECTS
NSAIDS	Nausea, epigastric pain, peptic ulcers, dizziness, rash, tinnitus
Beta-blockers	Hypotension, bradycardia, fatigue, sleep disturbance, depression
Ergotamine	Hypertension, transient tachycardia or bradycardia, weakness, vomiting, vertigo
Calcium channel blockers	Constipation, dizziness, nausea, hypotension, peripheral edema
Tricyclic antidepressants	Constipation, dry mouth, blurred vision, orthostatic hypotension
Sumatriptan	Arrhythmias, angina, dizziness, vertigo, paresthesia
Muscle relaxants	Lightheadedness, dizziness, drowsiness, nausea, allergic manifestations

13. Describe the treatment for tension headaches in athletes.

NSAIDs and acetaminophen have been the traditional medications for tension headaches in both athletes and nonathletes. Because of the inordinate amount of stress placed on competitive athletes by coaches, family, and the athletes themselves to gain the winning edge, psychotherapy and biofeedback have been incorporated in the treatment of tension headaches. Other adjuvant therapy includes cervical massage, hydrotherapy, iontophorosis, preactivity dosing with acetaminophen or NSAIDs, and hypnosis. Besides the use of analgesics and NSAIDs, anxiolytics and antidepressants are useful in some athletes experiencing psychogenic tension headaches.

14. Other than medications, what can be used to prevent headaches in the athlete?

Conditioning plays an important role in prevention of headaches. The better conditioned an athlete, the smaller the likelihood of developing exercise headaches. The conditioning period can be used as a diagnostic tool to reproduce the athlete's headache in relation to heart rate and maximal effort during exercise. Athletes who develop headaches may be able to control recurrence by a slow, steady warm-up period before practice and competition. Behavior modification has been used for relief of refractory forms of exercise-induced headaches.

15. What common substances may produce headache in athletes?

Alcohol, analgesic abuse, anabolic steroids, nitrate or nitrite compounds, monosodium glutamate, caffeine, nicotine, and other stimulants are commonly misused and may precipitate headaches. The physician must be aware of commonly prescribed medications for headaches as well as over-the-counter preparations and illegal substances in the community. A complete history of substance use must be taken and close monitoring for signs and symptoms should be done at all levels of athletic involvement.

16. Are all exercise-induced headaches benign?

A small percentage of athletes experiencing exercise-induced headaches have intracranial lesions that exhibit similar signs and symptoms as exertional headaches. Therefore, it is imperative to evaluate the athlete's neurologic status systematically through a complete history and physical examination. Many intracranial lesions, such as posterior fossa tumors, arteriovenous anomalies, Arnold-Chiari malformations, aneurysms, and subdural hematomas, have similar characteristics to exercise-induced headaches.

17. What symptoms should signal concern for possible intracranial pathology in benign exertional headaches?

A change in the intensity or pattern of a headache warrants further evaluation. Headaches associated with recurrent memory loss, inability to concentrate, decrease in attention span, speech difficulty, visual field deficits, neck stiffness, and gait abnormalities indicate the need to repeat the neurologic examination. If focal neurologic signs are noted, the athlete needs immediate hospital evaluation. In athletes, the cardinal sign of head and neck pathology after trauma is a headache.

18. What is the role of cervical spine radiographs in the evaluation of exertional headaches?
Cervical spine radiographs may be used as a diagnostic tool to help detect osseous abnormalities and ligamentous instabilities. Cervical views assess subluxation, cervical lordosis, neuroforaminal canals for osteophyte impingement, and congenital fusion of vertebral bodies. Included in the cervical series are anteroposterior, lateral, oblique, open-mouth, and full flexion and extension views.

19. Describe the differences in the use of computed tomography (CT) and magnetic resonance imaging (MRI) in the evaluation of exertional headaches.
MRI is now considered far superior to CT in studying soft tissue lesions indicating ischemia, infarction, and tumors, especially in the posterior fossa. CT scanning offers one specific advantage in remaining the modality of choice for evaluating bony detail of the cervical skeleton and calvarium. The advantages of MRI compared with CT include avoiding radiation exposure and an allergic reaction to the contrast material needed to enhance epidural and subdural hematomas. CT is still more widely available than MRI. Other imaging techniques, such as single-photon emission CT may provide future pathogenic and diagnostic information.

BIBLIOGRAPHY

1. Basoglu T, Ozbenli T, Bernay I, et al: Demonstration of frontal hypoperfusion in benign exertional headache by technetium-99m-HMPAO SPECT. J Nucl Med 37:1172–1174.
2. Bennett DR: The athlete with headache. In Mellion MB, Walsh WM, Shelton GL (eds): The Team Physician's Handbook, 2nd ed. Philadelphia, Hanley & Belfus, 1997.
3. Cacayorin ED, Petro GR, Hochhauser L: Headache in the athlete and radiographic evaluation. Clin Sports Med 6:739–749, 1987.
4. Diamond S, Soloman GD, Freitag FG: Headache in sports. In Jordan BC, Tsairis P, Warren RF (eds): Sports Neurology. Rockville, MD, Aspen Publishers, 1989.
5. Dimeff RJ: Headaches in the athlete. Clin Sports Med 11:339–349, 1992.
6. Garfinkel D: Headache in athletes. Phys Sportsmed 11(1):67–75, 1983.
7. Lambert RW, Burnet DL: Prevention of exercise induced migraine by quantitative warm-up. Headache 25:317–319, 1985.
8. Massey EW: Effort headache in runners. Headache 22:99–100, 1982.
9. Matthews WB: Footballer's migraine. BMJ 2:326–327, 1972.
10. McCarthy P: Athletes' headaches: Not necessarily "little" problems. Phys Sportsmed 16(10):169–173, 1988.
11. Pascual J, Iglesias F, Oterino A, et al: Cough, exertional, and sexual headaches: An analysis of 72 benign and symptomatic cases. Neurology 46:1520–1524, 1996.
12. Paulson GW: Weightlifter's headache. Headache 23:193–194, 1983.
13. Perry WJ: Exertional headache. Phys Sportsmed 13(10):95–99, 1985.
14. Rooke ED: Benign exertional headache. Med Clin North Am 52:801–809, 1968.
15. Yetter JF III, Butcher JD, Uyemura MC: Neurologic injuries. In Lillegard WS, Rucker KS (eds): Handbook of Sports Medicine: A Symptom-Oriented Approach. Boston, Butterworth-Heinemann, 1993.

45. SPORTS DERMATOLOGY

Richard Levandowski, M.D., Gary Keogh, M.D., MRCGP, DA(UK), and Joseph P. Mullane, M.D.

1. What is the cause of red marks and blisters on the area where a brace or pads are in contact with the skin?
This irritation is typical of contact dermatitis. The area is reddened where contact has taken place (where the knee brace was in contact with the skin), but this must be differentiated from irritation due to chaffing from sweat, a fungal infection, or a bacterial infection. Usually 0.5–1% hydrocortisone cream or 0.1% triamcinolone applied daily relieves itching and rash.

2. Is poison ivy contagious? Can it be spread by contact?

No. Poison ivy is not spread by scratching or person-to-person contact. Once the oil from the poison ivy plant makes contact with the skin, antibodies to allergens in the oil bind within a half hour, and this histaminic reaction causes the itch. The later eruptions are due to a smaller amount of oil and thus less inoculum, causing a less severe delayed reaction.

3. Which are the most common infections that preclude wrestling participation?

Herpes simplex (herpes gladiatorum), impetigo, pustular acne, fungal infections (e.g., ringworm), and open wounds.

4. What should be done about blisters on the foot?

First, prevent them. Wear properly fitted shoes along with a pair of "wicking" socks under regular socks and use foot powders, moleskin, and Second Skin to reduce shearing forces (especially when wearing new shoes or starting a new sport after having been inactive for awhile). This protects skin as long as the area is not overused before building up a callus. The participant can usually feel the blister being formed as a "hot spot." Prevention is the key.

If a blister is formed and it is over 2 cm, drain it using sterile technique. Keep the roof of the blister intact (this will form an anatomic barrier and help start a callus). Cover the area with mupirocin cream or ointment (Bactroban) and a dressing. Hydrophilic dressings for protection of the area also are available and they may allow the athlete to participate.

5. If lesions are seen that look like herpes blisters with a crusted yellow appearance and a red weeping base, is this impetigo?

Most commonly it is. Impetigo is a bacterial infection caused primarily be streptococci or staphylococci. During the weeping phase, it is extremely contagious. An athlete cannot participate until the lesions dry, which most commonly occurs in 3–5 days but can be as long as 10 days.

6. How is impetigo treated?

Impetigo may be treated with oral antibiotics (most commonly erythromycin) or an oral cephalosporin, which are equally effective. Also, a penicillinase-resistant penicillin such as dicloxacillin or cloxacillin will be efficacious. Remove the crusts and treat with topical mupirocin cream or ointment (Bactroban) twice a day. Both treatments should be for 10 days. The athlete should be on antibiotics for at least 3 days and the lesions must be dry 2 days before athletic contact is resumed.

7. How can impetigo be differentiated from herpes infection?

The important differentiation between impetigo and herpes is that impetiginous lesions usually become pustular within a few days after appearance and cause regional lymphadenopathy without constitutional symptoms. Herpes starts as redness followed by vesicles on an erythematous base. Culture is necessary for definitive diagnosis.

8. Explain what type of herpes affects wrestlers and what the recommendations are for participation and treatment.

The characteristic appearance of herpes simplex virus infection (herpes gladiatorum) is a cluster of vesicles on an erythematous base. Herpes gladiatorum is somewhat unusual in its presentation. It can present in a linear fashion with multiple lesions or appear as a single lesion of contact anywhere on the body. There are fluid-filled vesicles that, when opened, do not usually appear reddened but weep. This is a most contagious lesion and participation cannot be permitted until the area crusts and dries. Crusting alone is not enough; the lesion must be dry for at least 2 days. The athlete should have a course of at least 5 days of acyclovir (Zovirax), 200–400 mg, 5 times/day for 5 days, or famciclovir (Famvir), 500 mg 2–3 times/day for 5 days.

9. What is herpetic whitlow?

Herpetic whitlow, which can be distinguished from bacterial infections around the nailbed by its vesicular/papular or bullous appearance without pustules, will usually accompany a herpes infection. The same precautions apply as in herpes gladiatorum with respect to participation.

10. Are sexually transmitted diseases such as crabs, also known as pediculosis pubis, and scabies (caused by *Sarcoptes scabiei*) contagious? Where are they normally seen? What is the treatment?

Crab lice are usually transmitted from person-to-person by intimate contact. Head and body lice are spread by the sharing of personal articles, i.e., clothing and hairbrushes. Pubic lice do not seem to spread as quickly and their movements are much slower. Sexual contact is the most common form of contact. And yes, in the case of pubic lice, you can catch it from a toilet seat! Several over-the-counter preparations are available. The most effective nonprescription products contain pyrethrins and piperonyl butoxide. One application should be effective in killing both the adult lice and nits. Kwell is the most common prescription drug used in the United States. This product contains lindane and should be avoided in small children and pregnant women.

In the transmission of scabies, evidence indicates that prolonged intimate contact is necessary as suggested by the high incidence of transmission among sexual partners and low transmissions that occur among family members and roommates. However, younger children who are frequently hugged are more likely to have the disease than older children.

Scabies usually presents as exquisitely pruritic papules and burrows in the region of the genitalia, waistline, fingerwebs, wrists, axillae, and buttocks. The definitive diagnosis can be made by visualizing the mite under the microscope. Microscopic identification is difficult, and if clinical symptoms persist treat empirically. The treatment is to apply 5% permethrin cream at bedtime and allow it to stay on overnight (at least 8 hours) and then it is rinsed off. All clothing and bed linen should be washed in hot water. The athlete may return to contact the day after treatment.

11. What is molluscum contagiosum? How is it spread?

Molluscum contagiosum is a viral infection that spreads through autoinoculation or person-to-person contact. The lesions are recognized by their firm papular umbilicated form and are white or skin colored. They are removed most commonly by curettage, trichloroacetic acid, electrodesiccation, tretinoin, or cryotherapy. Athletes may resume contact sports 48 hours after lesions are gone.

12. How do you prevent athlete's foot?

Athlete's foot is a fungal infection spread from person-to-person or by contact—for example, by a contaminated towel or mat. Preventive measures include:
1. Keep the feet dry.
2. Avoid occlusive footwear or synthetic stockings, rubber-soled shoes, or plastic insoles.
3. Use cotton and wool or polypropolene socks, and change them one to three times per day.
4. Use shower clogs.
5. Use fungicidal spray, powders, creams, or lotions.
6. Alternate pairs of sneakers if available.
7. Disinfect shower rooms and locker rooms daily.

13. What causes folliculitis?

It is a low-grade infection occurring in areas with short, coarse hairs. Folliculitis that affects the deeper layers of the skin is normally called pyoderma or impetigo. If this occurs, furuncles (boils) occur and possibly carbuncles. Carbuncles are caused by communication between infected follicles.

14. Is folliculitis contagious?

Yes. Conditions increasing the spread are communal contact with contaminated fomites, the use of occlusive equipment, and conditions that produce wet, hot, macerated skin.

15. Do certain factors predispose one to folliculitis?

Predispositions to folliculitis include diabetes and also certain occupational exposures such as tars and oils, especially combined with skin occlusion. A condition called hot tub folliculitis is a pseudomonal infection. It is usually self-limited and resolves within 7–10 days.

16. Are fungal skin infections contagious?

Yes. Circumstances increasing the chances of spread include contact sports and communal facilities; for example, locker rooms and sharing of towels and clothing.

17. When can an athlete with a fungal infection compete?

The athlete may participate in a contact sport after 3 days of treatment with oral and topical agents if the affected area of skin can be securely and confidently covered. For example, athletes with jock itch (tinea cruris) can often play if the affected area is covered. Treat with topical agents.

18. Is acne a problem in sports?

Acne is a skin disorder resulting from dysfunction of the pilosebaceous unit. It is associated with androgen stimulation, bacterial growth, disordered keratinization, and mechanical irritation. In contact sports, the friction associated with athletic gear, such as football helmets, as well as the increased sweating and humidity involved in activity, can make matters worse. Psychological stress seems to exacerbate this condition. A generalized increase in the formation of acne lesions is associated with the use of androgenic/anabolic steroids.

19. How can acne be helped in the athlete?

The wearing of clean, dry, loose-fitting, absorbent cotton clothing decreases the problem. Wet clothing should be changed as often as possible. The environment is important—working out in minimal clothing and in a cool, well-ventilated environment can help. In an athlete with large, cystic acne vulgaris, contact sports or even the protective gear can lead to rupture of the comedones and cysts. This situation can lead to enlarged lesions, a delay in healing, and more scarring. The athlete should be advised regarding this, and the decision as to whether or not he or she should take part in the activity has to be made by the physician. Remember that in a nodulo-cystic or conglobate type of acne, the open sores place the athlete (e.g., a wrestler) at risk for other infectious and contagious diseases, such as herpes or impetigo.

20. For which skin conditions are topical steroids used?

Topical steroids are used for inflammatory skin conditions such as contact, atopic, and sebor-rheic dermatitides and also in hyperplastic disorders, such as psoriasis. They are used commonly in granulomatous diseases such as sarcoid or connective tissue diseases such as cutaneous discoid lupus erythematosus. At least 20 brands are marketed that are available in different vehicles and strengths. A weak formulation of 1% hydrocortisone is available over-the-counter without a pre-scription. The most common reason that a prescribed corticosteroid is ineffective is that it is given for the wrong diagnosis or in too small an amount. Treatment of choice is based on diagnosis; cu-taneous fungal or bacterial infections would be inappropriately treated using topical steroids.

21. For which skin conditions are topical steroids contraindicated?

Some other conditions that are generally not treated with topical corticosteroids include herpes simplex, impetigo, acne, urticaria, ichthyosis, and rosacea.

Hydrocortisone is absorbed six times as well to the forehead as to the forearm, and 42 times as well through scrotal skin. To avoid adverse effects, a low-potency agent is used. An alternative approach is to choose a more potent medication for short-term treatment and then either discon-tinue it or substitute a low-potency agent for maintenance or long-term use , depending on the diag-nosis and the area involved. For example, in the axilla, where occlusion occurs, a weak corticosteroid such as Cortistan 1 percent results in a middle-strength effect.

Familiarize yourself with one or two creams, ointments, or lotions in each of the major potency classes:

- 6 and 7 being mild
- 4 and 5 intermediate
- 2 and 3 potent
- 1 is a new group of superpotent agents that are not commonly used.

The least expensive full-strength topical steroid is triamcinolone, which is available as a generic preparation in amounts up to 240 gm.

22. How do you decide which vehicle to use for the steroid medication?

You may need a certain type of ointment or cream depending on the patient's tolerance or allergies. For example, he or she may be allergic to preservatives. Also, it depends on the location of the skin problem and whether it is weeping and wet or dry and scaly. Creams are used for acute and subacute dermatitis where there is oozing, because creams are miscible with serous fluids. Ointments can be used for chronic dermatitis with scaling or itching. Steroid solutions, lotions, or gels are useful in hairy or intertriginous regions or in the ear canals.

23. Discuss the side effects of topical steroids.

Avoiding side effects of corticosteroids is important. Systemic effects from topical corticosteroids are rare in dermatologic use, but the potent topical steroids produce atrophy of the epidermis and dermis in 3 weeks or less. If atrophy is to be avoided, there is only one class of drugs to use—hydrocortisone alcohol or acetate 1%. Lesions on the eyelids are an exception to this. Hydrocortisone valerate 0.2% is much less atrophogenic than other corticosteroids.

Occlusion increases the effectiveness of the corticosteroid but side effects appear more rapidly. Prolonged use of corticosteroids is associated with rosacea, dilated blood vessels, and perioral dermatitis resembling acne. Again, prolonged use around the eyes has been associated with glaucoma and cataract formation.

Systemic effects from absorbed corticosteroids in adults do not develop unless more than half the body is treated with high-potency corticosteroids under plastic occlusions and for several months. The effects include hypertension, glucose intolerance, glaucoma, salt and water retention, and depressed pituitary adrenal responsiveness. However, in small children without occlusion after use of potent topical steroids, growth retardation and hypertension have been reported.

Because of tachyphylaxis, a good approach is to use a more potent steroid initially to control the situation, and then change to a low-potency steroid if needed.

BIBLIOGRAPHY

1. Arndt K, Korizzo J: Patient Care May 30, 1992, pp 115–120.
2. Barker LR, et al: Principles of Ambulatory Medicine. Baltimore, Williams & Wilkins, 1986.
3. Billstein SA, Mattaliano VJ: Med Clin North Am 74:1487–1505, 1990.
4. Fitzpatrick TB, et al: Color Atlas and Synopsis of Clinical Dermatology. New York, McGraw Hill, 1990.
5. Lillegard WA: Dermatologic problems in the athlete. Sports Medicine Review. Kansas City, MO, American Academy of Family Physicians, 1993.
6. Wilson JD, et al: Harrison's Principles of Internal Medicine, 13th ed. New York, McGraw Hill, 1994.

46. ANEMIA, ATHLETIC PSEUDOANEMIA, AND SICKLE CELL DISEASE

E. *Randy Eichner*, M.D., FACSM

ATHLETIC PSEUDOANEMIA

1. What is sports anemia?

Athletes, especially endurance athletes, tend to have lower hematocrits and hemoglobin concentrations than do sedentary people. In other words, athletes tend to be judged as slightly "anemic" when compared with norms from the general population. This has been called sports anemia. Sports anemia, however, is a misnomer because the most common cause of a low hematocrit in an athlete is a false anemia. This false anemia is due to regular aerobic exercise, which expands the baseline plasma volume, diluting the red blood cells and thus the hematocrit and hemoglobin concentration. In other words, the naturally lower hematocrit of the endurance athlete is a dilutional pseudoanemia.

2. How does aerobic exercise expand the plasma volume?

It expands it as an adaptation to the acute loss of plasma volume, or hemoconcentration, that accompanies each workout. Vigorous exercise reduces plasma volume by (1) increasing mean arterial blood pressure and thus capillary hydrostatic pressure; (2) generating lactic acid and other metabolites in working muscle that increase tissue osmotic pressure; and (3) producing sweat. To adapt, the body releases renin, aldosterone, and vasopressin to conserve water and salt. Also, albumin is added to the blood. As a result, the baseline plasma volume expands.

3. What good is the expanded plasma volume?

It confers two benefits: (1) better athleticism and (2) better health. The athletic pseudoanemia is a cardinal part of aerobic fitness. The rise in plasma volume increases the cardiac stroke volume. This increase more than offsets the fall in hemoglobin concentration per unit of blood so that more oxygen is delivered to muscles. Also, the athlete's blood is "thinned" in a healthful way: both hemoglobin and fibrinogen are diluted. This makes blood flow more easily and clot less readily and thus helps prevent heart attack and stroke. The "unhealthy mirror image" of the athlete is the sedentary, obese man with "stress erythrocytosis" or "thick blood," owing to a subnormal plasma volume.

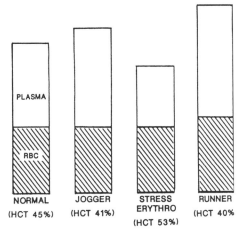

Schematic hematocrit for a normal man, a male jogger, a man with stress erythrocytosis, and a male elite runner. Note that the differences in the first three examples are in plasma volume and that the elite runner has a small expansion of red cell mass but a large expansion of plasma volume, which keeps his hematocrit low.

TRUE ANEMIA IN ATHLETES

4. What is the most common true anemia in athletes?

As in the general population, it is iron deficiency anemia. "Foot-strike hemolysis," or exertional hemolysis, occurs in some athletes, but generally does not cause anemia.

5. Are athletes uniquely prone to iron deficiency anemia?

Probably not. The claim that women athletes, as a group, are prone to iron deficiency anemia is unwarranted, because many studies lack proper control groups or fail to consider athletic pseudoanemia. Only minute amounts of iron are lost in sweat, so the preeminent cause of iron deficiency in athletic women—as in nonathletic women—is too little iron in their diet to meet physiologic needs. Many athletic women, especially "low-weight" athletes like distance runners, gymnasts, and ballet dancers, cut back on calories and thus iron. Also, because many women athletes are modified vegetarians, much iron in their diet is not highly bioavailable.

6. What about gastrointestinal bleeding in athletes?

Gastrointestinal bleeding—usually occult, minor, and brief and more common during racing than routine training—occurs in some endurance athletes, like distance runners, cyclists, and triathletes. Seldom is the bleeding frequent or severe enough to cause iron deficiency anemia, although rare athletes have had major bleeds. The bleeding site usually is the stomach, apparently from superficial "stress ulcers"; occasionally the site is the colon, apparently from "ischemic colitis," as blood during strenuous exertion is diverted away from the gut and to the working muscles. These ulcers heal in a few days.

7. What is foot-strike hemolysis?

Foot-strike hemolysis is intravascular hemolysis, or the bursting of red blood cells in the blood stream as the foot strikes the ground. Originally described in marchers and runners, it was attributed to impact. But the recent finding of mild intravascular hemolysis in swimmers and rowers suggests that impact is not always key in the genesis of exertional hemolysis.

8. How is foot-strike hemolysis diagnosed and treated?

Foot-strike, or exertional, hemolysis is characterized by a subnormal serum or plasma concentration of haptoglobin, the protein that picks up free hemoglobin in the plasma and delivers it to the liver for salvage. The peripheral blood smear is usually normal. The reticulocyte count may be slightly elevated, as the bone marrow compensates for the mild hemolysis. The mean red cell volume (MCV) may also be slightly elevated, reflecting the preferential hemolysis of older red cells, which are smaller than normal, and their replacement by reticulocytes, which are larger than normal. Foot-strike hemolysis is more salient in heavy runners with "stomping" gaits in thin shoes on hard roads and can thus be mitigated by "cushioning"; that is, by attention to weight, gait, shoes, and terrain.

9. How is iron deficiency anemia diagnosed in athletes?

Classically, the MCV is low, the peripheral blood smear shows hypochromic, microcytic red cells, and the serum ferritin concentration is subnormal.

10. How can iron deficiency anemia by prevented in athletes?

Iron deficiency can be prevented in most athletes by paying attention to their diets. To increase dietary iron absorption, athletes should (1) eat more lean red meat or dark meat of chicken; (2) improve iron absorption from bread and cereal by avoiding coffee or tea with meals and drinking instead a source of vitamin C, such as orange juice; (3) cook occasionally in cast-iron skillets and pans; acidic foods especially—such as vegetable soup and tomato sauce—will leach iron from the cookware; and (4) eat poultry or seafood with dried beans or peas; the animal protein increases absorption of iron in the vegetables.

11. When do iron supplements come into play?

Only when, for example, a female athlete repeatedly develops iron deficiency anemia despite the above dietary advice. One might reasonably treat such an athlete preventively with, for example, ferrous sulfate, 325 mg two or three times a week.

12. Does a marginal or low serum ferritin value, in the absence of anemia, limit athletic performance?

No. This notion has been proven to be a myth. The ferritin value is only an inert marker of iron stores. On the other hand, even very mild anemia from iron deficiency curbs athletic performance, and it is sometimes difficult to distinguish mild iron deficiency anemia from athletic pseudoanemia. When in doubt, an empirical trial of iron therapy—ferrous sulfate, 325 mg three times a day for 2 months—is prudent. A rise in hemoglobin concentration of at least 1 gm/dl "proves" that the mild anemia was at least in part due to iron deficiency.

SICKLE CELL DISEASE

13. Does sickle cell trait pose any harm to athletes?

With rare exceptions, no. Sickle cell trait, present in 8% of American blacks and in about 1 in 10,000 whites, is usually covert and benign. People with sickle cell trait have no anemia, no blood smear abnormalities, and few or no clinical consequences. Sickle cell trait is consistent with elite athletic performance. There are the expected number of athletes with sickle cell trait in the National Football League, in high school football, and in young elite athletes and runners from Africa.

14. Are there any complications associated with the presence of sickle cell trait?

For practical purposes, there are three: (1) hematuria and hyposthenuria; (2) splenic infarction at moderate altitude; and (3) a rare syndrome of exertional sickling, fulminant rhabdomyolysis, and collapse.

15. How do these complications affect athletes?

The hematuria, which is due to sickling and papillary necrosis deep in the renal medulla, is not necessarily caused by sports play but calls for rest until it clears. The hyposthenuria, also due to sickling in the medulla, may foster dehydration. Splenic infarction occurs mainly because of hypoxia, but exercise at altitude may contribute. Physicians should suspect splenic infarction when any person, black or white, suffers acute abdominal pain or distress when new at altitude. Early diagnosis may obviate splenectomy; bed rest, oxygen, and hydration may suffice. The dire threat in sickle cell trait is from the rare syndrome of fulminant exertional rhabdomyolysis.

16. What is fulminant exertional rhabdomyolysis?

Emerging evidence suggests that, in some military recruits and athletes with sickle cell trait, maximal exercise, especially in hot weather or when new at altitude, can evoke a life-threatening syndrome of sickling in working limbs, fulminant rhabdomyolysis, lactic acidosis, collapse, acute renal failure, and hyperkalemia. In the past two decades, about 30 such cases, many fatal, have been reported. Physicians and coaches must know that this syndrome can mimic other causes of sudden collapse, and that prompt diagnosis can save lives. To avoid this syndrome, all athletes—with or without sickle cell trait—should train wisely, stay hydrated, rest when sick, heed environmental stress and early symptoms, and never charge recklessly into heroic exercise.

BIBLIOGRAPHY

1. Eichner ER: Runner's macrocytosis: A clue to footstrike hemolysis. Am J Med 78:321–325, 1985.
2. Eichner ER: The anemias of athletes. Phys Sportsmed 14(9):122–130, 1986.
3. Eichner ER: Anemia in female athletes. Your Patient & Fitness 3(2):3–11, 1989.

 4. Eichner ER: Gastrointestinal bleeding in athletes. Phys Sportsmed 17(5):128–140, 1989.
 5. Eichner ER: Hematology of inactivity. Rheum Dis Clin North Am 16:815–825, 1990.
 6. Eichner ER: Hematuria—A diagnostic challenge. Phys Sportsmed 18(11):53–63, 1990.
 7. Eichner ER: Sickle cell trait, heroic exercise, and fatal collapse. Phys Sportsmed 21(7):51–64, 1993.
 8. Kark JA, Posey DM, Schumacher HR, Ruehle CJ: Sickle cell trait as a risk factor for sudden death in physical training. N Engl J Med 317:781–787, 1987.
 9. Lane PA, Githens JH: Splenic syndrome at mountain altitudes in sickle cell trait. Its occurrence in non-black persons. JAMA 253:2251–2254, 1985.
10. Martin TW, Weisman IM, Zeballos RJ, Stephenson SR: Exercise and hypoxia increase sickling in venous blood from an exercising limb in individuals with sickle cell trait. Am J Med 87:48–56, 1989.
11. Selby GB, Eichner ER: Endurance swimming, intravascular hemolysis, anemia, and iron depletion: A new perspective on athlete's anemia. Am J Med 81:791–794, 1986.

47. PROTEINURIA, HEMATURIA, AND ATHLETIC PSEUDONEPHRITIS

Michele Helzer-Julin, PA-C, M.S.

1. What is athletic pseudonephritis?

Athletic pseudonephritis is a benign genitourinary condition in which any combination of red blood cells (RBCs), white blood cells (WBCs), hemoglobin, myoglobin, protein, and various casts are observed in the urine of athletes following exercise. It has also been called stress hematuria, marathoner's hematuria, 10,000 meter hematuria, and march hemoglobinuria. The major difference between this and potentially serious renal disease such as glomerulonephritis is that abnormal urinary sediment following exercise will clear after the athlete rests or reduces strenuous activity for 24–48 hours.

2. What athletes are typically affected with pseudonephritis?

Athletic pseudonephritis is prevalent in sporting events that require high oxygen uptake and with distances of 10,000 meters or longer. Although most frequently seen in the running population, it has also been reported in basketball, football, baseball, cross-country skiing, rowing, lacrosse, swimming, hockey, and badminton.

3. Is athletic pseudonephritis rare or common?

Abnormal urine following exercise appears to be the rule and not the exception. Proteinuria seems to be the most consistent abnormality, with a reported incidence of 70–100% in runners. Hematuria has been reported in 10–25% of runners. Urinary casts have been reported in more than 50% of runners.

4. What are the usual formed elements of urinary sediment in athletic pseudonephritis?

The first voided specimen after exercise may contain any or all of the following: RBCs, WBCs, hemoglobin, myoglobin, protein, and various casts. Hematuria may be either gross or microscopic, and proteinuria is almost always present.

5. Is athletic pseudonephritis only evident microscopically?

No. Although routinely urinary abnormalities are only detected microscopically, occasionally gross hematuria also is observed. Gross blood urination is sometimes preceded by urinary frequency and tenesmus. Painless blood clots as large as 0.5×1.0 cm have been reported. In both male and female runners, early cystoscopies have revealed localized bladder contusions with loss of bladder epithelium and the presence of fibrinous exudates. This is a benign condition and follow-up recommendations are outlined in question 9.

6. Are any physical symptoms associated with athletic pseudonephritis?
The vast majority of patients are urologically asymptomatic; however, mild suprapubic and flank discomfort, as well as initial dysuria, may be present on occasion.

7. How are urinary abnormalities caused by athletic pseudonephritis distinguished from those caused by serious genitourinary abnormalities?
The abnormal urinary findings apparent in athletic pseudonephritis are similar to those found in serious renal diseases such as acute glomerulonephritis, pyelonephritis, acute tubular necrosis, and other degenerative or infective renal disorders. The major difference between exercise-related abnormalities and potentially serious renal disease is that abnormal urinary findings in athletic pseudonephritis will decrease or disappear after the athlete rests or reduces strenuous activity for several days. In addition, fevers and trauma are not associated with athletic pseudonephritis.

8. What findings warrant further diagnostic workup and urology referral?
1. Progressive symptoms: colic or flank pain
2. Persistence of hematuria or proteinuria beyond 48 hours after exercise
3. Positive urine culture
4. Oliguria after prolonged strenuous exercise

9. What follow-up is necessary for athletic pseudonephritis?
Proof of reversion to a normal urine after exercise-induced hematuria/proteinuria is important to exclude serious renal diseases. Repeat urinalysis is recommended after 24 to 48 hours of rest. Urine culture may be obtained if infection is suspected. If repeat urinalyses are negative, no further tests are indicated.

10. Following exercise, what is the typical time required for urinary abnormalities to return to baseline?
Rapid resolution is an important feature. Routinely urinary abnormalities should return to normal within 24–48 hours following exercise.

11. Is there any need to restrict exercise in athletes with pseudonephritis?
Exercise should be restricted for 24–48 hours in order to obtain a follow-up urinalysis. Otherwise, no exercise restrictions are required because to date no long-term deleterious effects have been associated with this condition.

12. Are there any sequelae or long-term detrimental effects from athletic pseudonephritis?
This appears to be a benign, transient, and reversible condition. Although hematuria is recurrent in as many as 50% of the patients, studies have shown renal function has remained normal on long-term follow-up. No series, thus far, has suggested an increased incidence of renal disease in athletes.

13. What are proposed etiologies for athletic pseudonephritis?
Various etiologies have been proposed to include both renal and bladder origins. Renal ischemia, increased glomerular filtration rate, increased glomerular permeability, decreased tubular reabsorption of protein, repetitive microtrauma to the kidneys, and bladder contusions have all been suggested. Exercise intensity, duration, and hydration also are factors.

BIBLIOGRAPHY

1. Abarbanel J, Benet AE, Lask D, Kimche D: Sports hematuria. J Urol 143:887–890, 1990.
2. Alyea EP, Parish HH: Renal response to exercise—urinary findings. JAMA 167:807–813, 1958.
3. Cianfiocco AJ: Renal complications of exercise. Clin Sports Med 11:437–451, 1992.
4. Clerico A, Giammattei C, Cecchini L, et al: Exercise-induced proteinuria in well-trained athletes. Clin Chem 36:562–564, 1990.

5. Elliot DL, Goldberg L, Eichner ER: Hematuria in a young recreational runner. Med Sci Sports Exerc 23:892–894, 1991.
6. Gambrell RC, Blount BW: Exercise-induced hematuria. Am Fam Physician 53:905–911, 1996.
7. Gardner KD: "Athletic pseudonephritis"—Alteration of urine sediment by athletic competition. JAMA 161:1613–1617, 1956.
8. Helzer MJ: Athletic pseudonephritis in the distance runner. Physician Assist 8:67–82, 1984.
9. Hoover DL, Cromie WJ: Theory and management of exercise-related hematuria. Physician Sportsmed 9(11):91–95, 1981.
10. Javitt NB, Miller AT: Mechanism of exercise proteinuria. J Appl Physiol 4:834–839, 1952.
11. Jones GR, Newhouse I: Sports-related hematuria: A review. Clin J Sport Med 7:119–125, 1997.
12. Kallmeyer JC: Urinary changes in ultra long-distance marathon runners. Nephron 64:119–121, 1993.
13. Poortmans JR: Exercise and renal function. Sports Med 1:125–153, 1984.
14. Poortmans JR, Geudvert C, Schorokoff, DePlaen P: Post exercise proteinuria in childhood and adolescence. Int J Sports Med 17:448–451, 1996.
15. Riess RW: Athletic hematuria and related phenomena. J Sports Med 19:381–388, 1979.
16. Robertshaw M, Cheung CK, Fairly I, Swaminathan R: Protein excretion after prolonged exercise. Ann Clin Biochem 30(Pt 1):34–37, 1993.

48. GASTROINTESTINAL PROBLEMS IN ATHLETES

James M. Lynch, M.D.

1. What effects do regular exercise have on the normal gastrointestinal (GI) tract?

Digestion is a physiologic process that takes place normally under resting conditions. Exercise causes a shifting of blood flow from the GI tract to the skeletal muscle. It is known that inactivity is associated with constipation. Regular physical activity has been assumed to have a beneficial effect on fecal elimination through easier evacuation. The amount of exercise needed to garner this benefit has not yet been delineated. Long-term effects of exercise are much more difficult to establish. Four of five large studies found that regular exercise was associated with a lower incidence of colon cancer. These studies are not conclusive, however, because of the difficulty of controlling diet in a large longitudinal study.

2. What general considerations should one be cognizant of with regard to exercise and GI disorders?

The influence of exercise on the motility of the GI tract seems to be the most common malady. GI blood loss as a result of physical activity is also a common complaint. Abdominal trauma will be seen by a sports medicine practitioner on a routine basis. Of utmost importance is the fact that athletes are subject to the same GI problems as the general population.

3. How is the upper GI tract affected by exercise?

Symptoms are reported by 10–24% of athletes. Heartburn, nausea and vomiting, and loss of appetite are most commonly reported. Heartburn seems to occur more often after intense runs, suggesting a dose response to increasing activity. Women seem to have more upper GI symptoms than men, and inexperienced athletes have more difficulty than the experienced. Exercise has profound results on esophageal motor activity and gastroesophageal reflux, both of which are intensity dependent. The amplitude, duration, and frequency of esophageal contractions decrease steadily as exercise intensity increases. Lower esophageal sphincter pressure may also decrease.

4. What is the mechanism for upper GI symptoms?

Research has focused on three main areas: gastric emptying time, gastroesophageal reflux, and gastric fluid content. Gastric emptying time is initially accelerated by exercise. When runners reach 75% VO$_2$max, gastric emptying times decrease. It has been suggested that light exercise increases gastric emptying through abdominal contractions. Increasing levels of endorphins and catecholamines, along with the reduced intestinal blood flow associated with intense exercise, may account for the decreasing emptying times. Gastroesophageal reflux seems to occur because of transient relaxations of the lower esophageal sphincter and increased swallowing of air during running. The decrease in peristaltic contractions may decrease the clearance of fluid volume from the esophagus, while the decrease in swallowing of saliva may lessen neutralization of residual acid. Gastric fluid content appears to be concentrated by exercise, although there does not seem to be any change in pH. Reflux and decreased gastric emptying seem to be the most common mechanisms for upper GI complaints.

5. What is the diagnostic work-up for an athlete with upper GI complaints?

Because these are such common complaints, many athletes accept the symptoms as being normal. For those who do seek medical attention, a thorough history is, as always, of paramount importance. The athlete should be questioned as to whether the symptoms occur without exercise. Peptic ulcer disease and disorders of the esophagus are considerations. Lactose intolerance may be a causative factor in GI complaints. Approximately 70% of the world's population loses some ability to digest lactose between the ages of 3 and 5. Nongastrointestinal causes must also be considered. Coronary artery disease may mimic gastroesophageal reflux. A physician should be mindful of this when symptoms occur only with exertion. Performance anxiety may also be a consideration.

6. What are the treatment options for an athlete with upper GI symptoms associated with exercise?

Several possibilities exist once other causes have been ruled out. Because symptoms are often related to intensity of exercise, reducing the level of exertion is a consideration, although it will not be a viable alternative in many cases. Since intense exercise slows gastric emptying, fatty high-caloric meals must be avoided. Easily digestible meals should be consumed prior to competition. Carbohydrate-rich liquids may be consumed prior to competition by athletes with severe symptoms. Antacids may be taken, but large doses may cause cramping during competition. H$_2$ blockers have been used, but questions remain as to their effects on exercise.

7. How is the lower GI tract affected by exercise?

Exercise-induced symptoms of the lower GI tract include the urge to defecate, lower abdominal cramping, increased frequency of bowel movements, diarrhea, and rectal bleeding. In surveys, 10–40% of athletes reports some lower GI symptoms. The pattern is similar to upper GI symptoms in that an increase in intensity of exercise increases symptoms. Between 10 and 35% of the general population have irritable bowel syndrome. One prospective study of 44 previously sedentary people training for a marathon for over 18 months showed only 18% had lower abdominal cramping and there were no reports of diarrhea, suggesting that the higher rates of complaints in the other studies may have been secondary to underlying disorders.

8. What are the mechanisms for lower GI symptoms associated with exercise?

Increased transit time through the lower GI tract has been an often considered mechanism. Light exercise decreases transit time from the mouth to the cecum, although this finding has been called into question more recently. The effects on the colon remain less clear. It is most commonly thought that exercise has minimal effect on the large intestine if the diet is kept constant. With the increasing caloric demands of exercise, most athletes augment their caloric intake and therefore their residue, which could contribute to changes in GI transit. Beta-endorphin production with exercise is a possible factor affecting intestinal activity. Naloxone has not been shown to change GI activity with exercise, however, which may disprove the endorphin theory, indicate that the involved receptors are naloxone-resistant, or suggest a catecholamine mechanism. Psoas muscle hypertrophy with compression of colon has been suggested as a contributing factor but seems unlikely. Others purport that athletes may have increased parasympathetic tone at rest, decreasing transit time. The most popular hypothesis is that of relative ischemia during heavy exercise. Fluid status seems to be involved since 80% of runners who have a greater than 4% loss of body weight report GI symptoms.

9. What is the diagnostic work-up for an athlete with lower GI complaints?

First and foremost, a proper diagnosis must be reached. Changes in bowel habits cannot always be blamed on exercise. Complaints of weight loss and anorexia should be evaluated. Infections, especially parasitic, can present insidiously. Inflammatory bowel disease is a consideration, as is colon cancer in an older athlete.

10. What are the treatment options for an athlete with lower GI complaints?

Several treatment options are available. Avoidance of foods that cause difficulty is an obvious intervention. Caffeine is a gastric stimulant and a diuretic, so limiting its intake should be helpful. Eating low residue foods prior to exercise should limit symptoms. Eating several hours before activity will stimulate the gastrocolic reflex and aid in bowel evacuation prior to exercise. Fluid status is very important and hydration should be a primary consideration. Attention to hydration should start prior to exertion before a fluid deficit has to be corrected. Pharmacologic manipulations are possible but the side effects can be detrimental to performance. These medications act through different mechanisms but all reduce gastrointestinal motility. Several medications cause drowsiness, whereas others act through an anticholinergic mechanism, which would also inhibit sweating, thereby reducing heat tolerance.

11. How often does GI bleeding occur in athletes? What is the cause?

Most studies have been done in runners. Seven to twenty percent of respondents have reported occult fecal blood loss following a marathon. In an ultramarathon, up to 85% of participants may have fecal blood loss. Frank hematochezia is much less common, so evaluation requires consideration of microscopic blood loss. Cyclists have been shown to have Hemoccult-positive stools at a rate of 8%. This was more likely to occur following competition rather than training. Areas of bleeding have been found in both the upper and lower GI tracts with fiberoptic evaluation. It is thought that the mucosa becomes susceptible to injury following a period of decreased perfusion and relative ischemia. Fluid status therefore remains of paramount importance in the athlete. These lesions appear to resolve quickly with the return of normal splanchnic circulation. Mechanical factors do not seem to be causative in GI bleeding and the "cecal slap syndrome" presently is in doubt. Aspirin and nonsteroidal antiinflammatory drugs (NSAIDs) have not been positively correlated with GI bleeding in athletes as of yet.

12. What is the diagnostic work-up for an athlete with GI bleeding?

Given the high prevalence of GI disease in the general population, a full evaluation is necessary in any athlete with GI bleeding. Frank hematochezia is of particular concern. Local causes such as hemorrhoids and rectal fissures should be ruled out on physical examination. A complete blood count should be obtained, with the presence of anemia substantiating the need for a complete evaluation. Inflammatory bowel disease is a concern in the younger population, whereas carcinoma is more common in older age groups.

13. What are the treatment options for an athlete with GI bleeding?

If all pathologic causes of GI bleeding have been ruled out via a diagnostic examination, attention should first be directed toward proper fluid status to decrease the relative ischemia as much as possible. If the athlete is taking aspirin or an NSAID on a routine basis, discontinuation is a reasonable option even though there has been no clear association with GI bleeding in athletes. Healing of established GI disease can be effective with H_2 blockers. Prophylactic treatment of ultramarathoners with cimetidine significantly reduced the incidence of Hemoccult-positive stools. H_2 blockers appear to protect the gastric mucosa from ischemic injury. A small amount of bleeding has not been shown to be detrimental to athletic performance, however, so the decision to treat prophylactically should be individualized. Use of prostaglandin inhibitors such as miso-prostol has been considered for the cytoprotective effects, but no studies have shown a benefit.

14. Which abdominal organs are most commonly injured through trauma?

The spleen is the most commonly injured solid organ in the abdomen. Its location below the ninth to eleventh ribs makes it susceptible to direct trauma and laceration by a rib fracture. Splenomegaly secondary to infectious mononucleosis (an acute self-limited viral infection) in-creases the risk of rupture and requires a period of inactivity. Trauma to the liver and pancreas can also occur but is more uncommon. Lacerations and contusions of the liver occur but have fewer clinical symptoms than a splenic injury. The pancreas is located deep in the abdominal cavity and is rarely injured. The close proximity of the pancreas to the retroperitoneum should make pancreatic injury a consideration when persistent abdominal pain radiates to the back. Traumatic injuries to the hollow organs are rare. The fixed areas of the bowel are most suscepti-ble to rupture. The presumed mechanism is crushing of the bowel against the spine. Abdominal muscle strains are also common. Rectus abdominis strains, usually at the pubic insertion, com-monly occur but the oblique and transverse muscles may also be strained. Rectus sheath hematomas may occur with rupture of the deep epigastric vessels. Contusions of the abdominal musculature usually respond to treatment, as do contusions located anywhere.

15. What should be done in the evaluation of suspected abdominal trauma?

A high index of suspicion must be maintained in evaluation of abdominal injuries. Early signs are often subtle. The key to proper management is careful repeated physical examinations. The patient should be kept NPO (nothing by mouth). Intraabdominal injuries have associated pain with loss of bowel sounds, guarding and rebound tenderness. A rigid or distended abdomen may be present. A splenic rupture may cause pain in the left upper quadrant and left neck or upper shoulder pain. A liver laceration can result in a painful right upper quadrant and right shoulder or neck pain. Both splenic and liver ruptures are associated with rib fractures. Signs of hypovolemia may be present. Serial hematocrit and white blood cell counts should be obtained along with re-peated serum amylase values. A urinalysis should be obtained for signs of hematuria. An ultra-sound or liver-spleen scan are considerations in the evaluation. A CT scan or arteriography may be needed. Peritoneal lavage should be considered when there is evidence of blood loss or ab-dominal tenderness. Appendicitis is always a consideration in a patient with abdominal pain.

16. What should be done with an athlete who has diarrhea while on a trip?

Acute gastroenteritis is second only to upper respiratory infections in young adults. The in-citing agents are most commonly the rotavirus and the Norwalk agent. Bacterial and protozoan infections may also occur. Traveler's diarrhea is defined as the passage of at least three unformed stools in a 24-hour period with nausea, abdominal cramping, tenesmus, or the passage of mucoid or bloody stools. The illness typically consists of 3–10 unformed stools per day for 3–5 days. Twenty percent of patients are confined to bed for 1–2 days. The diarrhea lasts more than 1 week in 10% of patients and more than 1 month in 2%. The degree of dehydration should be assessed prior to any decisions concerning practice or play. Replacement of fluids and electrolytes is of primary importance in any patient with diarrhea. An attempt should be made to replace the lost fluid liter for liter. Many patients will require no additional therapy. Symptomatic treatment is also a consideration. Bismuth subsalicylate will reduce the number of unformed stools by ap-proximately 50%; loperamide reduces diarrhea by 80%. Loperamide is to be avoided in the pa-tient with fever or dysentery because of the rare exacerbation of disease with invasive organisms. Antimicrobial therapy is recommended in traveler's diarrhea after the passage of the third un-formed stool in a 24-hour period; for diarrhea associated with moderate to severe pain or cramps, fever, or dysentery; and for symptoms that recur when symptomatic treatment is discontinued. A fluoroquinolone antibiotic is the drug of choice in most parts of the world, but trimethoprim-sul-famethoxazole may also be appropriate in some parts of the world. After initiation of antimicro-bial therapy, diarrhea will last 16–30 hours.

17. Should prophylactic therapy for diarrhea be initiated in athletes traveling to areas of risk?

Traveling athletes should be counseled as to proper food and beverage choices while traveling. Travelers should consume only foods that are freshly prepared and served steaming hot; fruits that can be peeled; vegetables that have been washed thoroughly with previously boiled or bottled water; and syrups, jellies, or breads. Tap water and ice should be considered contaminated. The antimicrobial medications and bismuth subsalicylate can be effective in preventing traveler's diarrhea but are not currently recommended for prophylaxis. The side effects of short-term bismuth administration are tinnitus and blackening of the tongue and stool, both of which are transient. The side effects of antimicrobial drugs include rashes, vaginal candidiasis, photosensitivity reactions, bone marrow hypoplasia, and antibiotic-associated colitis. Severe reactions may include anaphylaxis and Stevens-Johnson syndrome. The development of antimicrobial resistance is also a consideration. The first consideration in the institution of prophylactic treatment is the underlying health of the patient. The second point is the importance of the trip and the ability of the traveler to tolerate a short period of discomfort. The next consideration is the athlete's own wishes regarding prophylaxis and the desire or ability to take medication diligently and appropriately. Finally, the athlete's willingness and ability to select appropriate foods must be assessed.

BIBLIOGRAPHY

1. Amaral JF: Thoracoabdominal injuries in the athlete. Clin Sports Med 16:739–753, 1997.
2. Brouns F, Beckers E: Is the gut an athletic organ? Digestion, absorption and exercise. Sports Medicine 15:242–257, 1993.
3. Convertino VA, Armstrong LE, Coyle EF, et al: ACSM position stand: Exercise and fluid replacement. Med Sci Sports Exerc 28:1–vii, 1996.
4. DuPont HL, Ericsson CD: Prevention and treatment of traveler's diarrhea. N Engl J Med 328:1821–1827, 1993.
5. Green GA: Gastrointestinal disorders in the athlete. Clin Sports Med 11:453–470, 1992.
6. Mellion MB, Walsh WM, Shelton GL: The Team Physician's Handbook, 2nd ed. Philadelphia, Hanley & Belfus, 1997.
7. Moses FM: The effect of exercise on the gastrointestinal tract. Sports Med 9:159–172, 1990.
8. Okano G, Sato Y, Takumi Y, Sugawara M: Effect of 4 h pre-exercise high carbohydrate and high fat meal ingestion on endurance performance and metabolism. Int J Sports Med 17:530–534, 1996.
9. Soffer EE, Merchant RK, Durthman G, et al: Effect of graded exercise on esophageal motility and gastroesophageal reflux in trained athletes. Dig Dis Sci 38:220–224, 1993.
10. Soffer EE, Summers RW, Gisolfi C: Effect of exercise on intestinal motility and transit in trained athletes. Am J Physiol 260(Pt I):G698–702, 1991.

49. THE ATHLETE'S HEART

Mark Batt, M.B., B. Chir., M.R.C.G.P. Dip. Sport Med.

1. What is athlete's heart syndrome?

The term athlete's heart syndrome refers to the cardiovascular manifestations of the normal physiologic adaptations to prolonged, intense physical training.

2. What constitutes the athlete's heart?

In response to repetitive exercise (both isotonic and isometric), a normal physiologic response of cardiac hypertrophy and resting bradycardia occurs. This produces a variable constellation of physical signs and apparently abnormal investigative findings in an asymptomatic athlete. The typical findings are biventricular cardiac enlargement, soft ejection systolic murmur, added heart sounds, resting sinus bradycardia, and indices of increased cardiac function.

3. Are the changes invariably seen in all athletes?

No. Changes generally occur only after periods of significant training; however, the cardiac enlargement has been noted after as little as a week of activity. The degree of physiologic adaption varies among individuals and may have a hereditary component. Both isotonic (endurance) and isometric (resistance) exercises induce an increased left ventricular mass (LVM); the former also produces an increased ventricular volume.

4. How does the cardiac enlargement occur?

By enlargement of myocardial muscle fiber size (hypertrophy) rather than number (hyperplasia). Unlike pathologic hypertrophy, there is no associated fibrosis, so the process is reversible.

5. How does the bradycardia arise?

This is probably a function of the combination of increased vagal tone and an intrinsic cardiac component related to the increased size of the heart. In addition, the athlete's heart also is less sensitive to sympathetic tone.

6. What changes may be found on physical examination?

1. Resting sinus bradycardia ± sinus arrhythmia
2. Displaced apex beat—palpable cardiac enlargement
3. Third and occasionally fourth heart sounds; hence a gallop rhythm
4. Soft ejection systolic murmur due to high stroke volume, which may occur in up to 40% of young male athletes

7. What EKG changes can be expected?

The range of changes reflect the alterations of cardiac chamber enlargement, rate and rhythm, and repolarization. These are bradycardia, sinus arrhythmia, first- and second-degree heart block, nodal escape rhythm, right bundle branch block, right and left ventricular hypertrophy, ST segment and T wave changes. Isometric (resistance) exercise may be associated with predominantly ST-T wave changes, whereas isotonic (endurance) exercise produces more pronounced voltage changes.

8. What are the uses of echocardiography?

The most important role of echocardiography is to help distinguish athlete's heart syndrome from hypertrophic cardiomyopathy. Unlike plain-film radiographs, the echocardiogram may distinguish specific cardiac structures such that the nature of the cardiac hypertrophy may be characterized.

9. What are the echocardiographic changes?

The echocardiographic measurements of athletes fall outside the normal range, and these changes may be noted after just a few weeks of training. There exists a "sports-specific hypothesis" regarding the nature of these changes. Endurance-trained athletes develop increased LVM from enlarged left ventricular internal dimensions (eccentric enlargement) resulting from volume overload, whereas resistance-trained athletes develop increased LVM from increased left ventricular wall thickness result from pressure overload while the internal dimensions remain unchanged (concentric enlargement). However, few exercise modalities are purely either isometric or isotonic, and once body parameters are normalized (body mass and surface area), this effect in resistance athletes is seen to be less pronounced. Cardiac enlargement may be related to a combination of body type and exercise intensity rather than be specific for exercise type. Echocardiographic changes seem to bear no absolute relationship to performance.

10. Is an exercise treadmill EKG a useful adjunct?

Although controversial, useful information may be obtained and it is often most valuable for the purposes of reassurance. However, it is important to be aware of the incidence of false-positive tests and their consequences. Unlike an echocardiogram, these tests do not provide indices of cardiac dimensions; however, they may show reproducible electrographic changes in athletes. In athletes the heart rate response to exercise is brisk but lower than the comparable heart rate for a given submaximal exercise load in untrained subjects. The recovery postexercise is more rapid and may be associated with a sinus arrhythmia. The most frequent test finding is for resting ST segment (ST elevation with J point shift) and T wave (inversion) changes, which may mimic ischemia, to normalize with exercise.

11. What other changes in cardiac parameters are evident in the athlete's heart?
The stroke volume increases, particularly in endurance-trained athletes, but the ejection fraction (reflecting myocardial contractility) remains unaltered. Coronary resistance and blood flow appear to remain unaltered. This change in endurance-trained athletes contributes to the elevated maximal aerobic power (VO_2max) and represents a central adaptation to endurance exercise.

12. Are endocrine factors important?
At present, no consensus of opinion exists as to the role of hormone secretion with exercise and its link to cardiac enlargement. Thyroxine, testosterone, and growth hormone have all been studied in addition to substances of abuse.

13. Are the findings similar for male and female athletes?
Similar changes in resting heart rate and EKG findings are seen, although the prevalence of added heart sounds is reduced. Cardiac dimensional changes occur in women in response to training; however, they seldom reach pathologic levels. It is likely that qualitative responses to exercise are similar but that quantitative differences exist. This may represent hormonal differences—notably the influence of estrogen and testosterone. This suggests that the diagnostic differentiation of athlete's heart and hypertrophic cardiomyopathy is practically limited to male athletes.

14. Are similar findings found in children?
Data are limited but suggest that these changes are not seen in children.

15. Are the changes of "athlete's heart" permanent?
Longitudinal studies in this area are required; however, it appears that once training ceases, over a period of years the cardiovascular parameters revert. The sinus bradycardia is lost initially, followed by EKG evidence of left ventricular hypertrophy, and finally the conduction changes revert to normal.

16. What diagnostic dilemmas exist?
Hypertrophic cardiomyopathy may produce changes similar to those in the athlete's heart syndrome. Unlike the systolic murmur of hypertrophic cardiomyopathy, the soft ejection systolic murmur of the athlete's heart reduces in intensity with standing or with a Valsalva maneuver. Echocardiography may provide a differentiation from hypertrophic cardiomyopathy; the most significant index is the ratio between septal thickness and ventricular end-systolic or end-diastolic diameter. In marginal cases, examination of first-degree relatives may be useful (asymmetrical hypertrophy being regarded as suspicious). Additionally, a diagnostic period of detraining may be required to document regression of cardiac changes in athletes with the athlete's heart syndrome.

CONTROVERSIES

17. Is screening for hypertrophic cardiomyopathy feasible?
At present, probably not, given the low incidence (2.5/100,000/year) and prevalence (20/100,000) of the condition, the lack of proven treatments that provide for a better prognosis, and the low sensitivity and specificity of available screening tests. Most important is a thorough review of systems of any athlete presenting for examination. Approximately half the cases of hypertrophic cardiomyopathy are familial, so testing of family members of known cases is an option. Sudden

death at a young age of a first-degree relative and symptoms of syncope or presyncope, palpitations, and a history of chest pain should all be regarded as suspicious and further investigated.

18. Does the athlete's heart syndrome have any recognized sequelae?

Probably not. However, a report of middle-aged patients involved in vigorous physical training suggested that athlete's bradycardia may develop into a condition similar to the sick sinus syndrome. Prospective studies of athlete's bradycardias are required, as the group cited may represent patients in whom bradyarrhythmias would have developed and that exercise training merely subjected them to increased vagal tone, hence unmasking the condition.

BIBLIOGRAPHY

1. Abdon N-J, et al: Athlete's bradycardia as an embolising disorder? Br Heart J 52:660–666, 1984.
2. Bryan G, et al: Athletic heart syndrome. Clin Sports Med 11:259–272, 1992.
3. Cantwell JD: The athlete's heart syndrome. Int J Cardiol 17:1–6, 1987.
4. Clark AL, et al: Screening for hyertrophic cardiomyopathy. Br Med J 306:409–410, 1993.
5. Ehsani AA, et al: Rapid changes in left ventricular dimensions and mass in response to physical conditioning and deconditioning. Am J Cardiol 42:52–56, 1978.
6. George KP, et al: The athletic heart syndrome. Sports Med 11:300–331, 1991.
7. Huston TP, et al: The athletic heart syndrome. N Engl J Med 313:24–32, 1985.
8. MacFarlane N, et al: A comparative study of left ventricular structure and function in elite athletes. Br J Sports Med 25:45–48, 1991.
9. Maron BJ: Structural features of the athletic heart as determined by echocardiography. J Am Coll Cardiol 7:190–203, 1986.
10. Maron BJ, et al: Reduction in left ventricular wall thickness after deconditioning in highly trained Olympic athletes. Br Heart J 69:125–128, 1993.
11. Morganroth J, et al: The athlete's heart syndrome: A new perspective. Ann NY Acad Sci 301:931–941, 1977.
12. Oakley DG, et al: Significance of abnormal electrocardiograms in highly trained athletes. Am J Cardiol 50:985–989, 1982.
13. Oakley GDG: The athletic heart. Cardiol Clin 5:319–329, 1987.
14. Pelliccia A, et al: Athlete's heart in women. Echocardiographic characterization of highly trained elite female athletes. JAMA 276:211–215, 1996.
15. Rowland TW, et al: Clinical manifestations of the athlete's heart in prepubertal male runners. Int J Sports Med 15:515–519, 1994.
16. Shephard RJ: The athlete's heart: Is big beautiful? Br J Sports Med 30:5–10, 1996.
17. Tunstall Pedoe D: Sports injuries. Cardiological problems. Br J Hosp Med 3:213–220, 1983.
18. Warren SE, et al: The athletic heart revisited. West J Med 131:441–447, 1979.
19. Zehender M, et al: ECG variants and cardiac arrhythmias in athletes: Clinical relevance and prognostic importance. Am Heart J 119:1378–1391, 1990.

---

50. SUDDEN DEATH IN HIGH SCHOOL AND COLLEGE ATHLETES

Kevin E. Burroughs, M.D., and Karl B. Fields, M.D., C.A.Q., SpMed.

---

1. Define sudden death.

A nontraumatic, nonviolent, unexpected death occurring instantaneously or within 6 hours of an event that changes the previously healthy state of an individual.

2. How many sudden deaths occur in high school and college athletes? What is the most common cause?

In a 10-year study of deaths in athletes, Van Camp et al. reported a total of 160 deaths, of which 126 were high school athletes (115 males and 11 females) and 34 were college athletes (31 males and 3 females). Cardiovascular conditions were the most common cause (73.5%). A similar pattern was later reported in another 10-year study in which 85% of the sudden deaths were due to cardiac causes. The majority of deaths occurred during or immediately after a training session or formal competition.

3. What are the less common causes of sudden death?

Commotio cordis, drug abuse, hyperthermia, rhabdomyolysis associated with sickle cell trait, pulmonary conditions such as status asthmaticus, and electrocution due to lightning are less common causes reported in catastrophic death registries.

4. What is commotio cordis?

Sudden death from cardiac arrest after a blunt trauma to the chest in the absence of structural cardiovascular disease. The apparent mechanism for death is ventricular dysrhythmia induced by an abrupt, blunt precordial blow during an electrically vulnerable period in the cardiac cycle.

5. Define sudden cardiac death.

Sudden cardiac death (SCD) is generally defined as death that is nontraumatic, nonviolent, unexpected, and resulting from cardiac arrest within 6 hours of onset of symptoms in an individual without previously recognized cardiac disease. Such occurrences usually attract attention because athletes are thought to exemplify the picture of good health.

6. What are the causes of SCD in athletes?

The most common cause in western athletes, as well as in the general population, is coronary artery disease. Coronary artery disease is the most common cause in people above the age of 35 years but not in high school and college athletes.

7. What is the most common cause of SCD in athletes less than 35 years of age?

Athletes from 13–35 who die from SCD typically have congenital heart disease. The differential diagnosis includes, in order of occurrence, hypertrophic cardiomyopathy (HCM) or unexplained cardiac hypertrophy, anomalies of coronary arteries, myocarditis, Marfan syndrome, aortic valvular stenosis, dilated cardiomyopathy, arrhythmogenic right ventricular dysplasia, dysrhythmias such as Wolf-Parkinson-White syndrome, and, rarely, mitral valve prolapse.

8. By what mechanism does SCD occur?

Dynamic (e.g., running) and static (e.g., weightlifting) exercise produces various hemodynamic and electrophysiologic changes in the heart (see figure, top of next page). Because of the increase in heart rate, wall tension, and contractility, myocardial oxygen demand is increased. If there is an underlying abnormality in either the coronary vessels or conduction system, the athlete is at risk for arrhythmias and/or ischemia. Uncontrolled arrhythmias may lead to ischemia; conversely, myocardial ischemia may induce electrical instability, which may trigger serious ventricular arrhythmias such as ventricular tachycardia and ventricular fibrillation. Without treatment, ventricular fibrillation leads to death.

9. How often does SCD occur?

Reported numbers vary with the population. Approximately 0.75 and 0.13 per 100,000 young male and female athletes and 6 per 100,000 middle-aged men die during exertion per year. In the specific stress of a marathon, Maron found that sudden death occurred at a rate of 1 in 50,000. Young military recruits, who are prescreened and generally physically active, have a dramatically lower risk; deaths are estimated at 1 of each 735,000 exercising men. The overall estimate for young athletes is approximately 1 per 250,000.

10. What is hypertrophic cardiomyopathy?

HCM is a primary cardiac disease in which the most common diagnostic finding is an asymmetrically hypertrophied and nondilated left ventricle in the absence of any other cardiac

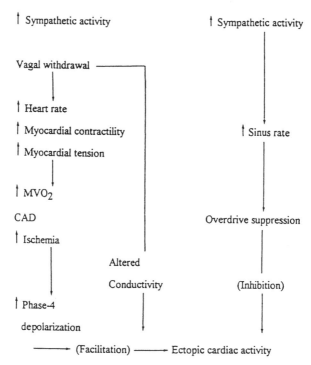

Physiologic alterations during exercise that promote (facilitation) and inhibit (inhibition) cardiac arrhythmias. HR = heart rate, MVO_2 = myocardial oxygen demand, CAD = coronary artery disease. (Adapted from Amsterdam EA, Laslet L, Holly R: Exercise and sudden death. Card Clin 5:337, 1987; with permission.)

or systemic disease that could be associated with similar findings. Gross pathologic changes include a disproportionate septal hypertrophy. Microscopic findings include swirling, disordered myocardial cells as opposed to a more organized hypertrophy of cells in general LVH.

11. How common is HCM?

In the evaluation of 4111 subjects aged 18–30 years, probable or definitive HCM was present in only 7. Demographic breakdown showed a frequency of 0.26% in men, 0.09% in women, 0.24% in blacks, and 0.10% in whites.

12. How is HCM diagnosed?

The history may suggest greater risk for HCM. At-risk individuals may have a family history of cardiac death before age 50, symptoms such as palpitations, syncope or near-syncope, and/or chest pain in relation to exercise. A positive history warrants further investigation.

Cardiovascular examination should begin with the character of the past medical illness. In auscultation, the murmur of HCM is typically systolic in nature and has unique characteristics. In normal valvular murmurs, increased flow across the valve causes an increase in the intensity of the murmur. The opposite is true in HCM. Increased flow in subvalvular stenosis widens the area, thus decreasing the intensity of the murmur; conversely, a decrease in flow allows the hypertrophied septum to encroach on the ventricular outlet. Therefore, any murmur that increases with standing or the Valsalva maneuver is suspicious for HCM.

Once HCM is suspected, EKG is the first diagnostic test; 70–90% of people with HCM show nonspecific abnormalities, including high voltages, prominent Q waves, and deeply inverted T waves. A chest radiograph does not differentiate HCM from benign cardiac enlargement in athletes. Echocardiography is the gold standard for diagnosis. Criteria are (1) left ventricular hypertrophy without dilation and in the absence of systemic disease or left-sided obstruction; (2) a ratio of the intraventricular septum to left ventricular free posterior wall thickness > 1.3; or (3) an intraventricular septum or left ventricular free wall thickness > 15 mm. The upper limit of normal thickness is 12 mm; thus a thickness of 13–14 mm places the athlete in an inconclusive gray zone. Further evaluation and clearance by a cardiologist are required before continuation in athletics.

13. Does the heart normally enlarge with activity?

Regular and consistent exercise produces physiologic changes in the heart and creates an entity known as athlete's heart syndrome (AHS). Physical findings consistent with AHS include sinus bradycardia, secondary to increased vagal tone (vagotonia); third heart sound, due to increased diastolic filling; heart block, again due to enhanced vagal tone; and ST-T wave changes, due to increased cardiac mass, vagal tone, and early repolarization. Morphologically there is concentric hypertrophy of the left ventricle.

14. Do women show findings consistent with athletic heart syndrome?

A study of 600 elite female athletes found cardiac dimensional changes due to exercise, although only 8% showed left ventricular enlargement that exceeded normal limits and only 1% were in the range of cardiomyopathy. Left ventricular wall thickness ranged from 6–12 mm, all within normal ranges (< 12 mm).

15. What are the most common coronary artery anomalies?

Although recognized as the second leading cause of SCD in young athletes, coronary artery anomalies are rare. The most common is anomalous origin of the left main coronary artery (LCA) from the right sinus of Valsalva. For unexplained reasons, affected people tolerate vigorous training without complications for long periods before succumbing to a fatal event. Although most athletes are asymptomatic, dizziness, syncope, or chest pain with exercise should mandate withdrawal from competition until further evaluation can be performed. Other congenital coronary anomalies include anomalous origin of the LCA from the pulmonary artery, hypoplasia of either the LCA or RCA, and coronary artery bridging.

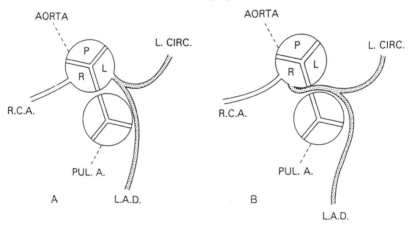

Congenital coronary artery anomalies capable of causing sudden death in young athletes. *A*, Normal anatomy is shown for comparison. *B*, Anomalous origin of the left main coronary artery from the right (anterior) sinus of Valsalva. The left coronary artery may have a separate or common ostium with the right coronary artery, which also arises from the right (R) sinus of Valsalva. Note the acute leftward bend of the left main coronary artery at its origin and its posterior course between the aorta and pulmonary trunk. L.A.D. = left anterior descending coronary artery; L. CIRC. = left circumflex coronary artery; P = posterior (noncoronary) cusp; PUL. A. = pulmonary artery; R.C.A. = right coronary artery. (From Maron BJ: Triggers for sudden cardiac death in the athlete. Cardiol Clin 14:195–210, 1996.)

16. Describe coronary artery bridging.

In coronary artery bridging a major coronary artery is "buried" or "tunnels" into and is completely surrounded by the myocardium. While noted as a cause of SCD, this condition is present in approximately 25% of hearts examined at necropsy. Therefore, in the rare situation that an athlete is identified with bridging, he or she can participate in all competitive sports if there is no evidence of myocardial ischemia at rest or during exercise.

17. How is myocarditis diagnosed? What is the most common cause?

Myocarditis is usually suspected by symptoms such as fatigue, exertional dyspnea, syncope, palpitations, arrhythmias, or acute congestive heart failure in the presence of left ventricular dilation. Echocardiography shows evidence of ventricular dysfunction. EKG shows ST-T wave changes and possibly a generalized decrease in voltage. Coxsackie B virus is the most common cause, followed by echoviruses, adenovirus, and influenza.

18. What should be done if myocarditis is suspected?

Withdrawal from practice or competition is advised for athletes with elevated temperatures, persistent tachycardia, myalgia, or unexpected fatigue. If myocarditis is confirmed, exercise should be avoided for 6 months. A full cardiac evaluation, including assessment of ventricular functioning at rest and during exercise, is necessary before return to athletics.

19. What is Marfan syndrome? How does it cause SCD?

Marfan syndrome is an inherited connective tissue disorder that presents with a constellation of findings that affect three main body systems:

1. Skeletal: tall stature, arachnodactyly, kyphosis, arm span greater than height, joint hypermobility, pectus excavatum or carinatum, pronated flattened arches, high arched palates

2. Cardiac: mitral or prolapse or other valvular changes

3. Ocular: myopia, ectopic lens

Death usually results from aortic dissection with or without rupture. Necropsy reveals separation and fragmentation of elastic components of the aorta.

20. Is mitral valve prolapse a cause of concern for SCD?

Mitral valve prolapse (MVP) is a generally benign disorder in which the mitral valve leaflets protrude back into the left atrium during systole. The classic physical finding is a midsystolic click on auscultation with or without an associated late systolic murmur. MVP is said to occur in approximately 5% of the general population. Some people with MVP have associated palpitations, dizziness, and abnormalities on EKG, including supraventricular and ventricular arrhythmias. Although cases of SCD in patients with MVP have been reported, they appear to be rare.

21. Describe arrhythmogenic right ventricular dysplasia and its contribution to SCD.

One of the more obscure causes of SCD, arrhythmogenic right ventricular dysplasia is associated with recurrent and often intractable ventricular and/or supraventricular arrhythmias. Morphologically, an unusual fibro-fatty infiltration replaces myocytes in the right ventricular wall. There is a strong genetic component, and the largest number of reported cases are among competitive athletes in an area of northern Italy. Classically there are T-wave inversions in V1 and V2, and a significant number show premature ventricular contractions as well as bundle-branch abnormalities.

22. Which arrhythmias are associated with SCD?

Wolff-Parkinson-White Syndrome (WPW) is a rare cause of SCD. In WPW an accessory pathway (bundle of Kent) from the atrium to the ventricle bypasses the AV node and predisposes the athlete to tachycardias. Death occurs from ventricular fibrillation after rapid atrial fibrillation causes ischemia. EKG studies show a shortened PR interval and a delta wave. Athletes may be asymptomatic or present with unexplained syncope or palpitations. Guidelines for athletic participation are found in the 26th Bethesda Conference Recommendations.

Long QT syndrome (LQTS) is a rare inherited condition characterized by a prolonged ventricular repolarization, which increases the risk for R-on-T phenomenon. R-on-T phenomenon may lead to ventricular arrhythmias and thus cause SCD. EKG studies show a corrected QT interval > 440 ms, and frequent T and U wave abnormalities. Again, unexplained syncope may be the only presenting symptom. The cause of syncope in LQTS is the polymorphic ventricular tachycardia torsades de pointes. The current recommendation from the Bethesda Conference is that all people affected by LQTS should be restricted from competitive sports.

Bradycardia secondary to increased vagal tone is a common finding in well-conditioned athletes. Recurrent exercise-induced syncope is believed to be caused by vasovagal-mediated hypotension and bradycardia. Although not a cause of cardiac death, it may inhibit athletic participation.

CONTROVERSIES AND NEW ADVANCES

23. What is new in the detection and diagnosis of HCM?
One of the main dilemmas of diagnosing HCM is that many athletes remain asymptomatic until death. Recent advances in genetic testing involving the beta myosin heavy chain may help to identify patients before SCD. Once HCM is suspected, more comprehensive evaluation may be possible using magnetic resonance (MR) imaging. In a study comparing the diagnostic value of spin-echo MR with echocardiography, MR was found to provide additional anatomic information as well as allow calculation of wall thickness.

24. What is tilt table testing?
Tilt table testing is a provocative test used in the diagnosis of athletes suffering from vasovagal syncope. With tilting of the patient from supine to up to 80° with and without isoproterenol infusion, the patient is monitored for syncope, bradycardia, and hypotension. A positive tilt table test is said to be diagnostic for vasovagal or neurocardiogenic syncope. Therapy for this condition includes beta-blockers, hydrofludrocortisone, disopyramide, and selective serotonin reuptake inhibitors (SSRIs).

25. Given the relative infrequency of sudden cardiac death, is a preparticipation screening examination of any use?
Various studies have shown only minimal efficacy in predetermining athletes at risk of sudden cardiac death. Maron et al. found that only 4 of 115 athletes had some aspect of the examination that aroused suspicion of cardiac disease. In a study of competitive athletes over 30 years in Italy, Pelliccia and Maron found that in a population of 125,408 athletes, 3,190 (2.5%) were disqualified; 51% were disqualified because of cardiovascular disorders. Four hundred eighty of 22,000 elite athletes were disqualified at least temporarily. A position paper by the American Heart Association suggests that hemodynamically significant aortic stenosis is the lesion most likely to be detected during routine screening. Hypertrophic cardiomyopathy is difficult to detect by the standard physical examination because most athletes have a nonobstructive form that causes a soft murmur or none at all.

Detection of HCM with screening echocardiograms is controversial. High expense and low prevalence of disease make such testing questionable. DNA screening for the genetic make-up of HCM may be an answer, but to date it is experimental and expensive. Screening EKGs have been proposed, but because of the high frequency of EKG changes secondary to physiologic adaptations to high-level exercise, abnormalities have a low specificity for HCM.

26. What is the position statement of the American Heart Association on preparticipation screening?
The AHA recommends both a history and physical examination before participation in organized high school (grades 9–12) and collegiate sports. Screening should be repeated every 2 years, with an interim history in the intervening years. Although the AHA acknowledges the inability of the preparticipation physical examination to predict SCD, hypertension, other medical

conditions, and orthopedic injuries merit screening. On rare occasions a significant cardiac finding such as aortic stenosis is detected. Currently, the AHA is modifying their position statement to incorporate the recommendations of the American College of Sports Medicine, the American Society of Sports Medicine, and other medical groups.

27. Can athletes with detected HCM participate if they undergo electrophysiologic studies and do not have inducible ventricular tachycardia?

Certain athletes with documented HCM have participated after electrophysiologic (EP) study. However, clinical studies suggesting that athletes with HCM and normal EP studies will not experience SCD are lacking.

28. Can athletes with Marfan syndrome continue to participate while undergoing serial echocardiogram determination of aortic root size?

The natural history of aortic dilation, dissection, and ultimate rupture in Marfan syndrome is unknown. Thus, although the physician may feel reassured by finding a normal aortic root diameter, no evidence suggests that dilation and rupture cannot occur acutely. Until more evidence helps to predict clinical outcomes, Marfan syndrome remains a contraindication to vigorous sports participation.

BIBLIOGRAPHY

1. Fields KB: Sudden cardiac death. In Halpern B, Bergfield J (eds): Textbook of Sports Medicine. Malden, MA, Blackwell Science, in press.
2. Grubb BP, Temesy-Armos PN, Samoil D, et al: Tilt table testing in the evaluation and management of athletes with recurrent exercise-induced syncope. Med Sci Sports Exerc 25(1):24–28, 1993.
3. Leonard RB, Alexander D, Byrum JE: An athlete dying young: Arrhythmogenic right ventricular dysplasia. N C Med J 55(4):110–112, 1994.
4. Maron BJ: Triggers for sudden cardiac death in the athlete. Cardiol Clin 14:195–210, 1996.
5. Maron BJ, Gardin JM, Flack JM, et al: Prevalence of hypertrophic cardiomyopathy in a general population of young adults. Circulation 92:785–789, 1995.
6. Maron BJ, Poliac LC, Kaplan JA, Mueller FO: Blunt impact to the chest leading to sudden death from cardiac arrest during sports activities. N Engl J Med 333:337–342, 1995.
7. Maron JB, Poliac LC, Roberts WO: Risk for sudden cardiac death associated with marathon running. J Am Coll Cardiol 28:428–431, 1996.
8. Maron BJ, Shirani J, Poliac LC, et al: Sudden death in young competitive athletes. JAMA 276:199–204, 1996.
9. Maron BJ, Thompson PD, Puffer JC, et al: Cardiovascular preparticipation screening of competitive athletes: A statement from the sudden death committee and congenital cardiac defects committee, American Heart Association, Circulation 94:850–856, 1996.
10. Pelliccia A, Maron BJ: Preparticipation cardiovascular evaluation of the competitive athlete: Perspectives from the 30-year Italian experience. Am J Cardiol 75:827–829, 1995.
11. Pelliccia A, Maron BJ, Culasso F, et al: Athlete's heart in women: Echocardiographic characterization of highly trained elite female athletes. JAMA 276:211–215, 1996.
12. Posma JL, et al: Assessment of quantitative hypertrophy scores in hypertrophic cardiomyopathy: Magnetic resonance imaging versus echocardiography. Am Heart J 132:1020–1027, 1996.
13. Rich BSE: Sudden cardiac death. In Fields UB, Fricker PA (eds): Medical Problems in Athletes. Malden, MA, Blackwell Science, 1997, pp 83–86.
14. Rich BSE: Sudden death screening. Med Clin North Am 78:267–288, 1994.
15. Roden DM, Lazzara R, Rosen M, et al: Multiple mechanisms in the long-QT syndrome: Current knowledge, gaps, and future directions. Circulation 94:1996–2012, 1996.
16. Smith BW: Marfan's syndrome. In Fields KB, Fricker P (eds): Medical Problems in Athletes. Malden, MA, Blackwell Science, 1997, pp 121–126.
17. Thompson PD: The cardiovascular complications of vigorous physical activity. Arch Intern Med 156:2297–2302, 1996.
18. Thompson PD, Klocke FJ, Levine BD, Van Camp SP: 26th Bethesda conference: Recommendations for determining eligibility for competition in athletes with cardiovascular abnormalities. Task Force 5: Coronary artery disease. J Am Coll Cardiol 24:888–892, 1994.
19. Van Camp SP, Bloor CM, Mueller FO, et al: Nontraumatic sports death in high school and college athletes. Med Sci Sports Exerc 27(5):641–647, 1995.
20. Zipes DG, Garson A Jr: 26th Bethesda Conference: Recommendations for determining eligibility for competition in athletes with cardiovascular abnormalities. Task Force 6: Arrhythmias. J Am Coll Cardiol 24:892–899, 1994.

51. SUDDEN CARDIAC DEATH IN ADULT ATHLETES

Robert J. Johnson, M.D.

1. Define sudden death.

Sudden death is nontraumatic, unexpected death occurring instantaneously or within minutes of an event that abruptly changes an individual's clinical status. Exertional sudden cardiac death is considered a subset of sudden death. During exercise, sudden death is defined as death that occurs in a medically unsupervised activity (exercise) during the actual activity or within 1 hour after completion of the activity.

2. What is the most common cause of sudden cardiac death in exercising adults?

In the young adult (under 35 years of age), structural abnormalities of the heart are the most common cause of sudden cardiac death. The number one cause in most studies is hypertrophic cardiomyopathy, with estimates ranging as high as 48%. Other cardiac abnormalities include concentric left ventricular hypertrophy, anomalous coronary arteries, aplastic coronary arteries, Marfan syndrome, and conduction abnormalities. Coronary artery disease has been responsible for about 10% of exertional sudden death in this age group. Myocarditis has also been implicated as a cause of sudden death in young adults. The exact incidence is difficult to establish because pathologic evaluation of the myocardium often shows inflammatory cells. Whether this inflammation is the exact cause of the death or a result of some other fatal event remains unclear. Nevertheless, exercise, practice, or competition should be discouraged in anyone with a febrile illness accompanied by myalgias.

In the exercising adult over 35 years of age, the usual cause of sudden death is coronary artery disease. In fact, most studies that examine all forms of exercise find that about 75% (range of coronary artery disease as a cause of sudden death is 54–81% based on available studies) of those who die during exercise have had coronary artery disease as the direct cause. As with the sedentary population, most exercisers have no symptoms prior to the event. Conduction abnormalities, HCM, and anomalous coronary arteries are also cited as causes, although infrequent, of sudden cardiac death in the over-35 age group.

3. What is the mechanism of sudden cardiac death in the exercising population?

Regardless of the underlying problem, either coronary artery disease or structural cardiac abnormalities, the inciting incident is usually myocardial ischemia, which leads to electrical instability and results in an arrhythmia. Most often the arrhythmia is ventricular tachycardia, which degenerates to ventricular fibrillation. Without intervention, ventricular fibrillation leads to death. Other events leading to sudden cardiac death include acute myocardial infarction, thrombus formation in the coronary arteries, and rupture of coronary artery plaques. Each of these episodes can cause ischemia and the subsequent electrical instability that causes the fatal event.

4. How frequent is exertional sudden death in adults?

In one study, there was 1 death for every 396,000 hours of exercise (running). Another study reported 1 death for every 15,000 to 18,000 exercisers each year. Coplan, in a study of 4 million runners, determined a mortality frequency of 3/10,000. This frequency can be interpreted in another way, expressing the overall incidence of death during athletic activity as a rate of 0.003–0.006 per year. Yet another study acknowledged the increased risk for all adults when they are physically active. The risk of death ranged from 4–56 times the risk at rest. The most crucial variable was the individual's normal activity pattern. Those with the highest intensity and most frequent activity level were the **least** likely to die at rest **and** during activity. Those who were sedentary (no regular physical activity) had the greatest risk of death during physical exertion **and** at rest. The actual risk for the regular exerciser is very, very low and should not discourage anyone from regular activity and recreation. In fact, the safety of regular activity is highlighted by its safety and efficacy in post-myocardial infarction patients as a critical part of their rehabilitation program.

5. How does this risk of sudden death compare to the general population?

The Framingham study yielded data showing a sudden death frequency in nonathletes to be 3/10,000 for ages 35–44 and 25/10,000 for ages 55–64. Compare this to Coplan's data for the exercising population of 3/10,000 for ages 20–59.

6. Is the incidence of sudden cardiac death the same for both men and women athletes?

Most of the data refer to men. The incidence of sudden death in women is thought to be 14 times less than in men. More information is necessary because the number of active women is on the rise as is the average age of these women.

7. What is hypertrophic cardiomyopathy (HCM)?

HCM is a condition in which the ventricular septum is uncharacteristically large. A ventricular septum greater than 15 mm in width is considered abnormal. This thickened septum adversely affects the hemodynamics of left ventricular function. Other important pathologic features contributing to sudden death include myocardial cellular disarray and abnormally thickened intramural coronary arteries with narrow lumens. Any of those abnormal features could contribute to either symptoms or ischemia and a fatal event. Unfortunately, most athletes with HCM are asymptomatic, as are most of these athletes with other structural cardiac abnormalities. Only about one-third of those with structural abnormalities will have prodromal symptoms. One-half of those affected with HCM will have a completely normal functional capacity as they perform their sport.

8. What are the screening tests for HCM?

The most effective screen for HCM is a good medical history. The most important historical questions include:
• Is there a family history of cardiac death prior to age 35?
• Have you ever fainted or had a near-fainting spell during exercise, a practice, or game?
• Do you have chest pain while exercising?
Positive responses to these questions, coupled with a cardiac exam that reveals a systolic murmur that increases in intensity during Valsalva maneuver or squatting, may be an indication for an echocardiogram, which is usually diagnostic of HCM. EKG abnormalities are also common but may not be specific; that is, a normal EKG is solid evidence **against** HCM. Any athlete who has confirmed HCM should avoid all moderate or vigorous forms of activity or sport. Routine screening for HCM with echocardiograms is prohibitively expensive.

9. What are common coronary artery anomalies?

Anomalous or aplastic coronary arteries are uncommon. The most common anomaly causing sudden death has been the anomalous origin of the left coronary artery from the right sinus of Valsalva. This causes the coronary artery to follow a course that takes a sharp turn from its origin and courses between the pulmonary artery and aortic trunk. Theoretically, during vigorous activity, the artery is "pinched" at its origin or between the two major arteries, causing ischemia. Hypoplastic or aplastic coronary arteries may eventually result in an ischemic event. Pete Maravich, the great NCAA and NBA basketball star, died of this cause at age 40 playing a "pick up" basketball game after a long and successful professional career. He had an absent right coronary artery.

10. Is myocardial bridging a cause of sudden death?

Myocardial bridging refers to the condition in which the normally epicardial coronary arteries dive into the myocardium. In theory, the contraction of the myocardium could constrict the arteries, leading to ischemia. The occurrence of myocardial bridges based on the results of autopsy studies determined an incidence of bridging as high as 84% of all autopsied hearts, far in excess of the attributed frequency of this cause. Consequently, this cause probably contributes little to the overall frequency of structural causes of cardiac death.

11. Which conduction abnormalities can cause sudden death?

Wolff-Parkinson-White (WPW) syndrome may be an infrequent cause of sudden death in athletes. WPW has an accessory pathway from the atrium to the ventricle. In bypassing the atrioventricular node, tachycardias may develop. Those that are potentially dangerous include those with a rapid atrial fibrillation with ventricular rates 190–300, which may degenerate into a fatal ventricular fibrillation. If the short PR interval disappears with exercise, the prognosis is usually very good and these athletes need not be restricted.

Prolonged Q-T syndrome, a corrected Q-T interval > 440 msec (inherited or drug-induced), also may lead to fatal arrhythmias.

Bradycardias are seldom a cause of sudden cardiac death. Bradycardias are common in well-trained athletes, occasionally with pauses of 2 seconds. Exceptions may be in those who have symptoms related to the slow rate or those in whom pauses exceed 4 seconds.

12. How does Marfan syndrome cause sudden death?

Marfan syndrome is an inherited disease of connective tissue that involves the cardiovascular, musculoskeletal, and ocular systems. The fatal event is usually aortic dissection and/or aortic rupture related to cystic medial necrosis of the aorta. Cardiac evaluation for aortic root abnormalities may be considered in athletes who are tall, have an armspan greater than their height, chest deformities such as pectus carinatum or excavatum, high-arched palate, and myopia or lens subluxation. A family history of early cardiac death or known Marfan syndrome confirms the need for screening of the athlete by history and physical exam, which may include evaluation of the aortic root by echocardiogram.

13. Does mitral valve prolapse (MVP) play a role as a structural cause of sudden death?

Early studies of the cause of sudden exertional death in athletes frequently cited MVP as a cause. Subsequent evaluation showed a possible contributory cause in 3% of all sudden cardiac death. Because the overall incidence of MVP in the asymptomatic population is 6–17%, far exceeding the 3% causation, MVP is unlikely to be a factor. Those with asymptomatic MVP have no need to restrict their activity level.

14. Is there a way of screening athletes over 35 years of age who may be at risk for sudden exertional death?

As in the younger age group, those over 35 can best be screened with an appropriate medical history. Critical risk factors for the exerciser over age 35 include:
- Family history of sudden cardiac death prior to age 50
- Sedentary lifestyle
- Diabetes mellitus (type I or II)
- Hypertension (systolic BP > 160 or diastolic BP > 90)
- Lipid disorders (LDL > 130 and/or HDL < 35)
- Current or former tobacco user

A physical exam should complement the history in the decision for further testing.

15. How effective is an exercise tolerance test (ETT) in screening a person who wants to begin an exercise program?

In a person with chest pain of any type, the ETT is a very effective diagnostic test. Sensitivity [true positives/(true positives + false negatives)] is reported as 55–70%. In the same patient, the specificity [true negatives/(true negatives + false positives)] is also highly accurate, with a specificity of 80–95% in men and 60–80% in women.

In symptom-free people who undergo an ETT, however, the test loses reliability. Both the sensitivity and specificity are low. A low sensitivity indicates that the test will not identify those with "silent" disease and, therefore, at risk for sudden death. A low specificity suggests a significant number of false positive tests that will create the dilemma of identifying those who may need to undergo more expensive and sophisticated testing, many unnecessarily. These tests carry a significant morbidity and mortality risk.

Study of the use of the ETT has identified two problems. The first is that **most** who die a sudden cardiac death have negative ETT results. Second, most of those testing "positive" do **not** have significant coronary artery disease (> 50% stenosis angiographically).

16. What, then, is the value of the ETT in asymptomatic people?

The ETT can be used for symptomatic and asymptomatic people as a prognostic test. For instance, McNeer found that **anyone** tolerating more than 12 minutes of the Bruce protocol (a commonly used graded exercise protocol progressing from light to vigorous walking) and/or exceeding a heart rate greater than 160 beats per minute had a 1-year mortality rate of 1% regardless of the presence or absence of angiographic abnormalities. Other nomograms and formulas may also be used to establish prognostic information. Additionally, many clinicians are using the ETT as a means of quantitating fitness levels, determining a true maximum heart rate for exercise prescription, and motivating the novice exerciser.

17. Are there current guidelines for ETT?

The American College of Sports Medicine has updated their recommendations regarding the use of ETT to minimize the over- or underdiagnosis of coronary artery disease.

The intensity of the planned exercise program is important to consider. If the program is one of moderate exercise (40–60% VO_2max or less than 70% of maximum heart rate) the suggestions are as follows:

	Apparently Healthy	Higher Risk		Known Disease
		No Symptoms	Symptoms	
Men < 40 and women < 50	No	No	Yes	Yes

If the intended program is vigorous (> 60% VO_2max or > 70% maximum heart rate), the recommendations are as follows:

	Apparently Healthy	Higher Risk		Known Disease
		No Symptoms	Symptoms	
Men 40 or > and women 50 or >	Yes	Yes	Yes	Yes

Some very qualified experts believe these recommendations are too inclusive and suggest even more relaxed guidelines, with the implication that too many people are being evaluated by the ETT.

18. What instructions should be given to adults who exercise on a regular schedule?

1. Encourage them to continue their exercise program for the proved health benefits of an exercise program.

2. Counsel exercising adults about properly interpreting warning signs. Any exertional symptom, whether it is the classic chest pain of angina, or a not-so-classic exertional lightheadedness, nausea, or shortness of breath, must be taken seriously as a potential sign of coronary ischemia and discussed with a physician to determine the appropriate evaluation or treatment.

BIBLIOGRAPHY

1. Coplan NL, Foster V: Limitations of the exercise test as a screen for acute cardiac events in asymptomatic patients. Am Heart J 119:987–990, 1990.
2. Epstein S, Maron B: Sudden death and the competitive athlete: Perspectives on preparticipation screening studies. J Am Coll Cardiol 7:220–230, 1986.
3. Gibbons L, Cooper K, Meyer B, Ellison C: The acute cardiac risk of strenuous exercise. JAMA 244:1799–1801, 1980.
4. Gordon NF, et al: Reassessment of the guidelines for exercise testing: What alterations to current recommendations are required? Sports Med 13:293–302, 1992.
5. Mark DB, et al: Prognostic value of a treadmill exercise score in outpatients with suspected coronary artery disease. N Engl J Med 325:849–853, 1991.
6. Maron B, Epstein S, Roberts W: Causes of sudden death in competitive athletes. J Am Coll Cardiol 7:204–214, 1986.
7. Maron B, Roberts W, McAllister H, et al: Sudden death in young athletes. Circulation 62:218–229, 1980.
8. McNeer JF, et al: The role of the exercise test in the evaluation of patients for ischemic heart disease. Circulation 57:64–70, 1978.
9. Myerburg RJ: A biological approach to sudden cardiac death: Structure, function, and cause. Am J Cardiol 63:1512–1516, 1989.
10. Siscovick DS, Weiss HS, Fletcher RH: The incidence of primary cardiac arrest during vigorous exercise. N Engl J Med 311:874–877, 1984.
11. Thompson PD, et al: Incidence of death during jogging in Rhode Island from 1975 through 1980. JAMA 147:2535–2538, 1980.
12. Van Camp SP: Exercise-related sudden death: Cardiovascular evaluation of exercisers. Phys Sportsmed 16(6):47–54, 1986.
13. Van Camp SP: Exercise-related sudden death: Risks and causes (part 1 of 2). Phys Sportsmed 16(5): 97–112, 1988.
14. Van Camp SP: Sudden death. Clin Sports Med 11:273–289, 1992.
15. Waller B, Roberts W: Sudden death while running in conditioned runners aged 40 years or over. Am J Coll Cardiol 45:1292–1300, 1980.

IX. Overuse and Trauma

52. ELECTROMYOGRAPHY AND NERVE CONDUCTION STUDIES

Reuben Sloan, M.D.

Athletic injuries often involve nerve entrapment, traction, and bruising. Consequently, it is important to understand the electrophysiologic evaluation techniques used to diagnose these injuries.

1. What is an EMG?

EMG stands for electromyography, an electrophysiologic test that evaluates the status and function of peripheral nerves, motor units, and muscle fibers. In other words, it is an objective measurement of the peripheral nervous system. For complete evaluation, a guided history and physical examination should accompany the EMG evaluation.

2. What is NCS/NCV?

NCS stands for nerve conduction studies; NCV stands for nerve conduction velocity. Nerve conduction studies are an integral part of the electrophysiologic evaluation. The process involves selecting the nerve in question and placing electrodes over a muscle innervated by that nerve. An evoked response is elicited by giving a gentle shock at a set distance, usually about 8 cm proximal to the recording electrodes. A second site, usually proximal to a potential entrapment, is frequently used. An example is testing for cubital tunnel syndrome, which involves entrapment of the ulnar nerve across the elbow. Recording electrodes are placed over the abductor digiti minimi muscle. A stimulus is given over the ulnar nerve 8 cm proximal to the recording electrode at the wrist, followed by a second stimulus just distal to the medial epicondyle, and a third stimulus about 10 cm above the elbow. This method assesses the velocity of the conducted impulse across the frequently entrapped area of the cubital tunnel. Nerve conduction study involves evaluation of both the motor and sensory nerves.

3. Who does electrophysiologic testing?

An electromyographer, most commonly a physician, performs the test. He or she is usually a physiatrist or neurologist but may be any physician with appropriate training. In addition, some certified physical therapists with special training in electrophysiology can perform the test.

4. What are common indications for an EMG?

Because the EMG gives information about the peripheral nervous system, any suspected pathology that involves either peripheral nerves or muscles is an indication for an EMG. Most frequently the EMG evaluates for a potential entrapment neuropathy such as carpal tunnel syndrome. Other reasons include evaluation for a potential peripheral or diffuse neuropathy or radiculopathy. Because the test also involves evaluation of the motor fibers, an EMG can be used to evaluate for a myopathy or myopathic process.

5. When is the best time to order an EMG?

The test should be delayed about 2–3 weeks after injury or onset of symptoms to gain the most information. Because the neuromuscular system has a window period in which no objective findings can be demonstrated, the test should be delayed to allow the objective findings to develop. The test can be ordered earlier if one is attempting to rule out a preexisting condition.

6. What information can an EMG/NCS give?

An EMG/NCS can give a lot of information, including the distribution of an abnormality; whether the lesion is diffuse, focal, or even multifocal; the temporal course of the disorder; and whether the lesion is acute or chronic. We can also tell whether a particular neuromuscular process is improving or progressing when a prior study is available for comparison. In addition, the test can separate a neuropathic from a myopathic lesion.

7. What information cannot be obtained from an EMG/NCS?

Because the test evaluates neurophysiologic function, it cannot give information about an anatomic or etiologic process. For example, even if the EMG is consistent with a peripheral neuropathy, it cannot discern the exact etiologic process. It can, however, break the differential of peripheral neuropathy into two large categories: demyelinating and axonal pathology. It cannot further differentiate the process; thus, clinical correlation is always required. Moreover, central lesions that involve processes of the central nervous system cannot be evaluated because the EMG tests only the peripheral nervous system.

8. What typical abnormalities may NCS reveal? What do they mean?

Three parameters are obtained with NCS:

1. **Distal latency:** the time required for an impulse to travel down a given nerve, usually expressed in milliseconds (msec). Prolongation of distal latency indicates a demyelinating process; thus, the impulse takes longer to travel.

2. **Amplitude:** a summation of all of the axons in the tested nerve. The units are either millivolts or microvolts. Amplitude is a summation of all of the action potentials of all of the given axons in a nerve. A decrease in amplitude implies axonal degeneration.

3. **Conduction velocity:** the time required for an impulse to travel down a nerve segment. This parameter is an extension of the distal latency. The difference is that we have a known distance and the units are expressed in meters/second. As with prolonged distal latency, prolongation or slowing of conduction velocity implies a demyelinating process. A selective loss of larger-diameter, faster-conducting axons also may lead to slowing of conduction velocity.

9. What effect does temperature have on NCS?

NCS should be done on a limb that is at least 31–32° C. A lower temperature has an adverse effect on conduction, velocity, and distal latency. In other words, a false-negative test may occur. Limbs must be warmed to at least 31–32° C at testing time.

10. What is temporal dispersion?

Because an action potential is a summation of all of the evoked responses from a diverse population of stimulated axons, the conduction times from all of the evoked axons are different. The smaller, less myelinated axons are slower, whereas the larger, myelinated axons are faster. Because of this electrophysiologic property, the time difference between the arrival of the evoked responses from the faster and slower conducted axons increases the duration of the waveform. This phenomenon is termed temporal dispersion. A certain amount of temporal dispersion is normal. Marked temporal dispersion should lead the electromyographer to think of processes that cause multifocal demyelination, such as Guillain-Barré syndrome or chronic inflammatory demyelinating polyradiculopathy (CIDP).

11. How are nerve injuries classified?

The most common classification was described by Seddon in the 1940s:

1. **Neurapraxia** is the mildest form of nerve injury, characterized by damage to the myelin sheath or Schwann cell without damage or change to axonal integrity. EMG manifestations of

neurapraxia include slowing of the evoked response across the injured segment and frequently complete loss of the response distal to the segment. Recovery usually takes place within 4–6 weeks but may take longer.

2. **Axonotmesis** is a disruption of the myelin sheath and axon with preservation of the supporting structures and connective tissue. Because there is axonal damage distal to the injury site, Wallerian degeneration takes place. Manifestations on EMG/NCS include conduction loss distal to the injured site and abnormal spontaneous activity on needle examination. The prognosis for axonotmesis is less favorable; however, some recovery may take place, usually in the form of regeneration or reinnervation secondary to collateral sprouting from intact neighboring motor units.

3. **Neurotmesis** is the most severe nerve injury. Part or all of the supporting structures are damaged or transected. Surgical anastomosis is almost always necessary to promote regeneration or reinnervation. EMG manifestations are similar to those of axonotmeses.

12. What are preganglionic lesions?

The term *ganglionic* refers to the dorsal root ganglion of the sensory nerve. Preganglionic lesions involve proximal structures. Examples include cervical or lumbar radiculopathy and motor neuron diseases such as amyotrophic lateral sclerosis (ALS).

13. How can one distinguish a preganglionic from a postganglionic lesion?

A postganglionic lesion is distal to the dorsal root ganglion (DRG). An example is any peripheral neuropathy or entrapment syndrome. The most effective way to distinguish the two is sensory NCS. In a preganglionic lesion, the sensory nerve studies should be normal. Because DRG and the entire distal nerve segment are unaffected, the sensory nerve action potentials and conduction should remain unaffected. This is not the case with lesions distal to the DRG.

14. What are late responses? How are they helpful?

An example of late responses are the F wave and H wave. The **F wave** is not completely understood, but it is believed to be an echo of the alpha motor neuron. It measures only motor fibers and can be elicited from most muscles. F waves are obtained in an attempt to gain information from the segments proximal to the DRG. They are helpful in the diagnosis of radiculopathy.

The **H wave**, originally described by Hoffman, is the electrophysiologic analog of the deep tendon reflex. In adults, it is reliably obtained only from the tibial nerve, which corresponds to the S1 route. The H wave measures both motor and sensory fibers. Abnormalities are most commonly associated with S1 radiculopathy, but the H wave is also abnormal in peripheral neuropathies. The H wave must always be compared with the contralateral side.

15. What are the components of the needle examination?

The needle examination is complementary to the NCS and evaluates the physiologic state of the individual fibers. There are four main parameters:

- **Insertional activity.** As the electrode is advanced through the muscle, it detects the transmembrane potential. Depolarization occurs normally secondary to the trauma of introducing the needle into the fiber. Increased activity indicates membrane instability, whereas decreased activity may indicate atrophic changes that have led to replacement of muscle with inactive tissue such as fat or fibrous tissue.
- **Spontaneous activity.** The muscle is normally electrically silent at rest. Spontaneous activity at rest may be secondary to membrane instability, motor endpoint noise caused by fortuitous placement, or poor relaxation and failure to achieve a resting state. If denervation is present, the muscle fibers fire spontaneously at rest.
- **Motor unit assessment and morphology.** This part of the examination is done with a voluntary muscle contraction. The motor unit action potential (MUAP) represents the summation of all of the electrical activity of the muscle fibers in a given motor unit. The electromyographer evaluates the size or amplitude, which is a measurement of fiber density; the duration of the MUAP; and, finally, the shape or form.

• **Recruitment pattern.** This parameter depends on the number of intact motor units. The patient is asked to contract maximally, and an interference pattern is obtained. A full or complete interference pattern represents a good effort. The electromyographer cannot identify individual motor units. A reduced or incomplete recruitment may be secondary to poor effort or a neurophysiologic process. The electromyographer is able to identify some MUAPs. A discrete recruitment pattern indicates a neurophysiologic process, and the electromyographer can identify each and every MUAP.

16. What are fibrillations? How are they graded?

A fibrillation is the spontaneous finding of a single muscle fiber. It is crisp-sounding, like the sound of rain on a tin roof. There is an initial downward or positive deflection. Fibrillations indicate a denervation process. They are graded on a 1+ to 4+ scale, depending on the number of quadrants in which they are present.

17. What is a positive sharp wave?

A positive sharp wave represents a blocked action potential in a damaged or denervated muscle fiber. It has a low, dull, popping sound and an initial positive deflection. The grading for positive sharp waves is the same as for fibrillations. Positive sharp waves tend to precede fibrillations in an acute, demyelinating process. They appear 2–6 weeks after injury. They appear and disappear in a proximal-to-distal orientation.

18. What are fasciculations?

Fasciculations are spontaneous, repetitive discharges of a single motor unit. They fire at irregular rates and have a loud, dull, popping sound. They are not pathognomonic for any disease process and may occur in normal subjects. They are, however, seen in neuropathic lesions, especially lesions affecting the motor neurons, such as ALS.

19. What is a complex repetitive discharge (CRD)?

CRDs are high-frequency discharges representing the action potential of a group of muscle fibers firing near synchrony. The waveforms remain identical during a single train of action potentials. They start and end abruptly. Because of their characteristics, they sound like dive-bombers.

20. How are neuropathic disorders differentiated from myopathic disorders on EMG?

Neuropathic disorders have increased muscle fiber density per given motor unit because of reinnervation and collateral sprouting. EMG manifestations include increased amplitude, increased duration, and polyphasic and/or satellite potentials on needle examination. The recruitment pattern is either reduced or discrete in nature.

Myopathic lesions have decreased muscle fiber density per motor unit and scattered single-fiber loss. The needle examination manifestations are a decrease in amplitude and duration and an increase in polyphasia or number of wave phases because the surviving fibers fire asynchronously. The recruitment pattern is full; however, the amplitude of the recruitment pattern is low.

21. What should one write on the referral form when ordering an EMG/NCS?

The referring practitioner should specify what he or she is trying to find or rule out and, if possible, include the differential diagnosis. Sometimes an EMG/NCS is ordered when the referring doctor is not clear what the process is or the clinical picture is confusing. It is always helpful to indicate this information on the referral form. In addition, if the referring physician is trying to chronicle the injury, it is important to indicate this goal so that the prospective electromyographer can be sensitive to the request.

BIBLIOGRAPHY

1. Feinberg J: Upper extremity nerve injuries in the athlete. Physical Medicine Lecture Series, Department of PM&R, Columbia-Presbyterian Medical Center, New York, New York, September 1996.
2. Katz RT: Nerve entrapments: An update. Orthopaedics 12:1097–1107, 1989.

3. Kimura J: Electrodiagnosis in Disease of the Nerve and Muscle, 2nd ed. Philadelphia, F.A. Davis, 1989.
4. MacLean IC: Electromyography. A guide for the referring physician. Clin Phys Med 1:1–42, 1990.
5. Webster R, Kahn J: Carpal tunnel syndrome and the focal compression neuropathies. Clin Phys Med Rehabil 1:69–89, 1990.

53. SPRAINS, STRAINS, TRIGGER POINTS, AND SOFT TISSUE INJURIES

Walter L. *Larimore,* M.D., D.A.B.F.P.

1. What is a sprain?

It is an acute traumatic injury to a ligament (a dense tissue band that connects the articular ends of bones).

2. How are sprains graded?

A **first-degree sprain** is the acute minor trauma of tearing a few ligamentous fibers, which results in mild pain, swelling, and disability, but no joint instability.

A **second-degree sprain** is the acute moderate trauma of tearing a moderate number of ligamentous fibers, which results in moderate pain, swelling, and disability but little to no joint instability.

A **third-degree sprain** is the acute and complete tear or rupture of a ligament. Swelling and pain may be minimal to severe. Disability, however, is severe, and the joint will be unstable.

3. How are third-degree sprains subclassified?

Some authorities classify third-degree sprains by how much the opposing joint surfaces can be displaced: 0–5 mm is classified as 1+, 6–10-mm as 2+, and greater than 10 mm as 3+. Obviously, the classification is more useful in larger joints.

4. What is a strain?

It is an acute traumatic injury to the muscle-tendon junction or unit (MTU) and is commonly called a **"pull."** The force of injury is indirect (e.g., overuse, misuse, hypercontraction) as opposed to direct (e.g., a blow, cut, puncture).

5. How are strains graded?

A **first-degree strain** is a minor trauma to the MTU resulting in mild pain, swelling, and disability but usually does not disrupt the athlete's ability to produce a normal (albeit painful) contraction of the involved muscle.

A **second-degree strain** is a moderate injury to the MTU, including the tearing or disruption of a moderate number of muscle and tendon fibers, which results in moderate pain, swelling, and disability in association with an abnormal (weak and painful) contraction of the involved muscle.

A **third-degree strain** is a complete tear or rupture of the MTU. Swelling and pain may be minimal to severe and an extremely abnormal (extremely weak to nonexistent and usually painless) contraction of the involved muscle.

6. What is a contusion?

It is an acute traumatic injury resulting from a direct but blunt trauma to a soft tissue (e.g., skin, adipose tissue, muscle, tendon, ligament, synovium), which is commonly called a bruise, and usually results in pain and edema (swelling). There can be and usually is mild-to-severe extravasation of blood into the surrounding tissues.

7. If sprains and strains are acute injuries, then what are subacute injuries to ligaments or muscle-tendon units?

Nonacute injuries to soft tissues can be described as **microtraumatic overuse injuries**. Macrotraumas can be acute or chronic fractures, avulsions, dislocations, and subluxations. Microtrauma, however, involves microscopic injury from chronic, repetitive overuse trauma.

8. What microscopic changes occur with overuse injuries?

Usually, local tissue breakdown occurs with tissue lysis, lymphocytic infiltration, and blood extravasation. These changes result in pain and dysfunction, but usually not classic tissue inflammation (neutrophil invasion).

9. What is overuse or overtraining?

Typically, these terms describe a lack of balance between training and recovery resulting in a catabolic tissue state and, at least initially, microtrauma to the soft tissues.

10. What are the preexisting factors for overuse injuries?

Intrinsic and extrinsic factors are generally considered equally important in the development of overuse injuries. Examples of intrinsic factors include age, gender, genetic and anatomic factors such as bone length discrepancy, muscle imbalances, malalignments of joints or extremities, fatigue, inflexibility, and muscle weakness. Examples of extrinsic factors include technique errors, training errors, poor equipment, poor environment, poor terrain, and overtraining.

11. How are overuse injuries classified?

Grade I: Pain after the activity only
Grade II: Pain with activity that does not restrict but may affect the performance
Grade III: Pain with activity that restricts and moderately to severely affects performance
Grade IV: Pain occurring with activity and at rest

12. What are some common overuse injuries of ligaments?

Common examples include pitcher's elbow (Little Leaguer's elbow), golfer's elbow (medial epicondylitis), tennis elbow (lateral epicondylitis), swimmer's knee (breast stroker's knee), iliotibial band syndrome, plantar fasciitis, and jumper's knee.

13. What are some common overuse injuries of the MTU?

Each part of the unit (muscle or tendon) or the entire unit can be injured. **Tendinitis, myositis, myotendinitis**, and **tenosynovitis** are terms used to describe overuse injuries of the muscle-tendon unit.

14. Is there a difference between tendinitis and tendonosis?

Probably not. Most microscopic studies of tendinitis show no neutrophil (acute) reaction but rather lymphocytic (chronic) infiltration consistent with degenerative (rather than acute) changes of the tissue. Therefore, many sports medicine authorities are beginning to use the term **tendonosis** instead of tendinitis. Common examples include tennis elbow (lateral epicondylitis), golfer's elbow (medial epicondylitis), shin splint, groin strain, and rotator cuff strain.

15. What are some common overuse injuries of tendons (tendonosis)?

Common examples include Achilles tendinitis, rotator cuff tendinitis, bicipital tendinitis, de Quervain's disease, suprapatellar tendinitis, peroneal tendinitis, and posterior tibial tendinitis.

16. What is tenosynovitis?

Overuse injury of the tissue surrounding the tendon, also called **peritendinitis** or **tenovaginitis**, displaying crepitance or a "squishy," "dry-cracking leather" sensation over the involved tendon. Common examples include iliopsoas tenosynovitis in children, wrist tenosynovitis, and anterior tibialis tenosynovitis.

17. What is myositis ossificans?

Also called **myositis ossificans traumatica**, this term describes heterotopic bone formation in the area of a deep contusion to a large muscle (such as biceps or quadriceps). Some have suggested that applying heat therapy to large muscle contusions serves as an etiologic factor in the formation of myositis ossificans; therefore, most sports medicine therapists apply ice to muscle injuries. Myositis ossificans usually follows significant deep muscle contusion by 3–6 weeks. The myositic bone mass may remain unchanged or shrink in size over a 3–6 month period. However, when it is near a muscle origin or insertion, it is less likely to be reabsorbed and more likely to cause impairment. Recurrent myositis ossificans should cause the practitioner to think of bleeding disorders and to obtain studies for clotting deficiencies.

18. Are there any special treatments for severe large muscle contusions?

It has been said that the severity of large muscle contusions is almost always underestimated. Initially, the athlete experiences little pain or discomfort; however, stiffness, pain, and swelling often develop quickly after the athlete cools down. For athletes receiving significant direct blunt blows to large muscle masses that result in pain, limping, or disability, the athlete should not be instructed to "run out" the injury. Heat, massage, and whirlpool treatments should not be used, as these therapies may initiate additional bleeding.

Mild deep-muscle contusions produce little swelling and pain with some tightness and normal joint motion above and below the muscle. Treatment of mild deep muscle contusions include ice, transcutaneous electrical nerve stimulation (TENS), muscle stretching, and compression with elastic wraps.

Moderate deep-muscle contusions produce moderate swelling and pain with limitation to the range of motion of a joint above or below the muscle. Usually the muscle is in spasm. Treatment includes the therapy as described above for mild deep-muscle contusions, along with immobilization of the muscle in a "stretched" posture. This may involve the use of crutches for thigh and quadriceps contusions.

For **severe deep-muscle contusions**, swelling is very rapid and can be extreme and secondary to hemorrhage. Aggressive therapy can include aspiration or surgical evacuation because some data indicate that removal of large blood extravasations from muscle minimizes subsequent fibrosis and disability. In addition, injection of local anesthetics, enzymes, and corticosteroids (or IV corticosteroids) have been advocated by some practitioners. However, controlled data as to their effectiveness are sparse. In addition, the threat of introducing infection exists. Severe deep-muscle contusions should be treated with compression, ice, and strict bed rest. The extremity circumference should be checked serially and frequently.

19. How can one remember the general primary therapies for soft tissue strains, sprains, and contusions?

By the mnemonic PRICES:

P Protection
R Rest
I Ice
C Compression
E Elevation
S Support

20. How can one remember the secondary therapies for soft tissue injuries?

By the mnemonic NIPED:

N NSAIDs (nonsteroidal antiinflammatory drugs)
I Injection—The most commonly used injections include corticosteroids with or without local anesthetic, saline, or long- and short-acting anesthetics. However, corticosteroid injections may weaken tendons and result in tendon rupture and are contraindicated in (1) young athletes, (2) large joints where there is not objective degenerative change, and

(3) major load-bearing tendons. Indications/locations for corticosteroid injections may include (1) bursa inflammation, (2) small non–weight-bearing joints, (3) alongside or peripheral to muscle-tendon units, (4) alongside or peripheral to ligament attachments to bone where subsequent rupture of the ligament would not be considered disastrous, (5) tendon sheaths, or (6) documented degenerative joints. Traditionally, corticosteroid injections have been used for trigger points; however, recent studies seem to indicate that local anesthetic (or even saline) injections work at least as well and have less potential for side effects.

P   Physical therapy, or physical modalities, including, but not limited to, cryotherapy, thermal therapy, ultrasound therapy, iontophoresis, galvanic stimulation, electrical stimulation, massage therapy, and manipulative therapy.

E   Exercise and stretching, which are said to be the most commonly underutilized means for treating musculoskeletal sports injuries.

D   Device or braces.

Put together, the mnemonics PRICES and NIPED can be useful when counseling athletes about soft tissue injury therapy.

21. What is a trigger point?

In sports medicine, these points are described as the traditional acupuncture sites, which are based on ancient (and usually Asian) concepts or meridians. Family physicians and rheumatologists also use the term *trigger point* to describe typical areas of the muscular anatomy that demonstrate consistent tenderness and nodularity in patients with fibromyalgia (myofibrositis) or myofascial pain syndrome.

22. What is the origin of the trigger point concept?

Sports medicine or acupuncture trigger points are said to be derived from ancient and empirical observations that brief and intense stimulation (such as pressure, puncture, burn, vibration) of certain anatomic points produces prolonged pain relief in other areas of the body.

23. How can trigger points be stimulated?

Options include pressure (acupressure), vibration, electrical stimulation (TENS), puncture (acupuncture or "dry-needle therapy"), cooling (ice rub or ethyl chloride spray), or injection (saline, anesthetic [lidocaine, bupivacaine], and corticosteroids).

24. By what mechanism does trigger-point stimulation work?

Some suggest that the effect is placebo, distraction, or suggestion. Others suggest that this stimulation mediates the release of local endorphins. Still others suggest a "central-biasing network" (CBN), based on the theory that the midbrain receives input from widespread body areas and that if certain midbrain sites are stimulated (as can be reproduced in animal models), then gradients of analgesia are produced that are maximal in relatively small areas of the body distant to the areas stimulated. Therefore, it is suggested that a CBN may exert inhibitory control of the pain-signaling system.

25. What is an abrasion?

Abrasions are acute injuries resulting from shearing forces between the epidermis or mucosa and another surface (e.g., road surface, floor, mat, skin). These injuries are commonly called **scrapes**.

26. How can abrasions be treated?

Abrasions, often viewed by athletes as being trivial, are often inadequately treated and can easily become infected owing to the environmental factors common to sports.

27. How can one remember the primary therapies for abrasions?

A useful treatment mnemonic is SID:

S Soak, soap, scrub
I Irrigate, irrigate, irrigate
D Dressing

28. What dressing options are available for treating abrasions?

Many controversies exist. Some recommend that minor or shallow abrasions be left dry after they are cleansed. For others, antibiotic ointments can be very useful. Neomycin ointments are nonprescription and inexpensive but can cause sensitivity reactions and inflammation. Mupirocin ointment is an expensive but excellent antibiotic treatment. It is even indicated for impetigo; some practitioners believe it to be equivalent to oral antibiotics for the treatment of impetigo.

29. How are deeper or larger abrasions treated?

Many sports medicine therapists are using bio-occlusive dressings for these types of injuries. These dressings come in two basic types: (1) The thinner and less expensive bio-occlusive dressings serve as "artificial epidermis." These hydrophobic but oxygen-permeable membranes may have adherent on one side, and they should be applied to clean, dry abrasions, and work better for smaller, more superficial abrasions; and (2) deeper abrasions can be covered with thicker hydrocolloid dressings, which are usually 1 to 3 mm thick and fairly elastic. These thicker dressings, although expensive, absorb exudate, provide additional skin protection, reduce infection, and ease debridement, all secondary to the excellent and moist healing environment that they create. In addition, they appear to speed the healing process, adhere in spite of sweating, increase tolerance to shearing or collision forces, and prevent exudate or blood transmission to other athletes.

30. Does massage help soft tissue injury?

Massage or soft tissue manipulation seems to benefit athletes therapeutically, prophylactically, mechanically, physiologically, and psychologically. It is used by many athletes both pre- and postcompetition, as well as during competitive rest or breaks.

31. How does massage therapy work?

Massage is said to vasodilate (and can be used to "warm up") extremities, reduce or treat spasm of muscles, reduce swelling, or reduce soreness. In addition, massage is said to promote relaxation, which may promote healing and recovery. Massage is said to be especially useful in rehabilitation after sprains, strains, or contusions and is said to work by stimulating blood flow, reducing edema, preventing or breaking apart undesired fibrosis, and relaxing muscle spasm. Subjectively, massage therapy is said to relieve discomfort, increase pain threshold, and even improve performance.

32. Are there different types of massage therapy?

Yes. Broadly speaking, the types include friction, stroking, kneading, percussion, and shaking. These methods go by a variety of (primarily Asian) names. Each type is touted to have particular benefits.

33. Are there any contraindications to massage therapy?

Yes. Massage techniques that are likely to increase or worsen new injuries are contraindicated. For example, deep-kneading massage over an acute deep-muscle contusion may increase bleeding and therefore cause additional tissue injury.

BIBLIOGRAPHY

1. Adamson C, Cymet T: Ankle sprains: Evaluation, treatment, rehabilitation. Md Med J 46:530–537, 1996.
2. Arrington ED, Miller MD: Skeletal muscle injuries. Orthop Clin North Am 26:411–422, 1995.
3. Bernhardt DT: General principles in treating soft-tissue injuries. Pediatr Ann 26:20–25, 1997.
4. Best TM: Muscle-tendon injuries in young athletes. Clin Sports Med 14:669–686, 1995.
5. Best TM: Soft-tissue injuries and muscle tears. Clin Sports Med 16:419–434, 1997.
6. Cantu RC, Micheli LJ: ACSM's Guidelines for the Team Physician. Philadelphia, Lea & Febiger, 1991.

7. Garrett WE Jr: Muscle strain injuries. Am J Sports Med 24(Suppl):S2–S8, 1996.
8. Hosie G, Bird H: The topical NSAID felbinac versus oral NSAIDs: A critical review. Eur J Rheumatol Inflamm 14:21–28, 1994.
9. Johannsen F, Langberg H: The treatment of acute soft tissue trauma in Danish emergency rooms. Scand J Med Sci Sports 7:178–181, 1997.
10. Kibler WB, Chandler TJ, Stracener S: Musculoskeletal adaptations in injuries due to overtraining. Exerc Sports Sci Rev 20:99–126, 1992.
11. Mellion MB, Walsh WM, Shelton GL: The Team Physician's Handbook, 2nd ed. Philadelphia, Hanley & Belfus, 1997.
12. Ogilvie-Harris DJ, Gilbart M: Treatment modalities for soft tissue injuries of the ankle: A critical review. Clin J Sport Med 5:175–186, 1995.
13. Puffer JC, Zachazewski JE: Management of overuse injuries. Am Fam Physician 38:225–232, 1988.
14. Risser WL: The acute management of minor soft tissue injuries. Pediatr Ann 21:170–172, 1992.
15. Rzonca EC, Lue BY: TEMPER: An acronym for ankle sprain rehabilitation. Clin Podiatr Med Surg 5:661–675, 1988.

54. HEAD INJURIES

Douglas G. Browning, M.D., A.T.C., and John M. Henderson, D.O.

> *"If ever I need a brain transplant, I want one from a sports writer, 'cause I know it's never been used."*
> —Joe Paterno, Penn State Nittany Lions Football Coach

1. Following a closed head injury, what signs and symptoms are indications that an athlete needs emergency evaluation?

I	1.	Impairment of consciousness (or changes in mental status or behavior, increasing or continued)
Need	2.	Nausea and vomiting, persistent
My	3.	Motor activity, decreased, unequal, or pathologic posturing
Very	4.	Vital signs (change in ventilation pattern, increasing blood pressure, or decreasing pulse rate)
Special	5.	Seizures
Head	6.	Headache, increasing
Protection	7.	Pupillary inequality

(Important! Remember, the forces that cause a head injury may also produce cervical spine injuries.)

2. Identify the difference between nerve cells of the central nervous system and the cells of the rest of the body that makes prevention and careful management of head injuries the highest priority.

The nerve cells of the brain and spinal cord, unlike most other cells in the body, are *incapable of regeneration*. Thus, when these cells die, they are lost forever and are unable to regrow or be transplanted or replaced.

3. What is a concussion?

A concussion is a retrospectively diagnosed clinical syndrome characterized by immediate and *transient* impairment of neurologic function (e.g., alteration of consciousness, mental status changes, disturbance of vision, vertigo) due to mechanical acceleration and deceleration forces acting on the brain. Concussions are usually graded based on the length and severity of neurologic impairment.

4. Name the components of a mental status examination that are appropriate to check following a head injury.
- Affect/appearance
- Orientation (time, day/date, place, situation)
- Memory (immediate recall, recent, remote)
- Intellect (calculations)
- Judgment

5. What is second impact syndrome?
Second impact syndrome is the rapid development of diffuse brain swelling in the setting of a recent head injury followed by a second impact to the head. Usually within seconds to minutes of the second impact, the initially conscious but stunned athlete precipitously collapses, with rapidly dilating pupils, loss of eye movement, and evidence of respiratory failure. This often fatal condition is one reason conservative guidelines should be followed in allowing athletes to return to play after a head injury.

6. Describe the immediate management of an athlete who has collapsed and is thought to have second impact syndrome.
1. Protect the cervical spine.
2. ABCs of cardiopulmonary resuscitation (CPR).
3. Hyperventilation to reduce CO_2.
4. Transport to medical facility.
5. Intravenous administration of an osmotic diuretic (e.g., 20% mannitol). (A Foley catheter will be necessary to handle the osmotic diuresis.)
6. Cranial computed tomographic (CT) or magnetic resonance imaging (MRI) scan.
7. Intravenous steroids to reduce intracranial swelling.

7. Describe the evaluation and treatment of a scalp laceration.
All scalp lacerations should be carefully examined for persistent bleeding, foreign bodies, leakage of cerebrospinal fluid, or depression of bone fragments. Lacerations should be thoroughly cleansed and closed with a single-layer suture using sterile technique. All abrasions, contusions, hematomas, and lacerations of the face and scalp should be evaluated for evidence of intracranial injury.

8. What is an epidural hematoma?
It is a an accumulation of blood between the skull and the outer dural covering of the brain.

9. What causes an epidural hematoma?
The most common cause is a tear in the middle meningeal artery, and it is usually associated with a skull fracture. Epidural hematoma may occur as a result of a high-velocity impact such as from a baseball or bat, especially to the temporoparietal region.

10. Describe the signs and symptoms of an epidural hematoma.
It classically follows an apparently mild head injury that produces a skull fracture and brief loss of consciousness, which is followed by a lucid interval lasting up to several hours. Then there is progressive rapid deterioration into coma. Pupil dilation, paralysis, and death may follow (may be fatal in 30 to 60 minutes).

11. How should an epidural hematoma be managed?
Morbidity and mortality are high if an epidural hematoma is left untreated, but it is easily diagnosed by CT scan. Permanent neurologic injury may be prevented with prompt surgical intervention.

12. What is a subdural hematoma?
If is an accumulation of blood in the subdural space, which is beneath the skull and outside of the brain between the arachnoid membrane and the dura.

13. What causes the formation of a subdural hematoma?
A tear in the dural sinus veins.

14. Describe the signs and symptoms of a subdural hematoma.
A subdural hematoma may present in a variety of ways, but is usually accompanied by headache. There is often immediate or progressive decline of consciousness, with eventual coma or death if left untreated.

15. How should a subdural hematoma be managed?
CT scan will diagnose acute and chronic types of subdural hematoma, although MRI may be superior in locating smaller injuries, especially subacute hematomas in their early stages. This lesion requires surgical drainage.

16. Name the three ways subdural hematomas may present and describe their management.
In the **acute** type, the blood clot usually occurs simultaneously with brain injury. There is immediate neurologic dysfunction. Acute subdural hematomas have much poorer prognosis because of associated high-velocity brain injury.

In the **subacute** type, the brain has usually not been injured substantially. It presents 24 hours or more after injury. MRI may be superior in finding early subacute subdural hematoma.

The **chronic** type is most often seen in the elderly. It also is seen in people who sustain frequent falls, including the elderly, alcoholics, or someone with syncope or vertigo. The lesion presents 2 or more weeks after injury. Chronic hematomas usually respond to treatment without associated or prolonged brain dysfunction. Any underlying problems such as atherosclerosis, arrhythmias, or ethanol abuse need to be treated.

17. What is a subarachnoid hemorrhage?
Intracranial hemorrhage confined to the surface of the brain.

18. What causes a subarachnoid hemorrhage?
It occurs as a result of disruption of tiny brain surface meningeal blood vessels. Blood acts as an irritant on the surface of the brain (brain parenchyma is not affected, as there is no bleeding within the brain itself).

19. What are the signs and symptoms of a subarachnoid hemorrhage?
It usually causes a headache and is often associated with a neurologic deficit. It may also precipitate a seizure.

20. How should a subarachnoid hemorrhage be managed?
Surgery is not usually required unless an associated congenital anomaly is present (e.g., cerebral aneurysm or atrioventricular malformation). If a seizure occurs, the best method to protect the patient's airway is to log-roll the athlete onto his or her side. The use of an antithrombolytic agent may be considered.

21. What is an intracerebral hemorrhage?
Bleeding within the substance of the brain itself.

22. What causes an intracerebral hemorrhage?
It occurs secondary to tearing of small blood vessels within the brain tissues.

23. What are the signs and symptoms of an intracerebral hemorrhage?
It is similar to cerebral contusion or subarachnoid hemorrhage (see above) but is more severe.

24. How should an intracerebral hemorrhage be managed?
It is readily diagnosed by CT scan. An intracerebral hemorrhage often requires surgical evacuation to reduce intracranial pressure.

25. Name the most rapidly progressive type of intracranial hemorrhage.

The epidural (or extradural) hematoma. (Remember, this usually results from a tear in the moderately sized middle meningeal artery, in which blood is pumping under much higher pressure than in the veins, and is located in the potential space between the dura and the skull. This artery lies just anterior and cephalad to the ear, where the temporoparietal part of the skull is its thinnest).

26. Describe the evaluation of acute head injuries in an unconscious athlete.

The most important part of the initial examination is following the ABCs of any trauma, evaluating the athlete's Airway, Breathing, and Circulation. An unconscious athlete should be assumed to have a cervical spine injury and should be treated as such until proved otherwise. Only after taking care of these initial life-threatening problems should evaluation of further disability be undertaken. Examination should then include evaluation of the athlete's level of consciousness, pupil size and reactivity, extremity movement and withdrawal from painful stimuli, and reflexes.

A Airway (protect cervical spine)
B Breathing
C Circulation
D Disability (neurologic evaluation)
E Exposure (for remainder of examination)

27. What are the signs of temporal lobe herniation?

1. General effects of increasing intracranial pressure (increasing blood pressure, decreasing pulse).
2. Contralateral hemiparesis and ipsilateral dilated pupil ("blown pupil") usually occur early in injury with unilateral temporal lobe herniation.
3. Bilateral pyramidal tract signs (with paresis/paralysis) and bilateral pupil dilation occur late in injury when bilateral temporal lobe herniation occurs.
4. Impairment of respiration and consciousness occur as brainstem herniation follows.

28. What signs and symptoms are suggestive of a basilar skull fracture?

Bruises or bleeding behind the ear, in the ear canal, and around the eye suggest a possible basilar skull fracture. Blood or cerebrospinal fluid exiting from the ear or nose may also occur with basilar skull fractures. Hearing loss, lack of smell, or facial paralysis may develop from basilar skull fractures as a result of damage to cranial nerves as they penetrate the base of the skull.

Athletes with basilar skull fractures should be considered for admission for observation, as cerebrospinal fluid may continue to leak after an injury and may require craniotomy to seal any defect. Plain radiographs and CT scans of the head are usually indicated if a skull fracture or significant brain injury is suspected. Cervical spine injury should also be ruled out by radiography on anyone with an injury this significant.

29. What is retrograde amnesia?

Retrograde amnesia is the inability to recall events before the injury. This may occur with even mild concussions. In more severe concussions, post-traumatic amnesia, or the inability to recall events that have occurred since the injury, may occur.

30. Describe the sideline evaluation of a concussion.

Listed below are several guidelines for evaluating the severity of concussions on the field. No guidelines are universally accepted at this point, and common sense and individual situations may dictate much of how each injury is managed.

Classification of Concussion

	MODIFIED CANTU*	COLORADO MEDICAL SOCIETY[†]	AMERICAN ACADEMY OF NEUROLOGY[‡]
Type	Signs and symptoms:	Signs and symptoms:	Signs and symptoms:
Grade 1	No LOC PTA < 30 min	Confusion without amnesia No LOC	Transient confusion No LOC Symptoms and mental status abnormalities resolve in < 15 minutes
Grade 2	LOC < 5 min or PTA > 30 min, but < 24 hr	Confusion with amnesia No LOC	Transient confusion No LOC Symptoms and mental status abnormalities resolve in > 15 minutes
Grade 3	LOC > 5 min or PTA > 24 hr	Any LOC	Any LOC, either brief (seconds) or prolonged (minutes)

LOC = loss of consciousness, PTA = posttraumatic amnesia.

* Modified from Cantu RC, Micheli LJ: American College of Sports Medicine's Guidelines for the Team Physician. Philadelphia, Lea & Febiger, 1991, with permission.

[†] Adapted from Guidelines for the Management of Concussion in Sports. Colorado Medical Society, Sports Medicine Committee, May 1990 (Revised May 1991), with permission.

[‡] Adapted from Practice Parameter: The management of concussion in sports (summary statement). Report of the Quality Standards Subcommittee. Neurology 48:581–585, 1997.

31. When should an athlete be allowed to return to play after a head injury?

This is one of the controversies that continue to rage in the world of sports medicine. Many team physicians used to follow the "1-2-3 rule": one concussion and the athlete is removed from the game; two concussions, out for the season; three concussions, no more play. Recently, other guidelines have been developed. When in doubt, always err on the conservative side.

Guidelines for Return after Concussion

	MODIFIED CANTU*	COLORADO MEDICAL SOCIETY[†]	AMERICAN ACADEMY OF NEUROLOGY[‡]
Concussion	May return if:	May return if:	May return if:
First			
Grade 1	Remove from event Asymptomatic for 1 wk	Amnesia does not develop No symptoms for 20 min	Mental status abnormalities or postconcussive symptoms resolve within 15 min
Grade 2	Remove from event Asymptomatic for 1 wk	Remove from event Hospital evaluation	Remove from event Asymptomatic for 1 wk
Grade 3	Remove from event Withhold minimum of 1 mo, then may return if asymptomatic for 1 wk	Remove from event Hospital evaluation is normal Asymptomatic for 2 wk	Remove from event Hospital evaluation Brief LOC (secs)— asymptomatic for 1 wk Prolonged LOC (min)— asymptomatic for 2 wk
Second			
Grade 1	Remove from event Return to play in 2 wk if asymptomatic for 1 wk		Remove from event Asymptomatic for 1 wk

(Table continued on following page.)

Guidelines for Return after Concussion (Continued)

	MODIFIED CANTU*	COLORADO MEDICAL SOCIETY[†]	AMERICAN ACADEMY OF NEUROLOGY[‡]
Second *(Cont.)*			
Grade 2	Remove from event		Remove from event
	Return to play in 1 mo if asymptomatic for 1 wk		Asymptomatic for 2 wk
	Consider terminating season		
Grade 3	Remove from event; terminate season		Remove from event
	Return next season if asymptomatic		Asymptomatic for 1 mo (or longer)
Third			
Grade 1	Terminate season		
	Return next season if asymptomatic		
Grade 2	Terminate season		
	Return next season if asymptomatic		

LOC = loss of consciousness.
Asymptomatic means no headache, dizziness, or impairment of orientation, concentration, or memory during rest or exertion.
* Modified from Cantu RC, Micheli LJ: American College of Sports Medicine's Guidelines for the Team Physician. Philadelphia, Lea & Febiger, 1991, with permission.
† Adapted from Guidelines for the Management of Concussion in Sports. Colorado Medical Society, Sports Medicine Committee, May 1990 (Revised May 1991), with permission.
‡ Adapted from Practice Parameter: The management of concussion in sports (summary statement). Report of the Quality Standards Subcommittee. Neurology 48:581–585, 1997.

32. Is an athlete who has sustained a concussion more susceptible to head injury in the future?

An athlete who has sustained one minor head injury has a fourfold increase in his or her risk of having another concussive injury. Until the athlete has been given fully adequate time to recuperate from the injury, the athlete is at risk for second impact syndrome.

33. Describe the Glasgow Coma Scale and its usefulness.

Eye Opening		+	Motor Response		+	Verbal Response	
Spontaneous	4		Obeys command	6		Oriented	5
To speech	3		Localizes painful stimuli	5		Confused conversation	4
To pain	2		Withdraws from painful stimuli	4		Inappropriate words	3
No response	1		Abnormal flexion response (decortication)	3		Incomprehensible sounds	2
			Abnormal extensor response (decerebration)	2		No response	1
			No response	1			

The Glasgow Coma Scale provides a scale for comparing serial examinations of an athlete with a head injury. The Glasgow Coma Scale score also correlates with the patient's prognosis. Of patients with a Glasgow score of 3 to 4, 80% die or remain in a vegetative state. The prognosis progressively improves as the Glasgow score improves; of patients with a Glasgow score > 11, only 6% die or remain in a vegetative state.

34. Name the layers of the scalp.

S Skin
C Connective tissue—dense strands and fat, nerves, arteries, and veins
A Aponeurosis—aponeurotic tendon connecting the fronto-occipital muscles anteriorly with the occipitalis muscle posteriorly
L Loose connective tissue
P Pericranium—periosteum covering cranial bone

35. What are the two sports with the highest incidence of serious closed head trauma?

Boxing and football. (Although almost every sport has some risk of head injury.)

36. Explain the significance of a "blown pupil" occurring in a closed head injury.

A unilateral fully dilated pupil that is unresponsive to light is one of the first signs of increasing intracranial pressure, which is the result of transtentorial herniation of the brain pushing against the oculomotor nerve (third cranial nerve) below it, causing the cessation of synaptic transmission through the nerve. Treatment to lower intracranial pressure at this stage is absolutely necessary before pressure on the brainstem increases, leading to dilation of both pupils, impairment of respiration, unconsciousness, and death due to brainstem herniation.

37. What is the leading cause of death from athletic head injury?

Intracranial hemorrhage.

38. Name the cranial nerves.

Out	I	Olfactory
On	II	Optic
Our	III	Oculomotor
Turf	IV	Trochlear
Timid	V	Trigeminal
Athletes	VI	Abducens
Face	VII	Facial
Another	VIII	Auditory (vestibulocochlear)
Game	IX	Glossopharyngeal
Vs the	X	Vagus
Saskatchewan	XI	Spinal accessory
Hamsters	XII	Hypoglossal

BIBLIOGRAPHY

1. American College of Surgeons: Advanced Trauma Life Supports Student Manual. Chicago, American College of Surgeons, 1989.
2. Cantu RC: Second impact syndrome: Immediate management. Physician Sportsmed 20:55–66, 1992.
3. Cantu RC, Micheli LJ (eds): American College of Sports Medicine's Guidelines for the Team Physician. Philadelphia, Lea & Febiger, 1991.
4. Henderson J: Head injuries. In Mellion MB, Walsh WM, Shelton GL (eds): The Team Physician's Handbook, 2nd ed. Philadelphia, Hanley & Belfus, 1997.
5. Kelly JP, Nichols JS, Filley CM, et al: Concussion in sports: Guidelines for prevention of catastrophic outcome. JAMA 266:2867–2869, 1991.
6. Kelly JP, Rosenberg JH: Diagnosis and management of concussion in sports. Neurology 48:575–580, 1997.
7. Lehman LB, Ravich SJ: Closed head injuries in athletes. Clin Sports Med 9:247–261, 1990.
8. Maroon JC, Bailes JE, Yates A, Norwig J: Assessing closed head injuries. Physician Sportsmed 20(4):37–44, 1992.
9. Plum F, Posner J: The Diagnosis and Stupor of Coma, 3rd ed. Philadelphia, F.A. Davis, 1980.
10. Practice Parameter: The management of concussion in sports [summary statement]. Report of the Quality Standards Subcommittee. Neurology 48:581–585, 1997.
11. Torg JS: Athletic Injuries to the Head, Neck, and Face. St. Louis, Mosby, 1991.

55. CERVICAL SPINE INJURIES

Jeffrey P. Anthony, D.O., and Richard A. Parker, D.O., FAOASM

CERVICAL STRAINS AND SPRAINS

1. After a whiplash injury, the patient complains of a severe headache, burning dysesthesias, and "cramps" of the scalp. the patient has point tenderness over the occipital notch. The diagnosis is occipital neuralgia. What is occipital neuralgia, and why does it occur?

Unlike other spinal nerves, the ganglia of the C2 spinal nerve root lies exposed on the vertebral arch of the axis, which makes them vulnerable to crush injuries between the bony arches of C1 and C2 during hyperextension. Also, the occipital nerve penetrates the semispinalis and trapezius muscles, and contracture or spasm of these muscles can cause these symptoms.

2. After a play, a football player is face down on the field and is unconscious, not breathing, and unarousable. What is your treatment in a step-wise fashion?

1. Assume cervical spine injury.
2. Try to arouse the player without moving him. If unarousable, immobilize the head and log roll him to face-up position.
3. Leaving the helmet and chin strap on, remove the mouthpiece and face mask.
4. If the player is not breathing, open his airway and check the pulse, following the current CPR protocol. If there is no pulse, remove the shoulder pads before implementing CPR.
5. Use the jaw-thrust method for respirations if possible; if not, use the head tilt/jaw lift cautiously without overextending the neck.
6. Transport the patient on a spine board, after stabilization, immobilizing the head and neck as much as possible.

3. A defensive back lies motionless on the ground following a tackle. After 5 minutes of anxious evaluation, he is able to walk and is neurologically intact. The diagnosis is cervical spinal cord neurapraxia (CSN) with transient quadriplegia. What is CSN? What are some of the predisposing factors?

CSN is an injury of the cervical spine resulting in a transient episode of the following neurologic phenomena: burning pain, numbness, tingling, or loss of sensation, along with motor weakness or even complete paralysis. Although relatively rare, this condition can be very unsettling to the patient and the medical team. Usually there is complete recovery in 10–15 minutes, although it may take up to 48 hours. Of note is the fact that the patient is usually conscious and has no complaints of neck pain. Predisposing factors are spinal stenosis, congenital fusion, cervical instability, and acute or chronic intervertebral disc disease.

4. After a 5-minute episode of transient quadriplegia sustained from a tackle, the patient completely recovers. The clinical examination is normal with full range of motion of the cervical spine and a normal neurologic examination. Radiographs and magnetic resonance imaging (MRI) are both within normal limits. Describe your thought processes for the possibility of returning this athlete to play.

This is a controversial issue and one that particularly underlines the importance of informed consent. If there is evidence of cervical stenosis, many studies support a higher risk of recurrence of this injury in a collision-type sport. However, there do not appear to be data that indicate a risk of a more permanent injury, even in these athletes with cervical stenosis.

If the examination is completely within normal limits and the radiologic studies are normal, including the absence of degenerative changes, spinal stenosis, or indications of instability, most studies indicate that there is no increased risk of recurrence. However, the risks and benefits of return to activity must be discussed with the patient and heavily weighed.

5. After an open-field tackle, a collegiate football player sustains a "burner"—a shooting pain from his right shoulder down to his hand. What are your criteria for return to play?
1. Resolution of symptoms (paresthesias, pain).
2. Full pain-free range of motion of the cervical spine and upper extremities.
3. Normal neurologic examination, including a detailed examination of the strength of the upper extremity.

6. The history is vitally important for accurate diagnosis of any injury. What is the most likely diagnosis for the following: (1) complete right arm burning lasting a few seconds after a hard tackle; and (2) tingling in the thumb and outer aspect of the forearm occurring during a golf swing follow-through, which also occasionally wakes the patient up at night.
1. Probable brachial plexus or upper trunk neurapraxia or burner.
2. Consider a herniated nucleus pulposus with a C6 radiculopathy.

7. Considering an injury to the nerves, differentiate neurapraxia, axonotmesis, and neurotmesis.
Neurapraxia, or grade 1 nerve damage, involves demyelination of the axon sheath that leads to a conduction block. This usually heals within 1 to 2 weeks.
Axonotmesis (grade 2 neuropathy) involves loss or disruption of the axon and the myelon sheath. The epineurium is still intact.
Neurotmesis is the most severe injury to the nerve (grade 3 neuropathy). This disruption of the endoneurium, the perineurium, and the epineurium usually results in a permanent neurologic deficit.

8. A football player comes out of a game with complaints of numbness and burning in his right shoulder extending to his arm and hand. The player was in a pile-up and his head was forced into extreme left side-bending. His neck muscles are tender diffusely to palpation and you suspect a brachial plexopathy. Describe your findings with grades 1, 2, and 3 brachial plexopathy and your concerns about return to competition.
Grade 1 (neurapraxia): History and physical examination may reveal the following: pain, numbness, and paresthesias unilaterally into one extremity. There may or may not be associated paresis. There may also be tenderness and muscle spasm in the cervicothoracic area. This condition usually resolves in 5–10 minutes with full cervical range of motion, full strength, and absence of symptoms. With quick, complete resolution, further competition may be allowed after attention to possible risk factors such as, for example, the use of a neck roll or strengthening exercises.
Grade 2 (axonotmesis): This is a more severe injury with symptoms that may last for weeks to months. It is particularly important to evaluate the weakness of the upper extremity, especially with the biceps, deltoids, and infraspinatus (elbow flexion, shoulder abduction, and external rotation, respectively), recognizing that the onset of weakness may be delayed up to 1 week. It is also important to rule out other pathologies, such as fractures, with radiographs and electromyographs (EMGs) if symptoms last more than 3 weeks. Treatment includes a strengthening program for the neck, shoulders, and arms. The athlete should not return to activity until full strength returns and the physical examination is completely normal, which many times occurs before evidence of a normal EMG. Again, attention must be given to preventive measures.
Grade 3 (neurotmesis): A severe neurologic injury that disrupts the entire nerve and usually leads to permanent neurologic deficit. Return to competition should be evaluated on an individual basis. Recommendation is for noncollision or noncontact sports.

9. What is the most common mechanism of a transient brachial plexopathy or burner? What muscles are most commonly affected?
Although there are reported cases of nerve root compression, the most common mechanism of injury for the burner is a traction injury where the shoulder is depressed and the head is side

bent to the opposite shoulder. This more commonly affects the upper trunk of the brachial plexus, more specifically, the C5 and C6 nerve roots, which produces a burning pain and tingling in the lateral arm, thumb, and index finger.

If there is paresis, it usually involves the deltoid, biceps, and infraspinatus. During evaluation, it is extremely important to evaluate the strength of these three muscles because the athlete during a competition may be reluctant to indicate any sensory changes. If there is weakness of elbow flexion, shoulder external rotation, or abduction, the athlete should not return to competition and should be followed closely. Full strength of these muscles, which may not be affected for up to a week after injury, is the prime indication for return to competition after a moderately severe injury since EMG findings may lag behind those found on physical examination.

RADIOGRAPHS

10. Regarding the cervical spine radiograph, what is the Mach effect?
On the open-mouth AP view, the posterior arch of C1 projects over the base of the odontoid process, simulating a fracture.

11. Regarding the cervical spine radiographs, what are the normal parameters for the soft tissue markings on the lateral view?
As with other areas of the body, it is possible to have a fracture of the spine that is not readily apparent on the radiographs but can be inferred by a change on the soft tissue markings. One method to assess this soft tissue swelling is on the lateral cervical spine radiographs at C3 and C6. At the C3 level, the soft tissue density between the posterior pharynx and the anterior vertebral body should be less than half of the anteroposterior width of the third cervical vertebral body. At the C6 level, that soft tissue density is about equal to or less than the anterior posterior width of the C6 vertebral body.

12. When looking at the lateral radiograph, it is important to recognize the four parallel longitudinal curvilinear lines down the cervical spine. If there is any disruption in these curves, then one should suspect, for example, a vertebral subluxation or fracture. These four lines follow each vertebral body successively at which landmarks?
The anterior and posterior borders of the vertebral bodies
The posterior cortices of the lateral masses
The spinolaminar lines
The spinous processes all seem to converge on one point posterior to the cervical spine, and a change of greater than 11° raises the suspicion of vertebral disruption.

13. What are radiologic indicators for cervical spinal stenosis?
• **Plain cervical radiographs, lateral**
   Standard method: Measure the posterior vertebra to spinal-laminar distance. However, also take into account the individual technique, the magnification, and the distance from the tube to the patient. If these are all standard, the normal measurement is usually greater than 12 mm. This technique has a low correlation with symptoms because of individual variability as well as the fact that it shows only osseous structures.
   Torg ratio: This is a ratio on the lateral cervical spine of the sagittal spinal canal diameter to the anteroposterior width of the vertebral body. This technique takes into consideration the different technique variabilities such as magnification and so forth. The normal ratio is > 0.8; that is, < 0.8 indicates spinal stenosis. However, in previous studies, up to 30% of asymptomatic people have a Torg ratio < 0.8.
• **MRI:** This gives a good estimate of the central canal measurements. It is noninvasive and the preferred diagnostic study at this time.
• **CT myelogram:** This is probably the most specific measurement which correlates with the spinal canal dimensions. It is invasive and may be technically more difficult than MRI.

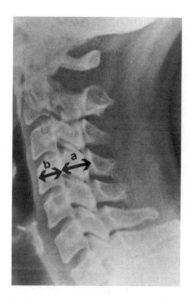

The Torg ratio. (From Pavlov H: Radiographic evaluation of the cervical spine and related structures. In Torg JS (ed): Athletic Injuries to the Head, Neck and Face, 2nd ed. St. Louis, Mosby, 1991, p 392, with permission.)

14. Is the spinal canal diameter diminished or expanded during cervical extension?

The spinal canal is narrowed during cervical extension because of approximation of the inferior posterior aspect of the vertebral body with the superior anterior aspect of the spinal laminar line. This "pincers" mechanism can be measured on a lateral cervical radiograph.

15. Which patients are at higher risk for having a diminished canal diameter?

Patients with spinal stenosis, degenerative disease, or osteophytes are at higher risk for a diminished canal diameter. However, the radiographs show only the osseous interferences and do not consider the canal narrowing secondary to the ligamenta flava or the posterior longitudinal ligament.

MECHANISM OF INJURY

16. What is the most commonly acknowledged mechanism responsible for fracture/dislocations of the cervical spine?

Axial loading in a slightly flexed position (flattening the normal cervical lordosis). The concepts of (1) the face mask of the helmet acting as a lever, forcing the head and neck into hyperflexion or (2) the implication of the posterior rim of the football helmet acting as a guillotine by causing forced hyperextension are without merit. (See figures, top of next page.)

17. What is the most common mechanism of injury in football resulting in permanent cervical quadriplegia?

Vertical compression (axial loading). Spearing is responsible for more than 50% of all injuries resulting in permanent cervical quadriplegia. It is followed by knee or thigh contact to the head in 15% of cases; collision, pile-up, or ground contact in 11%; and hyperflexion in 10% of cases. Hyperextension injuries account for only about 3% of these cervical injuries.

18. Which position in football is considered to pose the highest risk for sustaining a cervical spine injury?

Defensive back. In one study of 209 severe cervical spine injuries that occurred between 1971 and 1975, defensive backs accounted for 52% of these injuries at the high school level and 73% at the college level. Of this group, 13% were on specialty teams, whereas 10% were linebackers who tackled by using their heads as the initial point of contact.

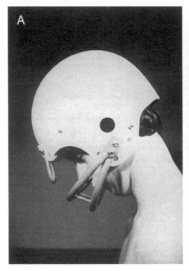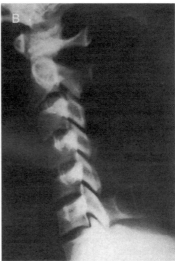

A and *B,* When the neck is flexed approximately 30°, the cervical spine becomes straight; from the standpoint of force, energy absorption, and the effect on tissue deformation and failure, the straightened cervical spine, when axially loaded, acts as a segmented column. (From Torg J: National Football Head and Neck Injuries Registry: Report on the cervical quadriplegia from 1971 to 1975. Am J Sports Med 7:127, 1979, with permission.)

CERVICAL FRACTURES AND INSTABILITY

19. When concerned about a C1 burst fracture, an AP open-mouth projection of C1–C2 is obtained. This view best demonstrates the lateral overhang of the C1 lateral masses in relationship to C2. At what point of combined lateral overhang should an instability associated with a transverse ligament rupture be suspected?

When the combined overhang is 7 mm or greater. The C1 burst fracture associated with disruption of the transverse ligament is considered unstable. It is generally treated with traction and halo immobilization to improve fracture fragment position. Surgery is occasionally necessary by way of posterior cervical fusion.

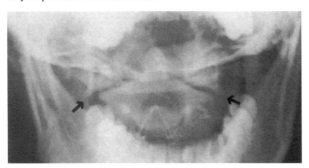

Open-mouth view illustrating an unstable C1 burst fracture with rupture of transverse ligament as indicated by lateral overhang greater than or equal to 7 mm *(black arrows).* (From Glasgow SG: Upper cervical spine injuries (C1 and C2). In Torg JS (ed): Athletic Injuries to the Head, Neck, and Face, 2nd ed. St. Louis, Mosby, 1991, p 459, with permission.)

20. Which is the most common type of C1 fracture, what is the cause, and how is it treated?

Fractures of the posterior arch. These fractures occur at the groove for the vertebral artery where the posterior arch is the thinnest. Posterior arch fractures result from an extension force causing a vertical compression of the C1 posterior ring by the occiput. These fractures are generally treated with a rigid cervical collar, as they are generally considered to be stable.

21. What is the most common type of odontoid fracture? How is it treated?

Type II—a fracture through the base at or just below the level of the superior articular process. This odontoid fracture is not only the most common but the most difficult to treat, as nonunion rates range from 17% in undisplaced fractures to as high as 64%. Undisplaced or minimally displaced (≤ 4 mm) type II odontoid fractures are treated with halo immobilization. In fractures significantly displaced (> 4 mm), attempted reduction with traction followed by halo immobilization versus primary posterior fusion is recommended.

22. In traumatic cervical flexion injuries, atlantoaxial instability can result from rupture of the transverse ligament and/or the alar ligaments. What measurement of the atlantodens interval (ADI), as demonstrated on lateral flexion/extension radiographs, indicates an instability of the atlantoaxial complex?

In adults > 3 mm and in children > 4 mm. The transverse ligament ruptures within a range of 3 to 5 mm. Greater than 5 mm generally involves a rupture of the alar ligaments as well. An ADI > 7.5 mm generally results in neurologic symptoms.

23. What is a hangman's fracture?

It is a fracture through the arch of the axis (C2) resulting in a traumatic spondylolisthesis.

24. When assessing the cervical spine radiographically for instability on the lateral flexion/extension view, horizontal translation of one vertebra relative to an adjacent segment should not exceed what distance?

3.5 mm.

25. What is a "teardrop" fracture?

A triangular fracture fragment at the anteroinferior corner of a cervical vertebral body. Teardrop fractures are actually just a part of two specific compression fractures occurring in the lower (C4–C7) cervical spine. The term burst fracture has also been used to describe these specific injuries. Unfortunately, the terms teardrop and burst give an incomplete description of the actual pathology and mechanism of injury involved in these fractures.

BIBLIOGRAPHY

1. Hensinger RN: Congenital anomalies of the atlantoaxial joint. In The Cervical Spine, 2nd ed. Philadelphia, J.B. Lippincott, 1989.
2. Hershman B: Brachial plexus injuries. Clin Sports Med 9(2):311–330, 1990.
3. Moore K: Clinically Oriented Anatomy. Baltimore, William & Wilkins, 1980.
4. Saal J (ed): Neck and Back Pain. Physical Medicine and Rehabilitation: State of the Art Reviews. 4(2):175–387, 1990. Philadelphia, Hanley & Belfus.
5. Torg JS: Athletic Injuries to the Head, Neck and Face, 2nd ed. St. Louis, C.V. Mosby, 1991.
6. Torg JS: (ed): Head and neck injuries. Clin Sports Med 6:1, 1987.
7. Torg JS: National Football Head and Neck Injuries Registry.
8. White AA, Johnson RM, et al: Biomechanical analysis of clinical stability in the C-spine. Clin Orthop 120:85, 1975.

56. SPORTS-RELATED EYE INJURIES

John B. Jeffers, D.V.M., M.D.

1. Which sports have the highest frequency of eye injuries? What is most apt to cause the injury in each sport?
1. Basketball: usually by fingers and elbows
2. Baseball: usually by the ball while batting, line drive, or flyball
3. Swimming and pool activities: usually by elbows, fingers, and feet

2. Which age groups and corresponding sports have the highest frequency of eye injuries?
1. 5–14 years of age: baseball (Little League age) and softball, usually fielding
2. 15–24 years of age: basketball
3. 25–64 years of age: basketball (used to be racquet sports—now fewer because of appropriate protective eyewear)

3. List the sports related to low risk, high risk, and very high risk for eye injuries.

Sports-related Risk of Eye Injury

Low-risk sports	Cycling, track and field, swimming, tennis (singles)
High-risk sports	Football, hockey (ice, roller, and street), basketball, baseball, softball, tennis (doubles), racquet sports (racquetball, squash, "handball," badminton, swimming and pool activities, water polo, fencing, men's lacrosse*)
Very-high-risk sports	Boxing, full-contact martial arts, wrestling

* In women's lacrosse and field hockey, eye protection is elective. However, mouth guards are mandated.

Note: Remember contact lenses and daily wear glasses offer *no protection.* For adequate protection, the athlete should wear appropriate, well-fitted, certified protective eyewear.

4. What are the danger signs and symptoms of a potentially serious eye injury?
1. Sudden decrease or loss of vision
2. Loss of field of vision
3. Pain or movement of the eye
4. Photophobia ("light sensitivity")
5. Diplopia (vs. "ghost image")
6. Protrusion of one eye
7. "Lightning flashes," often with large floaters
8. Irregularly shaped pupil
9. Foreign body sensation
10. "Red eye"
11. Blood in anterior chamber
12. Halos around lights (cornea edema)

5. Define diplopia.
Seeing two images of the same object. Usually this occurs when both eyes are open—therefore when either eye is covered, one image disappears. Monocular diplopia is *rare*—it is most often related to a refractive error (i.e., astigmatism) and looks like a "ghost image" on a television set.

6. What are the important aspects of a preparticipation history?
1. Refractive error:
   - Needing glasses or contact lenses (contact lenses offer **no protection!**)
   - Highly nearsighted—may be more prone to retinal detachment
   - History of refractive surgery (i.e., radial keratotomy [RK]); incisional RK weakens cornea and excimer laser probably does not (but possible glare)

 2. Strabismus (i.e., crossed eyes)
   • Muscle surgery
   • Amblyopia or "lazy eye"
 3. Intraocular surgery (cataract extraction, retinal detachment) or eye trauma (traumatic hyphema, laceration of eye). Radial keratotomy, an extraocular surgical procedure to correct refractive errors, weakens the cornea.

7. What are the important aspects of the evaluation of the player with an eye injury?
 1. Obtain an adequate history to attempt to determine the force and direction of the force (i.e., baseball line drive, flyball, pitched ball, slapshot, street hockey ball or puck).
 2. Obtain a visual acuity before any manipulation (penlight or manual) of the eye. *Exception:* chemical (field markings) injury—immediately flush eye for 30 minutes!
 3. Determine severity of the injury and, if any doubt, refer to an opthalmologist.
 4. Use appropriate first aid: crushed ice, shield, "moist chamber."

8. What are the most common types of sports-related eye injuries?
 1. Corneal abrasion   3. Traumatic hyphema   5. "Black eye" (ecchymosis
 2. Traumatic iritis   4. Orbital fractures   and edema)

9. How do you examine the injured athlete following a "poke" in the eye?
 Pain and lid squeezing (blepharospasm) may make it difficult to open the lids; therefore, use one or two drops of topical anesthesia. To check for a corneal abrasion, "touch" a moistened strip of fluorescein paper to the *inside* of the lower lid. With a blue filter on a penlight, the abrasion will "light up" green. **Do not use topical anesthesia to prolong play!**

10. The athlete has severely edematous eyelids—what do you do?
 Use a small amount (size of a golfball) of crushed ice in a plastic sandwich bag, secure top, wrap in gauze, and tape to forehead. Avoid ice cubes or commercial ice packs, which may cause further damage because of the weight.

11. The eye may be so severely contused that edematous conjunctiva "pouches" through the eyelids. What is the easiest (and cheapest) way to handle this (prevent drying)?
 Use a sheet of plastic wrap or a sheet from the plastic sandwich bag and tape all edges around the eye to provide a "moist chamber" to protect the exposed mucous membrane. Using an antibiotic ointment to keep the tissue moist makes it difficult for further evaluation. Any therapy can be administered in drop form.

12. What do you do if you suspect a laceration of the eyeball?
 After obtaining an appropriate history, always try to obtain a visual acuity (a near vision card or the ability to count fingers at a certain distance) and document. Then tape a plastic shield over the eye to prevent any further pressure being placed on the globe. If no plastic shield is available, use the bottom of a styrofoam cup or milk carton. **Never** instill an ointment if an open globe is suspected!

13. What is the definition of the *functionally* one-eyed athlete?
 Any athlete with best-corrected vision of worse than 20/40 in one eye and 20/40 or better best-corrected vision in the good eye. **Both** eyes must be protected with polycarbonate lenses **all waking hours**. The important message is that any injury to the "good eye" would adversely affect the athlete's future athletic endeavors, lifestyle, and work.

14. Should the functionally one-eyed athlete be prohibited from participation in all sports?
 The only sports a one-eyed athlete should avoid are the high eye-risk sports such as boxing, wrestling, and full contact martial arts in which no eye protection is available. Participation in all

other sports may be allowed as long as the appropriate, certified, properly fitting eye protection is worn. In the case of a sport in which a helmet is being worn, a mask, cage, or face guard should be worn as well as polycarbonate sports goggles ("belt and suspenders").

15. What are the specifications of appropriate sports eye protectors?

1. Polycarbonate lenses with 3-mm center thickness (if prescription is too high for polycarbonate, CR39 [registered trademark PPG industrial] plastic may be used). For low-eye risk sports (e.g., cycling, track, swimming), polycarbonate lenses 2 mm thick are acceptable.

2. A sturdy frame with a posterior rim so the lens is less apt to be dislodged posteriorly *into* the eye. A polycarbonate frame with a molded temple is the strongest. The best available sports eye protectors for baseball and softball fielders are those that have passed the American Society for Testing and Materials (ASTM) standard F803-88. When impacted with a high-speed projectile like a baseball line drive, the frame may break at the temple or nosepiece; however, the polycarbonate lens will not break. Therefore, the eye is saved!

3. Antifog lens treatment.

4. Sports eye protectors should be fit by an experienced optometrist or optician. Most complaints about protective eyewear are due to a poor fit.

Eye Protection for Sports

MODEL	PRESCRIPTION CAPABLE	COMPANY NAME, ADDRESS, AND TELEPHONE NUMBER
Jr. Rec-Specs ("Neon Colors, Wraparound")* (small and large)	Yes	Liberty Optical
		380 Verona Avenue
Pro-Guard	Yes	Newark NJ 07104
All-Pro	Yes	800-444-5010
Sports Goggle	Yes	
Swim Goggles	Yes	
Sport-Lok (small & large)	Yes	
New Yorker	No	LSP Leader Sports Product, Inc.
Troy	Yes	One Trans Border Dr.
Dallas†	No	Chamlin, NY 12919
Westport Jr. Champ (Swim)	No	800-847-2001
Vizion II (over the glasses) (Lacrosse)†	No	
Vision Plus (Football shield)	No	
Polycarbonate Face Guard (Football, Hockey)	No	OneXcel, Inc.
		99 Rosewood Drive
		Suite 260
		Danvers, MA 01923
		978-777-5730
Polycarbonate Face Guard (Football, Hockey)	No	Itech Sport Products Inc.
		825 F, rue Tecumseh St.
		Dollard-des-Ormeaux
		Quebec H9R 4T8
		1-800-361-5595
Polycarbonate Face Guard (Baseball)	No	Face Guard Inc.
		P.O. Box 901
		Salem, VA 24153
		800-336-9683
Metal Face Guard (Baseball)	No	Shutt Sports Group
		1200 East Union
		Litchfield, IL 62056

(Table continued on following page.)

Eye Protection for Sports (Continued)

MODEL	PRESCRIPTION CAPABLE	COMPANY NAME, ADDRESS, AND TELEPHONE NUMBER
R.E.P. (small and large)	Yes	Eagle Eyewear Distributor of Ambassador Eyewear Group 1010 Arch St., 3rd floor Philadelphia, PA 19107 800-257-7878
Regent	No	Ektelon
Swim Goggles	No	1 Sportsystem Plaza
Interceptor	No	Bordentown, NJ 08505-9630
Olympus	Yes	800-283-2635
Odyssey	Yes	
Spector	No	
Mirage	No	
Action Eyes	Yes	Black Knight USA (formerly Viking Sports) 5355 Sierra Road San Jose, CA 95132 800-535-3300

* Kids love the bright "neon" nose and temple cushion; "wraparound"-cushioning covering rim of the frame.
† Passed impact test with women's lacrosse ball.
Note: Lensless eyeguards offer no protection!

16. Which organizations set the standards for eye protection for sports?

Standards for Eye Injury Protection (Meet or Exceed Standards)

Sports goggles for racquet sports:
  American Society for Testing & Materials (ASTM)
  (F803-88)
  100 Barr Harbour Dr.
  W. Conshohocken, PA 19428
	Baseball polycarbonate face guards:
	  ASTM (F910-86)
	
	Industrial safety glasses:
	  American National Standards Institute
	  (ANSI Z87)

Hockey helmets and face guards:
  American Hockey Association of United States
  Canadian Amateur Hockey Association
  Canadian Standards Association
	1430 Broadway
	New York, NY 10018
	(212) 642-4900

17. When can an athlete with an injured eye return to play?

1. When the ocular tissue has healed sufficiently to sustain a blow to the head or body that produces a "Valsalva maneuver," thereby increasing the pressure inside the eye.

2. When the eye is comfortable with adequate return of vision. Appropriate, well-fitting eye protectors *must* be worn!

3. During the game, immediate return to play is dependent on the complaint (i.e., blurred vision, pain) and the team physician's objective findings. *Never* use topical anesthesia to prolong play!

18. What are the "essentials" of an emergency kit for eye injuries?

1. Near vision card
2. Penlight (with blue filter)
3. Fluorescein strips
4. Commercial eye wash (plastic squeeze bottle)
5. Eye shields (plastic/metal)
6. Topical anesthesia (i.e., proparacaine)
7. Lid retractor (bent large paper clip)
8. Applicator sticks
9. Eye medication (your choice)
10. Plastic sandwich bags
11. Tape (eye patch optional)

BIBLIOGRAPHY

1. 1995 Sports and Recreational Eye Injuries. Chicago, Prevent Blindness America (PBA) (formerly National Society to Prevent Blindness), 1996.
2. Caveness LS: Ocular and facial injuries in baseball. Int Ophthalmol Clin 28:238, 241, 1988.
3. Easterbrook M: Ocular injuries in racquet sports. Int Ophthalmol Clin:232, 237, 1988.
4. Erie JC: Eye Injuries: Prevention, evaluation and treatment. Phys Sportsmed 19:108, 122, 1991.
5. Jeffers JB: An on-going tragedy: Pediatric sports-related eye injuries. Semin Ophthalmol 5:216, 223, 1990.
6. Jeffers JB: Pediatric eye safety. In Cibis GW, Tongue AC, Stass-Isern MI (eds): Decision Making in Pediatric Ophthalmology. St. Louis, Mosby-Year Book, 1993, pp 226, 269.
7. Larrison WI, Hersh PS, Kunzwerler T, Shingleton BJ: Sports-related ocular trauma. Ophthalmology 97:1265–1269, 1990.
8. Napier SM, Baker RS, Sanford DG, Easterbrook M: Eye injuries in athletics and recreation. Surv Ophthalmol 41:229–244, 1996.
9. Pashby DJ: Ocular injuries in hockey. Int Ophthalmol Clin 28:228–231, 1988.
10. Pashby TJ, Pashby RC, Chisholm LDL, Crawford JS: Eye injuries in Canadian hockey. Can Med Assoc J 113:663–674, 1975.
11. Strahlman E, Sommer A: The epidemiology of sports-related ocular trauma. Int Ophthalmol Clin 28:199–202, 1988.
12. Vinger PF: The eye and sports medicine. In Duane TD, Jaeger EA (eds): Clinical Ophthalmology, vol 5. Philadelphia, J.B. Lippincott, 1994, ch. 45.
13. Wichmann S, Martin DR: Single-organ patients: Balancing sports with safety. Phys Sportsmed 20:176–182, 1992.

57. MAXILLOFACIAL INJURIES

Mathew C. Gordon, M.D., D.D.S., and Harold Kai Tu, M.D., D.M.D., FACS

GENERAL CONSIDERATIONS

1. What are the three major categories of maxillofacial injuries?

Soft tissue injuries, dentoalveolar trauma, and facial skeletal trauma.

2. What are the general treatment objectives in maxillofacial injuries?

Overall treatment objectives are the restoration of function and facial appearance. Treatment priorities should be consistent with monitoring airway, control of hemorrhage, treatment of shock, and management of associated injuries (e.g., cervical spine).

3. Assuming the patient has a pulse, what are the initial treatment objectives?

Immediate control of the airway, hemorrhage, and cervical spine injuries is essential.

In the conscious patient without evidence of neck injury, airway maintenance can be accomplished by sitting the patient upright and slightly forward. The oral cavity and oral pharynx should be freed of all foreign bodies (i.e., finger sweep). It may be necessary to put outward traction on the tongue if the patient has bilateral mandibular fractures and standard methods are ineffective. Maintaining airway in the unconscious patient or suspected cervical spine injury requires the use of jaw thrust, oral airway, endotracheal tube, or tracheostomy.

Cervical spine injuries must be suspected in all athletes with maxillofacial injuries or who are unconscious. Constant cervical traction or the use of sandbags or a cervical collar to immobilize the neck during any manipulation or transportation is required. Direct pressure is indicated for initial hemorrhage control.

4. What are the signs and symptoms of cervical spine injuries?

Check for neck pain, limited motion, and neurologic deficits. A change in voice (e.g., hoarseness), cervical emphysema, or loss of thyroid cartilage prominence should suggest laryngeal injury.

5. How are facial fractures evaluated?

In general, facial fractures are evaluated by symptoms, observation, and palpation. Facial asymmetry, point tenderness, bony steps, mobility, ecchymosis, and paresthesia are all suggestive of facial fractures. Occlusal (bite) discrepancy, pain, and limitation of mouth opening suggest fractures of the jaws, teeth, and alveolus.

6. What radiographs are diagnostic in facial injuries?

A facial series and panoramic radiography are good screening studies. Tomograms, computed tomography (CT), and magnetic resonance imaging (MRI) may be indicated in complex facial injuries.

7. What are the classifications of soft tissue injuries?

Contusions, abrasions, and lacerations.

8. How should the soft tissue wound be treated intraorally?

Following control of hemorrhage, complete exploration with copious irrigation is accomplished and the wounds are then closed primarily.

DENTOFACIAL INJURIES

9. What are dentoalveolar injuries?

Dentoalveolar injuries involve the teeth and supporting structures. Individual teeth may be impacted, luxated, and partially or totally avulsed. Alveolar fractures involving single or multiple teeth are usually seen in the anterior dentition. Intraoral soft tissue injuries are sometimes extensive in their appearance; however, careful debridement and meticulous closure will achieve anatomic reapproximation and minimal scarring.

10. What preliminary examinations can be performed in dentoalveolar injuries?

A complete regional examination should be done to rule out any associated facial injuries. An intraoral examination to determine the presence of missing and fractured teeth, occlusal (bite) discrepancy, lacerations, and foreign objects should be accomplished. If an avulsed tooth cannot be found, a chest radiograph should be done to rule out aspiration. Panoramic radiography or additional dental films may provide more detail.

11. What are the general treatment objectives in dentoalveolar injuries?

1. Replace avulsed teeth.
2. Close intraoral lacerations.
3. Reestablish premorbid occlusion.
4. Stabilize and fixate any fractured alveolar segment.
5. Place patient on a nonchewing diet for 2–3 weeks.
6. Recommend the use of a mouth guard on return to sports.

12. How should an avulsed tooth be immediately managed?

The tooth should be reimplanted into the socket as quickly as possible. Debris should be conservatively removed with milk, saline, or water without traumatizing the root surface. Instruct the patient to bite down on a gauze to keep the tooth stable and in place. If the tooth cannot be replaced in the tooth socket, place the tooth in milk or in the patient's mouth until a dentist can be reached. Oral penicillin V (or equivalent), 500 mg, four times a day for 10 days should be prescribed.

NASAL FRACTURES

13. What is a nasal fracture?
It is a fracture of the nasal bones and cartilage and represents the most common sports injury related to the face.

Frontal view of the skull showing common isolated nasal fractures.

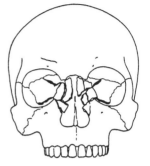

14. What are the common signs and symptoms of a nasal fracture?
The common signs and symptoms include epistaxis (bleeding), nasal airway obstruction, nasal asymmetry, crepitus over the nasal bridge, periorbital and subconjunctival ecchymosis, and septal hematoma.

15. What are the treatment objectives in a nasal fracture?
1. Secure the airway.
2. Control the bleeding by external pressure and if necessary intranasal packing.
3. Protect from further injury and transport for definitive diagnosis and treatment.
4. The athlete should be restricted to noncontact drills and competition for the first 3–4 weeks. Protective headgear should be worn for 2–3 months.

MAXILLARY FRACTURES

16. What is a maxillary fracture?
It is a fracture involving the upper jaw and associated bony supporting structures. Maxillary fractures are classified as Le Fort I, II, and III, depending on whether the nasal or cheek bones are involved. A maxillary fracture is usually caused by direct trauma to the middle portion of the face.

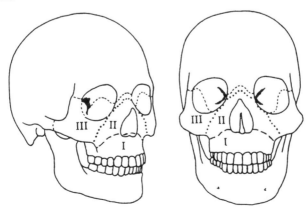

Left and frontal views of the skull showing Le Fort I, II, and III fractures of the upper jaw.

17. What are the common signs and symptoms of a maxillary fracture?

The common signs and symptoms include lengthening of face; mobility of maxilla or mid-face; malocclusion, especially open bite; ecchymosis (bruising) in the buccal vestibule; epistaxis (nasal bleeding); and nasal deformity and flattening or splaying of naso-orbital region.

18. What are the treatment objectives in a maxillary fracture?

1. Secure the airway. In the conscious patient, a forward-sitting position to allow dependent drainage of saliva and blood is helpful.

2. Cervical spine injuries should be suspected and precautions taken.

3. Nasal packing to control bleeding should be carried out by properly trained health professionals.

4. Immediate transportation for definitive diagnosis and treatment.

MANDIBULAR FRACTURES

19. What is a mandibular fracture?

It is a fracture of the lower jaw and represents the third most common facial bone fracture related to sports. Mandibular fractures are classified according to anatomic location; approximately 50% involve multiple fractures, with the most common sites being the condyle (jaw joint) and mandibular angle.

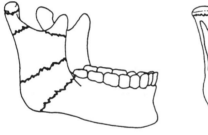 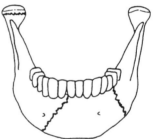

Left and frontal view of the mandible showing common mandibular fracture or an injury to the temporo-mandibular joint.

20. What are the common signs and symptoms of a mandibular fracture?

The common signs and symptoms include changes in occlusion (bite), mobility of mandibular segments, pain with function, inability to chew or open the mouth widely, numbness or paresthesia of lower lip, ecchymosis of the gums and the floor-of-mouth, and deviation of the lower jaw on opening.

21. What are the treatment objectives in a mandibular fracture?

1. Secure the airway.

2. Immobilize the lower jaw. A Barton bandage (see figure) or an Ace wrap from under the chin to around the back of the head can be used.

3. Transport the patient for definitive diagnosis and treatment.

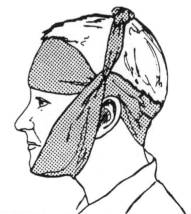

Barton (barrel) bandage for temporary immobilization in the treatment of a mandibular fracture or an injury to the temporo-mandibular joint.

22. What are some rehabilitation concerns with intermaxillary fixation (IMF) (jaws wired together)?

A major concern during IMF is nutrition. The patient will require a high-protein, carbohydrate liquid diet during IMF. Close monitoring of the patient's weight is required. A 5–10% weight loss is commonly seen, and loss over 10% requires nutritional supplementation. Activities such as weightlifting, running, and contact workouts should be avoided during IMF, as it may be difficult to breathe and the fracture may be displaced. Light activities such as stationary biking, swimming, and light weights are acceptable to maintain tone and condition. Direct contact sports (e.g., boxing, football) should be delayed generally for 1 month after release of IMF. Customized headgear and mouth guard should be worn to provide further protection. When rigid external fixation (bone plates) is used, full activity may be resumed much earlier.

Mandibular condylar fractures are treated with a shorter length of IMF (2–3 weeks) with earlier physical therapies. Condyle fractures should be followed closely in children and adolescents, because they may affect jaw growth.

ZYGOMATIC COMPLEX FRACTURES

23. What is a zygomatic complex (ZMC) fracture?

IT is the detachment of the zygoma or cheek bone usually at the front zygomatic, zygomaticotemporal, and zygomatic maxillary sutures. It is usually caused by direct blows to the cheekbone, and it is the second most common sports-related facial fracture.

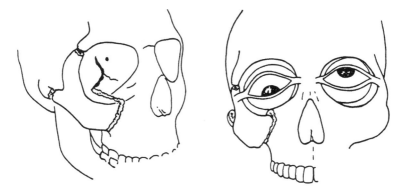

Left and frontal views showing a zygomatic complex fracture.

24. What are the common signs and symptoms of a ZMC fracture?

Physical examination may reveal flatness of the cheek, limited mandibular opening, paresthesia or anesthesia of the affected cheek, periorbital swelling and ecchymosis or emphysema, subconjunctival hemorrhage, enophthalmos, diplopia, step defects at the inferior and lateral orbital rims and zygomatic buttress, intraoral buccal ecchymosis, and limited ocular movement or pupillary height discrepancy.

25. How is a ZMC fracture treated?

1. Assess any visual changes.
2. Protect from further injury.
3. Transport the patient for definitive diagnosis and treatment.
4. Special headgear should be worn following reduction of the fracture for approximately 2 months. Visual disturbances may be a complication of a ZMC fracture. This may delay athletic rehabilitation, and an ophthalmologist should be consulted.

ORBITAL FLOOR FRACTURE (BLOWOUT FRACTURE)

26. What is an orbital fracture?
This is an isolated fracture of the orbital floor (eye socket). Orbital fat and muscle may herniate into the maxillary sinus. The orbital rim is intact in a pure blowout fracture. It is caused by a rapid increase in intraorbital pressure. The force is usually by a blunt object (e.g., tennis ball) slightly larger than the orbital bony aperture (opening).

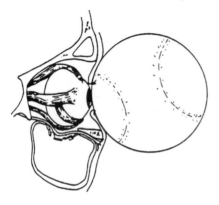

Orbital floor fracture (blowout fracture) caused by the force of the baseball striking the eye. The orbital rim is left intact.

27. What are the common signs and symptoms of an orbital fracture?
Clinical examination may reveal decreased ocular range of motion; diplopia (double vision); periorbital swelling, ecchymosis, or emphysema; subconjunctival hemorrhage; enophthalmos; unilateral epistaxis; and unequal pupillary height.

28. What are the treatment objectives in an orbital fracture?
Initial management consists of protecting the eye from further injury and referral of the patient for definitive care. Definitive care is directed toward correcting anatomic abnormalities and restoring normal ocular function.

29. What are rehabilitation concerns in an orbital fracture?
Rehabilitation is similar to that for a ZMC fracture.

TEMPOROMANDIBULAR JOINT INJURIES

30. What are temporomandibular joint (TMJ) injuries?
Injury is usually a result of a blow to the mandible with forces being transmitted to the TMJ. The injury can include hemarthrosis (intracapsule bleeding), capsulitis (inflammation of capsule ligaments), internal derangement (meniscal displacement), subluxation/dislocation, or fracture.

31. What are the common signs and symptoms of TMJ injuries?
Clinical examination may reveal limitation of mouth opening, pain or deviation in opening, change in occlusion, joint noise (clicking, popping, crepitus), or an inability to close the mouth.

32. What are the treatment concerns in TMJ injuries?
Initial management should immobilize the mandible using an Ace or Barton bandage. The patient should be referred for definitive diagnosis and treatment. This usually consists of limited function, soft diet, moist heat, and nonsteroidal inflammatory drugs (NSAIDs) for 7–10 days. Dislocation can be reduced manually by grasping each side of the jaw with the thumb hooked inside the mouth (away from the teeth) and exerting firm downward and posterior force (see figure, top of next page). Local anesthetic or sedation may be required.

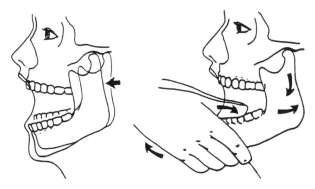

Manual reduction of a TMJ dislocation. Using both hands, hook thumbs inside the mouth, away from the teeth, and exert firm downward and posterior force. Anesthetic may be necessary.

33. What are rehabilitation concerns in TMJ injuries?
Rehabilitation consists of repetitive, passive mouth-opening exercises. Tongue blades may be used as an aid and to monitor progress. Thermotherapy, electrical stimulation, massage, and relaxation therapy can all be useful adjunctive therapy. Physical activities should be restricted until acute signs and symptoms diminish in approximately 7–10 days. Athletes on muscle relaxants should be restricted from workouts and competition. If surgery (arthroplasty) is involved, 4–6 weeks of recovery before returning to conditioning and light drills should be expected. Resumption of direct contact sports should be delayed an additional 2–3 months depending on the patient's response to therapy. Mouth guards are a requirement when the athlete returns to contact sports.

BIBLIOGRAPHY

1. Converse JM: Reconstructive Plastic Surgery, vol 2, 2nd ed. Philadelphia,W.B. Saunders, 1964.
2. Hawkins RW, Lyne ED: Skateboarding fractures. Am J Sports Med 9:99, 1981.
3. Kendrick RW: Some "sporting" injuries. Int J Oral Surg 1(Suppl 10):245, 1981.
4. Koplich B, Koplik M: Mouthguards prevent most oral injuries in contact sports. NY J Dent 44:84, 1974.
5. Morton JG, Burton JF: An evaluation of the effectiveness of mouthguards in high-school rugby players. NZ Dent J 75:151, 1979.
6. Rowe NL, Williams JL: Maxillofacial Injuries, vol 1. New York, Churchill Livingstone, 1985.
7. Rowe NL, Killey HC: Fractures of the Facial Skeleton, 2nd ed. Edinburgh, Churchill Livingstone, 1968.

---

58. SHOULDER AND CLAVICLE TRAUMA

Kirk S. Hutton, M.D., and John W. McClellan, III, M.D.

DISLOCATIONS

1. What is the difference between a dislocation and a shoulder separation?
It is quite common for patients to use the two terms interchangeably, but generally a dislocation is regarded as a glenohumeral injury, in which the articular surface of the humeral head and articular surface of the glenoid are not in contact with each other any longer. Lesser degrees of glenohumeral dislocation are actually termed subluxations and involve an abnormal movement of the humeral head on the glenoid, short of complete dislocation. Separations, on the other hand, are disruptions of the acromioclavicular joint.

2. How are glenohumeral dislocations classified?

Numerous classification systems have been published in the literature for shoulder dislocations. Hawkins describes multiple factors that are important to the treatment and cause of shoulder dislocations, including direction, degree, onset, and volition. The most common direction is
anterior; posterior and multidirectional instability are the common variants. The degree of instability is described in question 1 as either being dislocation or subluxation. Onset of instability is
related to whether the incident was traumatic or atraumatic, and volition (the ability to dislocate
and relocate the shoulder voluntarily) can generally be seen in patients with posterior instability,
although many patients with multidirectional instability (MDI) also show volition.

Two mnemonics devised by Matson help to remember the types of shoulder dislocations:
TUBS and **AMBRI**, which recently was expanded to **AMBRII**. The **TUBS** variety of instability
related to a **t**raumatic condition that is **u**nidirectional (usually anterior). A **B**ankart lesion, which
is a separation of the glenohumeral ligaments from the glenoid, is usually seen in traumatic episodes and typically is treated by **s**urgery. **AMBRII** instability refers to **a**traumatic onset, usually
multidirectional and involving **b**ilateral shoulders. Treatment is generally **r**ehabilitation, but for
patients who fail rehabilitation, surgery involves an **i**nferior capsular shift with attention to the interval lesion (abnormally wide separation between the supraspinatus and subscapularis tendon).

T	Traumatic	A	Atraumatic
U	Unidirectional	M	Multidirectional
B	Bankart	B	Bilateral
S	Surgery	R	Rehabilitation
		I	Inferior capsule shift
		I	Interval lesion

3. How can the physical examination differentiate an anterior from posterior dislocation?

The physical examination of an anterior shoulder dislocation is generally diagnostic. The patient is in obvious pain and shows significant muscle spasm. The humeral head often can be palpated anteriorly. The arm is held with slight external rotation and abduction, and the patient has
difficulty with internal rotation of the arm. Often, there is a hollow beneath the acromion with a
squared-off appearance of the shoulder. Posterior dislocations, on the other hand, may have no
obvious deformity because the arm is generally held across the abdomen in a position of adduction and internal rotation. Classic features include limited external rotation of the shoulder, with
forward flexion less than 90°, and a posterior prominence with slight rounding of the shoulder
compared with normal. In thin patients, a prominent coracoid process also may be seen.

4. Describe a Bankart and a Hill-Sachs lesion.

A Bankart lesion is an injury involving the anterior glenohumeral ligaments and glenoid
labrum, which become separated from the articular surface of the anterior glenoid neck during a
traumatic anterior dislocation. It is often possible to have a fragment of bone, which causes a bony
Bankart lesion in some severe traumatic episodes. A Hill-Sachs lesion is a defect in the posterolateral humeral head that occurs in a traumatic anterior dislocation when the posterolateral aspect of
the humeral head is abraded by the anterior rim of the glenoid. This lesion is often seen on the axillary radiograph, but other special x-ray views can be obtained to look for this lesion specifically.

5. What radiographs are important in evaluating a shoulder dislocation or suspected dis-location?

The most common error in diagnosing shoulder dislocation is not obtaining orthogonal
views of the glenohumeral joint. The common misconception is that anteroposterior (AP) views
of the humerus in internal and external rotation are sufficient, but they do not completely evaluate
the glenohumeral joint. An AP view of the shoulder and either an axillary lateral or transscapular
lateral view are the minimal requirements for evaluating a dislocated shoulder. The West Point
modification of the axillary view can be obtained to look specifically for bony Bankart lesions,
whereas the Stryker notch view can be obtained to look for humeral head or Hill-Sachs defects.

6. What structures are important to the stability of the glenohumeral joint?

There has been a long-term argument about what is the "essential lesion," or lesion responsible for causing shoulder instability. Numerous components are important to the overall stability of the shoulder. It is generally accepted that the glenohumeral ligaments as well as the rotator cuff and other large shoulder muscles contribute to the overall stability of the shoulder joint. The superior glenohumeral ligament prevents inferior translation with the arm at the side in 0° of abduction, whereas at 45–90° of abduction both the middle and inferior glenohumeral ligaments provide support and prevent anterior translation of the humeral head. The rotator cuff and large muscles of the shoulder obviously provide dynamic control by helping to compress the humeral head in the glenoid socket. This phenomenon has been called concavity compression. Other factors contributing to glenohumeral instability include the orientation of the glenoid as well as the collagen characteristics of the tissue and the possible effect of negative intraarticular pressure.

7. What types of problems can an unstable shoulder cause in athletes?

The obvious problem with an unstable shoulder is the potential for recurrent dislocations. In athletes with recurrent dislocations unresponsive to conservative treatment, surgery should be considered. In an overhead athlete, subtle anterior instability may cause significant problems, such as recurrent pain and secondary impingement, as shown by Jobe and others. This subtle anterior instability allows abnormal anterior posterior translation of the humeral head, thus fatiguing the rotator cuff and allowing impingement, which causes pain and prohibits the athlete from throwing.

8. What is the recurrence rate for an anterior dislocation?

The recurrence rate of an anterior dislocation seems to be most highly correlated with the age of the patient. For patients under the age of 20 years old, Rowe reported a recurrence rate of approximately 83%. For ages 20–40 years, the recurrence rate has been reported between 40% and 60%, and for patients older than 40 years, the recurrence rate is much lower. With patients over 40 years of age, however, the likelihood of a rotator cuff tear increases.

9. How is an acute traumatic anterior dislocation treated?

The first concern is atraumatic reduction of the dislocation. After the appropriate history and physical examination, an experienced physician may wish to proceed with the reduction maneuver if he or she is sure of the direction and type of dislocation. If the type of dislocation or the presence of additional injuries is uncertain, radiographs may be obtained before attempting the reduction maneuver. The most important factor in allowing a gentle reduction is appropriate patient relaxation, which is usually accomplished with intramuscular or intravenous narcotics as well as diazepam or midazolam to relax the patient completely and prevent further muscle spasm. As always, monitoring of the patient is necessary when narcotics and anxiolytic agents are used. Many maneuvers are available for the reduction of an anterior dislocation, and if the patient is appropriately relaxed, gentle traction with slight abduction and rotation of the humerus may allow the humeral head to reduce into the glenoid fossa. Postreduction AP and axillary lateral or transscapular lateral radiographs are needed to document the completeness of the reduction to look for any postreduction fractures. Once the dislocation has been appropriately reduced, the patient may be placed in a sling.

Immobilization has not been shown to decrease the recurrence rates after a first-time dislocation. Therefore, one may want to start gentle, protected range-of-motion exercises and isometric muscle strengthening early in the recovery course.

Whether a first-time traumatic dislocator should be treated surgically or conservatively is controversial. But most people still favor rehabilitation for the first-time dislocator. For a patient with multiple recurrences who has been treated with an appropriate rehabilitation program, surgical stabilization should be considered. Most surgeons agree that an anatomic reconstruction of the Bankart type is the best surgical procedure. The recurrence rate is low; the complications are low; and this type of reconstruction seems to limit external rotation much less than other procedures, such as the Putti-Platt, Magnuson-Stack, or Bristow procedure.

10. How are posterior and multidirectional instability treated?

As with anterior instability, after reduction of an acute dislocation, patients with posterior dislocations and patients with MDI are treated with a rehabilitation program. In patients who have failed an aggressive rehabilitation program and have unidirectional posterior instability, a posterior reconstruction may be indicated. Patients with multidirectional instability who continue to have symptoms may respond well to an inferior capsular shift procedure.

11. How are acromioclavicular separations classified?

The traditional classification of acromioclavicular (AC) joint injuries is types I–III. Type I is a simple sprain of the AC ligament; the AC joint remains intact. Type II is complete disruption of the AC ligament, but the coracoclavicular ligaments are uninvolved. The AC joint may be slightly wider with slight vertical separation compared with the normal shoulder. Type III involves complete disruption of the AC ligament as well as the coracoclavicular ligament with a coracoclavicular interspace between 25–100% greater than the normal shoulder.

Rockwood added types IV, V, and VI. Type IV involves complete separation of the distal clavicle from the acromion with the distal clavicle anatomically displaced posteriorly into or through the trapezius muscle. The posterior displacement of a clavicle may be such that it tents the skin on the posterior aspect of the shoulder. Type V is an exaggerated type III injury with complete rupture of the AC and coracoclavicular ligaments as well as detachment of the deltoid and trapezius muscles from the distal third of the clavicle. There is usually 100–300% difference in the distance between the clavicle and the scapula. Type VI injury is secondary to a traumatic abduction force of the upper extremity and involves dislocation of the distal end of the clavicle under the coracoid process and the conjoined tendon.

12. How are AC separations treated?

Types I, II, and III are generally treated with the **PRICES** principle: **p**rotection, **r**est, **i**ce, **c**ompression, **e**levation, and **s**upport. The arm is protected in a sling, and the patient is started on gentle range-of-motion exercises as soon as pain allows. There is some controversy in the literature about treatment of types II and III injuries. Unless the injury involves the dominant shoulder of a throwing athlete or heavy laborer, conservative treatment is still the initial choice. For patients with chronic symptoms related to types II and III injuries, surgery such as a Weaver-Dunn procedure may be indicated. Orthopedic referral and surgery are generally indicated for types IV, V, and VI, because the deformity is significant and does not respond well to conservative treatment.

13. What is the mechanism of injury for a sternoclavicular dislocation?

A sternoclavicular dislocation is the dislocation of the medial end of the clavicle from the sternum; the dislocation may be either anterior or posterior. Mechanism of injury is either a direct or an indirect force. For the direct mechanism, a force is applied to the anterior medial aspect of the clavicle, pushing the clavicle posteriorly behind the sternum and possibly into the mediastinum. This injury may occur in an athlete who is lying on his or her back on the ground and is jumped on or in an athlete who is kicked directly in the sternoclavicular area. The indirect mechanism, however, is the more common form of injury to the sternoclavicular joint; it occurs in an athlete who is lying on one side with the upper shoulder compressed. If the upper shoulder is rolled backward, an ipsilateral anterior dislocation results. If the upper shoulder is compressed and rolled forward, an ipsilateral posterior dislocation occurs, as in a pile-on in a football game.

14. Are radiographs helpful in the diagnosis of sternoclavicular joint injuries?

Radiographs are helpful in evaluating the sternoclavicular joint, but standard techniques are difficult to interpret. Standard posteroanterior (PA) and lateral chest radiographs have too much overlap of other bones and make it difficult to determine whether there is a sternoclavicular joint injury. Slight asymmetry may be noted on the AP or PA view, but this finding does not give a firm diagnosis. Rockwood has coined the term for a special x-ray technique that he calls the "serendipity view." This 40° cephalic tilt view shows whether there is significant anterior or posterior displacement of the medial clavicle. Other techniques, such as tomograms or CT scans, are also significantly helpful in further diagnosis.

15. What type of muscle injuries are common in the shoulder?

Complete muscle tears or tendon tears in the shoulder of young athletes are uncommon. It is more common to have a contusion in the rotator cuff in a younger athlete. In older athletes with traumatic episodes, a complete rotator cuff or even a proximal tear of the long head of the biceps tendon is possible. Complete tears of the rotator cuff need to be treated surgically in athletes, whereas proximal tears of the long head of the biceps tendon are treated according to the patient's age and activity level. Unless the patient is very young and the dominant arm of a throwing athlete is involved, long-head biceps tendon injuries are treated conservatively.

16. What common nerve injuries may occur in the shoulder?

The most common nerve injury in the shoulder is a stinger or burner, which is described in Chapter 55. It is common in football players but also may occur in hockey, soccer, and wrestling. The axillary nerve may be injured during an anterior shoulder dislocation, which may cause numbness in the lateral arm and forearm as well as weakness in the deltoid muscle. A less commonly injured nerve is the suprascapular nerve, which gives motor function into the supraspinatus and infraspinatus muscles. This nerve can be damaged by fractures through the glenoid and suprascapular notch or from direct trauma to the nerve. Ganglion cysts are another cause of compression of the suprascapular nerve in the shoulder.

FRACTURES

17. What is the most common clavicle fracture?

Clavicle fractures are common injuries, accounting for 5–10% of all instances of adult trauma. Middle third clavicle fractures account for 80% of all clavicle fractures.

18. How are clavicle fractures classified?

Allmann divided clavicle fractures into three basic groups. Middle third clavicle fractures, the most common type, are classified as group I. Group II fractures involve the lateral third of the clavicle and are the second most common. Group III are medial third clavicle fractures.

Neer subdivided group II (lateral third) fractures into five subtypes. Type 1 includes minimally displaced interligamentous fractures; type 2, displaced fractures with the fracture line medial to the coracoclavicular ligament insertion; type 3, fractures that enter the acromioclavicular joint; and type 4, childhood injuries. Type 4 fractures are displaced, but the coracoclavicular ligament remains attached to a periosteal sleeve. Type 5 fractures are displaced comminuted fractures with the coracoclavicular ligament attached to a separate inferior butterfly fragment.

19. What is the treatment of a clavicle fracture?

Most clavicle fractures are treated with figure-of-eight harness or shoulder sling until pain begins to resolve. Surgical treatment consists of open reduction and internal fixation using dynamic compression plating and screws. Indications for surgical intervention include neurovascular symptoms, skin breakdown due to bony prominence, and nonunion.

20. What is the cause of scapula fractures?

The scapula is well protected, sandwiched between a thick muscle mass posteriorly and the thoracic cavity anteriorly. Because of its anatomic location, scapular fractures are uncommon, constituting only 1% of all fractures. They usually result from direct high-energy trauma. Because of the mechanism of injury, up to 95% of scapular fractures are associated with other injuries.

21. How are scapula fractures evaluated radiographically?

True scapular AP and lateral views and glenohumeral axillary projection should be ordered. The radiographs should be evaluated for fractures of the scapular body and spine, coracoid, glenoid, acromioclavicular joint, glenohumeral joint, and scapulothoracic articulation. Computed tomography (CT) is often necessary to evaluate the extent of the fracture.

22. What is the classification of scapula fractures?

Scapula fractures are grouped into glenoid, acromion, coracoid, and scapular body fractures. Glenoid fractures are further divided into glenoid rim, glenoid neck, and fractures through the glenoid cavity. Any fracture line that runs from the posterior scapular spine or acromion to the undersurface of the acromion and the spinoglenoid interval is considered an acromial fracture.

23. What is the most common treatment of scapula fractures?

More than 90% of all scapula fractures are treated nonoperatively. Symptomatic treatment includes sling and swathe for comfort. Range-of-motion exercises are initiated early. Return of full function takes several months. The prognosis, in general, is excellent.

Surgical indications for glenoid rim fractures include fractures that will result in persistent subluxation of the humeral head. Such fractures have 10 mm or more displacement with involvement of one-fourth of the anterior or one-third of the posterior glenoid rim.

Surgical indications for glenoid neck fractures include translational displacement of 1 cm or greater and/or angulatory displacement 40° or greater in either the transverse or coronal planes. Significant displacement has been associated with loss of shoulder abduction, weakness, pain, and increased incidence of poor functional outcome.

Isolated fractures of the coracoid and acromion are generally treated nonoperatively, as above. Surgical indications include significant displacement resulting in functional compromise.

24. How are proximal humerus fractures classified?

The most accepted classification system in North America is the system devised by Neer. The proximal humerus can be divided into four bone segments: humeral head, lesser and greater tuberosities, and humeral shaft. A segment is considered displaced if it is separated from its neighboring segment by more than 1 cm or is angled more than 45° from its anatomic position. The fracture pattern refers to the number of displaced segments, not to the number of fragments or lines.

25. How are proximal fractures treated?

- Eighty-five percent of proximal humerus fractures are minimally or nondisplaced and can be treated with early functional exercises.
- Two-part anatomic neck fractures are difficult to treat with closed reduction. Open reduction with internal fixation is difficult because of inadequate bone purchase for screws. Most authors agree that hemiarthroplasty gives the most predictable results for displaced fractures.
- Displaced two-part greater tuberosity fractures may cause impingement under the acromion. Displacement of greater than 0.5 cm is associated with persistent pain. Open reduction with internal fixation is recommended with displacement greater than 1 cm.
- Two-part surgical neck fractures require 3–4 weeks of sling immobilization if they are minimally displaced. Angulation often occurs after closed reduction without internal fixation. Several forms of internal fixation have been described, including percutaneous pin, intramedullary fixation, tension band wire, and plate fixation.
- Three-part fractures in active, young patients are generally best treated with open reduction and internal fixation.
- Four-part fractures are associated with avascular necrosis in up to 90% of patients. Immediate hemiarthroplasty has become the accepted method of treatment.

BIBLIOGRAPHY

1. Boublik M, Hawkins RJ: Clinical examination of the shoulder complex. J Orthop Sports Phys Ther 18:379–386, 1993.
2. Gerber C, Krushell RJ: Isolated rupture of the tendon of the subscapularis muscle. J Bone Joint Surg 73B:389–394, 1991.

3. Hawkins RJ: Musculoskeletal Examination. St. Louis, Mosby, 1995.
4. Hawkins RJ, Hobeika PE: Impingement syndrome in the athletic shoulder. Clin Sports Med 2:391–405, 1983.
5. Hawkins RJ, Mohtadi NG: Clinical evaluation of shoulder instability. Clin J Sports Med 1:59, 1991.
6. Matsen FA, Arntz CT: Subacromial impingement. In Rockwood CA, Matsen FA (eds): The Shoulder, 2nd ed. Philadelphia, W.B. Saunders, 1998, pp 623–646.
7. Matsen FA, Thomas SC, Rockwood CA: Anterior glenohumeral instability. In Rockwood CA, Matsen FA (eds): The Shoulder, 2nd ed. Philadelphia, W.B. Saunders, 1998, pp 526–622.

59. OVERUSE INJURIES OF THE SHOULDER

Wade A. Lillegard, M.D., and Lucy Patti, M.D.

1. What should one look for on physical examination of the painful shoulder?

Findings and Their Significance on Physical Examination of the Shoulder

PHYSICAL FINDING	INTERPRETATION
Inspection	
Muscle wasting	
Deltoid	Axillary nerve damage, C5 nerve root compression
Supraspinatous and/or infraspinatous	RC tear, suprascapular nerve injury, C5 nerve root injury
Deformities	
Prominent scapular spine	Supra- or infraspinatous atrophy
High riding lateral clavicle	AC separation
Scapular winging	Serratous anterior weakness (long thoracic nerve)
Bulging biceps muscle belly proximally	Rupture long head of biceps
Loss of axillary fold	Pectoralis major tendon rupture
Palpation	
Acromioclavicular (AC) joint tenderness	AC sprain or separation, osteolysis of distal clavicle, AC arthritis
Periscapular trigger points	Consider spasm from cervical radiculopathy
Anterior/inferior acromion tenderness or crepitus	Subacromial impingement (tendinitis, bursitis)
Greater tuberosity tenderness	Supraspinatus tendinitis, RC tear, fracture
Bicipital groove tenderness	Bicipital tendinitis
Tenderness in suprascapular fossa	Transcapular notch ganglion, trigger point
Range of motion	
Difference between active and passive ROM	Severe pain, RC tear, neurologic deficit
Restricted active and passive ROM	Adhesive capsulitis (frozen shoulder)
Painful arc between 70–130° abduction	Impingement (RC tendinitis, bursitis)
Painful arc between 90–180° abduction	AC arthralgia or arthritis
Unable to initiate abduction	Complete RC tear, severe pain from partial tear
Weak abduction, elevation, external rotation	Large RC tear, nerve injury (C5–C6, suprascapular nerve)
Strength (compared with opposite side)	
Weak abduction (deltoid, supraspinatous)	Pain from RC tear, axillary or C5–C6 nerve injury
Weak supraspinatous (arm abducted 90°, forward-flexed 30°, thumb down)	Pain from RC tear, suprascapular or C5–C6 nerve injury
Weak external rotation (infraspinatous, teres minor)	Pain from RC tear, suprascapular or axillary nerve injury

(Table continued on following page.)

Findings and Their Significance on Physical Examination of the Shoulder (Continued)

PHYSICAL FINDING	INTERPRETATION
Provocative testing	
Neer's impingement test (passive forward flexion of the internally rotated arm)	Pain when inflamed supraspinatous tendon is impinged between humerus and acromion
Hawkins' test (passively internally rotating the humerus while it is forward flexed 90°)	Pain when inflamed supraspinatous rubs against coracoacromial arch
Yergason's test (patient attempts to flex elbow and supinate wrist against resistance with arm to side and elbow at 90°)	Anterior shoulder pain with bicipital tendinitis
Speed's test (the straight arm with hand supinated is forward flexed against resistance at 60°)	Anterior shoulder pain with bicipital tendinitis, labral tear involving biceps tendon anchor
Cross arm test (arm forward flexed with hand on front of contralateral shoulder; elbow is pushed up against examiner's hand)	AC arthralgia/sprain
Stability testing	
Load and shift test (examiner grasps the humeral head, pushes it into the glenoid, and applies both anterior and posterior stress)	Assesses for anterior and posterior instability (must be compared with opposite shoulder to interpret). Excessive translation indicates instability in direction in which patient becomes apprehensive or complains of pain
Apprehension test (supine position, arm is abducted 90°, elbow flexed 90°, external rotation is applied)	due to the humeral head slipping anteriorly (anterior instability and/or labral tear). Posterior directed pressure applied to the anterior proximal humerus relieves pain.
Push-pull test (patient supine, arm abducted, forearm pointed up. Examiner holds wrist with one hand and pushes posteriorly on the proximal humerus.)	Posterior shift or pain indicates posterior instability and/or labral tear.
Jerk test (axial pressure applied to the elbow while at side. The arm is then forward-flexed and adducted.)	As above
Crank test (arm abducted 160°. Examiner rotates arm internally and externally.)	Snap or clunk indicates labral tear.
Sulcus test (axial traction applied to the hanging arm)	A gap or sulcus forms between acromion and humerus indicates inferior instability.
Spurling's maneuver (axial pressure applied to the head while the head is rotated toward the painful shoulder)	Increased shoulder pain or radicular symptoms indicate cervical nerve root irritation at neuroforamen.

2. What radiographic studies should be ordered for patients with shoulder pain?

Radiographic Views of the Shoulder Based on Suspected Pathology

INDICATION	STUDY	FINDINGS
Shoulder trauma	Plain radiographs	
	True anteroposterior (AP) (45° lateral)	Profile of glenoid, separates glenoid from humeral head, assesses for dislocations and fractures
	Axillary lateral	Glenoid and humeral head relationship, direction of dislocation, glenoid fracture, anterior and posterior glenoid rim fracture

(Table continued on following page.)

Radiographic Views of the Shoulder Based on Suspected Pathology (Continued)

INDICATION	STUDY	FINDINGS
Acromioclavicular trauma	Plain radiographs	
	AP	AC separation
	AP stress (10–20°)	Partial vs. complete separation (coracoacromial distance > 25% difference)
	Axillary lateral	AP displacement, intraarticular fracture
Sternoclavicular trauma	Plain radiographs	
	40° cephalic tilt	Distinguish between anterior or posterior displacement
	CT scan	Subluxation, dislocation, medial clavicular fracture, arthritis
Impingement syndrome	Plain radiographs	
	AP, internal, external external rotation	Calcific tendinitis, superior migration of humeral head, cystic or sclerotic changes of greater tuberosity, AC degenerative joint disease, sclerotic changes under surface of acromion
	AP, 30° caudal tilt	Anterior acromial spur, coracoclavicular ligament ossification, subacromial spurs
	Scapular outlet view (lateral, 10° caudal tilt)	AC arch deformity, acromial spurs
	Arthrogram	Full-thickness RC tears
	Ultrasound	Full-thickness RC tear, partial tears > 1 cm
	MRI	Partial and complete RC tears, AC spurs, AC arch deformities
Instability	Plain radiographs	
	True AP (45° lateral)	Bone damage or soft tissue; calcium on glenoid rim
	AP, internal rotation	Hill-Sachs lesion behind lateral humeral head (from anterior dislocation)
	Stryker notch view	Hill-Sachs lesion behind lateral humeral head (from anterior dislocation)
	West Point axillary lateral	Anterior-inferior glenoid rim, glenoid defect from anterior dislocation
	CT scan	Size of Hill-Sachs lesion, fracture, fracture dislocations
	Arthrogram	Capsular volume (laxity), some labral tears
	MRI arthrogram	Labral tear, capsular integrity and volume

3. What is the rotator cuff?

The rotator cuff consists of the four **SITS** muscles: **s**upraspinatous, **i**nfraspinatous, **t**eres minor, and **s**ubscapularis muscles. It stabilizes the shoulder joint dynamically and assists in rotation and abduction. The supraspinatous originates in the supraspinous fossa, inserts onto the greater tuberosity, and serves to pull the humeral head into the glenoid fossa, allowing smooth glenohumeral articulation. The infraspinatous arises from the infraspinous fossa and the teres minor from the lateral border of the scapula. Both insert onto the posterior aspect of the greater tuberosity and serve as humeral head depressors and external rotators. The subscapularis originates on the anterior surface of the scapula, inserts onto the lesser tuberosity (anterior on the humerus), and internally rotates and depresses the humerus.

4. How does the rotator cuff become injured?

Rotator cuff injuries may result from both macrotrauma or repetitive microtrauma (overuse). In macrotrauma, one or more of the rotator cuff tendons (usually the supraspinatous) partially or completely tear when they are stretched as the humerus pulls away from the glenoid fossa. Tears are often subsequent to dislocation or longitudinal traction injury. With overuse, excessive demands are placed on the rotator cuff muscles. In throwing sports particularly, the supraspinatous and external rotators undergo repetitive eccentric contractions as they decelerate the arm. This generates considerable force on the tendon, which leads to small tears and tendinitis. Underlying instabilities also require the rotator muscles to work harder in an effort to control the glenohumeral joint, eventually resulting in cuff fatigue, tears, and tendinitis.

5. What is impingement syndrome?

Impingement is a general term used to describe pain originating from compression of inflamed tissue between the humeral head and coracoacromial arch. Any condition that causes a narrowing of the subacromial space (structural abnormalities, physiologic abnormalities, or both) may lead to impingement. Structural abnormalities that predispose to impingement include a curved (type II) or hooked (type III) acromion, acromioclavicular spurring, thickened coracoacromial ligament, or calcium deposits. Physiologic causes include overdemand on the rotator cuff muscles, which lead to partial tears that, in turn, lead to inflammation of both the tendon and overlying subacromial bursa. Inflamed tissues then become painful with any activity that narrows the subacromial space (e.g., overhead activity) or stresses the involved tendon (e.g., decelerating the arm after throwing, backhand tennis strokes). The subacromial bursa is almost always involved in impingement, but it is usually inflamed secondary to tendinitis. Underlying shoulder instabilities force the rotator cuff muscles to work harder to control the glenohumeral joint motion, which may lead to tendinitis and impingement. People predisposed to impingement are involved with repetitive overhead or throwing activities, such as mailroom personnel, carpenters, grocery clerks, throwing athletes, and swimmers. One-third of patients with impingement, however, have no identifiable etiologic activity. Patients usually present with insidious onset of pain, stiffness, weakness, catching, and in severe cases, difficulty with sleeping.

6. How does a rotator cuff tear differ from impingement?

Rotator cuff (RC) tears are associated with impingement in 95% of cases. Impingement lesions are classically described by Neer as having three progressive stages: (1) edema and hemorrhage, (2) fibrosis and tendinitis, and (3) rotator cuff tears, biceps tendon ruptures, and bony changes. RC tears are most common in patients over the age of 40. It is believed that prolonged and repeated impingement between the humeral head and coracoacromial arch wears out the rotator cuff, predisposing the cuff to complete tears with acute injury. Furthermore, any weakness of the rotator cuff musculature allows upward riding of the humerus against the acromion, exacerbating impingement symptoms and increasing cuff wear over time. The term *impingement* is specific for rotator cuff pathology associated with actual mechanical abutment of the rotator cuff. Rotator cuff tendinitis implies pathologic changes in the tendon. Pain results from inflammation of the rotator cuff rather than mechanical abutment.

7. How does bicipital tendinitis relate to impingement?

Inflammation of the tendon of the long head of the biceps results from the same mechanisms responsible for impingement; thus, it rarely exists as an isolated occurrence. With elevation and rotation of the arm, the biceps tendon may be compressed between the head of the humerus, acromion, and coracoacromial ligament. The following factors help to differentiate among these entities:

1. Speed's test is generally the most helpful in diagnosing bicipital tendinitis.
2. Location of pain often changes with motion in bicipital tendinitis, whereas there is generally no significant change in location with impingement.
3. Isolated bicipital tendinitis may or may not show impingement signs.
4. Point tenderness in the biceps groove (with isolated bicipital tendinitis) vs. a more diffuse tenderness in the deltoid region and upper arm (more consistent with impingement).

8. How should proximal biceps tendon ruptures be treated?

Treatment of biceps tendon ruptures depends largely on the patient's age and level of physical activity. Sedentary patients over 50 should be treated initially with short-term immobilization, antiinflammatory and analgesic medications, and moist heat for several weeks.

Patients younger than 50, patients who are physically active, or patients whose work requires repetitive supination should be treated more aggressively—first with diagnostic ultrasound or magnetic resonance imaging to evaluate for associated rotator cuff tears and then with early surgical correction. Mariani et al. compared surgical and nonsurgical treatment of biceps tendon rupture and reported residual arm pain to be infrequent in both groups. Surgically treated patients returned to work later than nonsurgical patients; however, 37% of the nonsurgical group compared with only 7% of the surgical group were not able to return to full work capacity. The nonsurgical group had lost a mean of 21% of supination strength and 8% of elbow flexion strength but had no weakness in grip, forearm pronation, or elbow extension. The surgical group had lost no strength in any of these parameters.

9. When should one suspect a glenoid labral tear?

A labral tear should be considered in patients who complain of pain with a clicking, catching, or popping sensation in the shoulder. These symptoms are often due to a labral flap interfering with the glenohumeral articulation. Labral tears or fraying also may cause ill-defined deep shoulder pain. Mechanisms of injury include repetitive overhead activity, sudden traction (avulsion) injury, or forceful entrapment of the labrum between the humeral head and glenoid rim (e.g., subluxation and dislocation). Assume the presence of glenohumeral instability until proved otherwise.

The following physical examination tests may be positive: Speed's, apprehension-reduction, load and shift, push-pull, jerk, and crank tests. Evaluation should include radiographs, and MRI arthrogram. In the absence of instability, partial arthroscopic labral resection has been reported to allow > 90% of patients to return to preinjury activity level with mild or no discomfort. This procedure, however, remains controversial because labral debridement may actually increase symptoms in an unstable shoulder by aggravating the preexisting instability. Indeed, a recent study by Tomlinson and Glousman reported good-to-excellent results in only 54% of patients (25 of 47, average age of 22 years) when followed 31 months after surgery. Rates of good-to-excellent results for professional baseball players and nonprofessional athletes were 75% and 43%, respectively. The authors concluded that aggressive, supervised therapy may be the most important factor in influencing the outcome of labral debridement in the absence of overt instability.

10. What should be the general approach to treating a shoulder injury?

1. **Relative rest.** Patients are instructed to avoid activity that aggravates symptoms.
2. **Decrease inflammation.**
   - Ice massage is performed 3 times daily after range-of-motion and stretching exercises.
   - NSAIDs of choice should be prescribed. More than one may be tried, because efficacy is often patient-specific and may take 3–4 weeks to be fully effective.
   - Steroid injections are indicated after 4–6 weeks if pain persists. Nine cc of 1% lidocaine is mixed with 6 mg of triamcinolone acetonide and injected in either the subacromial space (for impingement), intraarticular joint (for suspected labral fraying, chondromalacia, undersurface cuff tears or bicipital tendinitis), or acromioclavicular joint. If pain abates with the lidocaine component, the compartment injected is the source of pain.
3. **Range of motion.** Restoration of normal flexibility is begun as acute symptoms abate, with attention to forward flexion, internal rotation, and cross-body adduction. Stretching should be done in a gentle, sustained manner 3 times/day.
4. **Restoration of strength.** Once painfree range of motion is attained, restoration of strength is begun through a rotator cuff and scapular stabilizer rehabilitation program. The exercises are designed to strengthen internal and external rotators in an attempt to pull the humeral head dynamically down and away from the acromion. These exercises are to be performed against resistance using rubber tubing or free weights. Full activity should not be resumed until the shoulder had full mobility and strength.

5. **Maintenance of cardiovascular fitness.** It is important for patients to maintain overall physical conditioning with cross-training while out of mainstream activities.

6. **Return to full activity.** To return to full activity, some analysis and modification of activity (e.g., a swimmer's stroke) should take place to prevent recurrent injuries.

7. **Referral criteria**
- Patients who have a complete rotator cuff tear.
- Patients who describe recurrent anterior dislocations with symptoms of instability and positive apprehension testing and have failed aggressive rehabilitation.
- A glenoid labral tear is suspected and rehabilitative exercises have failed.
- Patients with evidence of significant soft tissue injury by arthrogram or magnetic resonance imaging who have not improved after 6 weeks of conservative therapy or in whom major symptoms persist beyond 3 months.
- Patients in whom the above studies are negative but activity-limiting impingement symptoms persist for more than 6 months.

BIBLIOGRAPHY

1. Andrews JR, Kupferman SP, Dillman CJ: Labral tears in throwing and racquet sports. Clin Sports Med 10:901, 1991.
2. Burkhead WA: The biceps tendon. In Rockwood CA, Matsen CR (eds): The Shoulder, 2nd ed. Philadelphia, W.B. Saunders, 1998, p 791.
3. Carson WG: Rehabilitation of the throwing shoulder. Clin Sports Med 8:657, 1989.
4. Cavello RJ, Spear KP: Shoulder instability and impingement in throwing athletes. Med Sci Sports Exerc 30(Suppl):18–25, 1998.
5. Glasgow SG, Bruce RA, Vacobucci GN, et al: Arthroscopic resection of glenoid labral tears: A report of 29 cases. Arthroscopy 8:48, 1992.
6. Gusmer P, Potter H, Schatz J, et al: Labral injuries: Accuracy of detection with unenhanced MR imaging of the shoulder. Radiology 200:519, 1996.
7. Hawkins RJ: Basic Science and clinical application in the athlete's shoulder. Clin Sports Med 10(4): 693–984, 1991.
8. Hurley JA, Anderson TE: Shoulder arthroscopy: Its role in evaluating shoulder disorders in the athlete. Am J Sports Med 18:480, 1990.
9. Lyons PM, Orwin JF: Rotator cuff tendinopathy and subacromial impingement syndrome. Med Sci Sports Exerc 30(Suppl):12–17, 1998.
10. Mariani EM, Cofield RH, Askew LJ, et al: Rupture of the tendon of the long head of the biceps brachii. Clin Orthop Rel Res 228:233, 1988.
11. Matsen FA, Arntz C: Subacromial impingement. In Rockwood CA, Matsen CR (eds): The Shoulder, 2nd ed. Philadelphia, W.B. Saunders, 1998.
12. Miniaci A, Fowler PJ: Impingement in the athlete. Clin Sports Med 12(1):91, 1993.13. Neer CS: Impingement lesions. Clin Orthop Rel Res 173:70, 1983.
13. Nicholas JA, Hershman EB (eds): The Upper Extremity in Sports Medicine. St. Louis, Mosby, 1990.
14. Tomlinson R, Glousman R: Arthroscopic debridement of glenoid labral tears in athletes. Arthroscopy 11:42, 1995.
15. Zuckerman JD, Mirabello SC, Newman D, et al: The painful shoulder. Part II: Intrinsic disorders and impingement syndrome. Am Fam Physician 43:497, 1991.

60. THE ELBOW IN ATHLETICS

James A. Whiteside, M.D., Gene A. Hannah, M.D., and Tony C. Roisom, M.D.

1. Explain the functional anatomy of the elbow.

The elbow is capable of flexion, extension, and rotation. Flexion and extension take place at the articulation of the trochlea of the distal humerus and the ulna. The elbow has a mild anatomic valgus angulation created by 6° valgus slope of the trochlea that, along with the proximal ulna, determines the "carrying angle" of the elbow. Rotation of the elbow takes place because of the radiocapitellar and radioulnar articulations. Stability of the elbow joint is afforded primarily by the ulnar collateral ligament. Secondary stabilizers include the flexor pronator muscle group, bony contributions from the olecranon-olecranon fossa complex, and the articulation of the radial head and capitellum.

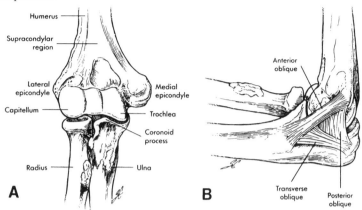

A, The elbow—anterior view. *B,* Medial view depicting the three components of the ulnar collateral ligament. (From Nicholas JA, Hershman EB: The Upper Extremity in Sports Medicine. St. Louis, Mosby, 1995, with permission.)

2. What forces act on the elbow to cause injuries in athletes?

Elbow injuries result from acute trauma and repetitive overuse as seen primarily in throwing sports, such as baseball, but also in the tennis serve and the volleyball spike. The common denominator is an acceleration phase during which the humerus is whipped forward ahead of the flexed elbow. This results in medial valgus tension and lateral compression. As forward momentum in the throwing motion is transferred from the humerus to the forearm and wrist, the elbow rapidly extends, causing posterior olecranon impingement. Medial tension and lateral compression also may occur in static positional activities such as the handstand in gymnastics.

3. Describe the physical examination of the elbow in the athlete.

With the athlete sitting, the neck, shoulder and arms, and trunk are exposed and visualized; muscular development and symmetry are noted. Look for ecchymoses, swelling or depression, and any area of skin atrophy (from steroid injections). Measurements of the carrying angle, flexion, extension, pronation, supination, and forearm circumferences should be made in both arms. Systematic palpation of the medial, lateral, posterior, and anterior aspects of the elbow focuses on areas of tenderness, crepitus, or soft tissue deficits. Search for medial epitrochlear lymphadenopathy. Next, with the distal forearm held at 20–30° of flexion, which allows for disengagement of the olecranon from its fossa, medial stability of the elbow is tested by placing a valgus pressure against the forearm. The examiner's hands are then reversed, and varus stress is applied to test for lateral stability. The ulnar nerve should be palpated for tenderness in the ulnar groove posterior to the medial epicondyle. Evidence of Tinel's sign and subluxation of the ulnar nerve over the medial epicondyle is recorded.

4. What normal variances may be seen in examination of the elbow in athletes?

Muscular hypertrophy may be exhibited in the triceps, biceps, and extensor and flexor forearm muscles of the sport-dominant arm. The dominant arm also may have a larger carrying angle and a mild flexion contracture. Flexion contracture in a young pitcher with medial elbow soreness should be regarded as abnormal and tested. Competitive gymnasts, by hyperextending their elbows, partially eliminate the stress across the elbow during handstands by hyperextending their elbows.

5. What common elbow problems are seen in athletes?

Anterior	Posterior
Biceps tendinitis	Triceps tendinitis
Distal biceps rupture	Valgus extension overload syndrome
Anterior capsule strain	Olecranon bursitis
	Dislocation

Lateral	Medial
Lateral epicondylitis	Medial epicondylitis
Radiocapitellar chondromalacia	Medial collateral ligament sprain
Osteochondritis dissecans capitellum	Medial epicondyle stress lesions
Radial head fracture	Ulnar nerve compression syndrome
Posterior interosseous nerve	Flexor pronator strain
compression syndrome	Cubital tunnel syndrome
	Stress fractures

6. What is biceps tendinitis?

Biceps tendinitis is an overuse syndrome that results from overloading of the biceps muscle, as seen in throwing sports and activities that require repetitive elbow flexion and supination. Usually, anterior elbow pain or aching presents after prolonged throwing or resisted forearm motion. There may be associated weakness. Examination reveals the distal biceps tendon to be tender to palpation in the antecubital fossa. The long head of the biceps tendon, by its adjunct position, serves as a humeral head depressor. Occasionally, overuse produces soreness in the deltopectoral groove.

7. Why do throwers get biceps tendinitis?

Although uncommon, biceps tendinitis occurs in the unconditioned athlete as a result of repetitive strain. The distal biceps functions to decelerate the elbow to prevent hyperextension produced by the enormous centrifugal forces generated at ball release. For prevention, an eccentric biceps strengthening program is mandatory for preseason conditioning in throwing athletes.

8. How is biceps tendinitis differentiated from distal biceps rupture?

A distal biceps rupture should be easily differentiated from biceps tendinitis. Biceps tendinitis has an insidious onset. Distal biceps rupture is described by the patient as a sudden, sharp, tearing pain in the antecubital fossa or lower anterior upper arm. With biceps tendon rupture, a visible deformity is noted with active flexion because of retraction of the muscle belly. Compared with the normal arm, there is a palpable defect in the antecubital fossa where the biceps tendon ordinarily inserts.

9. Is treatment of distal biceps tendinitis different from that of distal biceps tendon rupture?

Yes. Biceps tendinitis is generally treated by relative rest, ice, nonsteroidal antiinflammatory drugs (NSAIDs), and modification of improper technique. Management of distal biceps tendon rupture is surgical reattachment of the biceps tendon to the radial tuberosity.

10. Describe the presentation of an athlete with an anterior capsular strain of the elbow.

The athlete presents with diffuse, poorly localized anterior elbow pain after an incidental hyperextension injury. Radiographs are usually normal but may reveal a small capsular fleck avulsion of the medial or lateral epicondyle. In time, heterotopic ossification of the capsule results in flexion contracture of the elbow.

11. How is anterior capsular strain treated?

Treatment involves relative rest followed by active range of motion and strengthening as allowed by pain. Throwing is permitted when objective measurements are comparable to the opposite arm.

12. What is the etiology and presentation of triceps tendinitis?

Triceps tendinitis develops as an overuse syndrome secondary to repetitive extension of the elbow. It presents as posterior elbow pain. Examination reveals tenderness proximal to or at the insertion of the triceps or pain with elbow extension against resistance. Radiographs are often normal but may reveal a traction spur at the insertion of the triceps tendon into the olecranon and hypertrophy of the ulna. As with other overuse injuries, triceps tendinitis is treated with relative rest, ice, and NSAIDs as needed and a graduated stretching and strengthening program. Improper technique needs to be corrected.

13. Define the valgus extension overload (VEO) syndrome.

VEO is an overuse syndrome caused by repetitive extension and uncontrolled valgus forces generated during the late acceleration and deceleration phases of throwing. Unlike triceps tendinitis, the VEO syndrome involves pathologic bony change in the posterior elbow. Repeated abutment of the posteromedial olecranon forcefully against the medial wall of the olecranon fossa causes osteophyte formation and loose body formation.

14. What are the findings in VEO syndrome?

Subjectively, the throwing athlete complains of posterior pain with catching or locking of the elbow in extension. Physical examination reveals tenderness and swelling posteriorly and loss of elbow extension. Forced elbow extension combined with valgus stress reproduces the posterior pain. Occasionally, loose bodies are palpable. Anteroposterior, lateral, and axial radiographs show loose bodies or osteophyte formation at the olecranon tip and posteromedial aspect of the olecranon and in the olecranon fossa.

15. What is the treatment for VEO syndrome?

Treatment is conservative with relative rest followed by a well-supervised rehabilitation program that involves the elbow and the shoulder. If relief is not obtained, arthroscopic or open debridement of the area is indicated. Improper throwing technique must be avoided.

16. What is the significance of olecranon bursitis in athletes?

Olecranon bursitis is often the result of repeated blows to the unpadded posterior elbow. It is treated by ice and compression and occasionally by aspiration. Olecranon bursitis rarely prevents competing. Elbow pads defend against hard, artificial turf. If symptoms persist, radiographic examination is needed to rule out olecranon stress fracture in the mature thrower and separation of an unfused olecranon apophysis in the immature athlete.

17. Describe the historical and physical findings associated with ulnar collateral ligament (UCL) injuries.

UCL injuries usually occur during the acceleration phase of throwing. This injury is associated with moderate-to-severe elbow pain and is often accompanied by a "pop" that is felt or heard and tingling in the fourth and fifth fingers. Persistent pain and loss of velocity and control limit throwing. Some report working through recent medial elbow discomfort. On examination, medial elbow ecchymosis may be present as well as tenderness over the anterior oblique fibers of the ulnar collateral ligament that stretches from the medial epicondyle to the coronoid process of the ulna. Valgus stress applied with the elbow flexed at 20–30° precipitates medial pain and reveals instability due to an ulnar collateral ligament tear.

18. What ancillary tests may help to evaluate ulnar collateral ligament (UCL) injuries?

Radiographs that include a lateral view at 90° of flexion, anteroposterior, right and left oblique, and axial views are performed initially. These films may reveal avulsions, loose bodies, and traction spurs in the area of the ulnar collateral ligament. The integrity of the ligament may be studied further by stress (Telos) radiographs, computed tomographic arthrograms, or magnetic resonance imaging (MRI). If in a saline- or gadolinium-enhanced MRI a T-sign is noted, there is a tear in the distal UCL attachment to the sublime tubercle. Surgical repair and augmentation with the palmaris longus tendon or similar structure are indicated. Return to previous athletic ability may require several months. Electromyograms (EMGs) are noncontributory.

19. How are ulnar collateral ligament injuries treated?

UCL sprains are treated by removing the athlete from all aggravating activities, instituting the use of ice and NSAIDs, and immediately beginning a supervised rehabilitation program that includes stretching and strengthening. When essentially pain-free and full flexibility and strength have returned, a distance interval throwing program is instituted. When it has been completed, a second formal throwing program off the mound is begun before attempting to pitch in a simulated game. Rehabilitation must be continued even after returning to full activity. UCL tears, if left untreated, consistently result in decreased athletic abilities and hence are often repaired.

20. What is the most common musculotendinous injury noted medially in the elbow? Why does it occur?

Overuse injury or strain of the flexor pronator muscle group is a common source of medial elbow pain in throwing athletes. Arising from the medial epicondyle, the flexor pronator muscle group serves as a secondary stabilizer to the ulnar collateral ligament. The large valgus force created during the late cocking and acceleration phases of throwing creates significant tensile forces in the flexor pronator muscle group. When fatigued, these muscles may exhibit microscopic or macroscopic tears. Healing with scarring may produce muscle contractures that prevent full elbow extension. Anterior interosseous nerve syndrome (AINS) may occur along with flexor pronator overuse injuries. Poor mechanical function of the thumb, index, and long fingers and weakness of the long flexors are characteristic. There is no sensory component. As with UCL sprains, treatment consists of relative rest, the use of ice, NSAIDs, and flexibility and strengthening exercises. Prevention entails adequate physical conditioning, appropriate pitching mechanics, avoidance of overexertion, and warm-up and cool-down measures.

21. What is golfer's elbow?

Medial epicondylitis, also known as golfer's elbow, results from an overuse injury to the tendinous origin of the flexor pronator muscle mass. This area is placed under valgus stress at or near the top of the back swing and proceeds through the downswing to just before impact with the golf ball.

22. What are the signs of medial epicondylitis?

Medial epicondylitis presents tenderness at the medial epicondyle and pain with resisted wrist flexion and forearm pronation. Tinel's sign is negative at the cubital tunnel.

23. What is the management of golfer's elbow?

Management consists of routine conservative measures, including relative rest, ice, NSAIDs, and use of a splint. Steroid injections are rarely required. Recalcitrant cases may require surgery.

24. What is Little Leaguer's elbow?

To the purist, Little Leaguer's elbow is a medial traction apophysitis seen predominantly in young throwers between the ages of 9 and 12 years. It occurs as a result of valgus stress that leads to hypertrophy of the medial epicondyle, microtearing of the flexor pronator muscle group, and fragmentation and even separation of the medial epicondylar apophysis compared with the uninvolved elbow.

As with most overuse injuries, training errors cause the majority of cases. Examples include excessive throwing, usually without proper preseason conditioning, poor pitching technique, inadequate warm-up, and attempting to throw breaking pitches. Physical factors such as anatomic abnormalities, lack of flexibility, and muscle imbalances may contribute as well.

Usually young players present with complaints of medial elbow pain that occurs with throwing. At times, the pain continues for a short time afterwards. Other symptoms may include diminished speed and/or control in throwing. Athletes are generally tender to palpation over the medial epicondyle of the involved elbow and may have visible swelling in that same area. Resisted wrist flexion may cause pain at the medial epicondyle. In advanced cases, incomplete extension of the elbow is present.

25. How is Little Leaguer's elbow managed?

If the medial epicondylar apophysis is not significantly displaced, little leaguer's elbow can be treated with rest for 2–3 weeks along with ice and antiinflammatories as indicated; no throwing is allowed for 6–12 weeks. Pitching is not allowed during the concurrent season. During the rest period, as pain subsides, attention should be turned to stretching and strengthening exercises for the forearm. Return to throwing includes a supervised, functional progression program allowing a gradual increase in number, length, and speed of throws. Training errors must be identified and corrected.

If the apophysis is displaced compared with the opposite side, if it is incarcerated within the elbow joint, or if valgus instability is present, screw fixation is performed. Shoulder motion must be included in the rehabilitation.

26. Describe the ulnar nerve compression syndrome.

Ulnar nerve compression syndrome, also known as cubital tunnel syndrome, refers to ulnar neuropathy due to direct trauma to the ulnar nerve in the cubital tunnel, repetitive elbow flexion, hypermobility of the ulnar nerve, excessive valgus of the elbow, and osteophyte or loose body impingement of the ulnar nerve.

27. What are the major distinguishing characteristics of cubital tunnel syndrome?

Distinguishing characteristics are aching posteromedial pain, episodic paresthesias along the ring and small fingers with or without motor deficits, a positive Tinel's sign, pain with forced full elbow flexion, possible weakness of the thumb-index finger pinch, and, in long-term cases, wasting of the intrinsic musculature of the hand. These findings may be exacerbated with multiple subluxations of the hypermobile ulnar nerve in activities such as racquet sports.

28. How is cubital tunnel syndrome treated?

Treatment consists of relative rest, NSAIDs, and protection of the elbow and modification of technique. In patients with motor weakness, failed conservative treatment, or a positive EMG, surgical decompression and transposition of the ulnar nerve are performed.

29. What is tennis elbow?

Tennis elbow refers to lateral epicondylitis. Some authors prefer to label tennis elbow extensor tendinitis, because the pathology is microtearing of the extensor carpi radialis brevis (ERCB) muscle that originates from the lateral epicondyle. Lateral epicondylitis occurs seven times more frequently than medial epicondylitis and is most frequently seen in racquet sports. It also occurs in golf, fencing, and throwing sports.

30. What factors lead to lateral epicondylitis?

The common denominators in the development of lateral epicondylitis, regardless of the sport, are overuse, poor mechanics, and insufficient muscle conditioning. With racquet sports, improper backhand stroke production, inappropriate grip size, and too-tight racquet string tension plus repetition contribute to the overload of the extensor tendons. In throwing sports, extreme forearm pronation and wrist flexion at ball release in the deceleration phase cause tensile stress at the lateral epicondyle.

31. Describe the physical examination of an athlete with lateral epicondylitis.

Tenderness to palpation is elicited over or just distal to the lateral epicondyle. The athlete complains of pain along the extensor or dorsal aspect of the forearm when shaking hands. Weakness of the hand grip is pain-related. Persistent dorsiflexion of the wrist and palmarly flexed long finger against resistance reproduce the symptoms.

32. Explain the treatment for lateral epicondylitis.

As in other overuse injuries, the treatment begins with relative rest, ice, and NSAIDs. Physical therapy includes stretching and strengthening exercises, use of electrical stimulation, iontophoresis, or other modalities. Many patients find relief with use of an adjustable forearm splint that initially is worn 23 hours/day. Occasionally, local steroid injections over the lateral epicondyle are beneficial. Finally, any precipitating factors should be altered by the athlete. In recalcitrant cases, surgery may be required to remove the inflammatory reactive tissue and reattach the ECRB and conjoined tendon.

33. What is radial tunnel syndrome (RTS)?

RTS is a radial nerve entrapment syndrome. It frequently involves the posterior interosseous branch of the radial nerve at the level of the proximal edge of the supinator muscle (arcade of Frohse). RTS can mimic or coexist with chronic lateral epicondylitis. A key physical sign of posterior interosseous neuropathy is impaired function of the extensor carpi ulnaris that allows the production of ulnar-directed wrist dorsiflexion without cutaneous sensory deficits. The posterior interosseous nerve has no cutaneous sensory fibers. Conservative therapy of RTS is similar to that of lateral epicondylitis with the exception of the counterforce brace. Surgical forearm decompression is seldom required.

34. What conditions result from lateral compression forces in throwing activities?

Lateral compression forces result in osteochondrosis of the capitellum (Panner's disease) in the young and osteochrondritis dissecans and osteochondral defects of the capitellum and radial head, loose bodies, and degenerative changes in the more mature athlete. Osteochondritis dissecans is the leading cause of permanent elbow disability in throwing athletes.

35. How does osteochondrosis of the capitellum (Panner's disease) differ from osteochondritis dissecans?

Panner's disease occurs in younger athletes, involves the ossification center of the capitellum, has no loose bodies, and is generally associated with slow, complete recovery. Osteochondritis dissecans occurs in the 9- to 15-year-olds and is associated with focal capitellar defects formation of loose bodies and may preclude the return to previous throwing activities.

36. What is the treatment of lateral compression injuries?

In the skeletally immature athlete, unless loose bodies prevent normal joint mobility, treatment is conservative with elimination of throwing until full pain-free range of motion and strength have returned. In the athlete with radiocapitellar pathology, removal of loose bodies and debridement of radiocapitellar chondromalacia can be performed arthroscopically to promote a fibrocartilaginous healing response. Early, controlled mobilization of the elbow is an integral part of recovery.

37. What about elbow dislocations?

A fall on the outstretched hand with the elbow slightly flexed is a common mechanism of elbow joint dislocation. Most dislocations are posterior and produce considerable pain, swelling, tenderness, and obvious deformity. They may be associated with neurologic and vascular compromise. Trained medical personnel should attempt immediate reduction. Otherwise, treat and transport as an emergency. Ultimately, medial stability must be assessed. If instability is found, surgical correction is warranted.

BIBLIOGRAPHY

1. Andrews JR: Bony injuries about the elbow in the throwing athlete. AAOS Symposium on Upper Extremity Injuries in Athletes. St. Louis, Mosby, 1984.
2. Andrews JR, Craven WM: Lesions of the posterior compartment of the elbow. Clin Sports Med 10:637, 1991.

3. Andrews JR, Schemmel SP, Whiteside JA, Timmerman LA: Evaluation, treatment, and prevention of elbow injury in the athlete, 2nd ed. In Nicholas JA, Hershman EB (eds): The Upper Extremity in Sports Medicine. St. Louis, Mosby, 1995.
4. Cabrera JM, McCue FC: Nonosseous athletic injuries of the elbow, forearm, and hand. Clin Sports Med 5:681, 1986.
5. Hotchkiss RN: Common disorders of the elbow in athletes and musicians. Hand Clin 6:507, 1990.
6. Lansinger O, Karlsson J, Körner L, Mare K: Dislocation of the elbow joint. Arch Orthop Trauma Surg 102:183, 1984.
7. Mellion MB, Walsh WM, Shelton GL (eds): The Team Physician's Handbook, 2nd ed. Philadelphia, Hanley & Belfus, 1997.
8. Morrey BF (ed): The Elbow and Its Disorders. Philadelphia, W.B. Saunders, 1985.
9. Nicholas JA, Hershman EB: The Upper Extremity in Sports Medicine. St. Louis, Mosby, 1990.
10. Pappas AM: Elbow problems associated with baseball during childhood and adolescence. Clin Orthop Rel Res 164:30, 1982.
11. Singler KM, Roy SP: Osteochondrosis of the humeral capitellum. Am J Sports Med 12:351, 1984.
12. Weinstein SM, Herring SA: Nerve problems and compartment syndromes in the hand, wrist, and forearm. Clin Sports Med 11:161, 1992.
13. Whiteside JA, Andrews JR: Common elbow problems in the recreational athlete. J Musculoskel Med 6(2);17, 1989.

61. WRIST AND FOREARM PROBLEMS

Ian D. Crabb, M.D.

WRIST INJURY

1. What are the main loading patterns of the wrist in sports injuries?

The four main loading patterns of the wrist are traction, weight-bearing, twisting, and impact.

2. What type of wrist injuries are common to ball-throwing or racquet-type sports?

A traction force is applied as the wrist moves from dorsal-radial to volar-ulnar position. While the wrist is maintained at the dorsal-radial position, the extensor carpi radialis tendons are contracted, as are the extensors to the thumb. As the wrist moves into a forcefully ulnarly deviated and volar flexed position, the radial extensors exert a decelerating force. The repetitive use of these tendons may cause irritation in the tendon sheath and tendinitis, as observed in athletes participating in tennis, golf, and all throwing activities.

3. What type of injuries can be expected in an athlete who bears weight on the wrist?

Sports such as weightlifting, gymnastics, and shot-putting place a large compressive load across the wrist. This load forces the carpus into a radially deviated and dorsiflexed position. Forcing the wrist into this position causes increased tension on the volar ligament and capsule of the wrist, including the volar radial carpal ligaments as well as the volar ulnar carpal ligaments. The triangular fibrocartilage complex (TFCC) and pisiform are also under tension in this position. These ligaments may suffer partial or complete avulsions with this type of activity.

4. Which joint is involved in severe twisting injuries to the wrist?

The joint most commonly injured with a severe twisting force across the wrist is the distal radioulnar joint. Although severe twisting injuries are relatively uncommon in sports, they may occur in such violent sports as rodeo riding when the hand and wrist are fixed in one position and the body rotates about that position. Hyperpronation injuries generally cause a dorsal dislocation of the ulna, which reflects an injury to the volar radioulnar ligament complex. Conversely, a hypersupination injury tends to cause a rupture of the dorsal radioulnar ligaments and a volar dis-location.

5. Does impaction injury to the wrist cause a reproducible injury pattern?

Impaction loading to the wrist causes a great variety of injuries that are hard to predict based on mechanism. The most common injury is a distal radius fracture with the fracture apex volar. Other common injuries include ulnar styloid fractures, scaphoid fractures, volar radial carpal lig-ament tears, scapholunate disruptions, or even capitate fractures and perilunate dislocations.

6. Other than radiographs, what is the best way to diagnose a fracture or carpal injury after a traumatic event?

Frequently in the heat of the sports event, the athlete is unable to remember the exact posi-tion of her or his body at the time of injury. Certain injuries are associated with particular sports. Football injuries commonly result in scaphoid fractures, skating falls often result in distal radius fractures, and stick-handling athletes commonly suffer hook of the hamate fractures. The best way to pinpoint the specific diagnosis, however, is a careful physical examination. Careful palpa-tion of the carpal anatomy, especially before significant swelling has occurred, often reveals the exact spot of pathology. A pencil eraser is a convenient way to palpate small areas around the wrist. Specifically, scaphoid, snuffbox, and tuberosity tenderness often can be distinguished from scapholunate tenderness and from tenderness at the hook of hamate or over the TFCC and exten-sor carpiulnaris (ECU) complex.

7. If a football player presents with exquisite snuffbox tenderness, but the initial radio-graphs are negative, what is the recommended treatment plan?

The current recommendations are to immobilize the wrist and thumb for two weeks and repeat the radiographs. The rationale is that a minimally displaced scaphoid fracture may be hard to see on initial radiographs. As the bone around the fracture site resorbs, the fracture becomes more apparent.

8. Why is it important to make the diagnosis of the scaphoid fracture early?

The scaphoid is a bone almost entirely covered with articular cartilage. The blood supply enters distally and courses proximally to the proximal pole of the scaphoid. Fractures tend to occur across the waist of the scaphoid, often impairing blood flow to the more proximal aspect. Impaired blood flow is thought to contribute to a high incidence of delayed and nonunion of the scaphoid with subsequent carpal collapse and radiographic arthritis. The more proximal the frac-ture on the scaphoid, the longer it takes for the fracture to heal.

9. What common ligament injury presents with signs and symptoms similar to scaphoid fracture?

Complete rupture of the scapholunate ligament complex. Rupture of the scapholunate liga-ment allows the capitate to settle and displace the scaphoid and lunate, leading to a collapse de-formity due to dorsal intercalated segmental instability (DISI). Early operative intervention is necessary. A high level of suspicion is necessary to identify this ligament disruption, which often is not visible on radiographs.

10. What are the classic radiographic signs of scapholunate dissociation?

Three signs can be seen on the anteroposterior (AP) view of the wrist: a widened scapholu-nate interval (> 4 mm), the scaphoid ring sign, and a pyramidal shape of the lunate. The most clearly diagnostic sign is seen on the lateral view of the wrist: an increase in the scapholunate angle (> 70°). Comparison views with the uninjured wrist may be helpful. A clenched fist radi-ograph forces the capitate down on the scapholunate interval and may reveal a significant scapholunate gap not seen on radiographs taken without load applied.

TENDON INJURY

11. What is de Quervain's disease?

De Quervain's stenosing tenosynovitis is a tendinitis that involves the abductor pollicis longus and extensor pollicis brevis tendons. The abductor pollicis longus tendon often has multiple insertion slips, and its particular anatomy makes it prone to synovitis, resulting in pain and restriction of motion. The Finkelstein test or forced flexion of the thumb with the wrist in ulnar deviation often elicits extreme pain. Treatment consists of conservative modalities, antiinflammatory drugs, and ice with splinting and rest, with subsequent steroid injection or surgical release if initial methods fail.

12. How are the tendons attached to the wrist? How do they maintain their position through a wide arc of pronation and supination?

The flexor tendons are stabilized by passing through the carpal tunnel at the level of the wrist, whereas the extensor tendons are stabilized by a series of six separate compartments that function as tunnels and allow gliding of the tendons by keeping them fixed to the dorsum of the wrist. Because the wrist and hand are called to function in a great many different positions of rotation and wrist flexion and extension, these tendon sheaths are not always in optimal alignment with the direction of pull of the tendon. The potential results are increased friction and synovitis.

13. Wrist dorsiflexion, commonly needed for racquet sports, may affect the extensor tendons distally in the forearm. What is the name of this syndrome?

The intersection syndrome refers to the anatomic area in which the abductor pollicis longus tendon and muscle belly overlie the extensor carpi radialis longus and brevis tendons. This intersection may cause synovitis or irritation. Conservative management with nonsteroidal antiinflammatories and stretching is often curative. Injections or surgery may be used for more recalcitrant cases.

14. If a patient presents with a painful snapping over the ulnar side of the wrist after a forceful swinging event, what is a possible diagnosis?

Snapping of the extensor carpi ulnaris (ECU) tendon may occur along the dorsal ulnar surface of the wrist. The ECU tendon makes an acute angle into its wrist tendon sheath, especially when the forearm is supinated. Forceful actions in this position may result in tearing of the tendon sheath. When this occurs, the ECU tendon may sublux and cause a painful snapping over the distal ulna. Acute cases may be treated with surgical repair of the sheath. Chronic cases may need a reconstructive procedure.

NERVE ENTRAPMENT

15. What are the classic signs and symptoms of carpal tunnel syndrome?

The median nerve, along with eight flexor tendons, runs through the carpal tunnel on the volar surface of the wrist. The median nerve supplies sensation to the radial three and one-half fingers of the hand as well as motor innervation to the thenar muscles. Any process that increases pressure within the carpal canal leads to compressive force on the median nerve and subsequent symptoms. Patients often report numbness and tingling and diffuse pain. They frequently complain of pain that wakes them from sleep at night and have the need to shake their hands before they are able to return to sleep. Conservative management usually begins with a neutral or cock-up wrist splint, especially at nighttime. Antiinflammatory agents should be tried but are not of great value. Nerve conduction velocity testing is used to confirm the diagnosis of significant median nerve compression at the wrist.

16. What nerve innervates the majority of small muscles in the hand?

The ulnar nerve innervates most of the intrinsic muscles of the hand. The ulnar nerve may be compressed at the level of the wrist. The ulnar nerve splits into a deep motor branch and superficial sensory branch at the level of the pisohamate ligament. The sensory branch supplies sensation to the small finger and the ulnar half of the ring finger. The motor branch dives deep into the hand and innervates the intrinsics and ulnar lumbricals as well as the adductor of the thumb. Motor function of the ulnar nerve can be tested by asking the patient to abduct the fingers forcibly against resistance. The most common sign of ulnar nerve compression occurs more proximally at the level of the elbow, where the nerve passes around the medial epicondyle. Sensory problems related to the ulnar nerve deserve prompt attention, because delayed treatment often does not lead to satisfactory results.

17. What nerve entrapment is known as recalcitrant tennis elbow?
Radial nerve entrapment in the proximal forearm.

WRIST SPLINTS AND BRACES

18. How do wrist braces affect experimentally produced distal radius fractures?
Sports such as skateboarding and in-line skating have been associated with a high incidence of distal radius fractures. Volar wrist braces have been used in an attempt to decrease injury. Experimental data derived from a wrist cadaver model using brace protection demonstrated decreased incidences of capsular and ligamentous injury to the wrist.

19. Does taping of the wrist and fingers increase grip strength in athletes?
Contrary to popular perception, taping of the wrist and fingers causes a statistically significant decrease in grip strength when objectively evaluated.

20. What type of injuries may be expected in the forearms of unpadded football players?
Direct contusion to the unprotected forearm may cause bruising and heterotopic ossification. Traumatic ossifying periostitis of the border of the ulna also has been reported and must be distinguished from malignancy. This distinction generally can be made with careful history and physical examination as well as adjunctive studies.

BIBLIOGRAPHY

1. Green OP: Operative Hand Surgery, 3rd ed. New York, Churchill Livingstone, 1993, pp 861–928.
2. Moore MS, Popovic NA, Daniel JN, et al: The effect of a wrist brace on injury patterns in experimentally produced distal radial fractures in a cadaveric model. Am J Sports Med 25:394–401, 1997.
3. Ohnishi N, Ryu J, Chung IS, et al: Analysis of wrist motion during basketball shooting. In Nakamura RL, Linscheid RL, Miura T (eds): Wrist Disorders: Current Concepts and Challenges. Tokyo, Springer-Verlag, 1992, pp 49–55.
4. Pappas AM, Zawacki RM, Sullivan TJ: Biomechanics of baseball pitching: A preliminary report. Am J Sports Med 13:216–222, 1985.
5. Rettig AC, Stube KS, Shelbourne KD: Effects of finger and wrist taping on grip strength. Am J Sports Med 25:96–98, 1997.
6. Riester JN, Baker BE, Mosher JF, et al: A review of scaphoid fracture healing in competitive athletes. Am J Sports Med 13:159–161, 1985.
7. Ward WG, Sekiya JK, Pope TL: Traumatic ossifying periostitis of the ulna masquerading as a malignancy in a football player. Am J Sports Med 24:852–856, 1996.
8. Whalen JL, Bishop AT, Linscheid RL: Nonoperative treatment of acute hamate hook fractures. J Hand Surg 17A:507–511, 1992.
9. Witt J, Pess G, Gelberman RH: Treatment of de Quervain tenosynovitis. J Bone Joint Surg 73A:219–222, 1991.

62. FINGER, THUMB, AND HAND INJURIES

Keith L. Stanley, M.D.

PHYSICAL EXAMINATION OF THE HAND

1. Describe the profundus test.
The flexor digitorum profundus tendon flexes the distal interphalangeal joint. With the metacarpophalangeal joint and the proximal interphalangeal joint held in extension by the examiner, the patient is asked to flex the distal interphalangeal joint. This determines any disruption in the flexor digitorum profundus tendon.

2. Describe the superficialis test.
The flexor digitorum superficialis tendon flexes the proximal interphalangeal joint. This test is performed by the examiner holding the adjacent fingers in full extension while asking the patient to flex the finger being tested. The proximal interphalangeal joint will flex while the distal interphalangeal joint remains in extension if the flexor system is functioning normally.

3. What are the sensory dermatomes of the hand?

Cervical Root	Sensory Dermatome
C6	Palmar side including thumb, index finger, and hyperthenar area
C7	Middle finger and center of palm
C8	Ring finger, fifth finger and hypothenar area

4. How can angulation or malrotation of a finger be determined on physical examination?
Each finger, individually and collectively, should point to the tuberosity of the scaphoid upon flexion. If there is malrotation or angulation, there will be crossover of the digits.

DISTAL INTERPHALANGEAL JOINT INJURIES

5. How is a patient likely to present with a mallet finger injury?
The patient likely will have pain over the dorsal aspect of the distal interphalangeal joint, possibly some bruising, and an inability to extend the distal interphalangeal joint. The mechanism of injury is usually an axial load stress on the distal end of the finger.

6. What is the recommended treatment for mallet finger injury?
In patients with extensor tendon avulsion only, without fracture or with an avulsion fracture in an adult involving less than 25% of the articular surface, extension splinting with a dorsal splint for 6–8 weeks is the recommended treatment. In mallet finger injuries with associated fractures involving more than 25% of the joint surface in adults or involving Salter III-type injuries in pediatric patients, referral to a hand surgeon for open reduction and internal fixation should be considered.

7. What is a jersey finger injury?
This is an avulsion of the flexor digitorum profundus tendon. It is commonly seen in a football player who is trying to tackle an opposing player by grabbing his jersey and most commonly occurs in the ring finger. It presents as inability to flex the distal interphalangeal joint. Treatment is surgical reattachment of the tendon.

PROXIMAL INTERPHALANGEAL JOINT INJURIES

8. What is the most common type of dislocation of the proximal interphalangeal joint?

It is dorsal dislocation. This injury involves the volar plate of the proximal interphalangeal joint. The following is a summary of recommended treatments:

1. Stable after reduction and no fracture	Splint in 30° extension block splint for 2–3 weeks
2. Stable after reduction with nondisplaced fracture	Same as above.
3. Unstable, no fracture	Extension block splint at 30° for 4–6 weeks
4. Unstable with displaced fracture	Open reduction and internal fixation
5. Comminuted fracture	Refer to hand surgeon for possible volar plate advancement to prevent redislocation

9. What is the cause of a boutonnière deformity?

It occurs with a rupture of the central slip of the extensor digitorum communis over the proximal interphalangeal joint with migration of the lateral bands volar to the axis of the joint. It leaves the patient with an inability to flex the distal joint.

10. What is the recommended treatment for boutonnière deformity?

A boutonnière deformity without associated fracture is treated by splinting the proximal interphalangeal joint in extension with the distal joint left free for flexion to prevent lateral band adherence and retinacular ligament contracture. Splinting should be 24 hours per day in full extension for 6–8 weeks.

11. How can one differentiate between a true boutonnière deformity versus a pseudoboutonnière deformity?

In a pseudoboutonnière deformity, the patient will be able to flex the distal interphalangeal joint.

12. Disruptions of the radial or ulnar collateral ligament of the proximal interphalangeal joint are most likely treated by what method?

Most collateral ligament tears of the proximal interphalangeal joint can be treated by buddy taping using adhesive tape or Velcro strips.

13. Do dislocations that easily reduce require any further follow-up?

All dislocations of the joints of the finger require radiographic evaluation and thorough stabilization evaluation. The type of dislocation should be identified, as this will determine the type of splinting and the length of splinting necessary.

METACARPOPHALANGEAL JOINT INJURIES

14. What is a boxer's knuckle?

It is a longitudinal tear in the extensor digitorum communis tendon or the sagittal bands that overlie the metacarpal heads. It most commonly occurs in the third metacarpophalangeal joint. It is diagnosed by pain to palpation over the metacarpal head, a palpable defect, and extensor lag or weakness. Treatment should include splinting in full extension if acute. Surgical repair may be indicated in some patients.

15. Metacarpophalangeal joint dislocations are most common in which metacarpophalangeal joint?

The most common metacarpal joint dislocated is that of the thumb. The second most common is that of the second metacarpophalangeal joint.

METACARPOPHALANGEAL JOINT INJURIES TO THE THUMB

16. What is the mechanism of injury in a gamekeeper's thumb?

The gamekeeper's thumb, otherwise known as a skier's thumb or rupture of the ulnar collateral ligament of the first metacarpophalangeal joint, is due to a forced lateral stress with the metacarpophalangeal joint in near full extension.

17. What are the typical physical findings of an ulnar collateral ligament disruption of the thumb?

Patients with a disruption of the ulnar collateral ligament of the thumb typically have tenderness over the ulnar aspect of the first metacarpophalangeal joint and have exquisite pain with abduction stress. With significant ligament disruption, there will be significant joint laxity with abduction stressing.

18. How is the instability of the first metacarpophalangeal joint best evaluated?

The abduction stress test of ulnar collateral ligament injuries to the thumb should be carried out with the metacarpophalangeal joint and the interphalangeal joint both in flexion.

19. What is a Stener lesion?

The Stener lesion is the interposition of the adductor aponeurosis between the torn collateral ligament ends in the gamekeeper's thumb. The following is a summary of recommended treatments:

Incomplete lesions, grades I and II	Thumb spica cast for 3 weeks followed by thumb spica removable splint for 3 more weeks
Complete ruptures	Consider primary surgical repair

20. What is the recommended treatment for radial collateral ligament injuries of the first metacarpophalangeal joint?

These injuries should also be treated with thumb spica casting, as in the treatment of ulnar collateral ligament injuries.

PENETRATING INJURIES

21. What are some of the concerns with penetrating injuries to the hand?

Penetrating injuries to the hand should be thoroughly assessed for retention of foreign bodies and also for injuries to tendons and nerves that may be away from the site of the actual penetration of the hand.

LACERATIONS

22. The patient presents with a laceration over the third metacarpophalangeal joint. By history, the patient was involved in an altercation. Should this laceration be closed with suture?

Lacerations over the metacarpophalangeal joints that involve a potential human bite are of major concern. These lacerations should not be closed to allow drainage of any infectious material introduced into the wound. Further, these lacerations should be inspected thoroughly with the metacarpophalangeal joints in flexion as well as extension. Thorough assessment of the extensor tendon and the joint capsule should be carried out. Parenteral antibiotics should be considered as well as oral antibiotics.

23. What are the surface anatomic boundaries of "no man's land"?

No man's land is marked proximally by the distal palmar crease and distally by the proximal interphalangeal crease on the volar surface or palmar surface of the hand.

24. What is the significance of "no man's land"?

Lacerations or penetrating injuries in this area should raise concern for injury to the flexor digitorum communis and flexor digitorum superficialis that run in a common sheath through this area. Any laceration in this no man's land requires thorough evaluation for possible tendinous injury. Transection of nerves in this area should also be considered for surgical repair in an attempt to restore normal sensation to that digit.

BIBLIOGRAPHY

1. Amadio PC: Hand injuries in sports and performing arts. Hand Clin 6(3):429–453, 1990.
2. Buscemi MJ, Page BJ: Flexor digitorum profundus avulsions with associated distal phalanx fractures. A report of four cases and review of the literature. Am J Sports Med 15:366–370, 1987.
3. Culver JE (ed): Injuries of the hand and wrist. Clin Sports Med 11(1):1–252, 1992.
4. Flyn JE: Hand Surgery, 3rd ed. Baltimore, Williams & Wilkins, 1982.
5. Green DP: Operative Hand Surgery, 2nd ed. New York, Churchill Livingstone, 1988.
6. Hunter JM, Schneider LH, Mackin EJ, Callahan AD (eds): Rehabilitation of the Hand, Surgery and Therapy, 3rd ed. St. Louis, C.V. Mosby, 1990.
7. Jones NF, Peterson J: Epidemiologic study of mallet finger deformity. J Hand Surg 13A:334–338, 1988.
8. McCue FC, Wooten SL: Closed tendon injuries in the hand in athletics. Clin Sports Med 5:741–756, 1986.
9. Rockwood CA, Green DP: Fractures in Adults, 2nd ed. Philadelphia, J.B. Lippincott, 1984.
10. Stern PJ, Kastrup JJ: Complications and prognosis of treatment of mallet finger. J Hand Surg 13A:329–333, 1988.

63. THORACIC AND ABDOMINAL PROBLEMS

Ross M. Patton, M.D.

CHEST WALL INJURIES

1. What is the significance of rib fractures?

At the least, rib fractures are a source of significant pain. Displaced rib fractures may cause internal trauma. Pneumothorax and hemothorax are common complications of displaced rib fractures in the chest. Splenic trauma has been reported in up to 20% of left lower rib fractures and liver trauma in up to 10% of right lower rib fractures. Multiple rib fractures may produce flail chest.

2. What limitations does the diagnosis of rib fracture place on sports participation?

The usual recommendation is avoidance of contact or collision sports until the fracture has healed. In selected cases of nondisplaced fracture, participation is sometimes allowed as long as the ribs are adequately protected. However, the decision should be weighed heavily against the risk of turning a nondisplaced fracture into a potentially serious displaced fracture.

3. What is the common mechanism of injury in costochondral sprain and separation?

Costochondral injury usually is associated with either forced compression of the rib cage or a stretching injury to the joint when the arm is forcefully pulled to the side.

4. Which radiograph is best for diagnosing sternal fracture?

A lateral chest film is best for viewing sternal fracture.

5. What is the significance of a sternal fracture?

Although the fracture itself is not usually a significant problem, the incidence of associated intrathoracic trauma is high. Patients are best observed in the hospital.

6. Which is the most serious type of sternoclavicular dislocation?

The posterior dislocation is the most serious because it may compress the trachea or rupture underlying blood vessels. Because it causes little physical deformity, it may be difficult to diagnose. Fortunately, posterior dislocations are rare.

7. What are the physical findings in rupture of the pectoralis major muscle?

Major findings include weakness in internal rotation, flexion, and adduction of the arm on the affected side. A muscle bulge is palpable with resisted adduction. When rupture occurs at the site of the tendon insertion, a defect in the anterior axillary fold may be palpable.

8. Is surgical repair indicated in rupture of the pectoralis major muscle of athletes?

Yes. Because rupture of the pectoralis muscle results in mild-to-moderate weakness, surgical repair is the treatment of choice. The results are generally very good.

9. What is "effort thrombosis"?

Effort thrombosis is traumatic thrombosis of the subclavian or axillary vein. The thrombosis may occur after a single traumatic event around the shoulder or clavicle but is more commonly associated with repetitive trauma to the vessel in relationship to motion. It may be classified as a type of thoracic outlet syndrome.

10. How is the diagnosis of effort thrombosis made?

The athlete complains of pain and swelling in the affected arm and may experience numbness, heaviness, and easy fatigability. Physical examination reveals edema, prominence of the superficial veins, and normal pulses. The test of choice for confirmation of the diagnosis is venography.

11. Which athletes are most susceptible to effort thrombosis?

Athletes who use repetitive overhead motions.

EVALUATION OF INTRATHORACIC CONDITIONS

12. What structures are at risk in blunt chest trauma?

The bronchopulmonary system, heart, esophagus, great vessels, and diaphragm are the main intrathoracic structures at risk.

13. What is the etiology of pneumothorax in the otherwise healthy athlete?

Trauma is the most common reason, with or without rib fractures. However, spontaneous pneumothorax may occur and is more common in tall, thin, young males.

14. How is the diagnosis of pneumothorax made?

Symptoms vary in severity but often involve sudden chest pain and dyspnea. Physical findings may include decreased breath sounds in the area of the pneumothorax and tachycardia, but neither is necessarily present. The diagnosis is confirmed with a chest radiograph.

15. What are the symptoms of a tension pneumothorax?

This medical emergency presents with dyspnea, tachypnea, tachycardia, neck vein distention, hypotension, and tracheal deviation toward the side opposite the pneumothorax. A large amount of air from a large-bore needle placed in the second anterior intercostal pleural space confirms the diagnosis.

16. What is pulmonary contusion?

Pulmonary contusion results from lung trauma. Blood and protein leak into the alveoli and interstitial spaces, leading to atelectasis and consolidation.

17. How is the diagnosis of pulmonary contusion made?

The patient may present with chest pain, shortness of breath, cough, and hemoptysis. Auscultation of the lung often reveals tachypnea and rales. Chest radiographic findings vary from patchy infiltrates to consolidation. The most sensitive test is computed tomography (CT) scan.

18. How common are tracheobronchial injuries in blunt chest trauma?

Injuries to the trachea and bronchi are rare in blunt chest trauma (< 1% of injuries secondary to blunt trauma).

19. What is the definition of cardiac contusion?

Pathologically, cardiac contusion is hemorrhage and cellular death from blunt trauma. Damage may range from microscopic changes only to gross anatomic findings of marked necrosis. Clinically, the criteria for diagnosis are so varied that the condition is difficult to define.

20. Which findings support the diagnosis of cardiac contusion?

Nonpleuritic chest pain relieved by oxygen but not by nitroglycerin is present in most patients. Tachycardia is common. Although cardiac examination is usually normal, the presence of a friction rub or evidence of valvular dysfunction should raise the examiner's suspicion. Electrocardiographic (EKG) findings are nonspecific, but are the best predictor of significant contusion. Creatine kinase (CK)-MB enzymes will miss 40% of contusions when used alone. Measurement of cardiac troponin I levels may be predictive. Echocardiography is best used to follow patients suspected of having contusion rather than as a tool to make the initial diagnosis.

21. Why are CK-MB enzymes not more helpful in the diagnosis of cardiac contusion?

Because the right ventricle comprises so much of the frontal surface of the heart, it is the area most commonly injured. However, it comprises relatively little of the total myocardium and may release only small amounts of CK-MB enzyme. Because this costly test is not predictive, it can be eliminated as a means of evaluating patients with suspected cardiac contusion.

22. Should all patients with suspicion of cardiac contusion be admitted to the intensive care unit?

No. Only patients who are clinically unstable, have significant EKG changes, or have a history of cardiac disease should be monitored intensively. Telemetry monitoring outside the unit is acceptable in stable, younger patients with normal or nonspecific EKG findings.

23. When are dysrhythmias most likely to follow cardiac contusion?
Most dysrhythmias occur in the first 24 hours after injury.

24. Is cardiac tamponade sometimes a sequela of cardiac contusion?

Yes. It may occur at the time of injury but also may develop as a late complication several weeks after injury.

25. List the signs and symptoms of cardiac tamponade.

Hypotension, dyspnea, weak pulse, pulsus paradoxus, distant heart sounds, distended neck veins, and low-voltage on the EKG should raise the possibility of cardiac tamponade.

26. What is commotio cordis?

Commotio cordis is a term describing a functional injury (as opposed to a structural injury) to the heart. It is synonymous with the term *cardiac concussion*. The injury follows blunt chest trauma and results in cardiac dysrhythmia that is usually fatal. The dysrhythmia appears to be resistant to standard cardiopulmonary resuscitation techniques. It is most commonly seen in hockey and baseball players and usually involves preadolescent and adolescent athletes.

27. Does protective padding to the chest eliminate the risk for commotio cordis?

Theoretically, the use of protective chest padding should reduce the risk of injury, but no prospective studies are available to answer this question. However, in a review of 25 cases of commotio cordis, 44% of competitive athletes were wearing standard protective chest padding at the time of injury.

28. What is the mechanism of injury in rupture of the thoracic aorta?

Aortic rupture generally results from a high-speed deceleration injury. Bicyclists and skiers are most susceptible to this trauma.

29. Is the epidemiology of snowboarding injuries similar to that of skiing injuries?

No. Although both involve speed and collision, thoracic trauma occurs much less frequently in snowboarding. Head and abdominal trauma predominate in this rapidly growing sport.

30. Which inherited problem is associated with nontraumatic dissection of the aorta?

Marfan syndrome. Prevention involves recognition of the potential for Marfan syndrome by history and physical findings during the preparticipation sports examination.

ABDOMINAL WALL INJURIES

31. What is the usual treatment for abdominal wall contusions?

Contusions to the abdominal wall result from traumatic bleeding into the subcutaneous tissue. Because the bleeding is superficial, application of an ice pack is usually sufficient.

32. Should rectus sheath hematoma be treated as a simple contusion?

No. Rectus sheath hematoma results from rupture of the deep epigastric vessels. Bleeding may be significant and may require surgical ligation of the torn vessel and evacuation of the clot.

33. Describe the mechanism of injury when an athlete "gets the wind knocked out."

A blow to the epigastric area affects the neural solar plexus, leading to temporary reflex spasm of the diaphragm and paralysis of respiration.

34. What is a Spigelian hernia?

This unusual hernia is a protrusion at the point where the vertical linea semilunaris joins the linea semicirularis at the lateral border of the rectus abdominis muscle.

35. What is herniography?

Herniography is a type of peritoneography used to evaluate the pelvic floor and inguinal structures. It is performed by introducing a nonirritating contrast medium via a catheter placed through the left lower quadrant. The contrast is allowed to flow gravitationally into the lower pelvis and is viewed fluoroscopically.

36. What is the role of herniography?

Herniography is useful in the evaluation of obscure groin pain. In a Swedish study, herniography was positive in 85% of 78 male athletes with obscure groin pain. Physical examination was positive in only 8% of the same athletes.

37. Who is most susceptible to iliac apophysitis?

Running athletes whose ossification centers at the iliac crest have not closed are most vulnerable.

38. What is the presentation of iliac apophysitis?

The athlete complains of pain along the anterior iliac crest with running. The pain can be reproduced by the examiner with resistance to abduction of the affected hip.

EVALUATION OF BLUNT ABDOMINAL TRAUMA

39. How reliable is the side-line physical examination in the evaluation of intraabdominal trauma?
Unfortunately, vital signs as well as inspection, auscultation, and palpation of the abdomen may be normal or nonspecific at the time of and for several hours after significant intraabdominal trauma. However, tenderness to palpation, rebound tenderness, decreased bowel sounds, back pain in the absence of back trauma, pain referred to the shoulder, hypotension, and tachycardia should alert one to the possibility of significant injury.

40. In blunt abdominal trauma, which structures are most likely to be injured?
The spleen is the most likely to be injured, followed by the liver.

41. What are the advantages of CT in the evaluation of intraabdominal trauma?
CT has a high sensitivity (90–95%), identifies subcapsular bleeding, evaluates retroperitoneal structures, and identifies the specific organ damaged.

42. What are the disadvantages of CT in the evaluation of intraabdominal trauma?
CT should not be used in unstable patients; it usually requires moving the patient out of the emergency department, may not be available, may require sedation, and has the potential risk of a reaction to contrast media.

43. What are the advantages of diagnostic peritoneal lavage (DPL) in the evaluation of intraabdominal trauma?
DPL is highly sensitive (> 95%), can be performed rapidly in the emergency department, and is the test of choice in unstable patients. Criteria for positive DPL include the following:
- Bacteria or bile in lavage fluid
- Return of lavage fluid into chest tube or urinary catheter
- Amylase in lavage (20 IU/L)
- White blood cell count, 500 cells/ml
- Red blood cell count, 100,000 cells/ml
- Aspiration of 10 ml of gross blood

44. What are the disadvantages of DPL in the evaluation of intraabdominal trauma?
DPL detects such small amounts of free blood that it may lead to unnecessary laparotomy; it cannot detect subcapsular or retroperitoneal bleeding and has the potential for causing damage to other intraperitoneal structures.

45. What is the role of ultrasound in the evaluation of intraabdominal trauma?
Ultrasound has been used more extensively in Europe for this purpose and is effective in finding free fluid in the peritoneal pouches. Recently, use of ultrasound as an alternative to DPL has been studied in the United States and compares favorably in terms of sensitivity and specificity in evaluation of unstable patients. As training in the emergency use of ultrasound in patients with abdominal trauma increases, this noninvasive test may replace DPL.

46. Is serum amylase or amylase from peritoneal lavage effective in predicting pancreatic trauma?
No. However, lavage amylase may be indicative of bowel injury.

47. What is the goal in the treatment of splenic injury?
The goal is twofold: (1) prevention of severe hypotension and death from splenic bleed and (2) preservation of all or some of the spleen. Fortunately, these dual purposes are usually compatible.

48. Is surgery always indicated in traumatic splenic bleed?

No. In selected cases of subcapsular hematoma, expectant management with bedrest is acceptable.

49. Which common infectious disease predisposes athletes to splenic rupture?

Mononucleosis is almost always associated with a transient splenomegaly and may predispose the athlete to splenic rupture days to weeks after onset of illness. Return to competition criteria are controversial, but authorities agree that contact and collision sports are to be avoided if the spleen is enlarged to palpation. Opinions vary about timing of return to play when splenomegaly has resolved by clinical examination.

GENITOURINARY INJURIES

50. What is the usual mechanism of sports injury in vulvar hematoma?

In sports, vulvar hematomas are usually the result of straddle injuries, often in gymnastics competition.

51. How is vulvar hematoma treated?

The physical examination should ensure that the hematoma does not extend into deeper perineal structures, that there is no significant periurethral or urethral injury, and that there are no associated pelvic bone or vaginal injuries. The injury is usually limited to the soft tissue and is treated with mild analgesia and ice packs to reduce swelling. Rarely, the hematoma is so extensive as to require evacuation. Significant associated lacerations should be repaired.

52. What is the usual mechanism of sports injury to the vagina?

Contact with water at high speed is the most common mechanism. Injuries have been reported in water skiing, jet skiing, and recreational water slides. Wearing a wet suit is one means of prevention.

53. What athletic participation restrictions are recommended for female athletes with only one ovary?

Because the ovary is so well protected within the pelvis, trauma is not a significant risk. No participation limits are necessary.

54. What is the significance of gross blood at the urethral meatus?

It is usually indicative of urethral trauma. Other physical findings associated with urethral injury are penile or perineal hematoma and a high-riding or absent prostate on rectal examination.

55. How should one evaluate the possibility of urethral trauma?

A retrograde urethrogram must be performed before any attempts are made to pass a urinary catheter.

56. Is penile trauma common in sports?

No. Because the nonerect penis is so mobile, it is not generally subject to injury from trauma.

57. What is the differential diagnosis in nonpainful scrotal masses?

The differential diagnosis include varicocele, hydrocele, spermatocele, inguinal hernia, and testicular tumor.

58. What is the differential diagnosis in painful scrotal masses?

The differential diagnosis includes epididymitis, testicular trauma with hematoma formation, strangulated hernia, and torsion of the testicle.

59. How should scrotal masses be evaluated?
   Palpation and transillumination may help to distinguish between scrotal masses. Nuclear scans and ultrasound may be helpful. However, it there is any suspicion of torsion of the testicle or hematoma from testicular trauma, immediate urologic consultation for probable surgical exploration is indicated.

60. What is the best prevention for scrotal trauma in sports?
   Athletic supporters (jock straps) and cups offer some protection. Baseball catchers understand this concept. Soccer players have learned to cross their hands in front of their groin when defending against the direct penalty kick. Gymnasts need to land with both feet in the center of the balance beam. Bicyclists need to stay on their seats. And kick-boxers are asking for it.

61. What athletic participation restrictions are recommended for male athletes with only one testicle?
   In the past, athletes with one testicle were restricted to noncontact sports. Although it is still advisable to avoid contact sports, many athletes choose to participate in contact sports against the advice of the team physician. Discussion of the risks of participation with the athlete and the parents of minors must be documented carefully.

62. What is runner's bladder?
   Runner's bladder is the presence of gross hematuria seen after long-distance running. Although it is a benign condition, other causes of gross hematuria must be considered. An appropriate work-up is indicated.

63. Is blunt trauma a common cause of renal injury?
   Yes. Renal injury is related to blunt trauma in approximately two-thirds of cases.

64. Which age group is most susceptible to renal trauma?
   Children are most susceptible to renal trauma. Explanations include relatively large renal size and an immature and weaker protective musculoskeletal system. Sports activities are the cause of approximately 30% of renal trauma in children.

65. True or false: The degree of hematuria after trauma is predictive of the degree of injury.
   False. Although hematuria is indicative of renal trauma, the degree of hematuria does not necessarily indicate the extent of the injury.

66. What is the work-up of microscopic hematuria after blunt trauma in the area of the kidney?
   Recommendations are controversial. Because fewer than 10% of patients with true renal trauma have injuries serious enough for consideration of surgical intervention, cautious watching is probably sufficient. If gross hematuria is present or if microscopic hematuria is associated with hypotension, decreasing hematocrit, or an increasing retroperitoneal mass, further studies are indicated. CT is the study of choice.

67. What restrictions on athletic participation are recommended for athletes with only one kidney?
   In the past, athletes with one kidney were restricted to noncontact sports. Although it is still advisable to avoid contact sports, the risk of serious injury is low. Many athletes choose to participate in contact sports against the advice of the team physician. Discussion of the risks of participation with the athlete and the parents of minors must be documented carefully.

68. Is routine urinalysis indicated as part of the preparticipation sports physical exam?
   No. It should be done in patients who have historical or physical findings suggestive of renal disease or systemic disease with potential renal involvement.

BIBLIOGRAPHY

1. Adams JE, Dávila-Román VG, Bessey PQ, et al: Improved detection of cardiac contusion with cardiac troponin I. Am Heart J 131:308–312, 1996.
2. Biffl WL, Moore FA, Moore EE, et al: Cardiac enzymes are irrelevant in the patient with suspected myocardial contusion. Am J Surg 169:523–528, 1994.
3. Bloomfield J, Fricker PA, Fitch KD (eds): Textbook of Science and Medicine in Sport. Champaign, IL, Human Kinetics, 1992.
4. Burns RK, Ross SE: Emergency: Blunt abdominal trauma. Hosp Med 29(2):73–86, 1993.
5. Feliciano DV, Marx JA, Sclafani SJA: Abdominal trauma. Patient Care 26(18):44–83, 1992.
6. Freitas JE: Renal imaging following blunt trauma. Physician Sportsmed 17:12, 1989.
7. George RB, Light RW, Matthay MA, Matthay RA (eds): Chest Medicine—Essentials of Pulmonary and Critical Care Medicine, 2nd ed. Baltimore, Williams & Wilkins, 1990.
8. Gullmo A, Broome A, Smedberg S: Herniography. Surg Clin North Am 64:229–244, 1984.
9. Hershman EB (ed): Neurovascular injuries. Clin Sports Med 9(2):383–388, 1990.
10. Kaplan JA, Karofsky PS, Volturo GA: Commotio cordis in two amature ice hockey players despite the use of commercial chest protectors: Case reports. J Trauma 34:151–153, 1993.
11. Kulund DN (ed): The Injured Athlete. Philadelphia, J.B. Lippincott, 1982.
12. Lentz KA, McKenney MG, Nuñez DB, Martin L: Evaluating blunt abdominal trauma: Role of ultrasonography. J Ultrasound Med 15:447–451, 1996.
13. Ma OJ, Mateer JR, Ogata M, et al: Prospective analysis of a rapid trauma ultrasound examination performed by emergency physicians. J Trauma 38:879–885, 1995.
14. Maron BJ, Poliac LC, Kaplan JA, Mueller FO: Blunt impact to the chest leading to sudden death from cardiac arrest during sports activities. N Engl J Med 333:337–341, 1995.
15. Marx JA (ed): Advances in trauma. Emerg Med Clin North Am 11(1):81–145, 1993.
16. Mushkat Y, Lessing JB, Jedwab GA, David MP: Vaginal trauma occurring while sliding down a water chute. Br J Obstet Gynaecol 102:933–934, 1995.
17. Paone RF, Peacock JB, Smith DLT: Diagnosis of myocardial contusion. South Med J 86:867–870, 1993.
18. Prall JA, Winston KR, Brennean R: Severe snowboarding injuries. Injury 26:539–542, 1995.
19. Prime HT, Doig SG, Hooper JC: Retrosternal dislocation of the clavicle—A case report. Am J Sports Med 19:1, 1991.
20. Puffer JC (ed): Medical problems. Clin Sports Med 11(2):437–451, 1990.
21. Ray RL (ed): Emergency treatment of the injured athlete. Clin Sports Med 8(1):91–99, 1989.
22. Roy S, Irvin R: Sports Medicine—Prevention, Evaluation, Management, and Rehabilitation. Englewood Cliffs, NJ, Prentice-Hall, 1983.
23. Smedberg SGG, Broome AEA, Gullmo A, Roos H: Herniography in athletes with groin pain. Am J Surg 149:378–382, 1985.
24. Vinger PF, Hoerner EF (eds): Sports Injuries—The Unthwarted Epidemic, 2nd ed. Littleton, MA, PSG Publishing, 1986.
25. York JP: Sports and the male genitourinary system: Kidneys and bladder. Physician Sportsmed 18(9):116–129, 1990.
26. York JP: Sports and the male genitourinary system: Genital injuries and sexually transmitted diseases. Physician Sportsmed 18(10):92–100, 1990.

64. LOW BACK PAIN

Joel M. Press, M.D., and Jeffrey L. Young, M.D., M.A.

1. How common is low back pain?

Low back pain occurs commonly with estimates of 60–90% lifetime prevalence and 5% annual incidence. Low back pain is the leading cause of disability under the age of 45 and the third leading cause of disability all totaled. Approximately 2.6 million Americans are totally disabled secondary to low back pain and the same number are partially disabled. Approximately 40% of Americans will have an episode of sciatica at some time in their lives. The cost of low back pain is greater than $60 billion annually.

2. What is the cause of low back pain?

There are many causes. To treat a patient with low back pain, it is critical to understand which structures are possible tissue pain generators—in other words, which anatomic structures in the low back, when injured or disrupted, have free nerve endings that can cause pain. The major pain-sensitive structures in the spine that can cause pain are the outer fibers of the annulus fibrosis, the capsule and synovium of the facet joints, numerous supporting ligaments, nerve fibers, fascia, and muscle.

An acute "back strain" is often thought to represent an acute injury to any of these structures. Which structure is injured often depends on the mechanism of injury; that is, flexion with rotation would stretch the outer annular fibers of the disc as well as some posterior muscles and ligaments. An injury with extension may cause more injury to the facet joints and adjoining structures.

Interestingly, the disc itself is aneural (and avascular). For the disc to cause injury, there is usually some disruption of the annulus fibrosis with migration of the mucoproteoglycans of the disc to the areas outside the disc containing nerve fibers or pain-sensitive ligaments.

3. What are important questions to ask when obtaining a history in a patient with low back pain?

When did the pain begin?
Is the pain worse with flexion or extension?
Is the pain better or worse with sitting? Standing?
Is there night pain?
What makes the pain less intense?
What makes the pain more intense?
Are there associated bowel or bladder symptoms?
Do the symptoms get worse with coughing, sneezing, or Valsalva maneuver?
Has the patient injured his or her back before?

4. What are important tests to perform during a physical examination in a patient with low back pain?

A complete neurologic examination including sensation, muscle stretch reflex (in particular the symmetry of responses, not only their presence or absence) and manual muscle testing (often requiring repetitive testing; e.g., repeatedly going up and down on one's toes to elicit weakness in the S1 root muscles, the plantar flexors)

Straight leg raise test
Lumbar spine motion—flexion, extension, side bending
Manual palpation of the spine
Lower extremity flexibility testing

5. What is a positive straight leg raise?

Straight leg raise tests are performed to see if there is any irritation in the lumbosacral spine at the level of the dura on any of the lower nerve roots, in particular L5 and S1. When the leg is raised from a supine position with the knee straight, tension is placed on the dura after about 30° of flexion. If the L5 or S1 nerve roots are irritated, such as from a herniated disc, the patient will experience pain or tingling down the leg in the distribution of the specific nerve involved. The presence of low back pain with straight leg testing is not considered a positive test, because it is not suggestive of true radiculopathy. The presence of a positive straight leg raise test, and even more so, a crossed straight leg raise test, that is, raising the contralateral leg produces symptomatic side radicular symptoms, is highly suggestive of a herniated disc as the cause of the pain.

6. What is sciatica?

Sciatica is irritation or inflammation of the sciatic nerve with pain and sensory symptoms (anesthesia, dysesthesia) into the dermatomal distribution of the nerve. A herniated disc in the lumbar spine, in particular at L4–L5 or L5–S1, often is the cause of sciatica. True sciatica will cause symptoms below the knee and into the leg and foot and present with a positive straight leg raise.

7. Do all patients with a herniated disc need surgery?

No. Most herniated discs can be treated nonsurgically and have total resolution of symptoms. Aggressive nonsurgical management of a herniated disc may include some restrictions in activity (but not necessarily bed rest!), antiinflammatory medication, possibly an epidural corticosteroid injection, but most importantly physical therapy to decrease the pain and to improve the mobility and strength of the back and lower extremity muscles, and education so that further injury to the back may be prevented.

8. What is an electromyogram (EMG)? When is it necessary to order an EMG in a patient with low back pain?

An EMG is a recording of electrical activity associated with muscular activity. Electromyography and nerve conduction studies look at the dynamic physiology of nerve and muscles. They can help to delineate at which level a nerve is being injured, for example, L5 or S1 radiculopathy, if any peripheral nerve entrapment is present that may cause symptoms, or if there is a peripheral neuropathy or myopathy present. These tests are helpful when combined with the clinical presentation, physical examination, and anatomic studies (radiologic tests) to correlate anatomy and pathophysiology to arrive at an appropriate diagnosis.

Not every patient with low back pain needs an EMG. An EMG is usually done at least 3 weeks after the onset of symptoms when the diagnosis is in question or the diagnosis is speculated but the severity of the nerve injury needs to be assessed.

9. When would you order radiologic tests in a patient with low back pain?

Diagnostic testing of all kinds should be done when the diagnosis is unclear and a specific test can give important information as to the etiology of the pain, or if the diagnosis is known but the results of the test will change the management. For instance, a patient with a clinical history and physical examination consistent with a lumbar radiculopathy who is getting better with appropriate medication and treatment probably does not need an imaging study of his or her back. However, a patient with a lumbar radiculopathy who is not getting better with the current treatment may need an imaging study to determine if an anatomic alteration correlates with the patient's symptoms and signs and whether surgery or some other form of treatment is necessary. Radiographic examination findings do not equal pain! A significant number of persons with significant anatomic abnormalities have no symptoms and vice versa. All imaging studies must be interpreted in light of the history, physical examination, and other laboratory or electrophysiologic studies.

10. What signs and symptoms differentiate benign from more serious causes of low back pain?

It is often difficult to distinguish benign from malignant causes of low back pain. Their presentation is initially quite similar. However, their course is often quite different. Unrelenting pain not changed by position or rest is often more serious. Night pain should always raise the suspicion of malignancy. Pain that is worse when the patient is recumbent can be related to spinal cord tumors. Any patient with fever and night chills with low back pain should be evaluated for spinal infections, tuberculosis, or retroperitoneal infection (i.e., kidney infection).

Low back pain related to musculoskeletal causes will usually resolve in a short period of time. In fact, 90% of all episodes of low back pain will resolve in approximately 4–12 weeks. When patients are not improving at a rate that approximates this, the physician needs to think about other possible diagnoses, including more malignant causes. One can think of all patients with low back pain as points on a bell-shaped curve with the median being about 6–8 weeks. Most people will be somewhere within 2 standard deviations from the mean. When the patient starts to "fall off the curve," one needs to reevaluate the diagnosis and treatment.

11. What type of exercises are good for low back pain?

No single group of exercises is right for everyone (despite what pamphlets say that are handed out in doctors' offices). Exercise in general, however, is important in any rehabilitation program for low back pain. Studies have shown that people who are more fit have less low back pain. They also show that when people who are more fit get low back pain, it tends to resolve much faster. There probably is some protective effect of exercise both in terms of maintaining strength of the spine and spinal segments and in terms of providing nutrition to the avascular disc that requires motion for imbibition of nutrients.

Flexion exercises (e.g., Williams' exercises) are often done to decrease the compressive load on the posteriorly located facet joints and open the intervertebral foramina. Extension exercises (e.g., MacKenzie's exercises) allow decreased compressive load on the intervertebral disc and are performed in patients with disc-related disorders; that is, radiculopathy due to a herniated disc or degenerative disc disease. Flexibility and strengthening of the lower extremities are important in most low back pain rehabilitation programs. Lower limb flexibility and strength are important for normal lumbopelvic motion and particularly for proper spine mechanics for certain work-related activities such as squatting, bending, and lifting below-waist level.

12. Who is most susceptible to low back pain?

Persons with either very heavy work demands or very sedentary lifestyles are at the greatest risk for low back pain. Low back pain often results from an excessive load on a normal back or a normal load on a weak or unprepared back. Those with very heavy work demands have increased number of exposures to overload of the structures of the spine and therefore more chance of "overloading" the spine. Those persons with sedentary lifestyles are more susceptible to slight or minimal loads causing symptoms.

In terms of sports, golfing, baseball, and bowling are the three most likely activities to cause lumbar disc problems, including herniation, probably related to the excessive torque on the spine that these activities require. Industrial factors that may be predictive for low back pain injury include low job satisfaction, monotonous or repetitive work, poor employer appraisal rating, and relatively recent employment.

13. What is the difference between neurogenic and vascular claudication?

It is extremely important, particularly in elderly patients complaining of back and leg pain, to determine whether pain is due to pressure on nerve tissue (neurogenic) or due to ischemia to the lower extremities (vascular). Both types of patients will appear to give symptoms of claudication and will have limited walking ability. In the patient with neurogenic claudication, typically from spinal stenosis (a narrowing of the central spinal canal), pain is exacerbated with walking and is not necessarily relieved by rest unless the patient leans forward. Extension of the spine makes symptoms worse as well, and these patients almost paradoxically find it easier to walk up a small hill than down the hill. In the patient with vascular claudication, typically from aortoiliac disease, pain is also exacerbated with walking, but it may disappear rapidly with rest. Extension of the spine does not make the pain worse in these patients, and their pain is almost worse walking uphill than downhill.

14. Why do women who are pregnant get back pain?

Back pain is one of the most common musculoskeletal complaints of women during pregnancy. Some causes may be related to changes in posture (increased lumbar lordosis/thoracic kyphosis), fetal positioning against lumbosacral nerve roots, and on rare occasions disc herniation. However, the most common cause is probably dysfunction of the sacroiliac joint. Under normal conditions, the tough fibrous ligaments about the sacroiliac joints allow relatively little movement. However, during pregnancy, as relaxin and other hormone levels rise, the ligaments become less taut and the joint becomes more mobile. This can lead to malrotation of the joint and pain in the low back and buttock regions. Abdominal slings, sacroiliac joint supports, and posture-corrective exercises may all be used when trying to address the issue of pregnancy-associated low back pain.

BIBLIOGRAPHY

1. Albanese M, Pizzutillo PD: Family study of spondylolysis and spondylolisthesis. J Pediatr Orthop 2:496–499, 1982.

2. Andersson GBJ: Epidemiologic aspects of low-back pain in industry. Spine 6:53–60, 1981.
3. Bergenudd H, Nilsson B: Back pain in middle ages; occupational workload and psychologic factors: An epidemiologic survey. Spine 13:58–60, 1988.
4. Biering-Sorenson F: Physical measurements as risk indicators for low-back trouble over a one year period. Spine 9:106–119, 1984.
5. Bigos SJ, Spengler DM, Martin NA, et al: Back injuries in industry; a retrospective study. III. Employee-related factors. Spine 11:252–256, 1986.
6. Cady LD, Thomas PC, Karwasky RJ: Program for increasing health and fitness of firefighters. J Occup Med 27:110–114, 1985.
7. Cole AJ, Herring SA: the Low Back Pain Handbook. Philadelphia, Hanley & Belfus, 1997.
8. Frymoyer JW, Pope MH, Clements JH, et al: Risk factors in low-back pain. An epidemiological survey. J Bone Joint Surg 65A:213–218, 1983.
9. Herring SA: Low back pain. Phys Med Rehabil Clin North Am 2:1, 1991.
10. Herzog RJ: Selection and utilization of imaging studies for disorders of the lumbar spine. Clin Phys Med Rehabil 2:7–59, 1991.
11. Malanga GA (ed): Low Back Pain. Occup Med State Art Rev 13:1–239, 1998.
12. Pope MH, Andersson GBJ, Frymoyer JW, Chaffin DB (eds): Occupational Low Back Pain. Assessment, Treatment and Prevention. St. Louis, C.V. Mosby, 1991.
13. Saal JA, Saal JS, Herzog RJ: The natural history of lumbar intervertebral disc extrusions treated nonoperatively. Spine 15:683–686, 1990.
14. Svensson H, Vedin A, Wihelmsson C, Andersson GBJ: Low-back pain in relation to other diseases and cardiovascular risk factors. Spine 8:277–285, 1983.
15. Weber H: Lumbar disc herniation: A controlled, prospective study with ten years of observation. Spine 8:131, 1983.

65. SPONDYLOLYSIS, SPONDYLOLISTHESIS, AND FACET SYNDROME

Stuart M. Weinstein, M.D.

1. Describe the functional anatomy of the facet (zygapophyseal) joint.

The lumbar zygapophyseal joint is a synovial joint formed by the articulating facets of the superior and inferior vertebrae. It has weight-bearing properties and is a major determinant of lumbar segmental motion. With normal lumbar lordosis, the facet joint bears approximately 20% of the compressive load, which increases with extension and with disc space narrowing. The range of motion available at any normal motion segment depends partly on the bony constraints imparted by the zygapophyseal joint orientation. Owing to the 90° orientation of the lumbar zygapophyseal joints, motion in the sagittal plane (i.e., flexion and extension) is intrinsically greater than motion in either the axial plane (i.e., rotation) or coronal plane (i.e., side bending).

Rotation in the lumbar spine motion segment is limited to 2° or 3°, which serves as a protective mechanism for the intervertebral disc. Rotation greater than 3° may result in tensile failure of the anular fibers. The zygapophyseal joint capsule, in conjunction with other midline ligamentous structures, also acts as a passive restraint against excessive lumbar flexion. The presence of zygapophyseal capsular fibrosis or laxity, muscle hypertonicity, or associated intervertebral disc injury may affect the quality and quantity of segmental range of motion.

2. Define the spinal motion segment and the posterior column structures.

The motion segment, or three-joint complex, is the basic kinematic unit of the spine and consists of one discovertebral joint anteriorly and two zygapophyseal joints posteriorly. Throughout the longitudinal axis of the spine, three distinct anatomic columns can be defined at any spinal motion segment: the anterior, middle, and posterior columns. The posterior column contains the so-called posterior elements, including the pars interarticularis (i.e., the bony connection between the pedicle and lamina), zygapophyseal joints, and spinous processes. The supporting tissues of the posterior column include the ligamentum flavum, zygapophyseal joint capsule, and interspinous ligaments, all of which are components of the midline ligamentous structures.

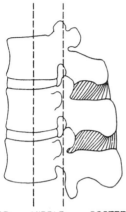

Anatomic columns of the spine. (From Mann DC: Spine fractures in children and adolescents. Spine: State of the Art Reviews 4:24–47, 1990, with permission.)

ANTERIOR:	MIDDLE:	POSTERIOR:
Ant. long. lig.	Post. long. lig.	Post. bony arch
Ant. annulus	Post. annulus	Ligaments:
Ant. body	Post. body wall	Supraspinous
		Interspinous
		Flavum
		Facet capsule

3. What is the most common mechanism leading to posterior element injury?

Posterior element injuries are more common among athletes—e.g., gymnastics, dancers, wrestlers, football players, pole vaulters, and divers—than in the general population. Pure extension and extension combined with rotation are the motions most commonly associated with pars interarticularis and zygapophyseal joint injury. These injuries typically result from chronic, repetitive loading of the posterior elements as opposed to acute, dynamic overloads. The pars interarticularis, for example, may fail at loads below the absolute tensile and shear strength of bone due to repetitive loading of the lumbosacral junction.[13] A rotational or torsional component may result in an ipsilateral compressive force to the pars, lamina, and/or zygapophyseal joint and contralateral tensile force to the zygapophyseal joint capsule. Hyperflexion injuries, usually acute, also may result in tensile or avulsion injury to the zygapophyseal joint capsule.

4. Does facet syndrome exist as a distinct clinical entity?

The existence of the facet syndrome is controversial. Theoretically, the zygapophyseal joint, like other synovial joints, has pain-generating capacity. Neuroanatomically, each zygapophyseal joint is innervated via the medial branch of the posterior primary rami of up to 3 adjacent spinal nerves. Immunohistologic studies in animals have demonstrated high- and low-threshold mechanosensitive afferent fibers serving as nociceptors and proprioceptors, respectively, in the zygapophyseal joint capsule.[1,19] The articular cartilage is not innervated, but a study of degenerative human lumbar zygapophyseal joints revealed substance P receptors, a known neuropeptide pain mediator, in subchondral bone and erosion channels as well as the joint capsule.[2]

Biomechanically, zygapophyseal joint injury may result in (1) hypomobility secondary to synovitis and capsular shortening or fibrosis or (2) hypermobility secondary to capsular laxity. The term *lumbar sprain syndrome* may reflect the most common clinical presentation of lumbar zygapophyseal joint-mediated pain. The symptoms and signs may include low back pain with or without a sclerotomal pain referral pattern (as opposed to a radicular pain pattern); pain that does not radiate below the knee; pain and/or dysrhythmia on recovery phase from forward bending to a standing position or with extension with or without rotation; local tenderness; and absence of dural tension signs. Although Mooney and Robertson's study of zygapophyseal joint-mediated pain suggested that pain referral patterns may closely mimic radiculopathies, critical review of their study design, with present knowledge of zygapophyseal joint anatomy, reveals that total volumes of injectate most likely exceeded the capacity of the joint capsule.[15] Thus, radicular pain patterns in fact may have resulted from direct irritation of the nerve roots following rupture of the capsule and extravasation of injected material. The concept of the motion segment also implies that chronic zygapophyseal joint dysfunction may lead to biomechanical alterations of the discovertebral joint with resultant disc and/or radicular symptoms and signs.

Schwarzer et al. determined that the prevalence of lumbar zygapophyseal joint pain was 15% by performing a double injection technique in which each of three joints was anesthetized (either intraarticularly or by medial branch block) with two local anesthetics of different duration. A zygapophyseal joint was considered a pain generator only when pain relief followed local blockade with each anesthetic and was concordant with its known half-life. Among subjects with zygapophyseal joint pain, no consistent clinical features were identified.[17] Lack of long-term benefit from intraarticular corticosteroid injection does not absolutely negate the existence of zygapophyseal joint syndrome. One study regarding zygapophyseal joint-mediated pain was a controlled, randomized evaluation of fluoroscopy-guided zygapophyseal joint injections in patients with chronic low back pain.[7] This study concluded that corticosteroid was no more efficacious than saline in controlling pain after several months. The premise of the study, however, was the use of injections as a single treatment tool, neglecting the conjunctive benefits of flexibility and strengthening exercises in unloading the posterior elements and maintaining the initial antiinflammatory response to the corticosteroid.

5. What are appropriate therapies for zygapophyseal joint-mediated pain?
As with any acute musculoskeletal injury, pain control, reduction in inflammation, and maintenance of mobility are the goals. These goals can be accomplished by relative rest; education in proper posture and body mechanics; oral antiinflammatory medications, typically nonsteroidal but occasionally steroidal; antiinflammatory modalities, initially ice, then superficial or deep heat and electrical stimulation techniques; traction to unload the zygapophyseal joints; and joint mobilization techniques[10] for pain control. Treatment of subacute joint pain and dysfunction includes single-level joint manipulation techniques for restoring proper joint glide; soft tissue mobilization as applied by myofascial releasing techniques[6] and stretching exercises, especially the anterior hip girdle to decrease excessive lumbar lordosis; strengthening and stabilization exercises for the trunk and spinal muscles; and sport-specific training. Other controversial treatments used for refractory zygapophyseal joint-mediated pain include intraarticular zygapophyseal joint injection with corticosteroid, particularly if bone scan with single-photon emission computerized tomography (SPECT) identifies a specific level; bracing with a rigid brace having a flexion bias; zygapophyseal joint nerve blocks; zygapophyseal joint rhizotomy for potentially long-term denervation of the joint; and spinal fusion.

6. Define and discuss the terms *spondylolysis*, *spondylolisthesis*, and *pars stress reaction*.
Spondylolysis is defined as a defect in the pars interarticularis. Anatomically, the pars is a thin (1–2 mm) bony bridge between the pedicle and lamina, consisting mainly of cortical bone. Isthmic spondylolysis is typically bilateral, with the pars defects manifesting as fibrous pseudoarthrosis as opposed to true bony union. Such pars defects are not congenital but have a genetic predisposition. The prevalence of spondylolysis in people older than 7 years of age is 5%, whereas in children younger than 5 years old the prevalence is negligible.

Pars defects also may result from excessive mechanical stress (i.e., traumatic spondylolysis); at least mechanical stress may cause a previously asymptomatic isthmic spondylolysis to become symptomatic. Biomechanically, the pars can be loaded with repetitive flexion, extension, and rotation as is common in athletics, and pars defects occur most commonly at L5, the site of maximal shear.

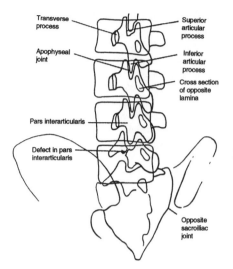

Spondylolysis. Defect of the pars interarticularis as demonstrated in this oblique representation of the lumbar spine (From Tachdjian MO: Pediatric Orthopedics, vol 3, 2nd ed. Philadelphia, W.B. Saunders, 1990, with permission).

Spondylolisthesis is defined as forward slippage of a superior vertebra on the one below. Isthmic spondylolisthesis typically occurs at L5–S1 if the spondylitic defects are bilateral. Isthmic spondylolisthesis does not usually progress beyond the end of adolescence, although progression of one stage (see below) associated with disc or zygapophyseal joint degeneration may occur. Any disruption of the posterior elements may result in slippage, including dysplasia of the L5 and/or S1 zygapophyseal joints (i.e., true congenital spondylolisthesis); acute fracture of the pars, pedicle, lamina, or zygapophyseal joint (i.e., traumatic spondylolisthesis); or erosion of the superior articular process of the caudal vertebra that allows the inferior articular process of the rostral vertebra to translate anteriorly (i.e., degenerative spondylolisthesis). Degenerative spondylolisthesis usually occurs at L4–L5 and is often associated with instability. The grades of slippage are usually defined as follows:

Grade I   Up to 25% displacement (of the rostral on the caudal vertebra)
Grade II   25–50% displacement
Grade III 50–75% displacement
Grade IV   75–100% displacement
Grade V   100% displacement; also known as spondyloptysis; the rostral vertebra drops off
           the caudal vertebra

Pars stress reaction is defined as a prespondylitic state with microfailure of the pars interarticularis without a true pars defect.[9] It may progress to a true spondylolysis with further loading. This stage is extremely important to recognize, because true bony healing is more likely with a pars stress reaction than with spondylolysis or certainly spondylolisthesis, if treatment is instituted early.

7. How does one determine whether a pars interarticularis abnormality is painful?

Some people with pars interarticularis defects may not be symptomatic. The presence of unilateral or even bilateral L5 pars defects on oblique lumbar spine radiographs, even in the clinical setting of acute low back pain, does not absolutely implicate them as the source of pain. This is especially true in young adults with acute low back pain, in whom the new onset of L5 spondylolysis is unlikely. A match between the mechanism of injury, clinical findings, and imaging studies is necessary to confirm that a spondylitic finding is acute and painful.

Symptomatic pars defects can be confirmed by bone scan imaging, particularly SPECT,[4,8] although even bone scans remain positive for a year or more after healing of an acute spondylitic injury. A negative bone scan, however, almost always rules out a spondylitic defect as the source of pain. Because pars defects indicate abnormal mechanical stress to a previously healthy or genetically predisposed spine, these same stresses may result in injury to the other components of the three-joint complex—namely, the zygapophyseal joints and disc.

CT imaging may confirm a spondylitic defect, either isthmic or pars stress reaction, in the setting of a positive bone scan, especially if oblique radiographs are equivocal. Occasionally, however, the CT image is parallel to the pars defect and thus yields a false-negative result. Injection of the pars defect with anesthetic under fluoroscopic guidance has been used to identify a painful structure, but precise localization is not always possible.

Determination of a healed pars defect is usually clinical but may be supported by specific imaging. Whereas plain radiographs may not reveal healing and bone scan may remain positive despite healing, CT is highly sensitive to bony healing. Although exposure to ionizing radiation should be minimized, especially in adolescents, repeat CT imaging with limited, thin sections through the known pars fracture should visualize whether true bony bridging has occurred. Standing lateral flexion and extension x-rays every 6 months through the adolescent growth spurt are indicated if spondylolysis or spondylolisthesis is present in children 10 years old or younger.[3]

8. Distinguish among the clinical features of spondylolysis and isthmic and degenerative spondylolisthesis.

Clinical Features of Spondylolysis and Isthmic and Degenerative Spondylolisthesis

	SPONDYLOLYSIS	ISTHMIC SPONDYLOLISTHESIS	DEGENERATIVE SPONDYLOLISTHESIS
Sex	Males more than females	Males more than females	Females much more than males
Age (yr)	7–14	7 to end of adolescence	> 40
Vertebral body/ segment	L5	L5–S1	L4–L5
Back pain	Acute—yes Chronic—?	Acute—yes, any stage Chronic—more likely if greater than grade II	? But more likely if unstable on flexion-extension radiograph
Radicular pain	Rarely (but if present, due to local irritation of the L5 nerve root from the fibrous mass)	L5, due to the fibrous mass or spur off the pars; in advanced stages, compression between the fibrous mass and vertebra	L5, due to marked facet degeneration and medial overgrowth
Examination	Hamstring tightness; pain on standing on single leg with lumbar extension	Step-off, muscle spasm; with or without L5 dural tension; L5 radiculopathy	Step-off; with or without L5 dural tension; L5 radiculopathy
Radiologic abnormality	Radiographs— obliques; SPECT bone scan; CT	Radiographs— flexion-extension instability	Radiographs— flexion-extension instability

9. When is immobilization used for spondylitic injury?

First, the spondylitic defect must be determined to be the source of pain (see question 7). Rigid immobilization, usually with a modified polypropylene brace, such as a neutral-degree Boston Overlap Brace (BOB), has been recommended for varying durations, ranging from waking hours to 23 hours per day and from 3 months to 6 months.[3,18] Absolute stabilization of the lumbosacral segment requires a thigh extension such as a hip spica, which is often not used because of potential noncompliance. Unilateral pars defects, pars stress reactions, young age (to early adolescence), and slippage up to 25% are criteria for longer periods of bracing to allow true bony healing or to prevent further slippage. One recent investigation demonstrated that nearly

40% of all spondylitic defects, the majority of which were in an early stage of development, healed successfully without the use of rigid immobilization.[16]

10. What are the return-to-play criteria after posterior element injuries?

The principles on which return to competition is considered include absence of symptoms; full pain-free range of motion; optimal lumbar and lower quadrant flexibility; normal strength and endurance; and sports-specific rehabilitation. All posterior element injuries require specific attention to flexibility of the anterior pelvic girdle muscles, particularly the psoas and rectus femoris. Stretching these muscles helps to unload the posterior elements by decreasing the lumbar lordosis. With spondylolysis requiring bracing, sporting activity in the brace may be allowed within 4–6 weeks if symptoms improve. Full unrestricted activity may be allowed in 3–6 months, depending on clinical improvement. Athletes with grade I spondylolisthesis may return to full activity if asymptomatic after completing a full course of bracing and rehabilitation. With grade II slips or greater, return to non–high-risk sports is allowed (see question 3 for examples of high-risk sports). Recurrent back pain, progressive slippage, or development of neurologic symptoms and/or signs may necessitate further bracing and possibly surgical consultation. The criteria for return to activity after surgery are less clear. In addition to the principles delineated for non-surgical treatment, the surgical procedure—that is, decompression alone for radiculopathy or fusion for back pain or instability—may determine which activities are permanently restricted.

BIBLIOGRAPHY

1. Avramov AI, Cavanaugh JM, Ozaktay CA, et al: The effects of controlled mechanical loading on group II, III and IV afferent units from the lumbar facet joint and surrounding tissue. An in vitro study. J Bone Joint Surg 74A:1464–1471, 1992.
2. Beamon DN, Graziano GP, Glover RA, et al: Substance P innervation of lumbar spine facet joints. Spine 18:1044–1049, 1993.
3. Bell DF, Ehrlich MG, Zaleske DJ: Brace treatment for symptomatic spondylolisthesis. Clin Orthop 236:192–198, 1988.
4. Bodner RJ, Heyman S, Drummond DS, Gregg JR: The use of single photon emission computerized tomography (SPECT) in the diagnosis of low-back pain in young patients. Spine 13:1155–1160, 1988.
5. Bogduk N, Twomey LT: Clinical Anatomy of the Lumbar Spine, 2nd ed. Melbourne, Churchill Livingstone, 1991.
6. Cantu RI, Grodin AJ: Myofascial Manipulation. Theory and Clinical Application. Gaithersburg, MD, Aspen, 1992.
7. Carrette S, Marcoux S, Truchon R, et al: A controlled trial of corticosteroid injections into facet joints for chronic low back pain. N Engl J Med 325:1002–1007, 1991.
8. Collier BD, Johnson RP, Carrera GF, et al: Painful spondylolysis or spondylolisthesis studied by single photon emission computerized tomography. Radiology 154:207–211, 1985.
9. Cuillo JV, Jackson DW: Pars interarticularis stress reaction, spondylolysis, and spondylolisthesis in gymnasts. Clin Sports Med 4:95–110, 1985.
10. Grieve GP: Modern Manual Therapy of the Vertebral Column. Edinburgh, Churchill Livingstone, 1986.
11. Jackson RP: The facet syndrome. Myth or reality? Clin Orthop 279:110–121, 1992.
12. Letts M, MacDonald P: Sports injuries to the pediatric spine. Spine State Art Rev 4:49–83, 1990.
13. Letts M, Smallman J, Afanasiev R, Goun G: Fractures of the pars interarticularis in adolescent athletes: A clinical-biomechanical analysis. J Pediatr Orthop 6:40–46, 1986.
14. Micheli LJ: Back injuries in gymnastics. Sports Med 2:473–484, 1983.
15. Mooney V, Robertson J: The facet syndrome. Clin Orthop 115:149–156, 1976.
16. Morita T, Ikata T, Katoh S, Miyake R: Lumbar spondylolysis in children and adolescents. J Bone Joint Surg 77B:620–625, 1995.
17. Schwarzer AC, Aprill CN, Derby R, et al: Clinical features of patients with pain stemming from the lumbar zygapophysial joints: Is the lumbar facet syndrome a clinical entity? Spine 19:1132–1137, 1994.
18. Steiner ME, Micheli LJ: Treatment of symptomatic spondylolysis and spondylolisthesis with the modified Boston brace. Spine 10:937–943, 1985.
19. Yamashita T, Cavanaugh JM, El-Bohy AA, et al: Mechanosensitive afferent units in the lumbar facet joint. J Bone Joint Surg 72A:865–870, 1990.

66. PELVIC AND BUTTOCK SYNDROMES

Kirk M. Peck, M.S., P.T.

HIP POINTER

1. What causes a hip pointer?

The term *hip pointer* is a loosely used diagnosis referring to a contusion of the iliac crest. Injury is generally the result of a direct blow to the iliac crest during collision and contact sports.

2. Discuss the symptoms and physical findings of a hip pointer.

Sudden, severe localized pain along with an audible pop or snap is common. The athlete often will be unable to walk because of the pain. Occasionally, the onset of pain is delayed. The physical evaluation reveals marked tenderness and often swelling. If hemorrhage is severe, ecchymosis will be present at the site or a small distance away from the injury. Ecchymosis migrates down the leg with time. Radiographs may be taken to rule out a fracture depending on the magnitude of the injury.

3. What is the appropriate treatment of a hip pointer?

Ice, analgesics, and a progressive supervised stretching program for the involved muscles should be started immediately or as soon as the symptoms allow.

ILIAC APOPHYSITIS

4. What is iliac crest apophysitis?

This syndrome involves pain and inflammation of the ossification centers of the iliac crests. The ossification centers first appear anterolaterally and then progress posteriorly until the athlete reaches maturity. Apophyseal closure occurs between the ages of 16 and 18 years in boys and between 14 and 18 years in girls. This syndrome is a tension apophysitis most commonly seen in adolescent runners, during a phase of rapid growth, when they increase their mileage. It is occasionally seen in baseball batters and pitchers as well. The increased repetitive contractions of the lower abdominal muscles cause an inflammatory response in the iliac crest apophysis characterized by pain and local tenderness. The radiograph is generally normal and is only necessary if a rare avulsion is suspected. The muscles most commonly involved and painful on palpation and/or a voluntary contraction include the tensor fascia lata, gluteus medius, and the internal and external obliques.

5. How is iliac crest apophysitis treated?

It is usually a self-limiting injury that responds well to relative rest. Abdominal muscle stretching and correcting the running technique, especially eliminating cross-body arm motion, may help.

PIRIFORMIS SYNDROME

6. What is piriformis syndrome?

The piriformis is a muscle with its origin on the anterior aspect of the sacrum from S2–S4 and insertion on the upper surface of the greater trochanter of the femur. The sciatic nerve travels underneath the piriformis and superior to the gemelli in 80% to 85% of the population. In 15% to

20% of the population, the nerve passes directly through the piriformis, leaving it susceptible to possible entrapment. A sciatic nerve entrapment may occur with any irritation that causes the piriformis to spasm and constrict the nerve. Symptoms may include a dull ache in the mid buttock region, pain walking up stairs or inclines, night pain, pain with prolonged sitting, or sciatic pain in the posterior aspect of the leg. Symptoms will often be magnified with sitting, walking, or running and lessen with lying supine.

7. Discuss the differential diagnoses of the piriformis syndrome.
Lumbar disc disease is most often confused with piriformis syndrome; but other differential diagnoses include spinal stenosis, facet syndrome, coccydynia, sacroiliac joint dysfunction, and ischial bursitis.

8. How is the piriformis syndrome treated?
Although surgically releasing the piriformis at its attachments has been popular in the past, the benefits of conservative treatment are now known. A supervised rehabilitation program emphasizing specific stretching exercises is generally successful. The use of nonsteroidal antiinflammatory drugs (NSAIDs), occasionally local steroid injections, aggressive massage, and a trial of ultrasound over the piriformis also may prove useful.

9. Are there other structures that may become entrapped because of piriformis irritation?
Yes. The superior gluteal nerve may become compressed at the superior edge of the piriformis muscle and present itself as a deep ache with tenderness on palpation. Passive internal rotation of the hip may exacerbate the symptoms. Weakness with hip abduction may be present, possibly due to pain inhibition, gluteal atrophy, or neurogenic weakness. A Trendelenburg gait may be evident.

10. How do you treat gluteal nerve entrapment?
The same as piriformis syndrome.

OSTEITIS PUBIS

11. What is osteitis pubis?
The pubic symphysis, although covered to a large extent by the groin and abdominal muscles, is composed only of periosteum and parietal fascia. This area of the symphysis is particularly susceptible to shear forces during athletic activities such as running, jumping, and kicking. During this time the symphysis actually can move up and down and even rotate slightly, leaving it prone to microtrauma. Because it has a poor blood supply, this area is not well equipped to handle such stress and in effect may develop a subacute periostitis.

12. What are the symptoms of osteitis pubis?
Osteitis pubis is most commonly an asymptomatic finding on pelvic films or a bone scan. Patients with symptoms, however, may have severe pain with localized tenderness. Stretching the groin muscles tends to aggravate the symptoms. Pain may radiate into the perineal and inguinal regions or along the adductor mass of the thigh. A loss of hip motion may further increase the stress to the symphysis.

13. Who is most susceptible to osteitis pubis?
It has been reported in a variety of settings, but most commonly occurs in soccer, ice hockey, track, and baseball athletes. It may also be present in elderly men after prostate surgery or in women after bladder neck and urethral surgery. Osteitis pubis also has been found in postpartum women often in conjunction with a widening and instability of the symphysis pubis.

Differential Diagnosis for Pelvic Disorders

TESTS	DESCRIPTION	SI JOINT	PIRIFORMIS	DISCOGENIC
Straight leg raise	Positive between 30°–70° of hip flexion	Negative	Negative	Positive
Reflexes	Knee jerk Ankle jerk	Negative	Negative	Positive/negative Diminished reflex if severe herniation
Lateral shift in standing	Observed in standing	Negative	Negative	Positive May either shift toward or away from painful side
Pain with sitting	Subjective	Negative	Positive	Positive Symptoms increase with prolonged sitting
Pain with standing	Subjective	Negative	Negative	Positive/negative Depends on degree of herniation
Pain with walking	Subjective	Positive Increased torsional stress	Positive/negative Contraction of piriformis	Positive/negative Increased torsional shearing of disc
One-leg hyperextension	Patient stands on one leg and bends backwards	Positive/negative May increase torsional stress	Negative	Positive/negative Depends on severity of herniation
Freiberg's	Pain with forced internal rotation of hip with patient in prone position	Positive/negative Pain with weight on affected side	Positive Specific for piriformis	Negative
Trendelenburg's	Balance on one leg. If the pelvis on the stance leg rises, the test is positive	Positive Torsional strain	Positive Pain on affected side	Negative
Patrick's (Faber)	Patient lies supine; foot of test leg placed on top of opposite knee, slowly lower test leg into abduction. Test is negative if leg falls to table or at least parallel with opposite leg.	Positive Rotational stress on affected side	Negative	Negative
Gaenslen's	Patient supine over edge of table, drop one leg over edge of table and pull opposite knee to chest	Positive Rotational stress on affected side	Negative	Positive/negative Torsional stress
Flexion in standing	Bend forward	Positive/negative Torsional stress	Negative	Positive Increases posterior disc herniation
Extension in standing	Bend backward	Positive/negative Torsional stress	Negative	Negative/positive May be positive if herniation is severe enough

14. What other symptoms have been used to describe osteitis pubis?

Rectus-adductor syndrome, traumatic inguino-leg syndrome, anterior pelvic joint syndrome, Pierson's syndrome, chondritis pubis, post-traumatic osteonecrosis of the pubis, and the gracilis syndrome.

15. Can other problems present as a periostitis of the pubic symphysis?

Ankylosing spondylitis. An HLA-B27 may be useful in diagnosing this systemic problem.

16. How intensive should treatment of osteitis pubis be?

If asymptomatic, no treatment is necessary. If mild symptoms do exist, the athlete should be instructed in a proper stretching program with activity modification until symptoms subside. Substitute activities may include water-running, cycling, and swimming. Return to running activities should be extremely slow to avoid aggravating the symptoms. Corticosteroids in a tapered dosage over a 10- to 14-day period may be tried. Steroid injections into the symphysis should be reserved for severe cases that are not responding to noninvasive therapy.

17. What do you do if all conservative treatment fails in osteitis pubis?

Quite often osteitis pubis has been known to become a chronic condition if not treated promptly and correctly. If this occurs and the athlete is unwilling to give up the offending sport, an arthrodesis (fusion) may be considered.

SACROILIAC DYSFUNCTION

18. What is sacroiliac (SI) dysfunction?

In general, any disruption in the mechanics of the SI joint that produces pain constitutes a dysfunction. Historically, much controversy has existed about identifying and treating the pathology of the SI joints. The SI joint was a commonly accepted source of low back pain well before Dr. James Cyriax identified disc pathology in the 1930s. It was Hippocrates who first observed that a woman's pelvis separated in first labor and remained so long after. In the last two decades, renewed interest and research have shed new light on SI dysfunction.

19. Are the SI joints a source of pain?

Yes. The ventral aspect is innervated primarily from L3 through S2 and the dorsal aspect from S1 and S2. Wide variances do exist, which account for diffuse pain patterns.

20. What lends stability to the SI joint?

Stability is inherent to the SI joint. The articulation between the sacrum and ilium is composed of many irregular bony ridges and valleys. Within the articulation lies the posterior interosseous ligament, considered by some to be the strongest ligament in the human body. The dorsal SI ligaments, along with the thoracolumbar fascia and its attachments to latissimus dorsi, gluteus maximus, transversus abdominis, and internal oblique muscles, provide dynamic stability to the posterior surface of the SI joints. Anterior stability is accomplished by the iliopsoas as it crosses over the SI joint. In addition, the sacrotuberous and sacrospinous ligaments provide static stability during weight bearing activities.

21. What movement is possible at the SI joint?

No single fixed axis of motion exists. Rather there is a wide number of axes and motions that are possible. SI movement is a combination of translation, flexion/extension, upward/downward or "nutation," and rotation. Controversy exists about the exact amount of motion that may occur at the joint. Although some still maintain that there is no motion in the adult SI joint, there is a growing general consensus that rotatory motion averages between 4° and 20° and translation in the anterior/posterior plane ranges from 0.5–7.0 mm.

22. What are the most common SI movements that occur?
- Anterior/posterior rotation of the ilia on the sacrum during flexion and extension
- Vertical upslips or downslips of the sacrum between the ilia
- Rotation of the sacrum between the ilia

23. Does age have any effect on the SI joint?

Yes. Extensive cadaver studies have concluded that the SI joints are mobile at least to the age of 40 for males and 60 for females. Extraarticular osteophyte formation is frequently seen after the age of 50 and is more commonly found in men. Statistics vary widely, but full bony ankylosis may not occur until 60–80 years of age. Some studies have found no bony ankylosis in females at any age.

24. Does pregnancy affect the mobility of the SI joint?

Yes. The hormone relaxin becomes elevated during pregnancy, especially in the last trimester, causing a decrease in the intrinsic strength and rigidity of collagen with a subsequent increase in ligamentous laxity around the pelvis. This increased laxity allows excessive movement at the pubic symphysis and SI joints, leaving them susceptible to injury.

25. Do SI joint dysfunctions create leg-length discrepancies?

Yes. This will be seen in the "long sitting test." A leg that shortens or lengthens as the patient rises from supine to a long-sit position indicates a rotational dysfunction in one of the SI joints. Asymmetric iliac crest heights in standing is a more "functional" test for leg-length discrepancy. Leg-length discrepancy caused by SI joint rotational dysfunctions is correctable by mobilization or manipulative techniques.

26. What other specific tests exist for the SI joint?

Many techniques have been used to test for SI joint pathology; however, only a few have proved reliable. The supine iliac distraction and side-lying iliac approximation tests demonstrate the greatest reliability as SI joint pain provocation maneuvers that stretch the anterior and posterior SI ligaments, respectively. Gaenslen's pelvic torsion and the posterior shear or "thigh thrust" test also have demonstrated high reliability. In addition, Patrick's (Faber) test is commonly used as a screening tool to rule out hip and SI joint pathology.

27. What treatments are appropriate for SI joint pain or dysfunction?

NSAIDs, appropriate activity restrictions, manipulative corrections, and/or SI joint mobilization exercises along with addressing strength and flexibility deficits. Occasionally, a shoe lift to correct true leg length discrepancies will help, but other measures should be tried first prior to going to this extreme.

28. Are radiographs needed?

In many cases, spine and/or pelvic radiographs will help to differentiate sacroiliac problems from other lumbosacral diseases. The most common finding is a transitional vertebra.

BIBLIOGRAPHY

1. Alderink GJ: The sacroiliac joint: Review of anatomy, mechanics, and function. J Orthop Sports Phys Ther 13(2):71, 1991.
2. Atwell EA, Jackson DW: Stress fractures of the sacrum in runners. Am J Sports Med 19:531, 1991.
3. Bowling RW, Erhard R: The recognition and management of the pelvic component of low back and sciatic pain. Bull Orthop Sec Am Phys Ther Assoc 2:4, 1977.
4. Cibulka MT: The treatment of the sacroiliac joint component to low back pain: A case report. Phys Ther 72:917, 1992.
5. Clancy WG, Foltz AS: Iliac apophysitis and stress fractures in adolescent runners. Am J Sports Med 4:214, 1976.
6. Coventry MB, Tapper EM: Pelvic instability, a consequence of removing iliac bone for grafting. J Bone Joint Surg 54A:83–101, 1972.

7. Cyriax J: Refresher course for general practitioners: The treatment of lumbar disk lesions. J Orthop Sports Phys Ther 12:163, 1990.
8. DonTigny RL: Anterior dysfunction of the sacroiliac joint as a major factor in the etiology of idiopathic low back pain syndrome. J Phys Ther 70(4):250, 1990.
9. DonTigny RL: Dysfunction of the sacroiliac joint and its treatment. J Orthop Sports Phys Ther 1:23, 1979.
10. DonTigny RL: Function and pathomechanics of the sacroiliac joint. J Phys Ther 65:35, 1985.
11. Estwanik JJ, Sloane B, Rosenberg MA: Groin strain and other possible causes of groin pain. Phys Sportsmed 18:54, 1990.
12. Garrick JC, Webb DR: Sports Injuries: Diagnosis and Management. Philadelphia, W.B. Saunders, 1990, p 175.
13. Gross J, Fetto J, Rosen E: Musculoskeletal Examination. Cambridge, MA, Blackwell Science, 1996.
14. Jackson DW, Wiltse LL, Dingeman RD, Hayes M: Stress reactions involving the pars interarticularis in young athletes. Am J Sports Med 9:304, 1981.
15. Jacobson T, Allen WC: Surgical correction of the snapping iliopsoas tendon. Am J Sports Med 138:470, 1990.
16. Kulund DN: Sports—accidents and injuries. In The Injured Athlete. Philadelphia, J.B. Lippincott, 1982, p 421.
17. Laslett M, Williams M: The reliability of selected pain provocation tests for sacroiliac joint pathology. Spine 19:1243, 1994.
18. Micheli LJ: Injuries in the young athlete. Clin Sports Med 7:513, 1988.
19. Micheli LJ: The pediatric athlete. Am Acad Orthop Surgeons Seminar 20:167–173, 1990.
20. Oldreive W: A critical review of the literature on tests of the sacroiliac joint. J Man Manip Ther 3(4):157, 1995.
21. Oldreive W: A critical review of the literature on the anatomy and biomechanics of the sacroiliac joint. J Man Manip Ther 4(4):157, 1996.
22. Pecina M, Bojanic I, Markiewitz AD: Nerve entrapment syndromes in athletes. Clin J Sports Med 3:36, 1992.
23. Porterfield J, DeRosa C: Mechanical Low Back Pain. Perspectives in Functional Anatomy. Philadelphia, W.B. Saunders, 1991.
24. Potter NA, Rothstein JM: Intertester reliability for selected clinical tests of the sacroiliac joint. J Phys Ther 65:1671, 1985.
25. Puranen M, Orava S: The hamstring syndrome. A new diagnosis of gluteal sciatic pain. Am J Sports Med 16(5):517, 1988.
26. Raether PM, Lutter LD: Recurrent compartment syndrome in the posterior thigh. Am J Sports Med 10(1):40, 1982.
27. Reid DC: Sports Injury Assessment and Rehabilitation. New York, Churchill Livingstone, 1992, p 651.
28. Rich BS, McKeag D: When sciatica is not disk disease. Phys Sportsmed 20:105, 1992.
29. Roosth HP: Low back and leg pain attributed to 'gluteal tendinosis.' Orthopedics Today 1991, p 10.
30. Taylor DC, Meyers WC, Moylan JA, et al: Abdominal musculature abnormalities as a cause of groin pain in athletes. Am J Sports Med 19:239, 1991.
31. Volk GJ, Hendrix MRG: The lumbar disk: Evaluating the causes of pain. Orthopedics 14:419–425, 1991.
32. Walker JM: The sacroiliac joint: A critical review. Phys Ther 72:903, 1992.
33. Walker JM: Age-related differences in the human sacroiliac joint: A histological study; implications for therapy. J Orthop Sports Ther 7:325, 1986.
34. Weisl H: The ligaments of the sacroiliac joint examined with particular reference to their function. Acta Anat 20(3):201–211, 1954.
35. Weismantel A: Evaluation and treatment of sacroiliac joint problems. Am Phys Ther Assoc 3:5, 1978.
36. Wiley JJ: Traumatic osteitis pubis: The gracilis syndrome. Am J Sports Med 11:360, 1983.
37. Zimmerman J: Sacro-iliac joint dysfunction. Phys Ther Forum 1991, vol. x, p 4.

67. HIP, GROIN, AND THIGH PROBLEMS

Mark E. Longacre, M.P.T.

AVULSION FRACTURES

1. What is the mechanism for an avulsion fracture?

It is caused by a sudden, violent muscle contraction (eccentric or concentric) or an increased muscular stretch across an open epiphysis. The injury often occurs in sprinters, jumpers, soccer players, football players, and gymnasts.

2. Give the common sites of an avulsion fracture.

Sartorius muscle from the anterior superior iliac spine (ASIS), hamstring muscle from the ischium, rectus femoris from the anterior inferior spine (AIIS), abdominal muscle from the iliac crest, iliopsoas insertion on the greater trochanter.

3. List the clinical findings of an avulsion fracture on examination.

1. **Hamstring avulsion:** Straight leg raise and manual muscle test of knee flexion increases pain; palpation of tuberosity increases pain; positive radiographs; patient complains of sudden pain in the buttock and cannot continue the activity.

2. **Rectus femoris avulsion from the anterior inferior iliac spine (AIIS):** Manual muscle test of the quadriceps increases pain; hip flexion or hip extension increases pain; patient relates a situation that caused a forced hip extension and knee flexion (e.g., hurdlers, soccer players).

3. **Sartorius avulsion:** Palpation of the anterior superior iliac spine increases pain: active range of motion of hip flexion and knee flexion increases pain.

4. What is the best treatment for an avulsion fracture?

Treatment consists of protected weight-bearing, ice, rest, and activity modification for 2–4 months. Resisted exercises can begin once full active range of motion is obtained. Return to sports is not permitted until full strength and function have returned. Surgery is required for a displaced apophysis.

BURSITIS

5. Give the three major sites of bursitis around the hip.

1. Psoas bursa
2. Greater trochanteric bursa
3. Ischial bursa

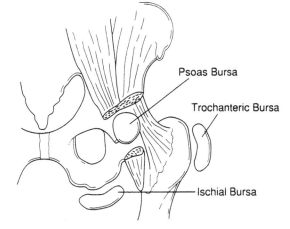

Locations of bursae around the hip. (From Reid DC: Problems of the hip, pelvis, and sacroiliac joint. In Sports Injury Assessment and Rehabilitation. New York, Churchill Livingstone, 1992, pp 626–661, with permission.)

6. List the classic signs of bursitis.

    1. Gradual onset of pain in the anatomic region of the involved bursa that becomes proportional to activity

    2. Pain present when first arising in the morning

    3. Walking often aggravates the problem

    4. Antalgic limp is often present when severe

7. Discuss the signs and symptoms distinguishing the major bursae.

Signs and Symptoms of Bursitis of the Hip

	PSOAS	GREATER TROCHANTER	ISCHIAL
Patient complaints	Symptoms worse with activity. Pain in inguinal area that radiates into femoral triangle	Burning or deep ache over or just posterior to greater trochanter. Pain with walking.	Admits to direct trauma such as a fall or from a hamstring pull.
Physical examination	Exquisite tenderness to palpation. Check for associated internal snapping hip syndrome.	Sharp pain as hip goes from flexion to extension in a weight-bearing position.	May be diagnosed as hamstring tear or epiphysitis.
Treatment	Relative rest, activity modification, NSAIDs, ice, possible corticosteroid injection, stretch hip flexors as symptoms improve.	Relative rest, NSAIDs, ice, stretch ITB, possible corticosteroid injection, assess increased supination at heel strike.	Relative rest, NSAIDs, ice, stretch hamstrings, possible corticosteroid injection, strengthen hip adductors, hamstrings, and gluteus maximus muscles

NSAIDs = nonsteroidal antiinflammatory drugs; ITB = iliotibial band.

SNAPPING (CLICKING) HIP SYNDROME

8. What is the etiology of a snapping hip?

Etiology of a Snapping Hip

SITE AND ASSOCIATED FACTORS	ETIOLOGY
Medial (internal)	Iliofemoral ligament over femoral head Iliopsoas tendon over iliopectineal eminence Iliopsoas tendon over lesser trochanter Subluxation of femoral head Suction phenomena in joint Iliopsoas tendon over anteroinferior iliac spine
Lateral (external)	Iliotibial band over greater trochanter Gluteus maximus tendon over trochanter
Contributing factors	Tight iliotibial band Narrow bi-iliac width Imbalanced flexibility Muscle imbalance Poor training techniques Biomechanical alignment

9. What are the clinical findings and treatment of a snapping hip?

    The patient reports sounds or sensations of clicking with hip flexion and extension. Very few patients ever complain of pain, and if pain is detected, it often derives from the associated bursa.

An internal snapping hip relates to the iliopsoas bursa and an external snapping hip relates to the trochanteric bursa. The appropriate treatment involves identifying the contributing factors and applying specific rehabilitative principles.

ILIOTIBIAL BAND SYNDROME

10. What are other terms used to denote iliotibial band (ITB) syndrome?

Iliotibial band friction syndrome and iliotibial band tendinitis.

11. Describe ITB syndrome.

An irritation of the iliotibial band due to friction at either the greater trochanter or the femoral condyle. It may be due to training errors (e.g., sudden increase in distance, speed work, hill running), leg length discrepancy, or biomechanical faults. Palpation of the distal iliotibial band increases pain.

12. What is the treatment for ITB syndrome?

Treatment consists of stretching the iliotibial band, ice, ultrasound, phonophoresis. An evaluation needs to include biomechanical faults, training, and exercise routines.

GLUTEUS MEDIUS SYNDROME

13. What is found on evaluation in the gluteus medius syndrome?

There is tenderness on palpation of the gluteus medius muscle. The patient may exhibit a Trendelenburg gait and weakness.

14. How can you distinguish between gluteus medius insertional tendinitis and trochanteric bursitis?

Gluteus medius insertional tendinitis demonstrates maximum tenderness proximal to the gluteus tendon and has pain on resisted hip abduction. Trochanteric bursitis demonstrates pain over the lateral aspect of the trochanter and no pain with resisted hip abduction.

15. Name the major cause of the gluteus medius syndrome.

Questionably, it is due to tilting of the pelvis with running; however, care needs to be taken in evaluating leg length for discrepancy.

GRACILIS SYNDROME

16. What is the cause of the gracilis syndrome?

It is most commonly due to repetitive microtrauma to the point of origin.

17. How can the gracilis syndrome be distinguished from osteitis pubis?

The gracilis syndrome involves the gracilis muscle at its origin on the pubic symphysis. Osteitis pubis is an inflammatory lesion of the bone with well-defined radiologic changes.

18. What is found on examination in the gracilis syndrome?

The patient complains of a gradual onset of pain in the perineal region. There is sharp pain with resisted hip adduction followed by a dull ache. Pain radiates distally through the medial thigh. Radiographs often are negative unless injury was traumatic.

19. Describe the usual management of the gracilis syndrome.

Activity modification, biomechanical evaluation, ice, modalities, NSAIDs, and steroid injections may be employed. If these approaches fail, surgery may be needed. Release of the gracilis and a small part of the adductor brevis may be considered.

THIGH STRAINS

20. What is the mechanism of adductor (groin) strains?
They commonly occur in sports requiring quick acceleration motions and sudden changes of direction.

21. Describe the symptoms of groin strains.
Symptoms include limping and pain during hip adduction or hip flexion with resistance. There is tenderness on palpation of the lesser trochanter, musculotendinous junction of hip adductor, or the ischiopubic ramus. The patient may develop edema and ecchymosis.

22. How should groin strains be treated?
The examiner must rule out disorders of bowel, bladder, testicles, kidney, and other soft tissue pathologies. If negative, use NSAIDs, PRICES principles (protection, rest, ice, compression, elevation, and support), hip spica wrap, and ultrasound if problem is chronic.

23. What is the mechanism of hamstring strain?
It may be caused by a sudden high-velocity movement seen in sprinters, hurdlers, high jumpers. Associated causative factors include poor flexibility, inadequate warm-up, fatigue, and quadriceps/hamstring muscle imbalance.

24. Describe the symptoms of hamstring strains.
the patient may have heard a "pop." There will be immediate pain, loss of function, and palpatory pain to muscle belly or origin of muscle. Pain may increase with straight leg raising.

25. How should hamstring strains be treated?
They should be treated with ice and wrap, and ice and ultrasound. Once soreness is gone, progression is made to hamstring curls, high-speed cycling, and stretching (including dural stretching).

26. What is the mechanism of a quadriceps strain?
Insufficient warm-up, poor stretching, tight quadriceps muscle, quadriceps muscle imbalance, leg length discrepancy, sudden acceleration.

27. Describe the symptoms of a quadriceps strain.
Pain down the entire length of the rectus femoris, localized tenderness, pain with an active quadriceps contraction, pain with passive stretching.

28. How should quadriceps strains be treated?
Use PRICE principles, with gradual progression into range of motion and strength exercises.

HIP DISLOCATIONS

29. What is the mechanism of hip dislocations?
Dislocation results from major trauma (from external forces) in high-speed sports (e.g., football, skiing).

30. How do you differentiate between anterior and posterior hip dislocations?
Approximately 90% of hip dislocations are posterior. Treatment involves splinting and transferring the patient to a hospital.

Hip Dislocations

SITE	POSTERIOR DISLOCATION	ANTERIOR DISLOCATION
Hip	Flexed Adducted Internally rotated Trochanter and buttock prominent	Slightly flexed Abducted Externally rotated Femoral head may be prominent
Thigh	Rests on contralateral leg	Lateral border rests on bed
Length	Appears short	Appears short
Foot	Points toward opposite leg	Points away from opposite leg

SLIPPED CAPITAL FEMORAL EPIPHYSIS

31. When might a slipped capital femoral epiphysis be present?
It should be considered when a young athlete (9–15 years old) presents with medial thigh pain, hip or knee pain, or a positive Trendelenburg gait. Special at-risk groups include obese, sedentary children and blacks.

32. What is found on examination in slipped capital femoral epiphysis?
The patient has pain with hip rotation. The hip is often held in flexion secondary to psoas spasms. As the hip is taken into flexion, it tends to rotate externally and abduct from midline. Radiographs will show widening of the epiphyseal line.

STRESS FRACTURE OF FEMORAL NECK

33. What are the causative factors of stress fractures of the femoral neck?
They occur secondary to repetitive microtrauma, sudden and rapid increase in training, training surface, or biomechanical abnormalities and are often seen in runners with persistent groin pain.

34. What are the findings on examination in stress fracture of the femoral neck?
Findings include tenderness on palpation of the inguinal area, pain at extremes of hip rotation, and limited range of motion into flexion and internal rotation. Often radiographs and laboratory tests are negative. Proceed with a bone scan if the patient is not getting better.

FEMORAL ANTEVERSION AND RETROVERSION

35. Define the term "femoral anteversion."
It is the angle the femoral neck makes with the femoral condyles. The angle decreases with age from 40° to 8° to 15°.

36. How can increased femoral anteversion cause problems in the lower extremity?
Excessive anteversion causes a "toe-in" gait. This leads to tight hip internal rotator muscles, internal rotation of the tibia, and flexion at the knee and hip, thus altering normal biomechanics. Excessive retroversion causes an out-toeing gait by external rotation of the femur and tibia and extension of the knee and hip. Sacroiliac joint pathologies are often found here. It is important to recognize biomechanical faults and the stresses they can put on the joints and soft tissue and refer the patient to appropriate physical therapy.

37. How can the presence of femoral anteversion or retroversion be determined?
The Craig test or Ryder method will give an approximation of the degree of anteversion. The athlete lies prone with the knee flexed to 90°. The greater trochanter is palpated and the hip

passively rotated until the trochanter is parallel to the surface. The degree of anteversion is the angle the lower leg makes with vertical. This test should be used only as an indicator of neck-shaft relation.

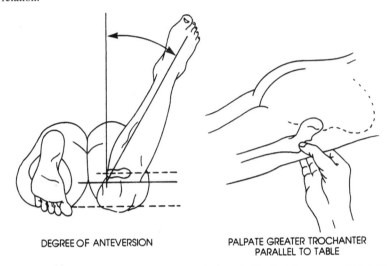

DEGREE OF ANTEVERSION   PALPATE GREATER TROCHANTER
                                                   PARALLEL TO TABLE

Craig test for femoral anteversion (From Magee DJ: Orthopedic Physical Assessment. Philadelphia, W.B. Saunders, 1987, p 252, with permission.)

QUADRICEPS CONTUSION

38. What is the mechanism for a quadriceps contusion?
A direct blow to the relaxed thigh compressing the muscle against the femur. The most common area is the anterior or anterolateral aspect of the quadriceps muscle.

39. What are the symptoms of a quadriceps contusion?
Local pain, stiffness, pain on passive stretching, tenderness, ecchymosis, hematoma formation, and loss of active extension.

40. How should a quadriceps contusion be treated?
Moderate-to-severe contusions need to be treated nonaggressively to prevent development of myositis ossificans. The most important period is the first 24 hours. During the acute phase avoid heat, massage, and forced stretching. Follow PRICE principles, active range of motion as tolerated, quadriceps sets, and prolonged knee flexion greater than 20 minutes. Pulsed ultrasound and electrical stimulation are possible treatment options.

BIBLIOGRAPHY

1. Andrews JR, Harrelson GL: Physical Rehabilitation of the Injured Athlete. Philadelphia, W.B. Saunders, 1991, pp 342–365.
2. Boker JM, Thibodeau GA: Athletic Injury Assessment, 3rd ed. St. Louis, Mosby, 1994, pp 509–541.
3. Brotzman SB: Clinical Orthopedic Rehabilitation. St. Louis, Mosby, 1996, pp 150–165.
4. Garrick J, Webb DR: Pelvis, hip, thigh injuries. Sports Injuries: Diagnosis and Management. Philadelphia, W.B. Saunders, 1990, pp 175–196.
5. Kalund DN: The Injured Athlete, 2nd ed. Philadelphia, W.B. Saunders, 1987, p 252.
6. Magee DJ: Orthopedic Physical Assessment. Philadelphia, W.B. Saunders, 1987, p 252.
7. Reid DC: Problems of the hip, pelvis, and sacroiliac joint. Sports Injury Assessment and Rehabilitation. New York, Churchill Livingstone, 1992, pp 626–661.
8. Starkey C, Ryan C: Evaluation of Orthopedic and Athletic Injuries. Philadelphia, F.A. Davis, 1996, pp 230–233.

9. Tomberlin JP, Saunders HD: Evaluation, Treatment and Prevention of Musculoskeletal Disorders, vol 2, 3rd ed. Chaska, MN, Saunders Group, 1994, pp 187–215.
10. Waters PM, Millis MB: Hip and pelvic injuries in the young athlete. Clin Sports Med 7:513–526, 1988.
11. Zachazewski JE, Magee DJ, Quillen WS: Athletic Injuries and Rehabilitation. Philadelphia, W.B. Saunders, 1996, pp 599–622.

68. TRAUMATIC KNEE INJURIES

Randall D. Neumann, M.D.

1. What is the most common cause of knee injuries?
Internal or external rotation.

2. Must contact occur to sustain ligamentous injury?
No. Commonly, anterior cruciate and medial collateral ligament injuries occur without contact, such as while cutting during basketball, cutting during football, and snow skiing.

3. What is the differential diagnosis of a traumatic hemarthrosis?
Meniscal tear, ligamentous tear, osteochondral fracture, and patellar dislocation.

4. What is the significance of fat globules found in the knee?
Their presence signifies osteochondral fracture, with the fat globules originating from the marrow components.

5. Explain why the timing of the development of a knee effusion helps in the diagnosis of knee injury.
Typically, bleeding is acute in ligamentous injuries, peripheral meniscal tears, and osteochondral fractures. Patients report that the bleeding started immediately and the effusion occurred within the first hour. Patients with meniscal tears typically have onset of effusion 12–18 hours after injury.

6. What are the components of the triad of O'Donahue?
This injury includes anterior cruciate ligament (ACL) tear, medial collateral ligament (MCL) tear, and medial meniscal tear.

7. What is the differential diagnosis of a locked knee?
Bucket-handle meniscal tear, loose body, ACL tear, and suprapatellar plica.

8. Describe the clinical tests for medial collateral ligament injury.
The **abduction stress test** at 30° of flexion is the most reliable test for MCL injury. The patient is placed in the supine position. The examiner places a hand under the thigh to support the thigh during testing. The other hand is used to cradle the foot or to hold the toe. The examiner applies valgus force at the foot with mild external rotation force. The supporting hand is then used as a fulcrum to lever the medial joint open. A test is considered positive if opening can be felt at the joint line level. The second test is the **anterior drawer test** with external rotation of the tibia. The patient is placed in the supine position and relaxed with the hip flexed approximately 45–60° and the knee flexed to 90°. The proximal tibia is then grasped with both hands and pulled toward the examiner. It is helpful to externally rotate the foot 30°. A positive test is excessive anterior rotation of the medial tibial condyle.

9. What is the treatment for MCL strains?

Most experts favor conservative treatment for isolated medial collateral ligament strains. Bracing should be done for partial (grade II) and complete (grade III) tears of the medial collateral ligament. For grade III, the knee should be braced for 4–6 weeks. Range of motion and weight-bearing should be protected.

10. Describe the clinical stress test for lateral collateral ligament injury.

Lateral ligaments are tested with the patient in the supine position. This is the same as the abduction stress test. The hand is reversed with the hand on the medial side of the knee. The test is performed with 30° of flexion. Stress is then placed in an abducted position so as to open the lateral joint line. A test is considered positive if opening can be felt on the lateral side.

11. Describe the anatomy and function of the anterior cruciate ligament (ACL).

The ACL is the prime restraint to anterior displacement of the tibia. The ACL is a fan-shaped structure composed of multiple fascicles that originate on the posterior lateral aspect of the femur and insert to a broad area between the spines of the tibia.

12. What complaints are typical of ACL injury?

Seventy percent of the patients report that they have heard a "pop." Most patients have immediate onset of effusion and are unable to continue their activity.

13. Describe an ACL tear.

It is a tear of part or all of the two major bundles of the knee—the posterior lateral and anterior medial bundles. Associated injuries include the medial or lateral collateral ligaments and meniscus. The anterior cruciate is usually torn in the mid-substance.

14. What is the mechanism of injury for ACL tears?

Hyperextension, varus or internal rotation, and extremes of valgus and external rotation are all possible causes.

15. Describe the instability found with ACL tears.

This is called anterior lateral rotatory instability. The lateral portion of the tibia rotates forward and anteriorly. The pivot shift test is used to reproduce the problem.

16. Describe the pivot shift test.

The patient is placed in supine position and relaxed. The knee is examined in full extension. The tibia is internally rotated, with one hand grasping the foot and the other hand applying mild valgus or abduction stress at the level of the joint. Then, with flexion in the knee to approximately 20–30°, a jerk is suddenly experienced at the anterior lateral corner of the proximal tibia. This shift is the anterior lateral subluxation of the lateral tibial condyle. A positive test is indicative of ACL injury.

17. What is Lachman's test?

The patient is in supine position. The examiner grasps the distal femur with one hand and the proximal tibia with the other. The knee is then flexed to 15–20°. Anterior force is applied to the proximal tibia. A positive test is excessive anterior translation of the tibia beneath the femur. This test is specific for ACL tears.

18. Describe the conservative treatment for ACL injuries.

Patients are treated with early range of motion, ambulation, and functional bracing. It is important to rehabilitate the hamstring muscles, which help to limit anterior subluxation of the tibia.

19. Is surgical repair of ACL injuries warranted?

Surgical repair of the anterior cruciate has been done in the past. About 50% of such repairs will fail, with gradual onset of instability, pain, swelling, and giving way. At this time, surgical repair is not the treatment of choice.

20. What are the long-term ramifications of the ACL-deficient knee?

Patients may develop chondromalacia of the patella and tibial condyles with multiple episodes of instability, pain, swelling, and effusion. Many patients subsequently develop meniscal tears. Degenerative changes are seen in approximately 40% of patients with ACL injury.

21. What are the surgical options for ACL-deficient knees?

Surgical options include open reconstruction, anthroscopically assisted reconstruction, and extra-articular procedures.

22. What grafts are used for ACL reconstruction?

The central one-third patellar tendon, semitendinosus and hamstring tendons, allografts, posterior tibialis tendon, fasica lata, and Achilles tendon.

23. Which allografts are used for ACL reconstruction?

Allografts can be used from frozen or freeze-dried patellar tendon bone, Achilles tendon, and posterior tibialis tendon.

24. Describe the surgical procedure for arthroscopically assisted patellar tendon bone reconstruction.

The arthroscope is used to diagnose the ACL tear. Meniscal lesions are addressed. The central one-third patellar tendon is harvested with bone plugs on each end from the patella and tibial tubercle. Drill holes, anatomic centers, and the femoral tibial attachment sites are then visualized and reamed on the tibial side from the anterior tibial cortex into the tibial spine. On the femoral side, reaming is done from the lateral femoral cortex to the intracondylar notch. The graft is then placed and held with screws on each end.

25. Describe the function and anatomy of the posterior cruciate ligament (PCL).

The PCL is the primary restraint to posterior subluxation of the tibia on the femur. It originates off the medial femoral condyle in broad origin, just posterior to the articular surface in the intercondylar notch. It traverses extrasynovially to the posterior lip of the tibia.

26. Describe the common causes of PCL injuries.

- Valgus injury to the knee
- Fall on the flexed knee with forces directed posteriorly
- Dashboard injuries to the knee

27. What history is given with a PCL injury?

There is usually little swelling in the acute phase. Chronically, patients get the feeling of the femur sliding anteriorly off the tibia, especially with decelerating or descending slopes or stairs.

28. Which clinical tests are used to detect PCL injuries?

Posterior drawer test and posterior sag test.

29. Describe the posterior drawer test and posterior sag test.

The **posterior drawer test** is performed in the same manner as the anterior drawer test. Posterior force is applied to the proximal tibia. A positive test is straight posterior displacement of both tibial condyles. The **gravity or sag test** is done with the patient in the supine or relaxed position. The hips are flexed 45° and the knees to 90° with the feet flat on the table. Observe for any posterior displacement of the tibial tuberosity. Then, flex through the hips to 90° and support both legs by the ankles and feet. With the quadriceps relaxed, observe for posterior displacement of the tuberosity.

30. What is the customary treatment for PCL injuries?

Arthroscopically assisted reconstruction is generally employed. Patellar tendon bone or Achilles tendon allograft is used to place a graft from the medial femoral condyle to the posterior lip of the tibia.

31. Describe the function and the anatomy of the meniscus.

The menisci function by resisting large, compressive loads. They absorb energy and reduce the shock that the underlying cartilage and subchrondral bone would otherwise endure. They increase the stability of the knee joint by deepening the articular surface of the tibial plateau and filling in the dead space that would otherwise exist at the periphery of the condyle. Anatomically the menisci are C-shaped wedges of fibrocartilage located between the condyles of the femur and the tibial plateau. The medial meniscus is somewhat more C-shaped than the circular lateral meniscus. Both the medial and lateral menisci have capsular components that firmly affix them.

32. What is a bucket-handle tear of the meniscus?

A bucket-handle tear of the meniscus is a vertical tear at the periphery. The meniscus remains intact anteriorly and posteriorly. This interior portion of the meniscus then dislocates into the interarticular notch, which then locks the knee and mechanically blocks from extension.

33. Describe the locking that results from meniscal tears.

The knee is usually locked at approximately 30° of flexion. Flexion can then go from 30° to 90°. Attempts at extending the knee cause severe pain. Patients generally have limited movement until the problem is corrected arthroscopically.

34. What is the mechanism for meniscal injuries?

Patients usually describe an injury that results from twisting or squatting or may not be associated with ligamentous injuries.

35. What clinical signs are found in meniscal injuries?

The medial joint is normally tender in medial meniscus tears. McMurray's test is positive, as is Apley's compression test.

36. What is McMurray's test?

McMurray's test is done by flexing the knee maximally with external tibial rotation and internal rotation. While maintaining the rotation, the knee is brought from a fully flexed position to a fully extended position. A positive test is a painful pop over the medial or lateral joint line, indicating a medial or lateral meniscal tear.

37. What is the most common physical finding in medial meniscal tears?

It is medial joint line tenderness, most notably at the posterior medial corner.

38. What traditional symptoms are found with meniscal tears?

Patients have episodic locking with bucket-handle tears. Most patients have pain along the medial side of the joint. A catching phenomenon may also be felt. Patients complain of pain while twisting, especially when changing directions, getting out of a car, or going up and down stairs.

39. Describe the difference between acute, traumatic meniscal injuries and degenerative medial meniscal tears.

Acute injuries are usually vertical and occur toward the periphery of the meniscus. Often they occur with ACL injuries and are amenable to meniscal repair. Degenerative meniscal tears are usually horizontal. Multiple tears called complex tears are generally present. They usually are not amenable to meniscal repair and must be partially resected arthroscopically.

40. **What are the indications for arthroscopy in meniscal tears?**
   • Typical symptoms of joint line catching and pain, effusions, locking, and giving way
   • Positive physical examination including localized joint line tenderness, effusion, limitation of motion
   • Failure to respond to nonsurgical treatment
   • Absence of articular causes for symptoms on radiographs

41. **What are the surgical goals in meniscal surgery?**
   Partial medial meniscectomy is performed by removing the torn tissue with mechanical and motorized instruments. The diseased portion is removed back to a stable and contoured rim. Preservation of the capsular rim of the meniscus helps to maintain joint stability.

42. **Where do meniscal cysts occur?**
   Meniscal cysts occur on the medial or lateral joint line and are associated with complex and chronic horizontal tears of the medial meniscus.

BIBLIOGRAPHY

1. Clancy WG Jr, et al: ACL reconstruction using one third of the patella ligament. J Bone Joint Surg 64A:352–359, 1982.
2. Feagin JA: The office diagnosis and documentation of common knee problems. Clin Orthop 147:29–38, 1980.
3. Indelicato PA: Non-operative treatment of complete tears of the medial collateral ligament of the knee. J Bone Joint Surg 65A:323–329, 1983.
4. Indelicato PA: Treatment of the anterior cruciate ligament-deficient knee. Clin Sports Med 7:803–812, 1988.
5. McGinty JB: Anterior cruciate reconstruction. In McGinty JB (ed): Operative Arthroscopy. New York, Raven Press, 1991.
6. Neuman RD: Traumatic knee injuries. In Mellion MB (ed): Sports Medicine: Musculoskeletal Problems. Philadelphia, W.B. Saunders, 1992, pp 351–376.
7. Noyes FR, Bassett RW, et al: Arthroscopy in acute traumatic hemarthrosis of the knee. J Bone Joint Surg 62A:687–695, 1980.
8. Torg JS, Conrad W, Kalen V: Clinical diagnosis of an anterior cruciate ligament instability in the athlete. Am J Sports Med 4:84, 1976.
9. Walsh WM: Knee injuries. In Mellion MB, Walsh WM, Shelton GL (eds): The Team Physician's Handbook, 2nd ed. Philadelphia, Hanley & Belfus, 1997, pp 414–439.

69. PATELLOFEMORAL PROBLEMS

W. Michael Walsh, M.D.

1. **What is the most common knee problem encountered in clinical practice?**
   Surprisingly, the most common knee problem encountered is a patellar problem, usually occurring from overuse, and not a traumatic injury such as a torn meniscus or torn ligaments.

2. **Why are patellar problems so common?**
   They are common because, for the most part, they are all based on inherent anatomic factors. This physical predisposition seems to be extremely widespread in the general population.

3. **List the anatomic factors that may contribute to patellofemoral disorders.**
   There are many different anatomic factors, both bony and soft tissue.

Anatomic Factors in Patellofemoral Disorders

BONY	SOFT TISSUE
Excessive torsional deformity of femur/tibia	Lack of vastus medialis obliquus (VMO) muscle
High and/or lateral position of patella	Overdeveloped vastus lateralis muscle
Shallow femoral trochlea	Increased quadriceps angle
Flat foot from bony causes	Tight lateral retinaculum
	Flat foot from soft tissue causes

4. Does that mean it is certain that a patient with these factors will have problems?

Not necessarily. The predisposition may lie dormant and patients may be asymptomatic for their entire life. However, without such predisposition, patients will likely never develop patellofemoral complaints. Often, there is a trigger that creates clinical complaints from asymptomatic predisposition.

5. What are some of those triggers?

The most common trigger is repetitive overuse, as so frequently occurs in sports. This could be running, jumping, swimming, biking, or any other repetitive use of the lower extremity. Other triggers may be traumatic, such as blunt trauma to the anterior aspect of the knee or an acute instability episode of the patella.

6. What types of clinical syndromes present?

Painful syndromes, instability syndromes, or a mixture of both.

7. Are there typical patellofemoral symptoms?

The most frequent symptom is pain around the anterior aspect of the knee. This can be increased by any physical activity. Most commonly, the pain is aggravated by repeated stair climbing (especially descending stairs) and a prolonged sitting posture with the knee flexed, the so-called theater sign. Swelling is usually not a prominent feature. Transient catching episodes may occur. With instability syndromes, the patient reports a feeling of the kneecap slipping, causing the knee to give way.

8. Describe the typical physical findings.

The most common physical findings are those listed as anatomic predispositions above. In addition, there may be patellofemoral pain on compression of the patella, crepitation seeming to emanate from the patellofemoral joint, and excessive hypermobility and/or apprehension on lateral displacement of the patella.

9. Are radiographs important in making this diagnosis?

They are not nearly as important as a complete history and physical examination. Many different techniques exist for imaging the patellofemoral joint. These may demonstrate some of the anatomic abnormalities. However, radiographs may appear perfectly normal in a patient with severe patellofemoral disability.

10. How do these problems relate to "chondromalacia" of the patella?

Unfortunately, chondromalacia of the patella has become a wastebasket term applied to any syndrome characterized by pain and/or crepitation around the anterior knee. This term should be reserved for cases with objective changes of articular cartilage damage on the patella. This diagnosis cannot be made with certainty from clinical examination. Other terms often seen in the literature referring to these problems are extensor mechanism malalignment, patellofemoral malalignment, patellofemoral pain syndrome, anterior knee pain, excessive lateral pressure syndrome, and subluxation of the patella.

11. Are these problems related to the common growth-related disorder known as Osgood-Schlatter disease?

We now know that Osgood-Schlatter disease is not a "disease." It is a mechanical disorder related to the same anatomic factors discussed above. It is aggravated by rapid growth, especially with resultant muscular tightness. The difference is that the focus of the excessive stress is at the patellar tendon insertion into the growing tibial tuberosity apophysis, causing it to enlarge and become painful.

12. What other clinical syndromes are related to these mechanical factors?

Patellar tendinitis (jumper's knee) is probably the most common. Less frequently seen are quadriceps tendinitis, painful accessory patellar ossification centers, and various avulsion fractures.

13. Describe the proper initial treatment for patellofemoral problems.

The most important aspect is a physical therapy rehabilitative exercise routine that emphasizes patellofemoral control rather than pure strengthening. Knee extension exercises must **not** be done, as these usually aggravate patellofemoral problems. Flexibility exercises are important. External bracing or patellofemoral taping is also very helpful. Less important are nonsteroidal antiinflammatory drugs (NSAIDs), modalities to inflamed areas, activity modification, and correction of foot deformities that may aggravate patellofemoral problems.

14. Does this stand much chance of curing the problem?

Nonsurgical treatment will **control** patellofemoral symptoms in 80–90% of cases. **Cure** is not the right word, because the anatomic factors will always be present. It is therefore important to have the patient understand that this is a potentially lifelong situation with which he or she may need to cope.

15. What happens to the other 10–20% of patients in whom this treatment program does not work?

Some may simply choose to modify their life-styles and put up with milder degrees of aggravation. In others, the disability is significant enough that they may consider surgical options.

16. Explain the surgical options.

There are techniques to help realign the forces on the patella. The simplest is that of arthroscopic lateral release of the patella, although this does not help in every case. The more extensive procedure is that of open reconstruction with not only lateral release but also advancement of the vastus medialis obliquus muscle and transfer of the patellar tendon insertion slightly medially and distally. Much less commonly used surgical options include anterior advancement of the tibial tuberosity to "decompress" the patellofemoral joint, derotational osteotomy of the limb, and patellectomy.

17. How long should nonsurgical treatment continue before these surgical options are considered?

There is no set length of time. Usually patients will have tried nonsurgical treatment for months to years. This probably depends more on the trend of symptom improvement rather than the absolute length of time. So long as the patient's disability is controlled, it is best to continue with nonsurgical treatment.

18. Will surgical treatment eliminate all future problems and give the patient a "normal" knee?

No! Surgical treatment may help a lot. It can help facilitate the patient's effort with rehabilitative exercises. However, the patient still has anatomic variations that may continue to cause problems later on. It is extremely difficult to provide the patient with a knee that feels like it did before problems began.

19. How is this situation changed when the patient has an acute, complete lateral dislocation of the patella?

The dislocation, of course, requires treatment in itself. This treatment often includes some period of immobilization. However, the current trend is away from 6 weeks of casting and more toward early functional rehabilitative treatment. Dislocations may also produce osteochondral fractures that require separate consideration. After treatment of the acute dislocation, however, treatment options appear to be about the same.

20. Will the patella dislocate again?

It will dislocate again in approximately half of patients. Others may go on to have minor subluxation episodes. Some will later develop more typical pain syndromes.

21. What activities typically continue to bother patients with extensor mechanism problems?

Most typically, activities that place high compressive loads across the patellofemoral joint such as squatting or stair climbing are bothersome. In other cases, patients may have difficulty with running, jumping, or cutting activities.

22. Is there anything that can be done to prevent these problems?

Choose your parents carefully! Seriously, because these conditions are based largely on inherited predisposition, one often sees patellofemoral problems running in families. On the other hand, in the course of preseason athletic screening examinations, the anatomic predisposing factors are seen in a large segment of the asymptomatic population. It would be difficult to imagine putting all of these individuals on a preventive program. However, it may make some sense to point out this predisposition, carefully ask about preexisting symptoms, and direct these athletes toward good stretching programs, quadriceps control exercises, and the use of some external support.

BIBLIOGRAPHY

1. Bourne MH, Hazel WA, Scott SG, Sim FH: Anterior knee pain. Mayo Clin Proc 63:482–491, 1988.
2. Carson WG, James SL, Larson RL, et al: Patellofemoral disorders: Physical and radiographic evaluation. I. Physical examination. Clin Orthop 185:165–177, 1984.
3. Carson WG, James SL, Larson RL, et al: Patellofemoral disorders: Physical and radiographic evaluation. II. Radiographic examination. Clin Orthop 185:178–186, 1984.
4. Dugdale TW, Barnett PR: Historical background: Patellofemoral pain in young people. Orthop Clin North Am 17:211–219, 1986.
5. Fisher RL: Conservative treatment of patellofemoral pain. Orthop Clin North Am 17:269–272, 1986.
6. Fox, JM, Del Pizzo W: The Patellofemoral Joint. New York, McGraw-Hill, 1993.
7. Franz WB III: Overuse syndromes in runners. In Mellion MB (ed): Office Management of Sports Injuries & Athletic Problems. Philadelphia, Hanley & Belfus, 1988, pp 289–309.
8. Fulkerson JP: Disorders of the Patellofemoral Joint. Baltimore, Williams & Wilkins, 1996.
9. Galland O, Walch G, Dejour H, Carret JP: An anatomical and radiological study of the femoropatellar articulation. Surg Radiol Anat 12:119–125, 1990.
10. Henry JH: Conservative treatment of patellofemoral subluxation. Clin Sports Med 8:261–278, 1989.
11. Hughston JC: Patellar subluxation: A recent history. Clin Sports Med 8:153–162, 1989.
12. Hughston JC, Walsh WM, Puddu G: Patellar Subluxation and Dislocation. Philadelphia, W.B. Saunders, 1984.
13. McConnell J: The management of chondromalacia patellae: A long term solution. Aust J Physiother 2:215–223, 1986.
14. Minkoff J, Fein L: The role of radiography in the evaluation and treatment of common anarthrotic disorders of the patellofemoral joint. Clin Sports Med 8:203–260, 1989.
15. Reider B, Marshall JL, Warren RF: Clinical characteristics of patellar disorders in young athletes. Am J Sports Med 9:270–274, 1981.
16. Shelton GL, Thigpen LK: Rehabilitation of patellofemoral dysfunction: A review of literature. J Orthop Sports Phys Ther 14:243–249, 1991.
17. Voight ML, Wieder DL: Comparative reflex response times of vastus medialis obliquus and vastus lateralis in normal subjects and subjects with extensor mechanism dysfunction; an electromyographic study. Am J Sports Med 19:131–137, 1991.
18. Walsh WM: Patellofemoral joint. In De Lee J, Drez D (eds): Orthopaedic Sports Medicine: Principles and Practice, vol II. Philadelphia, W.B. Saunders, 1993.
19. Walsh WM, Helzer-Julin MJ: Patellar tracking problems in athletes. Prim Care 19:303–330, 1992.

70. OTHER KNEE CONDITIONS

Kirk S. Hutton, M.D.

1. Explain the difference between bursitis and tendinitis.
Bursitis is inflammation of a bursa, which is a fluid-filled sac lined with a membrane that resembles synovium. Tendinitis is inflammation around a tendon involving the tendon sheath and surrounding soft tissue. A tendon, by definition, is a structure connecting muscle to bone.

2. What is the normal function of bursae?
Bursae are usually located near joints, especially where soft tissue structures such as skin, tendon, and muscle cross over a bony prominence. Bursae function to decrease friction over the bone in order to protect delicate structures.

3. Name some causes of bursitis.
Bursitis has many causes that are categorized by mechanism of injury.
- Acute trauma such as a direct blow
- Chronic trauma as seen with overuse syndromes
- Pyogenic infection secondary to a puncture wound
- Miscellaneous inflammatory processes, including gout, rheumatoid arthritis, tuberculosis, and syphilis

4. How many bursae surround the knee? What are they called?
At least eight major bursae can be found around the knee, as seen below.

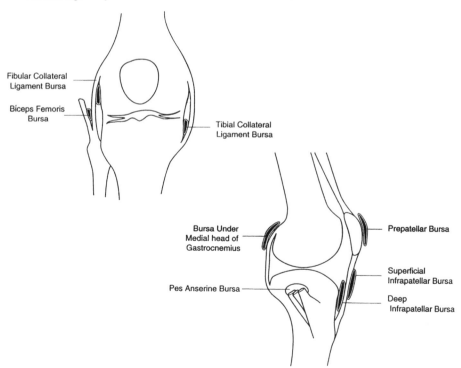

5. What are the physical findings in a patient with prepatellar bursitis?

The prepatellar bursa, which lies between the skin and anterior patella, becomes swollen as it fills with fluid. This fluid is usually blood in an acute injury such as direct trauma or synovial fluid in a chronic overuse injury as seen with "housemaid's" knee. The anterior knee will also be erythematous, warm, and painful to the touch. Flexion will be decreased secondary to increased tension in the skin as it is stretched over the swollen bursa. It is important always to rule out infection as a cause of swollen, painful knee.

6. Describe the features of deep infrapatellar bursitis.

Deep infrapatellar bursitis usually presents as a fluctuant swelling of the anterior knee that obliterates the depression on either side of the patellar tendon just superior to the tibial tuberosity. Again, bursal infection or septic arthritis must be ruled out, because the symptoms are similar. These symptoms include loss of full flexion and extension as well as maximum pain to palpation near the patellar tendon.

7. What is superficial infrapatellar bursitis?

The superficial infrapatellar bursa, as its name suggests, lies between the skin and infrapatellar tendon. It usually becomes inflamed secondary to a direct blow to the patella tendon and tibial tuberosity, causing pain and swelling in this area. The condition may be difficult to distinguish from Osgood-Schlatter disease; therefore, take into account the patient's age, mechanism of injury, and radiographic findings to help make the correct diagnosis.

8. List a differential diagnosis for medial knee pain.

Discoid medial meniscus synovial plica, metabolic conditions such as gout and chondrocalcinosis, infections including osteomyelitis and septic arthritis, tumors, trauma to any part of the knee causing fractures, medial collateral ligament sprains and bursitis, pes anserinus tendinitis, medial meniscus tears, and semimembranosus tendinitis, to name just a few. A good mnemonic to help make a differential diagnosis is Chocolate MINT:

Chocolate	Congenital
M	Metabolic
I	Infectious
N	Neoplastic
T	Traumatic

9. What are the signs and symptoms of tibial collateral ligament bursitis?

Bursae may be found in as many as five locations on the medial knee, most commonly between the longitudinal portion of the tibial collateral ligament and the knee capsule. The pain characteristically is on the medial aspect of the knee **below** the joint line and above the tibial insertion of the ligament. Some practitioners actually consider this condition to be fibrositis of the tibial collateral ligament. The diagnosis of bursitis/fibrositis should be considered in any patient with medial knee pain who does not have symptoms of joint instability or mechanical symptoms due to meniscal pathology. The treatment of this condition is nonsteroidal antiinflammatory drugs (NSAIDs) and rehabilitation. Occasionally, a corticosteroid injection is necessary.

10. Describe a condition similar to tibial collateral ligament bursitis that affects the lateral aspect of the knee.

Fibular collateral ligament bursitis has been described by Hendryson.[2] The bursa can be located at a variety of positions around the fibular collateral ligament and is extrasynovial. Pain is usually present over the lateral aspect of the knee and is increased when a varus stress is applied. The differential diagnosis for lateral knee pain includes biceps femoris tendinitis or partial avulsion, fibular collateral ligament sprain, popliteus tendinitis, meniscal pathology, as well as biceps femoris bursitis secondary to inflammation of the bursa between the fibular collateral ligament and the biceps femoris tendon.

11. Name the muscle insertions that form the pes anserinus.

Three tendons insert into an area of the anteromedial proximal tibia forming the pes anserinus. The muscles are the **S**artorius, **G**racilis, and the semi**T**endinosus. A helpful mnemonic is **S**ay **G**race before **T**ea.

12. How are the symptoms of pes anserinus bursitis different from those of other conditions affecting the medial knee?

The pes bursa is located between the medial collateral ligament and the pes tendons at approximately 2 cm distal to the anteromedial joint line. Pes bursitis presents with maximal pain directly over the anteromedial, proximal tibia and not the joint line, as with meniscal tears. The pain with tibial collateral ligament bursitis is actually more posterior than pes bursitis. A valgus stress can be used to differentiate a tibial collateral ligament sprain, which is usually painful with this maneuver, from pes bursitis. Rotational motion and contraction of the pes muscle group cause increased pain in the area of the pes bursa, thus confirming a diagnosis of pes anserinus bursitis. Another finding on physical examination that will aid in the diagnosis of bursitis is palpable crepitus over the affected bursa.

13. What is a baker's cyst?

A baker's cyst or popliteal cyst presents as a painful swelling in the popliteal fossa. It is usually caused by distention of the knee joint capsule owing to effusion. A new, synovial-lined sac may be formed in the popliteal fossa. Treatment should be directed at the primary intraarticular pathology that caused the effusion.

14. Is there a difference between a baker's cyst in an adolescent as compared with an adult?

An obvious difference in etiology as well as treatment does exist between adolescents and adults with popliteal cysts. In younger patients, the swelling and pain in the popliteal fossa may wax and wane and is usually not secondary to intraarticular pathology. Most investigators report that treating the adolescent patient with "benign neglect" is usually satisfactory. In adults, as previously mentioned, the cysts are usually secondary to intraarticular pathology and are likely to recur unless this pathologic lesion has been treated by arthroscopy or arthrotomy. Other causes of popliteal fossa and upper leg swelling that must be considered include infection, aneurysms, and deep venous thrombosis.

15. What is iliotibial band friction syndrome (ITBFS)?

ITBFS is an acute inflammatory condition that occurs when the iliotibial band repeatedly rubs over the lateral femoral epicondyle. This repeated trauma to the soft tissues in that area creates swelling and pain that is aggravated by further knee motion. It is commonly seen in runners who incorporate excessive downhill running into their training program as well as in bicyclists who are not conditioned for long rides.

As the knee flexes, the iliotibial band moves posteriorly and rubs over the lateral femoral epicondyle causing inflammation and pain after prolonged activity. This syndrome can be exacerbated in a runner with a varus knee deformity or one who "supinates" the foot, both of which cause increased force in the lateral knee. A helpful point in treating the symptomatic cyclist is to check the position of the foot in the pedals as well as raising the height of the seat to decrease the degree of knee flexion with each revolution.

16. What are the diagnostic features of semimembranosus tendinitis?

The diagnosis of semimembranosus tendinitis is usually made by finding point tenderness on the posteromedial corner of the knee slightly distal to the joint line. The pain is usually increased by flexing the knee to 90 degrees and resisting internal rotation of the tibia. As with all conditions, it is necessary to rule out intraarticular pathology.

17. Describe the difference between primary and secondary semimembranosus tendinitis.

Ray et al.[5] found that primary semimembranosus tendinitis generally occurs in the younger athlete with an overuse injury, whereas secondary tendinitis occurs in the older age group of patients who have intraarticular pathology such as chondromalacia patella, medial meniscus degenerative tears, or osteoarthritis of the medial compartment. The treatment of young patients is obviously rest and antiinflammatory agents, whereas the treatment of the older patient addresses the intraarticular pathology.

18. What is osteochondritis dissecans (OCD)?

OCD is a disease process by which subchondral bone loses its blood supply as a result of a form of avascular necrosis. Subsequently, the overlying articular cartilage becomes damaged secondary to loss of support from the avascular subchondral bone. In long-standing cases, the articular cartilage may become loose and thus forms a crater of exposed bone and a cartilaginous loose body in the knee joint.

19. Is there a definite etiology for OCD?

Many theories have been proposed as to the cause of OCD, but there is no proven, single causative factor. The proposed causes include ischemia, abnormal ossification in the epiphysis, genetic abnormalities, trauma, and a combination of all of the above. Currently, more attention is being paid to the role of trauma and recurrent microtrauma in the pathogenesis of OCD.

20. What are the symptoms of OCD?

OCD usually occurs in patients between the ages of 6 and 50. Males outnumber females two to one. The patient usually complains of a diffuse pain in the knee that may have been present for many weeks. A history of significant trauma is usually not obtained. Because OCD is the most common cause of loose bodies in the knee, the patient may present with symptoms of locking, popping, or even a palpable loose body within the knee joint or the suprapatellar pouch. Occasionally, these symptoms are incorrectly attributed to meniscal pathology.

21. Describe the radiographic findings of OCD.

The standard work-up of a suspected OCD lesion includes AP, lateral, and notch views of the knee. Because nearly 70% of OCD lesions are on the lateral wall of the medial femoral condyle, the notch or tunnel view is helpful in making the diagnosis. A loose body is commonly only articular cartilage and will not be well visualized on plain radiographs. Other studies that are of benefit include arthrograms and tomograms. Recently, magnetic resonance imaging (MRI) has been documented to be very helpful with the diagnosis as well as the treatment plan of OCD. An MRI scan will show the size of the lesion, the exact location, the condition of the cartilage, and will even show if the fragment is loose by detecting joint fluid on the subchondral side of the bone.

22. What are the treatment alternatives for OCD?

Treatment depends on the age of the patient and the degree of cartilage damage. Most children with open growth plates can be immobilized or simply watched with close observation. Older patients presenting with symptoms should have routine radiographs and in selected cases an MRI scan prior to arthroscopy. If the articular cartilage is in good condition, the fragment can be bone grafted and fixed with Herbert screws or newer absorbable pegs. If the articular cartilage is severely damaged, new techniques to transfer allograft osteochondral cores may be used. Research continues on the growth of hyaline cartilage cells to transplant into the defect.

BIBLIOGRAPHY

1. Athletic Training and Sports Medicine, 2nd ed. Parkridge, IL, American Academy of Orthopaedic Surgeons, 1991.
2. Bobič V: Arthroscopic osteochondral autograft transplantation in anterior cruciate ligament reconstruction: A preliminary study. Knee Surg Sports Traumatol Arthrosc 3:262–264, 1996.
3. Hendryson IE: Bursitis in the region of the fibular collateral ligament. J Bone Joint Surg 28:446, 1946.
4. Kerlan RK, Glousman RE: Tibial collateral ligament bursitis. Am J Sports Med 16:334, 1988.
5. Minas T, Nehrer S: Current concepts in the treatment of articular cartilage defects. Orthopedics 20:525–544, 1997.
6. Phillips B: Nontraumatic disorders. In Crenshaw AH (ed): Campbell's Operative Orthopaedics, 8th ed. St. Louis, Mosby-Year Book, 1992, pp 1939–1955.
7. Ray JM, Clancy WG, Lemon RA: Semimembranosus tendinitis: An overlooked cause of medial knee pain. Am J Sports Med 16:347, 1988.

8. Scott WN, Insall JN: Injuries of the knee. In Rockwood CA, Green DP, Bucholz RW (eds): Fractures in Adults, 3rd ed. Philadelphia, J.B. Lippincott, 1991, pp 1839–1844.
9. Waters P, Kasser J: Infection of the infrapatellar bursa: A report of two cases. J Bone Joint Surg 72A:1095, 1990.

71. LOWER LEG SYNDROMES

David E. Brown, M.D.

1. What is the differential diagnosis of chronic exertional leg pain?
- Medial tibial stress syndrome
- Chronic exertional compartment syndrome
- Stress fracture
- Vascular claudication
- Referred discogenic leg pain
- True shin splints (myositis or tendinitis of the anterior or lateral compartment muscles)

2. What are "shin splints"?
"Shin splint" is a descriptive term for an inflammatory condition of one or more of the musculotendinous units of the leg. It is most common in the anterior compartment muscles. Repetitive loading of the anterior compartment results in overloading and fatigue. This is often the result of early season conditioning and training errors that may result from running on hard surfaces, overly rapid increase in training intensity, weak ankle dorsiflexors (anterior compartment), poor shoes, or running technique.

3. How are common shin splints treated?
Treatment involves relative rest, icing, antiinflammatory medication, and stretching of the antagonist muscle groups. This is followed by a gradual return to athletics and activity. Cross-training activities may be necessary during the initial treatment phase. Immobilization is not recommended. All training errors, biomechanical abnormalities, and improper equipment should be evaluated and corrected.

4. Describe the medial tibial stress syndrome (MTSS).
MTSS is an inflammatory condition involving the periosteum of the deep posterior compartment. Pain usually starts after exercise and is relieved by rest. Symptoms may persist for hours or days after cessation of the exercise. On examination, there is a localized area of tenderness over the posterior medial edge of the distal third of the tibia. Evaluation of the foot may reveal excessive pronation. The remainder of the examination is usually normal. Radiographs are usually normal.

5. How is MTSS treated?
Rest is the primary treatment for this condition. Cross training is required, often for an extended period of time until the stress periostitis resolves. Strength and flexibility of the deep posterior compartment should be emphasized. Abnormal hindfoot and forefoot alignment should be corrected. Recurrences are common.

6. Where is the most common location for stress fractures in the leg?
Stress fractures of the tibia are most common in the proximal third or at the junction of the middle and distal thirds along the posterior medial margin. Fibular stress fractures are most common in the supramalleolar region.

An uncommon tibial stress fracture occurs in the anterior tibial cortex, usually in the middle third of the tibia. However, it is important to recognize that it is much more likely to progress to a delayed or nonunion. Prolonged immobilization and relative rest are required. In rare cases, bone grafting of the anterior tibial stress fracture is required to obtain union.

7. Name the various compartments and the muscles within each compartment.

The four compartments include the anterior, lateral, superficial posterior, and deep posterior. The anterior compartment consists of the tibialis anterior, extensor digitorum longus, extensor hallucis longus, and peroneus tertius. The lateral compartment includes the peroneus longus and brevis. The superficial posterior has the gastrocnemius-soleus complex, whereas the deep posterior compartment includes the posterior tibialis, flexor hallucis longus, and flexor digitorum longus.

8. What is acute compartment syndrome? What are its primary causes?

There is an acute increase in tissue pressure within the enclosed anatomic space (muscle compartment bounded by semirigid fascia). This results in increased local venous pressure that leads to a decrease in the arteriovenous gradient and thus a decrease in arterial inflow. Eighty-five percent of cases of acute compartment syndrome are caused by severe trauma associated with fractures or dislocations of the leg. The remainder are generally caused by marked and prolonged increase in exercise intensity such as a forced prolonged run in a military recruit. A small number are caused by vascular injury or prolonged externally applied pressure.

9. Give the primary symptoms of acute compartment syndrome.

Early symptoms: Pain with passive stretch of the muscles in the compartment and tenderness and extreme tightness of the compartment.

Late symptoms: Hypesthesia of nerves traversing the compartment and weakness of the muscles in the involved compartment.

10. What is a normal intramuscular compartment pressure measurement at rest?

0–10 mmHg.

11. At what pressure does acute compartment syndrome exist?

Any resting pressure above 40 mmHg is indicative of a compartment syndrome. Patients with values between 30 and 40 mmHg may have an impending compartment syndrome and need to be monitored very closely, often with continuous compartment pressure measurements.

12. What is the treatment of acute compartment syndrome?

1. Remove rigid circular dressings.
2. Position leg at the level of the heart.
3. Decompress compartment if there is not **prompt** resolution of symptoms and compartment pressures. Surgical decompression should be performed within 6–8 hours of onset and includes wide release of the skin, subcutaneous tissues, and fascia of the involved compartment.

13. Define *chronic* exertional compartment syndrome.

It is intermittent excessive pressure within an enclosed fascial compartment that occurs only during exercise. Pressures then slowly fall to normal following cessation of exercise but the pressure falls much more slowly than in a normal patient.

14. How does chronic exertional compartment syndrome present?

Athletes typically have pain in the involved compartment that begins at a consistent time into their exercise sessions. Symptoms may then slowly subside after cessation of exercise. They may note numbness in the top of the foot and weakness of ankle dorsiflexion.

15. How is chronic exertional compartment syndrome diagnosed by pressure criteria?

In the presence of appropriate clinical findings, the diagnosis of chronic compartment syndrome exists if (1) there is a preexercise pressure ≥ 15 mmHg; (2) there is a 1-minute postexercise pressure ≥ 30 mmHg; or (3) there is a 5-minute postexercise pressure ≥ 20 mmHg.

16. What is the incidence of bilaterality in chronic exertional compartment syndrome?

50–60%.

17. What is the incidence of muscle hernia in patients with chronic exertional compartment syndrome? What nerve can be compressed by these muscle hernias?

There is a 45% incidence of muscle hernia that usually occurs in the distal third of the anterior compartment where the superficial peroneal nerve exits the compartment and becomes subcutaneous.

18. How do you differentiate between a complete Achilles tendon rupture and a gastrocnemius muscle tear?

The Achilles tendon rupture consists of a complete disruption of the tendon portion of the gastrocnemius-soleus complex, whereas the gastrocnemius muscle tear usually occurs in the medial head of the gastrocnemius more proximally. Both occur most commonly in the 30- to 50-year-old male age group. Examination of the patient with an Achilles tendon rupture reveals weak ankle plantar flexion and a palpable defect in the tendon. The Thompson test demonstrates no plantar flexion of the ankle when the calf is squeezed. In the gastrocnemius muscle tear, there is no defect in the tendon and the Thompson test is normal. (Plantar flexion does occur when the calf is squeezed.)

19. What is the treatment of gastrocnemius muscle tear?

Treatment consists of the use of a heel lift and calf sleeve, avoidance of running, jumping, and push-off activities for approximately 4 to 6 weeks, ice massage, and gentle stretching as tolerated.

20. Give the advantages and disadvantages of surgical treatment of the acute complete Achilles tendon rupture.

Repair of the Achilles tendon rupture results in improvement in maximum ankle plantar flexion strength that is primarily noted in the aggressive athlete. The risk of rerupture is much less (2% rerupture rate in the surgically treated group compared with 8% rerupture in the nonoperative group). However, surgical treatment carries the risk of anesthetic complication, skin and soft tissue breakdown problems, and neuroma of the sural nerve.

21. Name the risk factors for the development of Achilles tendinitis.

1. Inflexibility of the tendo Achillis
2. Overpronation
3. Recent change in shoe wear
4. Recent increase in training, especially if it includes hill running.

BIBLIOGRAPHY

1. Holen KJ, Engebretsen, Grontvendt T, et al: Surgical treatment of medial tibial stien syndrome (shin splint) by fasciotomy of the superficial posterior compartment of the leg. Scand J Med Sci Sports 5:40–543, 1995.
2. Incavo SJ, Alvarez RG, Trevino SG: Occurrence of the plantaris tendon in patients sustaining subcutaneous rupture of the Achilles tendon. Foot Ankle 8:110, 1987.
3. Mubarak SJ, et al: The medial tibial stress syndrome: A cause of shin splints. Am J Sports Med 10:201, 1992.
4. Nelen G, Martens M, Burssens A: Surgical treatment of chronic Achilles tendinitis. Am J Sports Med 17:754, 1989.
5. Nistor L: Surgical and non-surgical treatment of Achilles tendon ruptures. J Bone Joint Surg 63A:394, 1981.
6. Pedowitz RA, Hargens AR, Murbarak SJ, et al: Modified criteria for the objective diagnosis of chronic compartment syndrome of the leg. Am J Sports Med 18:35, 1990.
7. Roberts JM, Goldstrom GL, Brown TD, et al: Comparison of unrepaired, primarily repaired, and polyglactin mesh-reinforced Achilles tendon lacerations in rabbits. Clin Orthop 181:244, 1993.
8. Shields CL, Redix L, Brewster CE: Acute tears of the medial head of the gastrocnemius. Foot Ankle 5:186, 1985.
9. Sommer HM, Valentine SW: Effect of foot posture on the incidence of medial tibial stress syndrome. Med Sci Sports Exerc 27:800–804, 1995.
10. Styf JR, Korner LM: Chronic anterior-compartment syndrome of the leg: Results of treatment by fasciotomy. J Bone Joint Surg 68A:1338, 1986.

72. ANKLE PROBLEMS

Curtis D. Reimer, M.D.

1. What is the most common injury to the ankle?
Sprains of the ligamentous structures are the most common injuries to the ankle. Sprains may consist of microscopic or complete tears of the ligaments.

2. Which sports are most frequently associated with ankle sprains?
Although ankle sprains may occur in any sport, they are associated most commonly with sports that involve jumping or sudden changes of direction. Ankle sprains have been estimated to account for 25–45% of all injuries in basketball, volleyball, soccer, and football.

3. What are the main ligaments involved with ankle sprains?
The ligaments of the ankle may be grouped into three complexes: lateral, medial, and interosseous. The **lateral complex** is composed of the anterior talofibular ligament (ATFL), calcaneofibular ligament (CFL), and posterior talofibular ligament (PTFL); it incorporates the majority of ankle sprains. Because the ATFL is the weakest of the lateral complex ligaments, it is the most frequently injured ankle ligament. The **medial ligamentous complex** is composed of four bands (three superficial and one deep) of the deltoid ligament. The **interosseous complex** is composed of the anterior tibiofibular ligament, posterior tibiofibular ligament, and interosseous ligament.

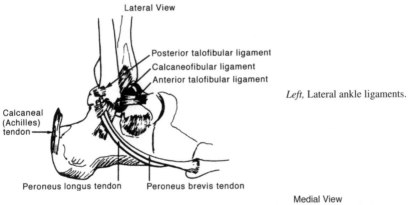

Lateral View

Posterior talofibular ligament
Calcaneofibular ligament
Anterior talofibular ligament

Left, Lateral ankle ligaments.

Calcaneal (Achilles) tendon

Peroneus longus tendon   Peroneus brevis tendon

Medial View

Posterior tibiotalar ligament – Deep deltoid

Superficial deltoid ligament
Tibiocalcaneal ligament
Tibionavicular ligament
Anterior tibiotalar ligament

Calcaneal (Achilles) tendon

Right, Medial ankle ligaments.

Tibialis anterior tendon   Tibialis posterior tendon

4. Which mechanism of injury most commonly produces ankle sprains?

Inversion injuries account for 70–85% of all ankle injuries. They occur when the foot is in a plantarflexed and supinated position. The mechanism of injury is often landing or stepping on another player's foot. Inversion injuries lead to sprains of the lateral ligamentous complex in the following order, from weakest to strongest: ATFL, CFL, and PTFL.

5. Describe the physical examination of ankle sprains.

The amount of ecchymosis and swelling may correlate with the severity of the sprain. Palpation for areas of maximal tenderness helps to define which ligaments are involved. In addition to palpating the individual ligaments, a complete evaluation should involve palpation of tendons, the fifth metatarsal base, the proximal fibula, and the medial and lateral malleoli to rule out other possible diagnoses.

6. What manual maneuvers aid in the diagnosis?

Mechanical stress testing evaluates the stability of the ankle. The **anterior drawer test** analyzes the integrity of the ATFL. It is performed by grasping the heel and pulling the foot anteriorly while applying a posterior force with the other hand to the tibia. Anterior excursion ≥ 5 mm more than the uninjured ankle and visible anterolateral dimpling (i.e., sulcus sign) are positive findings. The **talar tilt test** examines for CFL instability. It is performed by grasping the lateral aspect of the calcaneus in one hand, supporting the medial aspect of the tibia with the other hand, and attempting to invert the talus on the tibia. A positive test is defined by a marked difference in the degree to which the injured ankle opens compared with the other ankle, lateral dimpling, or lack of a firm endpoint.

7. How are ankle sprains classified?

Ankle sprains are typically classified as grade I, II, or III. **Grade I** sprains have stretching of the ligaments without macroscopic tear; physical exam elicits tenderness of the ligament but no swelling, instability, or loss of function. **Grade II** sprains involve a partial macroscopic tear, and exam shows moderate swelling and tenderness with decreased functional ability and mild laxity. **Grade III** sprains are severe injuries with complete rupture of the ligament; exam reveals diffuse swelling and ecchymosis, gross instability, and almost complete loss of function.

8. When are radiographs indicated in the initial evaluation?

Radiographs are needed when the patient is unable to bear weight or has point tenderness over a bony prominence, especially the posterior edge of either malleoli, the base of the fifth metatarsal, the tarsal navicular, or the proximal fibula. Repeat radiographic studies should be ordered in 7–10 days if improvement does not progress appropriately.

9. List the key radiographic findings to be ruled out.

Anteroposterior, lateral, and mortise views are required for accurate radiologic evaluation. Key findings are fractures, widening of the ankle mortise ≥ 2 mm (i.e., tibiofibular clear space), and osteochondral lesions of the medial or lateral corners of the talar dome.

10. Describe the timing, technique, and significance of stress radiographs.

Stress radiographs may be helpful in the acute evaluation of a suspected Grade III injury as well as in the work-up of chronic instability. The anterior drawer stress radiograph is a lateral view taken while the examiner performs an anterior drawer stress test. Anterior subluxation ≥ 5 mm is a positive test. The talar tilt stress radiograph is performed with the ankle in a neutral mortise-view position. If the ankle opens $> 25°$ or $> 10°$ compared with the opposite ankle, the test is considered positive and indicates mechanical instability.

11. Describe the initial treatment of ankle sprains.

Initially, treatment centers on the acronym **RICE: Rest** involves the use of crutches until the patient can ambulate without a limp. **Ice** is applied for 20 minutes 3–5 times daily until the effusion resolves. **Compression** with an Ace bandage and/or an ankle-stabilizing brace and **elevation** above the level of the heart also help to decrease swelling. Analgesic medicines such as acetaminophen or NSAIDs may aid in pain management.

12. What are the phases of functional rehabilitation?

Adequate rehabilitation is necessary to prevent chronic functional instability and recurring ankle sprains. **Phase I** consists of RICE (see above) and usually lasts 1–3 days until the patient is able to bear weight comfortably and swelling and tenderness have significantly decreased. **Phase II** focuses on restoring normal active range of motion and strengthening the dynamic stabilizers of the ankle. Achilles tendon stretching and strengthening of the ankle evertors and dorsiflexors help to attain these goals, usually requiring several days to weeks. **Phase III** is initiated when motion is near normal and pain and swelling are almost absent. Phase III emphasizes reestablishing motor coordination through proprioception exercises, functional conditioning, and endurance training. Functional activities progress from running on curves (i.e., figure of eight), to zig-zag running with cutting.

13. When can athletes safely return to participation?

Athletes can safely return to participation when they can perform sport-specific maneuvers, with or without a brace, without evidence of instability or significant pain. Functional support braces or taping is recommended for the remainder of the current season or 2–3 months. On average, return to play for grade I injuries is 0–5 days; for grade II injuries, 7–14 days; for grade III injuries, 21–35 days; and for syndesmotic injuries, 21–56 days.

14. Discuss injuries to the medial ligaments of the ankle.

The medial ligamentous complex is injured when an athlete suffers an eversion injury, usually associated with external rotation of the lower extremity while the foot is planted. Because the deltoid ligament is rarely injured in an isolated fashion, the clinician must have a high index of suspicion for an accompanying injury. When the deep deltoid is torn, the ankle mortise widens, and the joint becomes susceptible to rapid degenerative arthritis if anatomic reduction, usually by surgery, is not achieved. In addition to fractures of the medial malleolus and distal fibula, widening of the ankle mortise must be evaluated by radiographs. More than 2 mm between the talus and tibia represents an unstable ankle and requires surgical anatomic reduction.

15. What is a Maisonneuve fracture?

Medial malleolus fractures or medial ligamentous complex injuries extending through the interosseous membrane and associated with a fracture of the proximal fibula are called Maisonneuve fractures. The mechanism of injury is the same as for medial ligamentous sprains but with greater forces. The clinician must palpate along the fibula to avoid missing this potentially unstable ankle injury.

16. What ligamentous injury to the ankle has a prolonged morbidity?

Another ankle injury associated with external rotation is the **syndesmosis sprain** (i.e., high ankle sprain), which occurs in 1–11% of ankle sprains. The anterior tibiofibular ligament is injured; thus swelling and tenderness on palpation are located superomedially to the lateral malleolus. Provocative tests include the squeeze test, in which the tibia and fibula are squeezed together at the distal calf region, and the external rotation test in which the foot is externally rotated on the fixed tibia. Both tests are positive if pain is elicited at the syndesmosis. These injuries have a significantly prolonged recovery time and may lead to diastasis of the ankle joint. Treatment is similar to that for lateral ankle sprains, but the patient should be warned that return to play may require 6–8 weeks.

17. Which tendon injury is associated with an acutely fallen arch?

Rupture of the posterior tibial tendon may lead to an acutely fallen arch. Rupture occurs with dorsiflexion and pronation forces. Physical findings include weakness of eversion vs. resistance, failure of the calcaneus to turn inward with tip-toe raise, and tenderness over the arch. Treatment is surgical.

18. What lateral structure may subluxate over the lateral malleolus?

Rupture of the peroneal retinaculum may lead to subluxation of the peroneus tendon. The mechanism of injury involves inversion of an extremely plantarflexed foot with sudden contraction of the peroneal muscles. The patient may present with an acute injury that involved a sudden painful "pop" or a chronic history of something "popping in and out of place." Diagnosis is confirmed by demonstrating subluxation of the tendons over the lateral malleolus while the patient everts the foot against resistance. Initial treatment is conservative with padded reduction followed by ankle rehabilitation, but surgical referral is often necessary.

19. Describe the anterolateral impingement syndrome.

In the anterolateral impingement syndrome the soft tissue about the ankle impinges on the talus. The inferior aspect of the anterior tibiofibular ligament or anterior capsule thickening after recurrent ankle trauma is the usual culprit. Symptoms include chronic vague ankle soreness and stiffness that is worsened with dorsiflexion, such as walking up an incline. Bony impingements involving anterior talar or tibial spurs have similar presentations and may coincide with soft tissue impingement.

20. How is anterolateral impingement treated?

NSAIDs and aggressive rehabilitative exercises are the initial treatment for anterolateral impingement. If this approach fails to relieve the symptoms, arthroscopy is indicated.

21. Discuss functional vs. mechanical instability in relation to chronic ankle instability.

Chronic ankle symptoms occur after 10–30% of acute lateral ankle injuries, with chronic instability a frequent complaint. **Functional instability** is a patient's subjective complaint that the ankle recurrently gives way not only during athletic events but also with daily activities. An occult talar dome fracture or other osteochondral loose bodies may masquerade as functional instability. **Mechanical instability** is an objective finding of increased ankle motion with stress testing, usually documented with radiographs (see question 10). No correlation exists between functional and mechanical instability.

22. Describe the treatment of chronic ankle instability.

Vigorous attempts at rehabilitation are the initial treatment. Both functional and mechanical instability show documented improvement after muscle strengthening and proprioception exercises. Ankle stabilization with bracing or taping is helpful in preventing future recurrent injuries. Surgical repair is indicated when conservative management fails.

23. Discuss the lesion that may cause chronic ankle pain associated with a history of locking, buckling, or swelling.

Osteochrondral lesions in the ankle may arise secondary to trauma or as a growth abnormality. Chronic ankle pain associated with locking, buckling, or swelling is the usual presentation. Plain radiographs may reveal a fracture fragment or a pseudocystic lesion at either corner of the talar dome on mortise view. Magnetic resonance imaging (MRI) is indicated if an osteochondral lesion is suspected. Referral to an orthopedic surgeon is warranted for identified lesions.

CONTROVERSIES

24. Which is preferred—immobilization or functional management of acute ankle injury?

Early immobilization with casting used to be a frequent treatment of ankle sprains and is still advocated by some clinicians for more severe injuries. Presently, however, functional management with early mobilization and rehabilitation is recommended for initial treatment of sprains. Functional management has similar long-term disability as immobilization but reduces pain earlier and allows faster return to work or participation.

25. Which is preferred—conservative or surgical treatment of grade III ankle injuries?
Currently, grade III ankle sprains should be treated conservatively with early mobilization and functional rehabilitation. Delayed operative repair yields excellent results and should be used in athletes who fail conservative management.

26. Which is preferred for prevention of ankle injuries in athletes with no previous injury—taping or bracing?
Taping provides the best initial support of the ankle, but loosening of the tape with athletic performance has been documented. Lace-up braces appear to provide a more constant amount of protection during competition. Lace-up braces are also easily retightened during breaks in exercise, have a cost-saving benefit in the long term, and are more convenient for the "weekend warrior."

BIBLIOGRAPHY

1. Bergfeld J, Halpern B: Sports Medicine: Functional Management of Ankle Injuries. AAFP Video CME Program, Kansas City, 1991.
2. Eiff MP, Smith AT, Smith GE: Early mobilization versus immobilization in the treatment of lateral ankle sprains. Am J Sports Med 22:83–88, 1994.
3. Konradsen L, Holmer P, Sondergaard L: Early mobilizing treatment for grade III ankle ligament injuries. Foot Ankle 12:69–73, 1991.
4. Lassiter TE, Malone TR, Garrett WE: Injury to the lateral ligaments of the ankle. Orthop Clin North Am 20:629–640, 1989.
5. Patterson JO: Ankle injuries. In Lillegard WA, Rucker KS (eds): Handbook of Sports Medicine. Boston, Andover, 1993, pp 172–183.
6. Reid DC: Sports Injury Assessment and Rehabilitation. New York, Churchill Livingstone, 1992, p 340.
7. Ryan JB, et al: Office management of the acute ankle sprain. Clin Sports Med 8:477–492, 1989.
8. Shrier I: Treatment of lateral collateral ligament sprains of the ankle: A critical appraisal of the literature. Clin J Sport Med 5:187–195, 1995.
9. Stiell IG, et al: Implementation of the Ottawa Ankle Rules. JAMA 271:827, 1994.
10. Torres JL: Ankle problems. In Mellion MB (ed): Sports Medicine Secrets. Philadelphia, Hanley & Belfus, 1992, p 307–309.
11. Trevino SG, Davis P, Hecht PJ: Management of acute and chronic lateral ligament injuries of the ankle. Orthop Clin North Am 25:1-15, 1994.

73. FOOT PROBLEMS IN ATHLETES

Timothy C. Fitzgibbons, M.D.

1. Is it true that many foot and ankle problems are treated surgically more often now than in the past?
Although the lay press and medical articles have emphasized surgical treatment, most foot and ankle problems and injuries can and should be treated nonsurgically. When one encounters career-ending complications of surgery, one appreciates why surgical procedures should not be undertaken lightly.

2. When the athlete asks, "What shoe should I buy?", how should you answer?
There is no perfect shoe. The most important factor is proper fit. Athletes must avoid shoes that are too tight for obvious reasons, whereas shoes that are too loose may cause shear-related friction injuries. Shoe requirements vary from sport to sport, depending on the type of forces exerted on the foot. Most specialty athletic shoe stores have specific shoes for specific sports.

3. How do we prescribe orthotics? When do we use them?
There probably has been too much emphasis on the use of orthotics in athletes. Soft plastazote inlays that serve as shock absorbers and as devices to take pressure off the ball of the foot

are usually most helpful. These devices are *not* used for corrective purposes. A possible exception is the semirigid orthotic for plantar fasciitis developed by the University of California at Berkeley's biomechanics laboratory.

FOREFOOT PROBLEMS (TARSOMETATARSAL JOINT TO TOES)

5. What causes ingrown toenails in athletes?

Most ingrown toenails in athletes are related to dynamic forces. A chronic force across the soft tissues on either side of the toenail promotes the formation of an ingrown toenail. On the fibular side of the great toenail, most ingrown toenails result from pressure of the great toe against the second toe. On the tibial side of the great toenail, ingrown toenails result from pronation of the great toe during pushoff.

6. What is nonsurgical treatment of ingrown toenails?

Nonsurgical Treatment of Ingrown Toenails

Tibial side	1. Soaking foot in warm water twice daily
	2. Soft tissue teasing technique
	3. Wide toe-box shoes
Fibular side	1. Soaking foot in warm water twice daily
	2. Soft tissue teasing technique
	3. Use of spacer between the first and second toe
	4. Wide toe-box shoes

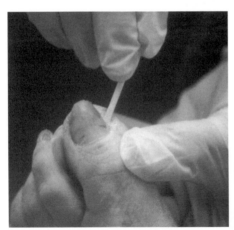

Left, Soak the foot for 20 minutes in plain warm water. The tissues will be soft and pliable to work with. Then "tease" the tissue back away from the nail with a manicure stick. (From Fitzgibbons TC, Keown BG, Sampson C, Burton D: Foot problems in Athletes. In Mellion MB (ed): Office Sports Medicine, 2nd ed. Philadelphia, Hanley & Belfus, 1996, p. 322, with permission.)

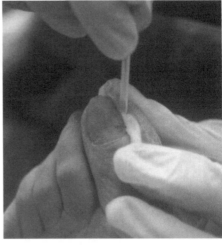

Right, Take a strand of a cottonball and wet it with plain warm water. Roll it slightly until cylindrical. Tuck cotton strand along the border of the nail. Blot out excess moisture and trim the ends if necessary. Do this twice daily until the inflammation settles down. (From Fitzgibbons TC, Keown BG, Sampson C, Burton D: Foot problems in Athletes. In Mellion MB (ed): Office Sports Medicine, 2nd ed. Philadelphia, Hanley & Belfus, 1996, p. 322, with permission.)

7. What are corns?
Corns are nature's response to pressure of the skin against a bony prominence. On the top of th toe, the so-called **hard corn** develops because of pressure of the toe against the top of shoe. Between the toes, the so-called **soft corn** develops because of pressure of the bony prominence of one toe against the bony prominence of an adjacent toe.

8. What is the treatment of corns?
Treatment is plain and simple—relieve the pressure on the corn. On the top of the toe this can be done with various types of corn pads and modification of shoes directly over the corn. Between the toes the soft corn can be treated with the use of lamb's wool and wider toe-box shoes. Surgery involving resection of the bone underlying the prominence is reserved for refractory cases and should rarely be done in the athlete.

9. What are callouses?
Callouses are a thickening of the skin on the plantar aspect of the foot secondary to excessive pressure against one or more metatarsal heads.

10. What is the treatment of callouses?
If one relieves the pressure on the plantar aspect of the foot, the callouses soften and diminish in size. Although periodic shaving of the callous is helpful and may be necessary, a plastazote or soft inlay in the shoe or an external metatarsal bar may alleviate the symptoms.

11. What is "turf toe"?
The turf toe is a sprain of the first metatarsal phalangeal joint and has received great notoriety in the sports medical and lay press.

12. What is the cause of turf toe?
The primary cause of turf toe is a hyperextension injury of the great toe metatarsophalangeal joint. Hyperflexion and valgus injuries to the great toe also may cause similar symptoms. The use of synthetic turfs has been highly incriminated as a cause of turf toe.

13. What is the treatment of turf toe?
Initial treatment consists of the usual forms of rest, ice, compression, and elevation, followed by shoe modifications to prevent recurrence. Taping of the toe to restrict dorsiflexion and stiffening of the sole of the shoe to prevent motion are commonly used.

14. What is a bunion?
A bunion is a painful bursa or bump caused by pressure of the shoes against the prominence of the medial first metatarsal head. The bunion usually occurs because of a congenital widening of the first and second intermetatarsal space with a secondary angulation of the toe.

15. What is the treatment of a bunion?
Initial treatment of a bunion involves the use of wide toe-box shoes, a spacer between the first and second toes, and appropriate antiinflammatory measures when indicated.

16. A 17-year-old senior track star asks whether he should have surgery for his severe bunion problem. What should you tell him?
Although surgery for bunions is justified in some adolescents, in high-intensity or elite athletes caution should be used. All bunion surgery involves exposing the great toe metatarsophalangeal (MTP) joint and subsequently guarantees some degree of permanent stiffness in the MTP joint after surgery. Therefore, it is highly likely that a running athlete will not be able to perform as well after a satisfactory bunion procedure.

17. A 35-year-old golfer states that he can no longer walk 18 holes without significant discomfort and stiffness in the great toe MTP joint. He has also developed a red bump on the top of his toe at the MTP joint. What is the problem?

The problem sounds like a classical dorsal bunion or hallux rigidis.

18. What is hallux rigidis?

Hallux rigidis is a premature degenerative arthritic condition that occurs most commonly in young males at the great toe MTP joint. A large spur develops on the dorsum of the distal metatarsal at the MTP joint, and when the shoe rubs against the spur, a prominence or bump develops on the top of the foot at the joint. Of more significance, however, is that the patient loses the ability to completely dorsiflex the great toe at the MTP joint.

19. What is the treatment of hallux rigidis?

Initial treatment involves stiffening the sole of the shoe at the MTP joint to prevent dorsiflexion of the great toe. This can be done with insertion of a steel plate in the sole of the shoe by a pedorthotist or by recommending a shoe with a stiffer Vibram sole, which is a commercially available lightweight, stiff shoe. Patients also may be helped with antiinflammatory medication, local corticosteroid injections, and physical therapy.

20. Is there a place for surgery in hallux rigidis?

Yes. The initial surgical treatment in most cases is aggressive resection of the distal portion of the metatarsal with the spur—the so-called cheilectomy. Ultimate surgical treatment is fusion of the great toe MTP joint. At present the orthopedic literature does *not* support the use of silastic implants—the so-called artificial joint.

21. What is plantar neuroma?

Plantar neuroma is a fibrosis or scarring around the distal branches of the posterior tibial nerve, right at the point where they bifurcate to send sensory branches to each toe. Plantar neuroma occurs between the metatarsal heads and the plantar aspect of the foot.

22. What are the symptoms of plantar neuroma?

The symptoms of plantar neuroma are usually numbness in the adjacent two toes. Many patients also feel a lump in the plantar aspect of their feet between the respective metatarsal heads.

23. What is the treatment of plantar neuroma?

Initial treatment is nonsurgical with the use of wide toe-box shoes and an external metatarsal bar or soft plastazote inlay. If the symptoms persist, an injection in the web space of the two involved toes for diagnostic and therapeutic purposes may be helpful. Surgery involves excision of the neuroma through a dorsal incision, but only after conservative measures have failed. One should be cautioned, however, that some apparent neuroma symptoms can be caused by more proximal problems such as radiculopathy.

MIDFOOT (TALONAVICULAR JOINT TO TARSOMETATARSAL JOINT)

24. What about athletes with pain in the middle portion of the foot?

Most problems in the midfoot tend to be soft tissue ligamentous type injuries, the so-called **midfoot sprain**. One also should be aware of the possibility of a stress fracture of the navicular bone, and in older athletes one should look for degenerative arthritis.

25. What is the treatment of midfoot sprains?

Most midfoot sprains can be treated initially with antiinflammatory medications and physical therapy. If symptoms persist, referral for more extensive testing and treatment may be necessary.

HINDFOOT (ANKLE JOINT TO TALONAVICULAR
AND CALCANEAL CUBOID JOINT)

26. What is the difference between plantar fasciitis and heel spur?

Plantar fasciitis is the inflammation of the plantar fascia either at its attachment to the calcaneus or, at times, more distal along the plantar fascia itself. It is an extremely common problem in both athletes and nonathletes. Its cause is unclear, but in athletes, it is most likely related to either one event or chronic stresses of the plantar fascia at the attachment to the calcaneus. The heel spur is the calcification that may occur at the attachment of the plantar fascia to the calcaneus—the so-called traction spur.

27. Is it true that pain is caused by stepping on the heel spur?

Except in the rare case in which a stress fracture occurs in the spur itself, most orthopedists agree that stepping on the spur is not the cause of pain. Rather, the pain occurs because of a pull on the inflamed plantar fascia.

28. What is the treatment of plantar fasciitis?

Plantar fasciitis is a common problem that takes a long time to resolve. A recent long-term study found that all patients eventually improved without surgery but that some patients took as long as 4 years to respond. Patients must be informed of this time frame. Treatment consists of antiinflammatory medication, local physical therapy measures, plantar fascial and Achilles tendon stretching, and heel lifts and protective pads to elevate the heel and relieve the tension on the plantar fascia and Achilles tendon. Local injections also may be of help.

29. Is there a place for surgery in plantar fasciitis?

As a last resort, release of the plantar fascia attachment to the calcaneus may be performed. Whether fascial release should be complete or partial remains controversial. Complete release tends to destabilize the lateral portion of the foot. Decompression of the first branch of the lateral plantar nerve as it dives into the deep fascia of the foot also should be considered. In some patients, compression of this nerve may cause some of the heel pain.

30. What is tarsal tunnel syndrome?

The tarsal tunnel is an area on the medial side of the hindfoot where the posterior tibial nerve passes from behind the medial malleolus to the point where it dives into the plantar aspect of the foot. In this area the retinaculum overlying the nerve as well as the abductor hallucis and flexor hallucis muscles may be tight enough to cause pressure on the posterior tibial nerve and its branches. Symptoms may be similar to those of plantar fasciitis, although patients tend to complain of significant burning pain and sometimes numbness in the plantar aspect of the foot.

31. What is the treatment of tarsal tunnel syndrome?

Treatment of tarsal tunnel syndrome is similar to treatment of plantar fasciitis. Recent studies have shown that the results of surgical decompression are equivocal; thus surgery is seldom indicated.

32. What about tendinitis in the foot?

The peroneal tendons on the lateral aspect of the foot and ankle and the posterior and flexor hallucis longus tendons on the medial side of the foot and ankle may become inflamed. Occasional inflammation also may occur in the anterior tibial tendon and extensor hallucis longus tendon. Initial treatment of tendinitis about the foot or ankle is basically the same—rest, antiinflammatory medication, and local physical therapy. If symptoms persist, some use of medial or lateral heel wedges in the hindfoot and stiffening of the sole in the mid and forefoot may be of benefit.

FRACTURES

33. What about toe fractures?
Displaced fractures of the great toe MTP joint are the one type of toe fracture that occasionally are treated with open reduction and internal fixation. Most other fractures involving the toes are treated nonsurgically with buddy taping of one toe to the other and forms of symptomatic treatment. A stiff sole or wooden-soled shoe may be used initially if necessary, but the decision about return to play usually depends on the symptoms and varies from 3–6 weeks.

BIBLIOGRAPHY

1. Arendt E, Teitz C: The lower extremities. In Teitz CC (ed): The Female Athlete. Rosemont, IL, American Academy of Orthopaedic Surgeons, 1997, pp 45–73.
2. Coker TP: Sports injuries to the foot and ankle. In Jahss MH (ed): Disorders of the Foot and Ankle, 2nd ed. Philadelphia, W.B. Saunders, 1991, pp 2415–2445.
3. Fitzgibbons T, Keown B, Sampson C, Burston D: Foot problems in athletes. In Mellion M (ed): Office Sports Medicine, 2nd ed. Philadelphia, Hanley & Belfus, 1996, pp 318–336.
4. Mann RA, Coughlin MJ (eds): Surgery of the Foot and Ankle, 6th ed. St. Louis, Mosby, 1992, pp 1095–1310.

74. STRESS FRACTURES

Donald Shell, M.D.

1. What is a stress fracture?
When forces applied to bone, including compressive, tensile, or rotational, exceed bone strength, the bone is irreversibly deformed until a microfracture or break occurs. These forces may be applied to the bone from repetitive smaller loads or from one very large load. Repetitive loading of the bone results in an overuse injury of the bone causing microfractures, which are propagated through the bone until a symptomatic stress fracture occurs.

2. What is the mechanism of damage in stress fractures?
With the repetitive loading of bone, the tensile and compressive forces result in fractures at the cement lines along the osteon or shear microfractures of bone, respectively. Bone will remodel in response to the stresses placed on it in predictable patterns. An increase in the stresses placed on bone will result in increased bone remodeling. Eventually, the concurrent osteoclastic resorption of bone will exceed osteoblastic new bone formation. When the osteoclastic resorption of bone outpaces bone formation, the weakened bone is much more susceptible to fracture if the causative forces are continued. These stress fractures, or microfractures, or fatigue fractures of bone resulting from small repetitive loading are influenced by the number of repetitions, frequency of repetitions, and the amount of load that is applied to the bone. If the weakened bone is allowed to rest, bone remodeling will occur with resultant healing.

3. Which radiographic imaging techniques can be used in the diagnosis of a stress fracture?
Plain radiographs are very specific for stress fractures, but they are not very sensitive. Two-thirds of plain radiographs are initially negative, and only one-half of these ever develop radiographic evidence of a stress fracture. The onset of pain can typically precede a positive radiographic finding in a stress fracture by 2–3 months. This varies depending on the bone that is injured; for example, there is typically a long delay of radiographic findings in stress fractures of

the tibia and femur, whereas negative radiographic findings are notorious throughout the course of a tarsal bone stress fracture. The characteristic radiographic findings include periosteal new bone formation and end osteal thickening or radiolucent line formation. Oblique views of the bone and carefully centered radiographs may elucidate subtle findings. The use of technetium bone scanning will generally show evidence of a stress fracture 2–8 days after the symptoms begin. The bone scan may be helpful in clinically differentiating stress fracture from other soft tissue abnormalities that may be included in the differential diagnosis for stress fractures. Shin splints, for example, may reveal a long linear tibial foci on the bone scan, and in the delayed-image phase of a triple-phase bone scan but negative for both the angiogram and blood pool portions of the studies. In the stress fracture, all three phases of the triple-phase bone scan will be positive, including the angiogram, blood pool, and delayed-image phase.

4. What are the essential components of the history of an athlete who presents with a stress fracture?

The athlete must be questioned in regard to a change in his or her training regimen, including an increase in distance or duration of training, training on a harder playing surface or track, and the acquisition of new footwear, all of which are important. In addition, female athletes must be questioned about menstrual status, history of smoking, and nutritional irregularities.

5. How do menstrual irregularities lead to the development of stress fractures in female athletes?

Oligomenorrheic or amenorrheic female athletes have a reduced ability to maintain bone density due to insufficient estrogen levels. This insufficient estrogen also upsets the normal hormonal balance between osteoclast and osteoblast via a lack of inhibition of interleukin-6, which stimulates osteoclast production.[7]

6. Explain the relation of the development of stress fractures to the late onset of menarche, history of smoking, and nutritional abnormalities in the female athlete.

Female athletes with late onset of menses or delayed menarche enter adulthood with a lower bone mineral density. This reduction of peak bone mass will lower the threshold for the development of stress fractures in the future. Cigarette smoking lowers serum estrogen levels in a dose-related fashion and therefore reduces bone mineral density in the same way. Research has shown that athletes with insufficient caloric intake may have a deficient calcium intake in addition. The inadequate calcium intake correlates very closely with a decreased bone mineral density. It has also been shown that athletes that weigh less than 75% of their ideal body weight have a much higher incidence of stress fractures than those athletes who maintain an ideal body weight and engage in the same athletic activity.

7. What biomechanical factors unique to female athletes place them at an increased risk of the development of stress fractures?

The wider gait as a result of the female pelvis and genu valgum, commonly seen in female athletes, increases the tendency toward foot pronation with resulting increased stresses placed on the tibia and fibula. This increased pronation decreases the ability of the structures to absorb impact loads and leads to the development of stress fractures. It has also been postulated that an undue amount of muscle fatigue will occur in the presence of these load stresses and therefore a greater force is transmitted to the bone rather than being absorbed by the muscle.

8. In what anatomic sites of the body do stress fractures occur and what are each site's unique characteristics and sport of occurrence?

The following table gives the anatomic sites in which stress fractures occur, their unique characteristics, and predisposing factors.

Sites of Stress Fractures and Unique Characteristics

SITE OF FRACTURE	PREDISPOSING FACTORS	PHYSICAL EXAM*	RADIOGRAPHIC CONSIDERATIONS	COMPLICATIONS	TREATMENT†	RETURN TO ACTIVITY‡
Coracoid process	Trapshooter	Pain with attempted active adduction and forward flexion against resistance	Plain radiograph with axillary view			
Clavicle-proximal humeral growth plate	Adolescent thrower					
Humerus	Throwing athlete, racquet sports, pole vaulter	Deep aching mid arm pain with pitching or at rest		Nonunion overt fracture	Relative rest, appropriate conditioning	Asymptomatic
Olecranon	Throwing athlete, diver			Nonunion	Immobilize early, no triceps use	
Ulnar	Racquet sports, volleyball, throwing, drummer, offensive lineman	Palpable callus			Avoid sport until healed	4–6 weeks
Radius	Gymnastics—dowel grip, drummer, offensive lineman	Pain on wrist weight-bearing and active dorsiflexion	Growth plate widening, beaked distal epiphysis, cystic change in the epiphyseal plate	Fracture of physis "epiphysiolysis"	Immobilization	Rest 6 weeks with gradual return to competition
Femoral neck transverse (superior cortex)	Older athlete, military recruits	Groin pain, painful hip ROM and walking, antalgic gait	Mandatory bone scan early; if radiograph negative, tomograms	Displacement with avascular necrosis, nonunion and malunion	Surgical correction whether displaced or not, internal fixation	
compression (inferior cortex)	Young individuals, athletes		Haze of internal callus at inferior cortex, bone scan, tomogram		Nonoperative, non–weight-bearing mandatory	Free hip motion
Femoral shaft subtrochanteric midshaft distal	Military recruit	Paucity of physical findings, mild deep thigh soreness, full hip ROM, antalgic gait ±	Oblique, spiral, or transverse fracture	Possible displacement of the distal injury	Nonoperative	

(Table continued on following page.)

Sites of Stress Fractures and Unique Characteristics (Continued)

SITE OF FRACTURE	PREDISPOSING FACTORS	PHYSICAL EXAM*	RADIOGRAPHIC CONSIDERATIONS	COMPLICATIONS	TREATMENT†	RETURN TO ACTIVITY‡
Patella	Athletes		Vertical or transverse fracture	Displacement of transverse fracture	Surgical treatment if if displaced	
Tibia plateau		Anteromedial tibial pain just below joint line, discomfort with weight-bearing	Early osteoporosis followed by endosteal callus or sclerosis		Conservative crutches	4 weeks
Tibia shaft	One-half of all stress fractures seen in athletes, Military—proximal; basketball, ballet, running—middle one-third; runner—junction of middle and distal one-third	Percussion tenderness away from fracture site	Oblique radiographs	"Dreaded black line"—midshaft anterior fracture with delayed nonunion	Relative rest, middle one-third: prolonged rest, TENS, excision bone grafts	4-6 weeks for medial lesions; several months for anterior lesions
Fibula lower one-third proximal one-third	Athletes Jumping exercises	Antalgic gait, localized tenderness	Bone scan early		Relative rest, ankle-foot orthosis	6 weeks
Medial malleolus	Basketball, long-distance running, football	Ankle swelling	Radiograph, bone scan	None	Bone scan positive but radiograph negative—immobilize with brace; unlimited ambulation with brace. Positive radiograph requires open reduction/internal fixation	Gradual return within 6 weeks
Os calcis	Military recruits, athletes rarely	Heel pain	Radiograph positive 1-2 weeks following injury	None	Relative rest	3 weeks
Tarsal navicular—uncommon	Basketball, athletes, cavus foot, flexible pes planus, or normal longitudinal arch, metatarsal adductus, limited ankle dorsiflexion, limited subtalar motion	Mild symptoms, vague dorsal pain in midfoot	Negative radiograph with positive bone scan requires tomograms to delineate fracture pattern	Delayed nonunion with delayed initial treatment can progress to displacement and ununited fracture	Displaced or nonunion fracture treated with internal fixation or bone grafting. Immobilization/non–weight-bearing cast 6 weeks	

Metatarsal 2nd and 3rd most common diaphyseal, neck or base	Military recruits, athletes, ballet	Pain in full "en pointe" ballet position	Bone scan or tomograms required	None	Diaphyseal or neck fracture	4–6 weeks
Jones fracture (5th metatarsal distal to the tuberosity)	Basketball, football		*Acute*—fracture line with sharp margin *nonunion*—obliteration of canal with sclerotic bone; *delayed union*—no intramedullary sclerosis	Failure of conservative treatment	*Acute*—cast, immobilization, non-weight-bearing; *nonunion*—surgical; *delayed union*—surgical	6–30 weeks
Great toe	Sprinter, fencer, rugby player, hallux valgus deformity	Metatarsophalangeal medial pain			Conservative or surgical correction of hallux valgus, rigid shoe orthotic	
Great toe sesamoids	Weightlifters, lumbermen, football linemen, tennis serve	Persistent local pain	Plain radiograph, bone scan to differentiate fracture from bipartate sesamoid		Walking cart, relative rest, metatarsal bar, rarely excision	
Pelvis—inferior pubic ramis	Military, runners	Groin pain in association with running. Possible buttocks or thigh pain. Exquisite pain with pubic ramis palpation	Plain radiograph, scintigraphy	Delayed nonunion	Discontinuation of running ± crutch ambulation	
Lumbar spine—pars interarticularis (spondylolysis)	Gymnast, dancer, repetitive cyclic flexion-hyper-extension, lateral flexion on extended spine.	Low back, posterior buttocks or thigh pain usually coincides with growth spurt. Gait abnormality secondary to hamstring tightness	Oblique views needed—"scotty dog," bone scan, CT rarely indicated	Adult—nerve root compression. Monitor for spondylolisthesis development	Conservative in long-standing injury. Cast or brace (TLSO), restriction of vigorous activity, back and abdominal strengthening, hamstring flexibility	Based on clinical response, may return to many activities in brace after asymptomatic several weeks

TENS, transcutaneous electrical nerve stimulation; TLSO, thoracic lumbosacral orthosis.
* All usually have tenderness at site; † Nonsteroidal antiinflammatory drugs may be useful; ‡ When symptom-free.

9. How does the shape of the foot play a role in the development of lower-extremity stress fractures?

The high-arched cavus foot is rigid and absorbs shock poorly. Individuals with cavus feet will therefore have a greater chance of sustaining impact-related lower-extremity trauma such as stress fractures.

10. Do stress fractures occur in children?

Stress fractures have been recognized in children but are much less common than nondisplaced fractures. Stress fractures in children have been seen in all age groups but primarily occur between the ages of 10 and 15 years. Sites of occurrence in children have included the proximal tibia metaphyses, fibula, patella, and iliac crest apophysis.

The diagnosis of a stress fracture in a child may be more difficult secondary to a poor history. Initial plain radiographs are usually taken later in the stage of the disease than in the adult population, and bone scans may be positive in the stress fracture but may also be positive in other diseases, such as infection, osteoid, osteoma, or malignancy, which must be differentiated in a child with bone pain. Diagnosis of a stress fracture in a child may require the use of tomograms and serial radiographs over a 6-week period to distinguish the stress fracture from malignant conditions.

11. Name the other abnormalities that should be included in the differential diagnosis of tibial shaft stress fractures.

Medial tibial stress syndrome (MTSS), shin splints, exertional compartment syndrome, and popliteal artery entrapment syndrome. Stress fractures are typified by sensation of pain with cessation of impact-loading activity, gradually occurring earlier in activity and eventually prohibiting participation, and distal percussion tenderness. The pain in exertional compartment syndrome is not restricted to impact-loading activity and may have associated parathesias or anesthesia. MTSS, as the name implies, results from stressful forces applied to the tibia not sufficient to cause a fracture but stimulate remodeling. Shin splints result from repetitive running on hard surfaces or forcible, excessive use of the foot dorsi flexors. Shin splints refer to musculocutaneous inflammations of the leg and exclude any fractures or ischemic disorders.

12. What form of treatment is recommended for a femoral neck stress fracture?

Internal fixation of a femoral neck stress fracture on the tension side (superior cortex) is recommended because of the high risk of displacement of an initially nondisplaced complete fracture. Some athletes will prefer to allow this fracture to heal on its own without surgery but are at increased risk of this complication.

13. Stress fractures of the distal radius in skeletally immature gymnasts have been associated with what complication?

Premature physeal closure of the distal radius among young gymnasts with stress fractures of the growth plate has been reported.

14. What is the basis of treatment of most stress fractures?

The athlete's activity must be reduced below the threshold for symptoms. This may be accomplished via cessation or reduction of the inciting sport, immobilization, non–weight-bearing of the lower extremity, or the use of orthotics. Alternative training activities may be used to maintain cardiovascular fitness, muscle tone, stamina, and prevent depression. Activities using the lower extremities will maintain conditioning more easily, and these include cross-country skiing machines, rowing machines, stationary bicycles, pool running, or swimming. Ice massage, nonsteroidal anti-inflammatory medication, stretching, and strengthening exercises are also recommended.

15. How may stress fractures be prevented?

Decreased estrogen levels in female athletes may be prevented by the use of oral contraceptive pills or decreasing the activity intensity or frequency of workouts to allow a return of menses.

A gradual increase in training load for individuals who are not physically fit also is recommended. Calcium supplementation in excess of the recommended daily allowance of 800 mg/day has also been shown to be of some value in increasing the mineral density in weight-bearing bones. Athletes must be counseled against overzealous dieting, and if an eating disorder is suspected, the athlete should be referred to a psychologist or psychiatrist for proper testing and treatment.

16. Is there any role for the use of computed tomographic (CT) scanning in the diagnosis of stress fractures?

CT may reveal the anatomic detail and bone alignment of a stress fracture. It will reveal the fracture position and any associated bony defect and therefore is useful in the diagnosis of stress fractures. The CT scan must be obtained in two planes but cannot be relied on to tell when a fracture is healed. CT scans may be used when bone scanning does not reveal conclusive results.

BIBLIOGRAPHY

1. Cahill BR: Stress fractures of the proximal tibial epiphysis: A case report. Am J Sports Med 5:186–187, 1977.
2. Cantu RC, Micheli LJ (eds): ACSM Guidelines for the Team Physician. Philadelphia, Lea & Febiger, 1991, p 248.
3. Carek PF, Fumich RM: Stress fracture of the distal radius not just a risk for elite gymnasts. Phys Sportsmed 20(5):115–118, 1992.
4. Carter SR, Aldridge MJ, Fitzgerald R, et al: Stress changes of the wrist in adolescent gymnasts. Br J Radiol 61:109–112, 1988.
5. Fick DS, Albright JP, Murray BP: Relieving painful shin splints. Phys Sportsmed 20(12):105–113, 1992.
6. Friedman MJ, Nicholas JA, Hershman EB (eds): Injuries to the Leg in Athletes. The Lower Extremity and Spine in Sports Medicine. St. Louis, C.V. Mosby, 1986.
7. Hackeling TA, Richmond JC: Women and stress fractures. Female Patient 18:63–80, 1993.
8. Hershman EG, Mailly T: Stress fractures. Clin Sports Med 9:183–214, 1990.
9. Li G, Zhang S, Chen G, et al: Radiographic and histologic analysis of stress fractures in rabbit tibias. Am J Sports Med 13:285–294, 1985.
10. Rupani MD, Molder LE, Espinola DA: Three phases of radionuclide bone imaging in sports medicine. Radiology 156:187–196, 1985.

X. Management Approaches and Techniques

75. INITIAL INJURY MANAGEMENT: P-R-I-C-E-S

Mark E. Shirley, D.O.

1. What does PRICES stand for?

P Protection—helps prevent further injury; examples include crutches, slings, and splints

R Rest—varies from complete rest (i.e., "absolute rest") to partial participation (i.e., "relative rest") depending on the severity of the injury

I Ice—cold therapy decreases pain, swelling, and inflammation

C Compression—gentle, even pressure used in conjunction with ice helps to limit swelling

E Elevation—placing the injured part above the level of the heart enhances venous return and extravascular fluid is drained away from the injured area

S Support—a functional type of protection, such as taping an ankle for a minor ankle sprain, used when an athlete has a minor injury without any significant symptoms and is going to return to play right away

2. When and who should implement the PRICES methods?

The PRICES methods should be implemented in the initial treatment of an acute musculoskeletal injury. These techniques are taught to the athlete, coach, athletic trainer, team physician, and any other individuals who may be involved in the initial first aid care of the injured athlete.

3. Under what circumstances should crutches be used?

In lower-extremity injury, crutches should be used if ambulation causes any pain, swelling, limping, or buckling of the extremity and should be continued until these symptoms are no longer present and more serious injury is ruled out. If a fracture is suspected or the athlete is in significant pain, an immobilizer or splint should be considered. Protective positioning instructions help the athlete avoid those positions that could cause additional stress to the injury.

4. How much rest is considered adequate?

This depends on the severity of the injury. In a more severe injury, the need for more rest is obvious; however, absolute rest in a minor injury is probably too strict.

5. When should relative rest be employed?

It should be used when an injury is not serious in nature. Since the goal of relative rest is to provide enough protection to keep the injury asymptomatic, the athlete is afforded the opportunity to minimize deconditioning through partial participation. For example, a mild lower extremity injury may not require crutches but may require refraining from running or cutting even if the athlete can walk without symptoms.

6. Should ice be used for the first 24 hours only and then heat thereafter?

No. Although many variations of the use of ice first then heat exist in medical textbooks, the thought that athletic injuries respond better to ice for the first day, then heat after is simply not true.

7. What are the physiological benefits to using ice?

Ice tends to reduce tissue swelling and bleeding, reduce inflammation, reduce the metabolic needs of injured tissue, and decreases firing of pain nerve receptors, helping to reduce muscle spasm.

8. What about heat?

Heat has little, if any, role in most acute injuries. Heat may increase tissue swelling and inflammation long after the initial injury or overuse process has occurred. There is a benefit of heat in relieving muscle spasm; however, in sprains, strains, and tendinitis, it is of minimal, if any, benefit. Any increase in swelling or other signs of inflammation as a result of applying heat indicate a need to stop the heating and apply cold immediately.

9. What about alternating heat and ice?

Contrast treatment is sometimes effective. The injured part is warmed for 1–4 minutes and then cooled for 1–2 minutes. The ratio of heat time to cool time is adjusted according to the likelihood of creating tissue swelling. Shorter heat times and longer cool times are used in an acute setting.

10. What are the different methods of applying ice?

The athlete should wrap the ice on with an Ace bandage, or hold it in place with bicycle shorts or compression shorts. Many methods of cooling tissue have been used. Ice cubes, crushed ice packs, and refreezable gel packs provide a better deep cooling effect than chemical cold packs and circulating freon gas. Ice massage with a block of ice directly on the skin provides local analgesia over a small area. Immersion of the injured part in ice water is effective, but hard to tolerate and elevation cannot be done at the same time.

11. What is the correct technique for using ice massage?

Freeze some water in a styrofoam cup. Tear the cup one-half way down and invert the ice over the injured area, using the remaining styrofoam portion to hold onto the ice. Leave the ice in a single position for 60–90 seconds or until an area of numbness directly underneath the ice to one-half an inch out from the ice exists. Gently massage the ice over the area, gradually expanding in a circular fashion underneath the cup but always staying within the numb area. Generally, an ice massage should last seven minutes for medium-sized injuries and ten minutes for large-sized injuries.

12. How many minutes should ice be applied?

A general rule is to apply ice 20 minutes out of an hour with a maximum of 30 minutes, followed by at least 30 minutes without cold packs; however, if a patient has a lower cold tolerance, then the treatment duration should be adjusted accordingly.

13. What are the benefits of compression with ice?

Used in conjunction with ice, compression provides a physical limitation to the space that swelling may occupy. It also helps disperse local edema, making it more readily available for reabsorption by the circulatory system.

14. How should compression bandages be applied?

The bandages should be wrapped distally to proximally, overlapping approximately one-half the width of the bandage.

15. How much pressure should a compression bandage apply?

An elastic bandage should apply enough consistent, even pressure to help reduce swelling in the area. The bandage should not be wrapped so tightly that constriction and reduction of venous return occur. Generally, one-fourth to one-third of the potential stretch of a new elastic bandage is adequate.

16. What about injuries that prevent application of consistent, even pressure?

Ankle injuries, for example, often prevent even pressure due to bony prominences. In these instances, a foam rubber or felt "horseshoe" or "donut"-shaped cut-out may be used to keep even compression over irregular areas. Though somewhat more expensive, pneumatic and hydraulic compression devices are also effective.

17. What should be used for support in an athlete who wants to return to play?

Lace-up ankle supports, stirrup splints such as an air cast or a gel cast, double upright knee braces, ankle taping, and slip-on neoprene braces have been used with much success.

18. Should an elastic bandage be used for support in an acute injury?

No. Particularly in lower extremity injuries, elastic bandages provide little support for a joint. The lever arm effect of upper body weight acting across the joint overrides the support an elastic bandage may provide. In addition, elastic bandages applied too tightly produce a tourniquet effect, resulting in further injury to the area.

BIBLIOGRAPHY

1. Shelton GL: Principles of musculoskeletal rehabilitation. In Mellion MB (ed): Office Management of Sports Injuries and Athletic Problems. Philadelphia, Hanley & Belfus, 1988, pp 161–162.
2. Shelton GL, Mellion MB: Preventing and rehabilitating sports injuries through patient education. In Patient Education Proceedings, vol 9. Kansas City, MO, American Academy of Family Physicians, 1987, pp 117–119.

76. REHABILITATION PRINCIPLES

Guy L. Shelton, M.A., P.T., A.T.C.

When carried out with good awareness of all factors involved, the process of rehabilitation will successfully return the athlete to participation in a majority of cases. In general, a functionally guided program with respect for the injury and the symptoms that the injury produces is the best formula to follow. Individual differences of each athlete and each injury also must be considered.

1. What is rehabilitation?

Rehabilitation is the process of restoring range of motion, flexibility, strength, endurance, agility, and sports skills following an injury or illness. The overall goal is to enable the injured athlete to resume participation at a level of skill and ability similar to that level of performance present prior to the injury in as short a period of time as is safe with respect to the injury.

2. Why is rehabilitation important?

The rehabilitation process is important for three reasons.

1. Without rehabilitation following the deconditioning process of an injury, it is extremely difficult for the athlete to return to previous levels of performance within a reasonable time. The importance of rehabilitation in this sense depends on the severity of the injury, other treatment methods, and the preexisting level of fitness of the athlete.

2. If an athlete attempts to resume a full level of participation with inadequate rehabilitation, the athlete is at greater risk for reinjury or injury to another area because of the relative conditioning deficit.

3. If an athlete allows the level of deconditioning following an injury to persist over a long period, the athlete is at greater risk for developing chronic, longer-term problems with regard to that injury.

3. Name the five components of a rehabilitation program.

1. Flexibility	3. Endurance	5. Agility and skills
2. Strength	4. Proprioception	

4. Describe the five components of a rehabilitation program.

Flexibility is the first component of rehabilitation. Generally following an injury, there is some loss of range of motion and in many cases, increased muscle guarding. This results in stiffness in the joints as well as lack of extensibility in the musculotendinous units. Exercises to improve flexibility might include active, active assisted, and passive joint range of motion, including joint mobilization, static stretching for the musculotendinous units and a variety of facilitated stretching techniques such as proprioceptive neuromuscular facilitation (PNF).

The second component of rehabilitation is **strength**. Strength exercises may be done in either isometric, isotonic, or isokinetic modes, with each mode having its advantages and disadvantages. Isometrics are particularly suited to the more acute injury stage because the intensity of the exercise can be adjusted by the patient athlete to avoid creating additional symptoms. The athlete may also exercise an injured joint in a position of relative comfort by avoidance of the extremes of the available range of motion. Disadvantages of isometrics are that they are static rather than dynamic in nature. The strength gains are also relatively specific to the position of the joint in which the exercises are performed.

Isotonic exercises are the most common strengthening techniques used in rehabilitation. These involve taking a joint through a specific range of motion against a fixed resistance. The resistance may be applied to the shortening contractions of the muscles (concentric exercise) or may be applied to the lengthening or controlling contraction of the muscles (eccentric contractions). Advantages are that the isotonic exercises are dynamic and have a wide variety of application to most sports skills. Disadvantages are that various joints have different efficiencies at different ranges of motion and with a fixed resistance, with a relatively inefficient exercise sometimes being the result.

Isokinetic exercise involves moving a joint through a range of motion against a device that controls the speed of movement rather than the resistance. The advantage here is that the resistance accommodates to the changes in the biomechanical efficiency of the joint through the range of motion. Isokinetic exercise can also be targeted to controlled higher speeds of contraction that can mimic speeds of more functional, sports-specific activities. Disadvantages of isokinetics include the cost and availability of exercise equipment and being somewhat limited in the functional patterns of movement available.

The third component of rehabilitation is **endurance**. Endurance includes increasing both anaerobic and aerobic muscular capacity as well as aerobic and anaerobic cardiovascular capacity. Increasing individual muscular endurance can be accomplished by adjusting the sets, number of repetitions, resistance, and pace of specific strength-training activities. Increasing cardiovascular endurance can be accomplished through traditional activities such as running, cycling, stair-stepper machines, swimming, upper extremity cycle ergometers, cross-country ski machines, and other means. The methods used here should be targeted toward the ultimate sport to which the athlete intends to return. However, there is certainly some merit for using a variety of exercise modes in a cross-training manner to avoid overstressing one area too much.

The fourth component of rehabilitation is **proprioception**. This involves basic activities to regain the ability of an injured muscle and joint to judge position in space. Devices and activities such as a single leg stance for balance, basic balance boards (uniaxial), advanced balance boards (multiaxial), and some of the commercially available balance machines can be used. Stress to the joint is applied very mildly at first with the injured area being protected from going to extreme ranges of motion. The athlete is encouraged to control the movement as well as possible. The amount of movement, the amount of weight-bearing on the injured limb, and complexity of the exercise are advanced as the injured area is able to tolerate. Upper extremity proprioceptive exercises also can be initiated on the balance board and both upper and lower extremity exercises can be advanced to activities such as the slide board to help improve the balance and reaction sense within the injured joint and muscle.

The fifth area of rehabilitation is **agility and skills drills**. This is the more advanced phase of rehabilitation that fine tunes an athlete's rehabilitation toward specifically the sport and activity that he or she wishes to resume. Here, the drills include fundamental drills for a given sport progressed from very basic to more complex as the athlete demonstrates he or she is handling these activities appropriately. This is a process of progressive motor learning and motor relearning. This can include general sports activities as well as very isolated fundamental and skill drills for the athlete.

5. Which of the five components of a rehabilitative program is most important?

No single component of rehabilitation is more important than the other in all circumstances. Depending on the initial level of condition of the athlete, the amount of deconditioning that has occurred since the injury, the competitive level of the athlete, and the specific sport or activity involved, any of these components could be deemed more important. For example, a gymnast might need to focus on flexibility and strength, a football player on strength and anaerobic conditioning, a marathon runner on cardiovascular conditioning, and a baseball pitcher on agility and skill for throwing. It should also be noted that the relative importance of each phase may change as the athlete progresses through his rehabilitative efforts. Rather than being looked at as completely independent phases, one could look at the phases or rehabilitation as a pyramid with each component relying on the other to allow the athlete a maximum level of conditioning and rehabilitatior to return to participation.

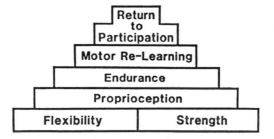

PYRAMID OF RECOVERY
(Therapeutic Exercise)

From Shelton GL: Comprehensive rehabilitation of the athlete. In Mellion MB, Walsh WM, Shelton GL (eds): The Team Physician's Handbook, 2nd ed. Philadelphia, Hanley & Belfus, 1997, p. 373, with permission.

6. How does rehabilitation differ from routine fitness and conditioning?

Even though the same components of conditioning are used in a routine fitness program, a routine fitness program basically tries to take something that is essentially normal (uninjured) and make it better in terms of the various components of rehabilitation. In rehabilitation, however, the injury itself must be respected as the phases of rehabilitation are progressed. Specifically, the rehabilitation activity should not create additional flareup of the injury (pain, swelling, favoring). The rehabilitation program must be progressed so that these symptoms, which are signs of additional stress to the injured area, are avoided.

7. What is the timetable for the rehabilitation program?

The most frequently asked question of an injured athlete or the parents and coach of an injured athlete is how long will it take the athlete's injury to recover so that he or she can return to participation. Unfortunately, this is an answer that we have relatively poor reliability in predicting with any great measure of success. In part, this is owing to the large number of variables and factors that interplay with the length of the healing, recovery, and rehabilitation. A functional timetable such as the one for ankle sprains shown in the graph below provides an example of functional milestones that can be adapted to most athletic situations. This functional timetable allows for the consideration of some of the other variables that affect the rate of healing, recovery, and rehabilitation.

Principles of Musculoskeletal Rehabilitation

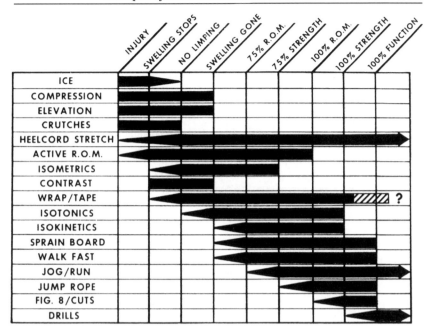

ANKLE SPRAIN REHABILITATION

Adapted from Garrick JG: A practical approach to rehabilitation. Am J Sports Med 9:67, 1981.

8. When is a rehabilitation program initiated following an injury?

The general answer to this question is **as soon as possible following the occurrence of the injury within the limits of the healing constraints**. In almost all injuries, the initial management could be construed to constitute the initiation of the rehabilitation program. Proper use of protection, rest, ice, compression, elevation, and support can greatly minimize the initial symptoms and improve the rate of recovery by minimizing the inflammation and irritation following the injury. In some injuries such as a fracture, some initial immobilization and healing may need to take place before significant rehabilitation can begin on the immobilized area. This may also be the case in some surgical problems. In other surgical problems, such as anterior cruciate ligament reconstruction, rehabilitation is initiated immediately following surgery, sometimes even the same day.

9. When is an injured athlete allowed to return to participation?

Return to participation is generally allowed once an athlete's injury is fully healed and once the athlete is fully rehabilitated. Fully healed means no pain, swelling, limping, favoring, or instability within the rehabilitation activities. Full rehabilitation is indicated by full range of motion and flexibility, normal strength, resumption of preinjury endurance levels, and good balance agility and skill ability. There are a number of specific tests for range of motion, strength, flexibility, endurance, and agility. These may be used to help guide the clinician in determining readiness for return to participation. However, the ultimate test for readiness to return to participation is the ability of the athlete functionally to perform the required skills and abilities of his or her desired sport at full speed and without any symptoms. The performance of these skills is best observed by the clinician. In some instances, however, the skilled observation of a knowledgeable coach is helpful. This is one area in which the athletic trainer is invaluable in being able to monitor and assess the athlete's functional progress.

10. What type of equipment is best for rehabilitation?

Many types of equipment on the market can be used for rehabilitation. These types of equipment are primarily for strengthening exercises and endurance exercises, although some specialized equipment may be available for flexibility training, proprioception, and skills training. No single type of equipment is ideal for rehabilitation of all types of athletic injuries. In many cases, a simple home program with ankle weights or rubber band resistance supplemented by good instruction and written handouts to which the athlete may refer is adequate. Particularly in the earlier stages of an injury when the injury is acute and may not tolerate the intensity of a running program or a traditional, heavy-duty strength-training program, many of the more traditional machines in the weight room will be too intense for the level of injury. In many instances, the skills and experience of the sports physical therapist or the certified athletic trainer come into play to create a rehabilitation activity best suited for a given athlete and his or her injury rather than always using a specific piece of exercise equipment. An athlete's access to the weight room at school is necessary only if the weight room contains the type of equipment best suited to the athlete at that particular stage of recovery and rehabilitation. By no means should an athlete be forced to use a piece of equipment for rehabilitation just because it is available if it is not the appropriate activity for the athlete at that particular stage of rehabilitation.

11. Discuss common pitfalls in the process of rehabilitation.

Pitfalls or problems that can interrupt or delay the rehabilitation process can be numerous. The first pitfall, and the one most frequently encountered, is having an athlete undergo a rehabilitation program that is "etched in stone" or a "cookbook." The exact same "recipe" for treating a given injury may not work in each individual because of individual variations in body chemistry, the care the athlete provides himself or herself, motivational factors, and other factors. A protocol may be used as an outline and framework for the rehabilitation process as long as the individual variations from patient athlete to patient athlete are considered.

A second pitfall is the injured athlete tries to force himself or herself to do too much too soon. Sometimes this zeal to return to participation outweighs the athlete's common sense and awareness of the injury. In some cases, coaches, teammates, or parents may put additional pressure on the athlete to return before he or she is ready.

The converse also is true. Sometimes an athlete, once injured, cannot muster the motivation to stick with a rehabilitation program long enough to attain full recovery. Such an athlete often drops out of athletic participation. This can be minimized to some degree by a more closely supervised rehabilitation program in which the athlete is seen on a more frequent basis by the therapist or trainer to provide guidance and motivation through critical phases of the rehabilitation process. Recreational athletes in particular may not have the motivation to return to the sport in which they were injured. In some cases, the athlete is "gun shy" about returning to an activity that created a painful injury. This is a valid choice for the athlete to make and should be supported by the clinician. However, it also is the clinician's responsibility to encourage a more full level of rehabilitation so that the injured area is not as vulnerable to reinjury in the future.

Many athletes, unfortunately, have the concept of "no pain, no gain" ingrained into their psyches from early in their sports careers. Whereas this might be an appropriate motivation to work hard and condition hard for a particular sport, it is all too often misinterpreted when it comes to an injury. The concept of "no pain, no gain" implies that athletes must work hard and feel the discomfort of exertion in order to condition and improve themselves. However, when the "pain" that is felt results in additional symptoms such as additional pain in the injured area, added swelling, or additional favoring of the injury, the injured area is getting worse rather than better. These athletes must be encouraged to focus on the symptoms, be aware of when they occur, and respect the symptoms by adjusting the activity accordingly.

One final pitfall encountered with injuries in all levels of sports competition is one of unreasonable expectations regarding recovery from an injury. Even if an injury is going to take only a few days to heal, this is generally longer than the athlete, and those associated with the athlete, want to endure. The athlete or the athlete's peers may pressure the athlete to participate "because the big game is this Friday night." In some instances, the same type of pressure is applied by the athlete's coaches, and the athlete at times is made to feel inferior because he or she cannot "suck it up and play." Even the athlete's parents may exert subtle pressure on the athlete to perform when it is in the athlete's best interest to refrain from performance until the injury has improved. The clinician should be aware of these pressures on the patient and try to intervene on the behalf of the athlete when possible.

BIBLIOGRAPHY

1. Anderson B: Stretching. Bolinas, CA, Shelter Publications, 1980.
2. Andrews JR, Harrelson GL: Physical Rehabilitation of the Athlete. Philadelphia, W.B. Saunders, 1991.
3. Arnheim D, Prentice W: Principles of Athletic Training, 8th ed. St. Louis, Mosby, 1993.
4. Curwin S, Stanish WD: Tendinitis: Its Etiology and Treatment. Lexington, MA, D.C. Heath, 1984.
5. Garrick JG: A practical approach to rehabilitation. Am J Sports Med 9:67, 1981.
6. Gould JA, Davies GJ (eds): Orthopaedic and Sports Physical Therapy, Vol. 2. St. Louis, Mosby, 1985.
7. Hunter LY, Funk FJ (eds): Rehabilitation of the Injured Knee. St. Louis, Mosby, 1984.
8. Prentice W: Rehabilitation Techniques in Sports Medicine. St. Louis, Mosby, 1990.
9. Prentice W: Therapeutic Modalities in Sports Medicine, 2nd ed. St. Louis, Mosby, 1990.
10. Shelton GL: Comprehensive rehabilitation of the athlete. In Mellion MB, Walsh WM, Shelton GL (eds): The Team Physician's Handbook, 2nd ed. Philadelphia, Hanley & Belfus, 1997.
11. Shelton GL: Principles of musculoskeletal rehabilitation. In Mellion MB (ed): Office Management of Sports Injuries and Athletic Problems. Philadelphia, Hanley & Belfus, 1988.

77. PHYSICAL THERAPY MODALITIES

Mark E. Longacre, M.P.T., and Kirk M. Peck, M.S., P.T.

CRYOTHERAPY

1. What is cryotherapy?

Cryotherapy is the treatment of an injury or a disease with cold. It is used for the immediate care and rehabilitation of soft tissue injuries and other musculoskeletal problems.

2. What types of cold therapy are typically used?

Ice packs, ice cup massage, cold water immersion baths, Cryotemp compression, vapocoolant sprays, and off-the-shelf cryocuffs. The optimal therapeutic temperature is 10–18°C (50–60°F).

3. What are the effects of cryotherapy on the human body?

1. Decreases metabolism
2. Produces vasoconstriction; decreases hematoma formation
3. Delays inflammation but does not eliminate the inflammatory response or decrease long-term chronic inflammation
4. Decreases pain by slowing nerve conduction and decreasing muscle spasms
5. Decreases muscle spasm by inhibiting the stretch reflex in the muscle spindle
6. Decreases tissue temperature to a depth of 4 cm

4. What are the indications for cryotherapy?

Cryotherapy is used for acute treatment of soft tissue injuries; for treatment of tendinitis, synovitis, etc.; for pain relief and acute/chronic phases or musculoskeletal injury during the rehabilitation phase; and for reducing swelling.

5. What are the contraindications of cryotherapy?

Raynaud's phenomenon	Systemic lupus erythematosus
Cardiovascular disease, because of pressor response to cold	Vasculitis
	Multiple myeloma
	Cold urticaria

HEAT

6. What are the main effects of therapeutic heat?

Therapeutic heat is indicated when the goal is to increase tissue temperature. In addition, heat increases blood flow to body tissues, edema formation, ligament capsular fiber and muscle elasticity, and leukocyte and phagocyte migration. Other therapeutic uses of heat include to decrease muscle tone and/or spasms, to accelerate the metabolic process, and to decrease pain.

7. Are there specific superficial and deep heat modalities?

Yes. Superficial heat modalities include warm whirlpools, paraffin baths, fluidotherapy, and moist heat from hydrocollator packs. Deep heating modalities include ultrasound and the diathermies (shortwave and microwave).

8. What are the indications for superficial heat?

Superficial heat is indicated for treatment of decreased joint range of motion (e.g., due to stiffness, contractures), hematomas, and increased pain.

9. What are the contraindications to therapeutic heat?

Therapeutic heat is contraindicated for patients with decreased pain or temperature sensation (e.g., diabetic neuropathy), impaired skin circulation, malignancy, acute inflammation, neurologic impairment, and poor thermal regulation.

IONTOPHORESIS

10. What is iontophoresis?

Iontophoresis produces direct current (DC) to drive ionized medications through the skin. Positive and negative surface electrodes are used to repel ions with positive and negative charges through the skin.

11. When is iontophoresis indicated?

Iontophoresis is generally used to treat acute and subacute localized tissue inflammation. Tissue pathologies commonly treated with iontophoresis include tendinitis, bursitis, superficial muscle strain, neuromas, and localized cysts.

12. What are the potential adverse reactions to iontophoresis?

Although iontophoresis involves a relatively painless and sterile application process, superficial burns may result from application of galvanic current to the skin surface. The most dangerous complication is an adverse reaction to the administered drug.

ULTRASOUND

13. What is ultrasound?

Ultrasound is the use of inaudible, acoustic, mechanical vibrations of high frequency that produce thermal and nonthermal physiologic effects in human tissue.

14. Distinguish between phonophoresis and ultrasound.

Phonophoresis is the use of ultrasound to drive an antiinflammatory medication through the skin to the underlying tissues.

15. What is the rationale for using continuous versus pulsed ultrasound?

Continuous ultrasound is used to increase tissue temperature and collagen extensibility, to decrease joint stiffness and spasm/pain, and to increase blood flow and produce some mild inflammatory reaction. Continuous ultrasound is most commonly used for its deep heating effects. Pulsed ultrasound is generally used to facilitate cellular metabolism through its nonthermal effects. Pulsed ultrasound is often indicated to treat acute injuries or when deep heating is contraindicated.

16. What are some of the guidelines to follow with the use of ultrasound?

Treatments should be limited to a maximum of 14 treatments per given condition. Acute injuries may best be treated with daily pulsed ultrasound for the first 6–8 days. Chronic injuries may receive ultrasound every other day. A 1-MHz ultrasound head penetrates to a depth of 5–6 cm and is typically used over fatty areas or deep tissues. A 3-MHz ultrasound head penetrates to a depth of 1–3 cm and is used primarily to treat superficial tissues.

17. What are the indications for ultrasound?

Because ultrasound is the best heating method for depths greater than 2 cm, it is indicated when deep, prompt tissue heating is needed. It can be used to increase joint range of motion, to treat heterotrophic scars and adhesion, to decrease pain of neuromas, and to decrease muscle spasms and increase blood flow.

18. What are the contraindications for ultrasound?

Ultrasound should not be used immediately following trauma when bleeding is present. It should not be used over a pacemaker, a suspected malignancy, growth plates in children, or in areas where there is decreased sensation. In addition, it should not be used when the patient has thrombophlebitis and should be avoided over joint replacements.

SHORT-WAVE DIATHERMY

19. What is diathermy?

Short-wave diathermy (SWD) is the use of high frequency electromagnetic currents to induce deep tissue heating by vibration and distortion of the tissue molecules. It typically will heat up to 3 to 5 cm, but this depends on the wave frequency and the electrical properties of the tissues. Most of the heat is dispersed superficially within the subcutaneous fat.

20. What are the indications for diathermy?

Osteoarthritis	Tendinitis	Neuritis	Contractions and muscle
Rheumatoid arthritis	Sprains	Joint capsule	guarding/spasms
Bursitis	Strains		

21. What are the contraindications for SWD?

A fresh hemorrhage	Pregnancy	Cardiac pacemakers
Sensory loss	Pelvic area in men-	Over the epiphyseal
Moist dressing	struating women	plates in children
Ischemia	Phlebitis	Someone with a tumor
Arteriosclerosis	Metallic implants	Someone who has an infection

TRACTION

22. What is mechanical traction used for?

Distraction of vertebral bodies	Widening of the intervertebral
Distraction and gliding of the facet joints	foramen
Tensing of ligament structures of the spinal segments	Stretching of spinal musculature

23. Who are candidates for mechanical traction?

Patients with disc herniations/protrusions, degenerative disc disease (DDD), degenerative joint disease (DJD), and joint hypomobility.

24. What are the general contraindications for the use of mechanical traction?

Contraindications for mechanical traction are tumors, vascular compromise, acute strain or sprain, pregnancy, osteoporosis, and hiatal hernia. In addition, mechanical traction should not be used if pain is elicited by manual traction. For this reason, a trial of manual traction should precede treatment with mechanical traction.

ELECTRICAL

25. What is transcutaneous electrical nerve stimulation?

Transcutaneous electrical nerve stimulation (TENS) administers electrical current through pads placed on the superficial surface of the skin. Electrical current may be used to stimulate peripheral sensory or motor nerves to cause a reduction in pain or to produce muscle contractions, respectively.

26. How does TENS work?

Two theories have been postulated. The first, based on Melzack and Wall's gate control theory, contends that TENS stimulates the large myelinated nerve fibers, which inhibit or block the transmission in small unmyelinated pain fibers at the spinal cord level. This process is immediately reversed once the stimulation is ceased.

The second theory is that TENS stimulates the release of opiates such as beta-endorphins at the spinal cord level, which decreases the perception of pain.

27. What is interferential current? How is it different from other TENS modalities?

Interferential current is produced by a type of TENS device that creates two separate AC sine waves from two different energy sources. The two sine waves are applied to body surfaces so that their paths cross in the tissues and thus create an interference pattern. It is hypothesized that interferential current penetrates tissues deeper than other TENS modalities. Some clinicians claim that it is more comfortable.

28. What is a Neuroprobe?

This tool is effective in both identifying and treating trigger points. With the use of a superficial point stimulator, trigger points may be found by measuring impedance values. Trigger points correspond to low resistant areas. Once these areas are found, brief but intense stimulation, utilizing a low-intensity, medium frequency (10,000 Hz) known as hyperstimulation, is applied to reduce pain.

29. What is neuromuscular stimulation?

Neuromuscular stimulation (NMS) is a technique by which motor nerves are stimulated with electrode pads placed directly on the skin. The stimulation of the large motor nerves causes a contraction of the desired muscle tissues.

30. What is the NMS used for?

Neuromuscular stimulation is frequently used to increase muscle strength, prevent muscle atrophy, and control edema. Through stimulation, the muscle acts as a pump to assist in the control of edema. Improved range of motion (ROM) at the site of a contracture may also be achieved through NMS, as well as atrophy prevention while an extremity is casted. Nonorthopedic uses include muscle reeducation for patients who have suffered a cerebrovascular accident (CVA), reduction of muscle spasticity, and facilitation of muscle recruitment in cases of upper motor neuron lesions.

31. What are the indications for NMS?

Candidates for NMS include patients who present with non-use muscle atrophy, postsurgical atrophy or weakness, or incomplete spinal cord injuries.

32. Who is not a candidate for NMS?

Neuromuscular stimulation will not have an effect on denervated muscles.

33. Are there various types of NMS?

Yes, Russian stimulation, developed by Dr. Kots, uses sinusoidal currents. This system has been used by Russian athletes to help develop bigger and quicker strength gains. It uses a 2,500-Hz current, which theoretically blocks small afferent fibers, thus activating large efferent nerve fibers and creating an anesthetic effect.

34. Are there any contraindications to the electrical modalities?

Yes. The following list should be viewed as general precautions to the use of any electrical modalities:

1. Patients with pacemakers or any significant cardiac history
2. Over the carotid sinuses
3. During pregnancy (safety not established)
4. Patients with any synaptic disease
5. Over any areas of peripheral vascular disorders
6. Over neoplasms or infections
7. Over open skin wounds
8. Infants
9. Senile patients with poor sensory perception

35. What are the uses for common electrical stimulation modalities?

Uses for Common Electrical Stimulation Modalities

USED FOR	NMS	TENS	INTER-FERENTIAL	HIGH VOLTAGE	MEDIUM FREQUENCY	MICROCURRENT STIMULATOR
Acute/chronic pain	No	Yes	Yes	Yes	No	Yes
Acute edema reduction	No	No	Yes	Yes	No	Yes
Enhancement of bone healing	No	No	Yes	Yes	No	Yes
Muscle strengthening	Yes	No	No	No	Yes	No
Muscle reeducation	Yes	No	Yes	No	No	No
Reduction of muscle spasm	Yes	Yes	Yes	Yes	Yes	No
Increase/maintain ROM contracture correction	Yes	No	No	No	No	No

CONTINUOUS PASSIVE MOTION

36. What is continuous passive motion (CPM)?

Continuous passive motion involves the application of an external force to take an involved extremity through a preset range of motion (ROM).

Specific devices are available for both the upper and lower extremities. Upper body ergometers and stationary bikes also fall into this category as the noninvolved extremity is used to apply the external force to move the involved extremity.

37. What is the purpose of CPM?

Clinical uses have been to relieve pain, to enhance nutrition of the involved joint (in particular, articular cartilage), and to prevent contractures/adhesions postoperatively. CPM has been found to be useful after total joint replacement to encourage early movement for healing and to relieve pain.

38. What is the rationale for CPM?

Several studies have shown the deleterious effects that immobilization has on articular cartilage. It has been documented that a build-up of fibrofatty tissue occurs within 30 days and destruction of cartilage occurs within 60 days. Possible ulceration of the articular cartilage with secondary changes in subchondral bone may also occur. The beneficial effects are increased clearance rate of effusion or hemarthrosis from synovial joints with joint motion, recovery of septic joints with less cartilage destruction, and improved healing of sutured tendons.

BIOFEEDBACK

39. What is biofeedback?

Biofeedback is used to detect muscle activity for the purpose of facilitating either muscle recruitment or muscle relaxation. Small electrodes are placed superficially on the surface of the skin to detect muscle activity. Electrical energy generated by muscle activity is converted to audio and visual signals through an EMG biofeedback unit. Visual and audio feedback allows an athlete to voluntarily alter muscle contractions.

40. How is biofeedback used in rehabilitation?

Biofeedback has become a popular modality to rehabilitate muscles that contract asynchronously or have atrophied from non-use or postsurgical procedures. Biofeedback is often used in conjunction with other therapeutic treatments in comprehensive rehabilitation programs. One example is to use biofeedback in the treatment of patellofemoral pain to facilitate the recruitment of the vastus medialis oblique and synchronize its contractions with the vastus lateralis muscle. In conjunction with biofeedback, specific patellar taping techniques are often used to help restore normal patellofemoral mechanics.

41. How does biofeedback work?

By receiving visual and auditory sensory input an athlete is able to alter muscle contractions voluntarily and thus facilitate normal function. Once desired muscle activity has been achieved, the sensory feedback is gradually reduced and eventually eliminated. Occasionally an athlete is able to achieve desired voluntary muscle contractions in one treatment session; however, multiple treatment sessions are not uncommon.

BIBLIOGRAPHY

1. Bare A, McAnaw M, Pritchard A, et al: Phonophoretic delivery of 10% hydrocortisone through the epidermis of humans as determined by serum cortisol concentrations. Phys Ther 76:738–749, 1996.
2. Byl N: The use of ultrasound as an enhancer for transcutaneous drug delivery: Phonophoresis. Phys Ther 75:539–553, 1995.
3. Costello C, Jeske A: Iontophoresis: Applications in transdermal medication delivery. Phys Ther 75:554–563, 1995.
4. DeLacerda F: A case study: Application of ultrasound to determine a stress fracture of the fibula. J Orthop Sports Phys Ther 2:134–136, 1981.
5. Drez D: Therapeutic Modalities for Sports Injuries. Chicago, Year Book Medical Publishers, 1989.
6. Dyson M, Suckling J: Stimulation of tissue repair by ultrasound: A survey of the mechanisms involved. Physiotherapy 64:105–108, 1978.
7. Fabrizio P, Schmidt J, Clemente R, et al: Acute effects of therapeutic ultrasound delivered at varying parameters on the blood flow velocity in a muscular distribution artery. J Orthop Sports Phys Ther 24:294–302, 1996.

8. Gann N: Ultrasound: Current concepts. Clin Management 11(4):64, 1991.
9. Gersh M: Electrotherapy in Rehabilitation. Philadelphia, F.A. Davis, 1992.
10. Hecox B, Mehreteab T, Weisber J: Physical Agents: A Comprehensive Text for Physical Therapists. Norwalk, CT, Appleton & Lange, 1994.
11. Howard J, Thomas D, Kellogg D: Effects of alternating current iontophoresis on drug delivery. Arch Phys Med Rehabil 76:463–466, 1995.
12. Mannheimer JS, Lampe GN: Clinical Transcutaneous Electrical Nerve Stimulation. Philadelphia, F.A. Davis, 1988.
13. Maxwell L: Therapeutic ultrasound and tumor metastasis. Physiotherapy 81:272–275, 1995.
14. Michlovitz, SL: Theramal Agents in Rehabilitation. Philadelphia, F.A. Davis, 1989.
15. Michlovitz S, Behrens B: Physical Agents: Theory and Practice for the Physical Therapist Assistant. Philadelphia, F.A. Davis, 1996.
16. Prentice W: Therapeutic Modalities in Sports Medicine. St. Louis, Mosby, 1994.
17. Snyder-Mackler L, Robinson AJ: Clinical Electrophysiology. Electrotherapy and Electrophysiologic Testing. Baltimore, Williams & Wilkins, 1989.
18. Weston M, Taber C, Casagranda L, Cornwall M: Changes in local blood volume during cold gel pack application to traumatized ankles. JOSPT 19:197–199, 1994.

78. THE USES OF MANUAL MEDICINE IN ATHLETES

R. Todd Dombroski, D.O.

1. Do providers of manual medicine diagnose musculoskeletal problems differently?

They use the same basic examination with a few added refinements. For example, a suspected rotator cuff strain is found by standard physical exam. Additional palpatory examinations of the shoulder musculature and the muscular insertions to the upper thoracic spine are fairly standard in manual medicine to help diagnose pathology. The exam also may evaluate the influence of possible cervical strain on neurovascular circulation to the shoulder. Assessment of such interconnections is the hallmark of osteopathic diagnosis; it also is fairly standard in all manual medicine approaches. Diagnosis in manual medicine should serve to complement, not replace, standard sports medicine diagnostic techniques.

The goal of palpatory diagnostic techniques is to find tenderness to palpation, asymmetry (of static structures), restriction of motion (in any plane), and tissue texture abnormalities (TART). Tenderness may be superficial or deep or may radiate according to trigger points. Asymmetry may be noted in the height of the iliac crests or atrophy of muscle or on deep palpation of the sacroiliac joints. Restriction of motion may be palpated as the joint is passively glided through all three planes of motion. This technique is different from the gross range of motion noted on a goniometer. The most sensitive palpatory findings involve soft tissue (fascia, muscle, tendon, ligament, and overlying skin). Different amounts of palpatory force are used to evaluate TART changes.

2. Define somatic dysfunction.

The palpatory findings noted in TART are categorized as somatic dysfunction, which is officially defined as "impaired or altered function of related components of the somatic (body framework) system: skeletal, arthrodial, and myofascial structures; and their related vascular, lymphatic and neural elements."[4] Somatic dysfunction describes the interconnection between a pathologic joint surface, which causes stiffness in the muscle, and impeded blood and lymphatic circulation, which results in local neural irritation noted as pain. Palpation of a restriction in a joint without a gross loss in range of motion is just one key finding. Atrophic changes in the skin from decreased circulation, bogginess of the tissue from lymphatic congestion, or hyperasthesias from light palpation are clues to somatic dysfunction.

3. How can palpatory findings in one area suggest pathology in other areas?

The concept of interconnection in manual medicine states that pathology in the body (sometimes called soma) can affect other areas of the neuromuscular system and/or associated viscera. These interconnections are not a new concept in medicine. Examples of somatic-somatic interconnections include chronic trapezius/rhomboid overuse due to rotator cuff injury and an anatomic short leg that causes back pain. Examples of somato-visceral interconnections include costochondral restrictions that decrease ventilation and thoracic strain that increases gastric acid output. Examples of visceral-somatic interconnections include cardiac dysfunction that causes left arm pain, and cholecystitis that causes shoulder pain. The finding that sympathetic nerves can carry afferent pain signals helps to explain the interconnections between the soma and the viscera. Therefore, by assessing the body framework as a whole, other clues to disease states may be found.

4. How is the barrier concept used in manual medicine?

Restriction of motion (the R in TART) must have a palpatory barrier that prohibits normal motion around the joint (in the spine or extremity). The barrier may be due to an inflamed facet joint capsule, a spasm in an injured muscle, edema surrounding a tendon sheath, or a combination of the above. The barrier may result in minimal restriction, not noted on gross range-of-motion testing.

The barrier concept is also used to classify the two general types of manual medicine. The first type is designed to move through the barrier to help achieve full range of motion (direct techniques). The second type works in the range of motion away from the restricted barrier (indirect techniques).

5. What neural inputs maintain a barrier to motion?

The spinal cord has many inputs from pain and mechanoreceptors in the joint capsule, periosteum, tendons and muscles. In addition, many interneurons interconnect contra- and ipsilateral spinal cord inputs. These inputs are sometimes processed at the cord level or may be influenced by higher brain centers. These afferent pathways have been documented; essentially their function is to restrict joint motion to help to prevent further injury. Irritation of the sympathetic nervous system increases neural output, affecting pain, circulation, and associated visceral functions. Changes in circulation may affect the lymphatics. Many of the known pathways are used to theorize how somatic dysfunction initiates. As the body heals, the reflexes are supposed to be reset (or shut off). If the reflexes are not shut off, they may become chronic patterns of restriction and somatic dysfunction.

6. Describe the major types of techniques and the theory behind their use.

1. The **high-velocity, low-amplitude (thrust) technique** is a quick, short thrust with low force. It is the classic "pop" technique common to both chiropractors and osteopaths. This quick direct technique through the barrier is thought to overstimulate mechanoreceptor input and thereby reset its normal tone.

2. **Muscle energy** uses a series of isometric contractions, each a little deeper through the barrier. This direct technique attempts specifically to decrease the input from the muscle spindles (a specific type of mechanoreceptor), thereby decreasing feedback tone in the muscle.

3. **Counterstrain** is an indirect technique that induces strain in the antagonist muscle to decrease interneuron or mechanoreceptor input.

4. **Myofascial release** is a direct or indirect technique for stretching the fascia that may be causing the barrier. Microscars in the fascia are theorized, but none has been seen on biopsy.

5. **Functional technique** is an indirect technique that uses available range of motion to retrace the pattern of injury and thus decrease pathologic motor patterns in the special cord or higher centers.

6. **Soft tissue technique** is a direct technique that involves deep stretching of soft tissue, including muscle, tendon and fascia. It attempts to improve circulation to these tissues and to increase lymphatic circulation.

There are many other techniques, but they are used less frequently. The above techniques may be used in combination on the same area or in related areas.

7. What are the contraindications to manual medicine?
Known instability of a joint is an absolute contraindication to manual medicine. High-velocity, low-amplitude techniques have several relative contraindications: bone tumors, metabolic bone disease, radicular compression syndromes, primary joint diseases (e.g., rheumatoid arthritis), congenital or acquired fixed deformities, hypermobility of the joint, and vertebral basilar artery insufficiency. Indirect techniques can be used with caution to treat patients with relative contraindications due to musculoskeletal disease.

8. Why is the facet joint so important in manual medicine?
Within millimeters of the facet joint are all of the components of somatic dysfunction. Each vertebral body has right and left, superior and inferior facet joint surfaces. The 24 vertebral (7 cervical + 12 thoracic + 5 lumbar) result in 96 joint surfaces that have to align perfectly with each other. Because nothing is perfect in the body, a bony asymmetry in the facet joint may cause somatic dysfunction. Arthrodial pathology is only one cause of somatic dysfunction. Synovial joints have capsules that may become edematous and restrict movement. Myriad short ligaments and short and long rotator muscles further restrict motion, thus decreasing the intervertebral foramen. A smaller intervertebral foramen irritates not only the somatic nerves but also the sympathetic nerves. This small area is ripe for somatic dysfunction and usually receives the most attention. All joints, including the pelvis and extremities, may have somatic dysfunction.

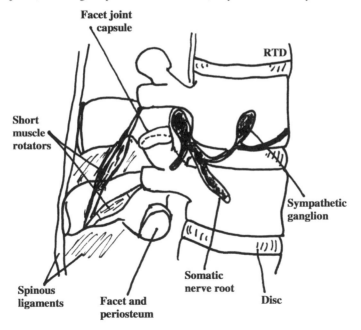

9. In which phase of athletic injury is manual medicine most useful?
In all phases of injury (acute, subacute, chronic) manual medicine can help the athlete recover. Even if the extremity is splinted, certain techniques can improve lymphatic drainage. Balancing muscle tension (decreasing restrictions) is the key for the subacute phase, especially after immobilization. The chronic or recurrent injury requires complete structural assessment. For example, chronic back pain has resulted from from an undiagnosed functional short leg, hamstring/quadriceps imbalance, or sacroiliac joint restriction.

10. How often can manual medicine treatment be used?

Frequency depends on severity, complexity, and chronicity of the injury. There are no specific rules, yet data suggest that the "right" amount of manipulation can improve outcome without increasing medical cost significantly. Before every manual medicine treatment, the patient should be rediagnosed by palpatory findings of somatic dysfunction; thus it is difficult to predict what the residual pathology might be on the next visit. It also stands to reason that too much mobilization of a joint may lead to hypermobility and instability.

11. Does research indicate that manual medicine works for low back pain?

Researching the efficacy of manual medicine is difficult because it does not fit the classical scientific model. Blinding of patients and physicians, designing of "sham" techniques, and interoperator standardization have been difficult. One review of the literature attempted to quantify the good points of all studies to date with a scoring system. Skekelle and others found 25 controlled trials from 1952 to 1992. The probability of recovery from uncomplicated low back pain in 3 weeks was 67% with manual medicine and 50% without. More recently, the Agency for Health Care Policy and Research reviewed the available studies and determined that the use of manipulation in nonradicular back pain within the first month can be of benefit.

12. What does an allopathic physician (M.D.) need to practice manual medicine techniques?

As fully licensed physicians, M.D.s may use manual medicine techniques and should document their use with osteopathic Current Procedural Terminology codes for manual medicine (739.0–739.9). To date, only osteopathic physicians are fully licensed to perform manual medicine techniques in addition to medicine and surgery. State and regional medical practices and certain health care plans may make it difficult to be reimbursed for manual medicine treatments. Allopaths can take classes from several sources (e.g., osteopathic colleges, the American Academy of Osteopathy). Whether an M.D. can become certified in manual medicine is not yet clearly defined.

BIBLIOGRAPHY

1. Bigos S, Bowyer O, Braen B, et al: Acute low back problems in adults. Agency for Health Care Policy and Research Publication 95-0642:26-28, 1994.
2. Carey TS, Garrett J, Jackson A: The outcomes and cost of care for acute low back pain among patients seen by primary care practitioners, chiropractors, and orthopedic surgeons. N Engl J Med 333:913–917, 1995.
3. Gilliar WG, Kuchera ML, Giulianetti DA: Neurological basis of manual medicine. Phys Med Rehabil Clin North Am 7:693–711, 1996.
4. Jones JM, et al: Glossary of Osteopathic Terminology. J Am Osteopath Acad 80:552–567, 1981.
5. Mein EA: Low back pain and manual medicine. Phys Med Rehabil Clin North Am 7:715–727, 1996.
6. Patterson MM, Howell JN (eds): Somatovisceral/Viserosomatic Interaction—1989, Indianapolis, International Symposium. American Academy of Osteopathy, 1989.
7. Skekelle PG, Adams AA, Chassin MR, et al: Spinal manipulation in low back pain. Ann Intern Med 117:590–598, 1992.
8. Travell JG, Simmons DG: Myofascial Pain and Dysfunction: The Trigger Point Manual. Baltimore, Williams and Wilkins, 1983.
9. Ward RC (ed): Foundation for Osteopathic Medicine. Baltimore, Williams & Wilkins, 1997, pp 53–82.

79. INJECTION AND ASPIRATION

John L. Pfenninger, M.D., FAAFP

1. What is the difference between joint aspiration and joint injection?

Joint aspiration indicates that fluid (pus, blood, serous effusion) will be withdrawn from a joint. Injection refers to the placement of some medication inside a joint, bursa, or around a tendon.

2. What are the common indications to "tap a joint"?

There are two broad indication categories: to make a diagnosis and to provide treatment. Aspirating a joint can provide synovial fluid to differentiate the cause of an effusion between infectious, rheumatic, or crystal-induced forms of arthritis. In a traumatic situation, fat cells in a bloody fluid can make a diagnosis of an occult fracture. Injecting an anesthetic such as lidocaine into a painful area also can be diagnostic. An example of this is injecting a trigger point in the back that resolves the pain being experienced by a patient. Further diagnostic work-up would not be needed.

Therapeutic benefits include removing purulent fluid from a septic joint, relieving pain by withdrawing fluid from a grossly swollen and distended joint, and injecting various medications (lidocaine, saline, or corticosteroids).

3. What are the conditions most helped by a steroid injection?

In general, the more inflammatory conditions (excluding infection) are helped most by steroid injections. These include rheumatoid arthritis, seronegative spondyloarthropathies (e.g., ankylosing spondylitis, arthritis associated with inflammatory bowel disease, psoriatic arthritis, Reiter's syndrome), crystal-induced arthritis such as gout and pseudogout, and periarticular inflammatory conditions (bursitis, tendinitis, nerve entrapments). Although not as inflammatory, osteoarthritic conditions also are symptomatically improved with steroid injections.

4. Which are the easiest joints to tap or inject?

Generally, the large joints are easier to enter. The prime example of this is the knee joint. If one compresses one side of the knee with the hand, the contralateral side will generally bulge if there is a significant effusion. The needle can simply be inserted into this area of the bulge beneath the patella. If there are multiple joints involved in a particular inflammatory process, tap the larger joints to obtain a diagnosis.

5. Should certain joints not be injected by the less experienced clinician?

Small joints and those joints located deeper in the body should probably be avoided by the inexperienced clinician. Examples of such joints would be the fingers, the hip joint, the sacroiliac joint, and the vertebral column joints. Joints with prostheses are more prone to infection and are best treated by other specialists. Some suggest withholding steroids in unstable joints, but at that point there is generally little to lose.

6. Is sterile technique used for aspiration and injection?

In the past, many clinicians did not use gloves and injected a joint after a mere alcohol wipe. Others will go through a full preparation with an antiseptic and use sterile gloves and sterile draping. The practical approach used by most physicians is to wear gloves, prepare with an alcohol or povidone-iodine (Betadine) wipe, and then inject. Sterile drapes are rarely used except in the immunocompromised patient.

7. What are the contraindications to entering a joint?

- Overlying cellulitis
- Severe coagulopathy

- Anticoagulation out of control
- Inaccessible joints
- Joint prosthesis (relative)
- Clinician unfamiliar with the risk, benefits, and possible complications

8. Are there additional contraindications for steroid injections?

Yes. The injection of steroids is definitely contraindicated with a septic effusion. Steroids should probably not be injected in a weight-bearing joint more than three times per year. Lack of response of any area after three or four injections should contraindicate further injections. Unless a particular joint is suspected as being the cause of fever, bacteremia is a contraindication, because bacteria may be introduced into the joint space. Some suggest that an unstable joint is a contraindication for steroids. However, by this time, most of the damage has been done, and little is lost by injecting steroids into a degenerated joint.

9. What are the common complications from the *technique* of joint injection?

Theoretically, one could inject medication into a vein or artery. This can be eliminated by simply withdrawing before injection. An injection into a tendon rather than around a tendon could cause weakening and subsequent rupture of that tendon. Similarly, one could cause trauma to nerves. Injection into the median nerve causes immediate pain and requires debridement. Being too forceful could cause articular cartilage damage from the needle tip. Pneumothorax has been reported after injection of trigger points in the thoracic area.

10. List the medical complications attributed to steroid injections.

Medical Complications of Steroid Injections

COMPLICATIONS	ESTIMATED PREVALENCE (%)
Flare	2–3
Arthropathy	0–8
Tendon rupture	< 1
Facial blushing	< 1
Skin atrophy, depigmentation	< 1
Iatrogenic infection	< 0.006
Transient paresis of injected extremity	Rare
Hypersensitivity reaction	Rare
Pericapsular calcification	43
Acceleration of cartilage attrition	Unknown

From Gray RG, Gottleib N: Intra-articular corticosteroids: An updated assessment. Clin Orthop 177:253–263, 1983, with permission.

11. Isn't infection after injection of steroids fairly common?

No. Hollander, using aseptic technique without sterile gloves or drapes, had only 18 infections out of 250,000 injections (0.072%). Gray's summary of various studies showed a rate less than 0.006%.

12. Do steroid injections universally cause cartilage destruction?

Studies of arthropathy with steroids have been based on subprimates. Primates have *not* been found to have long-term significant problems unless an excessive number of injections or an excessive amount of steroid is used in weight-bearing joints. Limiting the number of injections to three to five per year, especially in weight-bearing joints, should eliminate these complications.

13. Name the bacterium that causes most cases of infectious olecranon bursitis and also is the culprit in the rare postinjection infection.

Staphylococcus aureus. Because 40–50% of patients with olecranon bursitis are infected with staphylococci and it is almost impossible to differentiate infected and noninfected cases, aspiration and culture are recommended prior to injection of steroids. Steroids promote faster and more long-term healing.

14. List the most cost-effective diagnostic tests to run on synovial fluid.

Although many laboratory studies have been proposed in the past, Schmerling, after studying 100 consecutive patients, concluded that only color of fluid, white blood cell count, percentage of polymorphonuclear leukocytes (PMNs), the presence or absence of crystals, Gram stain, and bacterial culture (possible fungal and mycobacterial if indicated) were helpful. Levels of glucose, protein, lactic dehydrogenase (LDH), complement fixation, rheumatoid factor, electrolytes, uric acid, protein and albumin, and antinuclear antibody (ANA) are rarely if ever indicated.

Synovial Fluid Test	Sensitivity	Specificity
WBCs	0.84	0.84
%PMNs	0.75	0.92
Glucose	0.20	0.84
Protein	0.52	0.56
LDH	0.83	0.71

15. Which steroids are used for injection?

Almost any injectable preparation can be used. They differ in onset, length of action, and potency. Certain physicians are adamant about the benefits of the particular steroid they use, but the bottom line is to become familiar with one or two preparations and use them consistently. No good double-blind studies are available to compare different drugs. (See also questions 16 and 21.) Fat-soluble drugs are longer-acting than water-soluble drugs.

16. Discuss the potency and the length of action of various steroids used for injection.

Characteristics of Corticosteroid Injection Therapy for Joint and Soft Tissue Maladies

CORTICOSTEROID	ONSET OF RELIEF*[†]	PEAK TIME OF RELIEF[†]	DURATION OF RELIEF	DOSE OF INJECTION (mg)[‡]	POTENCY OF STEROID
Betamethasone sodium phosphate with beta-methasone acetate	Rapid	—	1–2 wk	0.25–2.0	25
Dexamethasone acetate	—	—	1–3 wk	0.8–16.0	25
Dexamethasone sodium phosphate	Rapid	—	3 days to 3 wk	0.4–6.0	25
Hydrocortisone acetate	—	24–48 hr	3 days to 4 wk	5–50	1
Methylprednisolone acetate	Very slow	7 days	1–5 wk	4–80	5
Prednisolone sodium phosphate	—	—	3 days to 3 wk	2–30	4
Prednisolone tebutate	Slow	—	1–3 wk	4–30	4
Triamcinolone acetonide	—	—	1–6 wk	2–20	5
Triamcinolone diacetate	—	—	1–8 wk	2–20	5
Triamcinolone hexacetonide	—	—	3–4 wk	2–20	5

Adapted from Birrer RB: Aspiration and corticosteroid injection. Phys Sportsmed 20(12):57–71, 1992.
* Very slow, 1–5 days; slow, 12–48 hr; rapid, 2–24 hour.
† Columns are incomplete because some values are highly variable.
‡ Dose depends, e.g., on size of lesion, joint bursa.

17. Are steroids the only type of medication ever injected?

Steroids are the most common medication injected but not the only one. Some studies have indicated that the volume of fluid injected is nearly as important as the injected material itself. The reason for this is unknown. Generally, steroids are combined with a local anesthetic such as lidocaine or bupivacaine in order to provide the volume necessary for optimal results. The larger the joint, the more volume injected. Some have used merely normal saline to inject over trigger points, for example, and have claimed excellent results.

18. Compare the risks and benefits of oral nonsteroidal antiinflammatory drugs (NSAIDs) to those of steroid injection.

Many consider the use of oral NSAIDs safer than the use of intra-articular steroids. However, one only has to recall how many patients on NSAIDs have been admitted because of gastrointestinal (GI) bleeds and the number of patients who have died either from sudden upper GI bleeds that were asymptomatic or from acute renal insufficiency (interstitial nephritis) to realize that NSAIDs are not without significant complications. One in five chronic users of NSAIDs will have gastric lesions. It seems illogical to risk complications throughout the body when many patients present with a single joint involvement. Focal treatment with an injection is the safer "more conservative" approach! Although NSAIDs are often used in conjunction with steroid injections, they can often be used for shorter periods of time.

19. Identify specific conditions improved with local corticosteroid therapy.

Conditions Improved with Local Corticosteroid Therapy

Articular conditions	Nonarticular disorders
Rheumatoid arthritis	Fibrositis
Seronegative spondyloarthropathies	Localized
Ankylosing spondylitis	Systemic
Arthritis associated with	Bursitis
inflammatory bowel disease	Subacromial
Psoriasis	Trochanteric
Reiter's syndrome	Anserine
Crystal-induced arthritis	Prepatellar
Gout	Periarthritis
Pseudogout	Adhesive capsulitis
Osteoarthritis	Tenosynovitis/tendinitis
	De Quervain's disease
	Trigger finger
	Bicipital
	Tennis elbow
	Golfer's elbow
	Plantar fasciitis
	Neuritis
	Carpal tunnel syndrome
	Tarsal tunnel syndrome
	Costochondritis
	Tietze's syndrome

From Pfenninger JL: Injections of joints and soft tissue: Part I. General guidelines. Am Fam Physician 44:1196–1202, 1991, with permission.

20. Discuss the problem of parabens preservatives with joint injection.

Multidose vials of lidocaine (Xylocaine) contain parabens as a preservative. Many steroids will precipitate when added to the anesthetic. Although they are still efficacious, these fine crystals may be responsible for a postinjection flare or for the small calcifications seen in joints after injection. If parabens are present, the fluid will be somewhat cloudy when mixed with the steroid. Parabens may also cause allergic reactions. Single-dose vials of lidocaine do not contain parabens. Alternatively, one can use bupivacaine (Marcaine), which also does not have parabens.

21. What are the common dosages of corticosteroids used for injecting various anatomic sites?

Dosages of Corticosteroid Preparations

CORTICOSTEROID	PREPARATION STRENGTH (mg/mL)	COMMON DOSAGES FOR SITE (mg)		
		TENDON SHEATHS AND BURSAE	SMALL JOINTS	LARGE JOINTS
Cortisone		20–50	10–25	50–125
Hydrocortisone acetate	25, 50	8–40	8–20	40–100
Prednisolone tebutate (Hydeltra-T.B.A.)	20	4–10	2–5	10–25
Triamcinolone				
Triamcinolone hexacetonide (Aristospan)	20	4–10	2–5	10–25
Triamcinolone diacetate (Aristocort)	40	4–10	2–5	10–25
Triamcinolone acetonide (Kenalog)	40	4–10	2–5	10–25
Methylprednisolone acetate (Depo-Medrol)	20, 40, 80	4–10	2–5	10–25
Dexamethasone				
Dexamethasone sodium phosphate (Decadron)	4	1.5–3.0	0.8–1.0	2–4
Dexamethasone acetate (Decadron-LA)	8	1.5–3.0	0.8–1.0	2–4
Betamethasone				
Betamethasone acetate (Celestone Soluspan)	6	1.5–3.0	0.8–1.0	2–4

Adapted from Leversee JH: Aspiration of joints and soft tissue injections. Prim Care 13:572–599, 1986.

22. Describe what is meant by a postinjection steroid flare.

A steroid flare consists of increased pain after injection. The exact etiology is unknown. Estimates range between 1% and 10% incidence. The pain will generally subside in 24–72 hours. Any pain or redness persisting after 72 hours should be considered an infection and requires further diagnostic tests. Treatment of a steroid flare includes NSAIDs, ice, and rest.

23. List some general guidelines to reduce complications from steroids and to "keep out of trouble."

1. Limit steroid injections to three per year in any particular area, especially in weight-bearing joints.
2. Withhold steroids if the patient cannot rest the area involved.
3. Withhold steroids if steroids are not helping after two or three injections.
4. Always use a "peritendon" injection not "intra" tendinous.
5. Be gentle—avoid cartilage trauma.
6. Avoid injecting difficult (deep or small) joints.
7. Be sure of the diagnosis before injection. Do not miss infection, tumor, fracture.
8. Withdraw on the syringe before injection.

24. Do steroids help slow the progression of inflammatory rheumatoid diseases?

No. Although symptomatic relief is unquestioned, the progression of disease is not altered with steroid injections.

25. What method of treatment is 90% effective for flexor tenosynovitis of the hand ("trigger finger")?

Corticosteroid injection(s).

26. What are the benefits of injecting "tennis elbow" (lateral epicondylitis)?

Short-term benefits (2–6 weeks) are better than long-term effects (> 6 weeks). Injections are associated with a significant risk of initial worsening of pain and atrophy over the injection site. Tendon rupture is rare. Important questions remain regarding optimal dosing, timing, technique, and volume.

27. What postinjection instructions should be given to the patient?

Generally only a Band-Aid is needed to cover the injection/aspiration site. This can be removed after 8 hours. Rest is generally advised in the acutely inflamed joints, especially if they are weight-bearing. However, this advice is variable. The difference between injecting a ganglion cyst versus the knee joint is obvious. NSAIDs are often used for 1–2 weeks in conjunction with the injection. This reduces postinjection flares as well as aids in reducing overall inflammation. Rehabilitation should not be forgotten. Passive exercises are certainly indicated and a gradual rehabilitation program should be initiated. The patient should call should pain persist after 72 hours or should there be any sign of fever, redness, or other unexpected signs or symptoms.

BIBLIOGRAPHY

1. Anderson B, Kaye S: Treatment of flexor tenosynovitis of the hand ("trigger finger") with corticosteroids. Arch Intern Med 151:153–156, 1991.
2. Assendelft WJJ, Hay EM, Ardshead R, Bouter LM: Corticosteroid injections for lateral epicondylitis: A systematic overview. Br J Gen Pract 46:209–216, 1996.
3. Birrer RB: Aspiration and corticosteroid injection. Phys Sportsmed 20(12):57–71, 1992.
4. Butcher JD, Solzman KL, Lillegard WA: Lower extremity bursitis. Am Fam Physician 53:2317–2325, 1996.
5. Gray RG, Gottlieb N: Intra-articular corticosteroids. An updated assessment. Clin Orthop 177:235–263, 1983.
6. Hollander JL: Intralesional corticosteroid therapy in arthritis. Maryland Med J 19:62–70, 1970.
7. Kasten SJ, Louis DS: Carpal tunnel syndrome: A case of median nerve injection injury and a safe and effective method for injecting the carpal tunnel. J Fam Pract 43:79–82, 1996.
8. Kowal CN, Schumacher HR Jr: Approach to arthrocentesis of the upper extremities. Hosp Med Feb:89–90, 1992.
9. Larsson LG, Baum J: The syndrome of anserine bursitis: An overlooked diagnosis. Arthritis Rheum 28:1062–1065, 1985.
10. Leversee JH: Aspiration of joints and soft tissue injections. Prim Care 13:592–599, 1986.
11. Oppliger I: Arthrocentesis: Lower extremity. Hospital Med March 1992, pp 121–129.
12. Owen DS, Irby R: Intra-articular and soft tissue aspiration and injection. Clin Rheum Pract March–May: 52–63, 1986.
13. Owen DS Jr, Weiss JJ, Wilke WS: When to aspirate and inject joints. Patient Care 24(14):128–145, 1990.
14. Pfenninger JL: Infections of joint and soft tissue: Part I. General guidelines. Am Fam Physician 44:1196–1202, 1991.
15. Pfenninger JL: Injections of joints and soft tissue: Part II. Guidelines for specific joints. Am Fam Physician 44:1690–1701, 1991.
16. Pfenninger JL: Joint and soft tissue aspiration and injection. In Pfenninger JL, Fowler GC (eds): Procedures for Primary Care Physicians. St. Louis, Mosby, 1994, pp 1036–1059.
17. Roth SH: Nonsteroidal anti-inflammatory drugs: Gastropathy, deaths, and medical practice. Ann Int Med 109:353–354, 1988.
18. Salzman KL, Lillegard WA, Butcher ID: Upper extremity bursitis. Am Fam Physician 58(7):1797–1806, 1997.
19. Samuelson CO Jr, Cannon GW, Ward JR: Arthrocentesis. J Fam Pract 20:179–184, 1985.
20. Shell D, Perkins R, Cosgavea A: Septic olecranon bursitis: Recognition and treatment. J Am Board Fam Pract 8:217–220, 1995.
21. Shmerling RH, Delbanco TL, Tosteson AN, Trentham DE: Synovial fluid tests. What should be ordered? JAMA 264:1009–1014, 1990.
22. Smith DL, et al: Treatment of nonseptic olecranon bursitis: A controlled, blinded prospective trial. Arch Intern Med 149:2527–2531, 1989.

23. Solomon DH: Toxicity of nonsteroidal anti-inflammatory drugs in the elderly: Is advanced age a risk factor? Am J Med 102:208–215, 1997.
24. Stefanich RJ: Intra-articular corticosteroids in treatment of osteoarthritis. Orthop Rev 19:65–71, 1986.
25. Wilke WS, Tuggle CJ: Optimal techniques for intra-articular and periarticular joint injections. Mod Med 96:58–72, 1988.
26. Zuckerman JD, Meislin RJ, Rothberg M: Injections for joint and soft tissue disorders: When and how to use them. Geriatrics 45(4):45–52, 1990.

80. FUNCTIONAL BRACING IN ATHLETICS

L. Christine Dunn, B.S., L.A.T.C., and Brian J. E. Jones, M.S., A.T.C.-R.

1. What is the purpose of wearing a functional ankle brace?

A functional ankle brace allows an athlete with an ankle injury to return to competition sooner by helping to prevent recurrent injuries. An athlete with a history of ankle sprains who is not wearing an ankle brace has at least 5 times the risk of sustaining another ankle injury as a braced athlete.[15]

2. What is the difference between wearing an ankle brace and having an ankle taped?

Although freshly applied tape has been shown to be more supportive than braces, braces retain their stability through the course of activity, whereas the support provided by tape degenerates during activity.[13]

3. What different types of ankle braces are available?

The different styles of available ankle braces include lace-up braces, stirrup braces, and stirrup braces with hinges. The lace-up braces are composed primarily of tough nylon; they are generally lightweight and thin but durable enough to last at least one competitive season. The stirrup ankle brace is composed of two pieces of plastic that are molded to fit on the sides of the ankle. The plastic pieces may have foam or air pads to enhance comfort; they are held to the joint by wrapping Velcro straps around the ankle. Stirrup braces are helpful immediately after injury, but they are not highly functional because they do not allow maximal plantarflexion and dorsiflexion. The newer version of the stirrup brace is the stirrup brace with hinges, which has a hinge mechanism that allows plantarflexion and dorsiflexion. The most highly recommended style of brace is the stirrup with hinge, which provides the most stability while allowing maximal mobility.[12] Since no one brace is right for all athletes, brace selection should be based on individual needs.

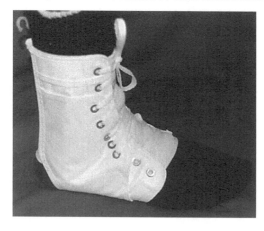

Lace-up ankle support.

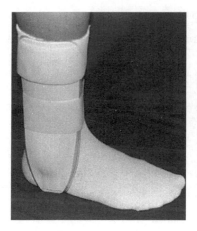
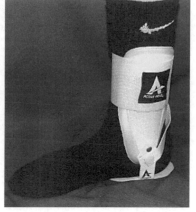

Stirrup ankle brace.   Stirrup with hinge ankle brace.

4. Will ankle braces restrict range of motion?

Most research indicates that the majority of ankle braces do not significantly reduce functional range of motion and do not affect normal running patterns.[7] It is the responsibility of the physician or the certified athletic trainer to examine an ankle brace before recommending it to an athlete. The brace should significantly reduce inversion, which is the most common mechanism for ankle sprains.[6] However, the brace should allow maximal plantarflexion and dorsiflexion.

5. How will an athlete's performance be affected by wearing an ankle brace?

Despite conflicting research, most studies indicate that ankle braces do not impede running patterns, agility, or vertical jump height.[11]

6. What are the criteria for selecting an ankle brace?

For people with chronic ankle instability, restriction of motion is a much greater concern than comfort. However, comfort is important if compliance is expected.[2] As with any other purchase, price and budget may be issues.

7. How much does an ankle brace cost?

Depending on the type of brace, an athlete may expect to spend $20–$40 on each brace. Although this may seem like a large out-of-pocket expense, when you consider that the cost of taping one ankle for an entire season may exceed $100, the cost advantage belongs to the brace.

8. Is the process of rehabilitation complete once the athlete returns to competition with a functional brace?

No. The athlete is not necessarily finished with rehabilitation once he or she returns to competition with the functional brace. The brace allows the athlete to return sooner, but he or she must still complete the rehabilitation protocol for the particular injury.

9. What is involved in the maintenance and upkeep of ankle braces?

The nylon lace-up braces may be cleaned in a washing machine. Replacement padding, air cells, and straps may be purchased at a minimal cost for the stirrup and stirrup braces with hinges. Proper maintenance increases the lifetime of the brace.

10. How many different types of knee braces are available?

Currently numerous types of braces are available for purchase either by written prescription from a physician or for over-the-counter purchase. Knee braces are divided into three categories based on their design and function[17]: rehabilitative braces, prophylactic braces, and functional braces.[10,17]

11. What is meant by the term *rehabilitative* knee brace?

A rehabilitative knee brace is designed to provide controlled motion early in the healing phase. Rehabilitative braces may be applied to injuries that have been treated operatively or non-operatively. Typical design features include:

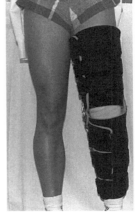

- Single axis or dual axis hinges
- Hinged arms that extend proximally along the thigh and distally along the lower leg
- Thigh and calf enclosures
- Straps that surround the hinged arms

Important characteristics of an ideal rehabilitative brace[10] include:

- Ability to control motion at the knee joint
- Adaptability to different leg sizes and shapes
- Durability
- Reasonable price
- Lack of migration
- Ease of application
- Availability

12. What is meant by the term *prophylactic* knee brace?

A prophylactic knee brace is designed to decrease the incidence and severity of valgus force injuries to the knee.[14] It is commonly used in high-risk collision sports such as football. The most common type of prophylactic knee brace is the lateral knee brace, which is designed to protect the knee from a contact load on the medial collateral ligament. Prophylactic braces are typically constructed with a single or double upright hinge and are usually strapped into place with Velcro straps or taped into place to secure the brace to the leg. A prophylactic brace may be purchased over-the-counter and generally costs around $20–$40.

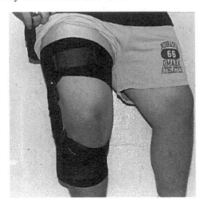

13. Is the routine use of a lateral prophylactic knee brace an effective means of preventing ligamentous injury to the knee?

This question has been debated continually over the past 10 years. During the mid 1980s, routine use of prophylactic knee braces was believed to decrease the incidence and severity of medial collateral ligament injuries. However, only a few studies have supported this belief,[1,14] whereas other studies have disputed the effectiveness of prophylactic bracing.[4,16] The American Academy of Orthopedic Surgeons warns that "routine use of prophylactic knee braces currently available has not been proven effective in reducing the number and severity of knee injuries."[9] Some studies even suggest that their use may actually increase the risk of medial collateral ligament, ankle sprains, and foot fractures.[4,5] It remains to be seen whether prophylactic knee braces are effective in reducing injuries to the medial collateral ligament of the knee. It may depend on the type of brace used, alignment of the player's leg, the ligamentous status of the athlete, position of the athlete, choice of footware, and surface interfaces.[17]

14. Will wearing a prophylactic knee brace affect performance and agility?

Once again, the answer depends on which study one reads. Most teams that use prophylactic braces require their use by offensive linemen, defensive linemen, and linebackers. One problem is that a prophylactic brace may loosen and slide down the leg. If this occurs, the brace will certainly affect performance and agility.

15. What is meant by the term *functional* knee brace?

A functional knee brace is designed to provide functional support to an unstable knee and to avoid further injury to a previously reconstructed knee joint.[17] The first functional knee brace was the Lennox Hill Derotational Brace, which was developed at Lennox Hill Hospital in New York in the early 1970s. Numerous types of functional knee derotational braces are now available. The most common use of a functional brace is after reconstructive surgery of the anterior cruciate ligament. Derotational braces typically incorporate similar designs; most use double-hinged uprights with range of motion stops, straps, or fitted cuffs or shells. These derotational braces may be a semicustom brace (below left) or a custom-fit brace[9] (below right).

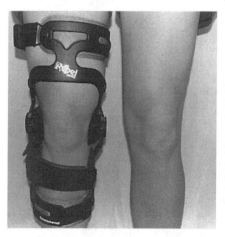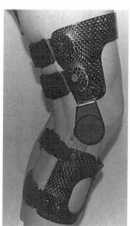

	SEMICUSTOM DEROTATIONAL BRACE	CUSTOM-FIT DEROTATIONAL BRACE
Advantages	Cheaper than a custom brace Typically costs around $500–$700 Ability to accommodate size changes of the affected leg Quick repair and service	Lightweight and durable Developed from a molded cast of the leg to help ensure a proper fit Good patient compliance
Disadvantages	May not fit well May migrate on the leg Poor durability Comes in standard sizes only (XS, S, M, L, XL, XXL)	High cost, typically around $1,200– $1,500 Inability to accommodate changes in leg size Slower turnaround time for repairs

16. Is the process of rehabilitation complete when an athlete begins to wear a functional knee brace?

No. The athlete needs to continue to develop strength and proprioception. The athlete probably needs to wear the brace for several months before returning to athletic activity. Some studies

suggest that athletes who wear a functional knee brace tend to lose muscular strength through muscle inhibition and a decrease in kinesthetic awareness. The primary concern of many clinicians is that the brace may provide a false sense of security.[17] Factors to consider before recommending a functional knee brace include:
- Joint stability after surgery
- Lower limb alignment
- Muscle girth
- Patient's strength and proprioception status
- Activity level of the patient
- Patient's psychological factors

17. How does a neoprene sleeve support the knee joint?

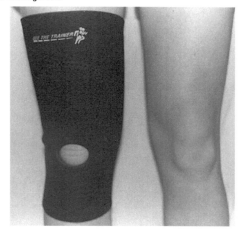

A neoprene sleeve may give no support to the knee, but it helps to increase the proprioception of the joint and provides warmth. Neoprene knee sleeves typically work well for the conservative management of general knee pain due to acute or chronic conditions. Patellofemoral problems generally require the use of a sleeve with a patellar cut-out as opposed to a closed patellar knee sleeve.

18. What other conditions may warrant the use of a neoprene knee sleeve?

A Palumbo lateral patella stabilizing brace (below, left), which is a neoprene knee brace with an open patella cut-out, may be used for the conservative or postoperative management of patellofemoral joint problems. It has a Y-shaped lateral buttress strap to decrease lateral patellar tracking.[8] Another type of neoprene knee sleeve has a double-hinged design to help protect the collateral ligaments of the knee (below, right). It is often indicated in the conservative treatment of injuries of the medial collateral ligament. The compression of the neoprene helps to reduce swelling, whereas the hinged action provides support to the injured knee.

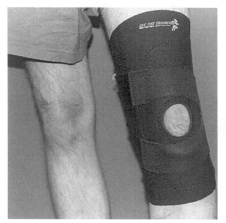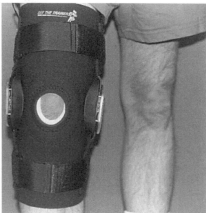

BIBLIOGRAPHY

1. Albright J, Powell J, Smith W, et al: Medial collateral ligament knee sprains in college football. Am J Sports Med 22:12–18, 1992.
2. Alves JW, Alday RV, Ketcham DL, Lentell GL: A comparison of the passive support provided by various ankle braces. J Orthop Sports Phys Ther 15:10–18, 1992.
3. Garrick J, Requa R: Prophylactic knee bracing. Am J Sports Med 15:471–476, 1987.
4. Grace T, Skipper B, Newberry J, et al: Prophylactic knee braces and injury to the lower extremity. J Bone Joint Surg 70A:422–427, 1988.
5. Hewson G, Mendin R, Wong J: Prophylactic knee bracing in college football. Am J Sports Med 14:262–266, 1991.
6. Kimura IF, Nawoczenski DA, Epler M, Owen MG: Effect of the AirStirrup in controlling ankle inversion stress. J Orthop Sports Phys Ther 9(5):190–193, 1987.
7. Lindley TR, Kernozek TW: Taping and semirigid bracing may not affect ankle functional range of motion. J Athlet Train 30(2):109–112, 1995.
8. Mellion M, Walsh W, Shelton G (eds): The Team Physician's Handbook, 2nd ed. Philadelphia, Hanley & Belfus, 1997.
9. Nash H: American Academy of Orthopedic Surgeons Report: Braces may not prevent knee injuries. Physician Sports Med 16:57, 1988.
10. Paulos LE, et al: The biomechanics of lateral knee bracing. Am J Sports Med 15:419–429, 1987.
11. Pienkowski D, McMorrow M, Shapiro R, et al: The effect of ankle stabilizers on athletic performance. Am J Sports Med 23:757–762, 1995.
12. Romaniello B: Functional ankle bracing. Sports Med Update 11(4):8–12, 1996.
13. Shapiro MS, Kabo M, Mitchell PW, et al: Ankle sprain prophylaxis: An analysis of the stabilizing effects of bracing and tape. Am J Sports Med 22:78–82, 1994.
14. Sitler M, Ryan J, Hopkinson W, et al: The efficiency of a prophylactic brace to reduce knee injuries in football. Am J Sports Med 18:310–315, 1990.
15. Surve I, Schwellnus MP, Noakes T, Lombard C: A fivefold reduction in the incidence of recurrent ankle sprains in soccer players using the sport-stirrup orthosis. Am J Sports Med 22:601–606, 1994.
16. Teitz C, Hermanson B, Kronamal R, et al: Evaluation of the use of braces to prevent injury to the knee in collegiate football players. J Bone Joint Surg 69A:510–521, 1987.
17. Wilk K: Is knee bracing effective? Sports Med Update 11(4):4–7, 1996.

81. ATHLETIC TAPING

Thomas A. Frette, M.A., ATC

Proper diagnosis, immediate care and treatment, and rehabilitation of sports-related injuries are of vital importance. The use of stabilizing and supporting measures (i.e., taping, bracing) assists the quick and safe return to play. Athletic taping or bracing, along with a treatment protocol, is an excellent tool to facilitate the injured athlete's return to play without placing him or her at greater risk of injury. Tape that is applied improperly or for no specific purpose may predispose an athlete to injury or add to the severity of an existing injury.

1. Why is taping used?
The application of athletic tape has two main goals: to promote a potentially faster return to play and to prevent further injury. Both goals can be accomplished by preventing a specific body part from being placed in a biomechanically compromised position that may be potentially harmful to the injured or noninjured athlete.

2. When is taping indicated?
Whether an injury is acute or chronic, athletic tape may be used when there is a need to add support and stability to an injured or weakened area. Keep in mind that the use of athletic tape must have a specific purpose. Taping for the sake of taping may place the athlete at a greater risk of injury.

3. What are the contraindications to the use of athletic tape?

If an athlete sustains an injury that may require an aggressive form of stabilization, athletic taping may not be sufficient; a more rigid form of support may be necessary. The use of athletic tape to restrict a joint's normal range of motion is also contraindicated; it may lead to a decrease in the function of the joint and possibly to secondary problems. Other contraindications include the presence of inflammation or effusion, skin allergies or reactions to the tape or tape adherent, and taping over skin lacerations.

4. Is the rehabilitation process complete once taping the injured area is initiated?

Using athletic tape is an excellent method to speed the athlete's return to play, but ultimately the athlete should strive to be independent of prophylactic taping. The appropriate use of rehabilitation associated with athletic taping facilitates functional return to activity. When using athletic tape as a means of injury prevention, the supporting structures must be considered. Athletes should be encouraged to engage in a training program that emphasizes strength, endurance, and proprioception to the affected area.

5. Is an Ace bandage an effective means of support?

The proper use of an Ace bandage is to compress an injured area; it is not a means of support. When used in conjunction with felt or foam padding, an Ace bandage helps to control or resolve localized edema or effusion. Another use of the Ace bandage is to hold protective padding in place. Spica wraps, used most frequently with shoulder, hip, and groin injuries, provide mild muscular support and help to prevent the body part from being forced beyond its normal range of motion.

6. How do you choose between athletic taping or bracing?

Although controversy surrounds the use of bracing, studies have demonstrated that braces are an effective means of support without diminishing an athlete's level of performance.[9] In choosing between taping and bracing, available resources must be taken into consideration. For taping, the athlete must have access to a certified athletic trainer or a person who has been proficiently trained in taping techniques. If such a person is not available, bracing may be the proper choice.

7. Do athletes have a preference for taping or bracing?

Although recommendations can be made, every athlete has an individual preference. Psychologically, emotional support may be gained from the person applying the tape. Tape also provides added physical comfort to the athlete compared with bracing. On the other hand, bracing has the ability to maintain support for extended periods as well as or better than tape.[3] In addition, bracing provides increased convenience through self-application.

8. Which is more cost-effective—taping or bracing?

Over the long term (i.e., athletic season), bracing is probably the more cost-effective choice. For example, a standard roll of athletic tape for the ankle, at university wholesale cost, is approximately $1.25 per roll. Taping one ankle should be completed with roughly ¾ of a roll of tape. The cost is about 94 cents. Taping one ankle, 6 times per week, costs $5.64. Over a 16-week season, the cost rises to $90.24. This price includes only the cost of the tape—not the cost of the prewrap, tape adherent, or heel and lace pads. Compare this price to that of one ankle brace ($15–$25), and the fiscal advantage of bracing is obvious.

9. Is there a proper method for the application of athletic tape?

Every certified athletic trainer or person with proficient taping skills has a unique style or technique for taping. Below are general guidelines for the application of athletic tape:

1. Place the area in need of support in a stabilizing, yet functional, position.
2. Surface to be taped should be clean, dry, and free of body hair.
3. Apply tape adherent to aid in the bonding properties of the tape.

4. If desired, a polyurethane foam underwrap can be applied between the adherent and the tape. The underwrap adds comfort, but certain precautions should be used:
   • A single layer of underwrap ensures proper tape adherence and reduction of friction.
   • Lubricants should be used on high-friction areas (i.e., the heel and lace areas of the ankle).
5. Apply anchor strips initially, if indicated.
6. Avoid the use of continuous strapping because of possible constriction of the vascular and neurologic supply to the affected area.
7. Each strip of tape should overlap the previous strip by one-half to prevent spaces that may result in blister formations.
8. Follow the surface contour of the taped area to allow a smooth appearance. Athletic tape does not possess the elastic qualities to conform to sharp angles; thus, the tape should not be forced in a specific direction but should be allowed to follow its natural path.
9. To allow for optimal form and function, elastic tape may be used over muscular areas.
10. The pressure of the tape should be equal throughout its application.

10. Once tape has been applied, how long should it be left in place as a means of support?

In general, the tape should be removed after the activity. The area then should be cleansed thoroughly, removing all tape residue. In certain cases, the tape may be left in place for extended periods (e.g., patellofemoral taping).

11. How long does it take to become a proficient taper?

There is no specific answer, although individual skill and amount of practice are essential factors. For example, taping the ankle 50 times is the estimated requirement to reach a minimal level of competence. Once again, the individual's skill level is a crucial factor. When taping competence has been achieved, skills must be maintained by regular practice.

12. Is taping of an injured knee an effective means of support?

Once used extensively for support of an injured knee, taping has been replaced almost entirely by commercially manufactured braces. Many braces are custom-fit and provide support for specific injuries to the knee. Although knee braces tend to be costly, they provide greater support and increased comfort. In acute knee injuries, athletic taping may still prove to be effective, especially in conjunction with a knee brace.

BIBLIOGRAPHY

1. American Academy of Orthopedic Surgeons: Athletic Training and Sports Medicine, 2nd ed. Parkridge, IL, American Academy of Orthopedic Surgeons, 1991.
2. Arnheim DD: Principles of Athletic Training, 8th ed. St. Louis, Mosby, 1993.
3. Bunch RP, Bednarski K, Holland D, Macinanti R: Ankle joint support: A comparison of reusable lace-on braces with taping and wrapping. Physician Sports Med 13(5):59–62, 1985.
4. Fandel D, Frette T: Taping and bracing. In Mellion MB (ed): The Team Physician's Handbook, 2nd ed. Philadelphia, Hanley & Belfus, 1997, pp 617–638.
5. Feuerbach JW, Grabiner MD: Effect of the Aircast on unilateral postural control: Amplitude and frequency variables. J Orthop Sports Phys Ther 7:149–154, 1993.
6. Greene TA, Wright CR: A competitive support evaluation of three ankle orthoses before, during and after exercise. J Orthop Sports Phys Ther 11:453–466, 1990.
7. Mellion MB: Office Management of Sports Injuries and Athletic Problems. Philadelphia, Hanley & Belfus, 1988.
8. Paris DL, Sullivan SJ: Isometric strength of rearfoot inversion and eversion in nonsupported, taped, and braced ankles assessed by a hand-held dynamometer. J Orthop Sports Phys Ther 15:229–255, 1992.
9. Paris DL: The effects of the Swede-O, New Cross, and McDavid ankle braces and adhesive ankle taping on speed, balance, agility, and vertical jump. J Athlet Train 27:253–256, 1992.
10. Roy S, Irvin R: Sports Medicine: Prevention, Evaluation, Management, and Rehabilitation. Englewood Cliffs, NJ, Prentice-Hall, 1993.

XI. Specific Sports

82. FOOTBALL

Kevin N. Waninger, M.D., and John A. Lombardo, M.D.

1. What are the most common injuries in football?

It is estimated that more than 300,000 high school players, 35,000 college players, and one-half of all National Football League (NFL) players are injured to some extent each football season. Lower extremity injuries account for approximately 50% of all football injuries, whereas upper extremity injuries account for 30%. The most frequently injured body parts are the knee (medial collateral ligament, followed by meniscus and anterior cruciate ligament), ankle, shoulder, and upper leg. In general, sprains and strains account for approximately 40% of injuries; contusions, 25%; fractures, 10%; dislocations, 5%; and concussions, 5%.

2. What are the major causes of nontraumatic deaths in football?

Arrhythmias, heart failure (myocarditis), heat stroke, sickle cell crisis, and asthma account for most of the nontraumatic deaths in football players on the playing fields or sidelines.

3. What about the use of ammonia capsules for the dazed athlete?

Ammonia capsules have no role in care of the head-injured athlete. In a dazed, semiconscious athlete, a controlled verbal arousal with cervical spine precautions should be undertaken until the athlete is coherent and a full assessment of injuries can be made.

4. Do players need supplemental water and salt replacement?

Players should have free access to water during both practice and games. Daily weights before and after practice may be used as an indicator of water loss and as a guide for water replacement. The specific gravity and color of the urine also may be used as a rough indicator of hydration status. No evidence supports any benefit from salt replacement tablets in players who consume a balanced diet. However, because many households have eliminated salt from cooking and dinner tables, inclusion of salty foods or moderate use of table salt by athletes during times of high heat and/or humidity may be helpful.

5. Discuss the need for on-field oxygen.

Professional football mandates the presence of on-field oxygen for players during the game. However, in athletes with no underlying pulmonary, hematologic, or cardiac problems, any additional benefit of supplemental oxygen is minimal, and routine use of supplemental oxygen for brief periods during recovery from exhaustive exercise has not been shown to hasten recovery or to improve subsequent exercise performance.[23] The measured pO_2 of the blood plasma may increase, but this increase does not translate into increased oxygen-carrying capacity, because the hemoglobin is near maximally saturated under normal conditions.

6. Do nasal strips have any documented value?

Nasal strips are small adhesive strips that, according to anecdotal reports from many athletes, mechanically open nasal passages and allow easier breathing. Although some initial studies claim success in improving snoring patterns, nasal congestion, and allergic rhinitis, no physiologic data suggest increased oxygen uptake or improved physical performance in athletes using nasal strips.

7. Discuss the on-field approach to the helmeted football player with head and neck injuries.

The algorithm below presents an organized, systematic approach to the helmeted football player with head or neck injuries. Athletes who regain consciousness after a brief episode of unconsciousness may enter the conscious algorithm if an experienced examining physician determines that the athlete's mental status will not compromise a reliable physical examination.

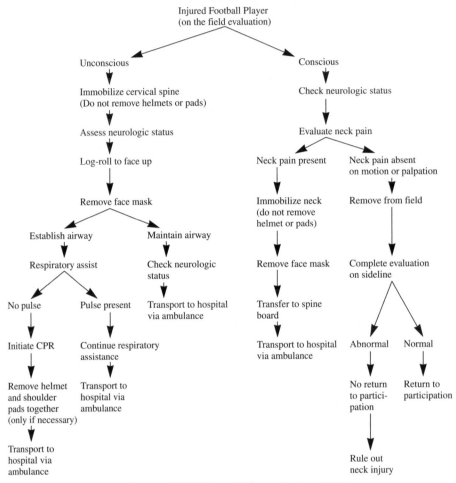

An algorithm for field decision making in head and neck injuries.

8. Discuss the management of a player with a head injury.

Concussions are the most common consequence of head injury in football, with an estimated annual incidence of 250,000. It is estimated that among high school football players one in five will experience a minor head injury each season. Several classification systems for the head-injured athlete have been published in the literature, but no universal agreement exists about the grading systems and subsequent management.

Team physicians are frequently faced with the question of when a player with a head injury may return to competition. In football, the chance of having a second concussion is estimated to be 4 times greater than the chance of sustaining a first concussion. Repeated concussions appear to cause cumulative damage, resulting in increasing severity and duration with each concussion. A second relatively minor head injury in players who are still symptomatic from a prior concussion may result in catastrophic brain swelling, the so-called second-impact syndrome. Thus, careful evaluation of the head-injured athlete is necessary before clearance for return to sports.

In the most common form of concussion the athlete suffers only momentary confusion without amnesia or loss of consciousness. This concussion is typified by the athlete who gets his or her "bell rung." Mild alterations in balance, coordination, and gait may be present. Such athletes should be removed from the game and evaluated serially for the development of amnesia or postconcussive symptoms (dizziness, headache, nausea, photophobia). The period of confusion and neurologic alteration is normally short, lasting from 5–15 minutes, before the athlete returns to baseline mental status. When all symptoms and signs *fully* resolve, the athlete may return to participation.

The literature offers limited scientific support for any of the rules for return to competition after a concussive head injury. Athletes who remain symptomatic or exhibit retrograde or post-traumatic amnesia and athletes who had loss of consciousness should not be allowed to return to participation on the day of injury. It is not uncommon for such athletes to suffer postconcussive symptoms consisting of persistent headache, irritability, fatigue, visual difficulties, dizziness, behavioral problems, or inability to concentrate. The athlete should not be allowed to return to participation until all symptoms have resolved and the physical examination is normal. If significant loss of consciousness and/or posttraumatic amnesia occurs, the time to return to competition may be delayed further.

The guidelines for return to competition after multiple head injuries are even more variable. The length of time before return to contact depends on the number of concussions as well as the timing and severity of each episode. Each athlete needs to be counseled individually about return to play, and factors such as level of play, importance of play to the athlete, and potential health risks and consequences need to be involved in the decision-making process.

9. How is the spearing technique implicated in cervical spine injuries?

Most cervical spine injuries result from excessive axial loading combined with flexion (more common) or extension.[20] Most injuries associated with quadriplegia occur during tackling; a "spearing" technique is implicated in over one-half of such incidents. Defensive backs, special team players, and linebackers play the most vulnerable positions. When a player lowers the head to ram an opponent (30° flexion), the cervical spine is straightened, converting a normally lordotic curve into a segmented column. At the time of collision, the head stops but the trunk keeps moving, compressing the cervical spine. When the compressive force cannot be dissipated by controlled motion in the spinal segments, the cervical spine flexes and buckles, with resulting fracture, subluxation, or dislocation.[19,20] Rule changes instituted in 1976 prohibiting use of the head as a primary and initial contact area of blocking and tackling have resulted in a dramatic decrease in the incidence of cervical spine injuries in football.

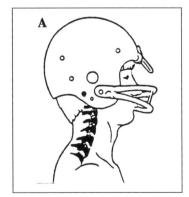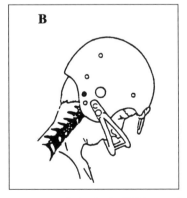

When the head and neck are in a normal upright position (*A*), the cervical spine is slightly extended because of neutral cervical lordosis. When the neck is flexed about 30° (*B*), the cervical spine is straightened, converting it to a segmented column. *(Figure continued on following page.)*

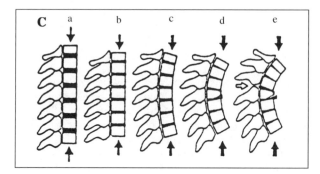

The straightened cervical spine behaves like a segmented column when it is subjected to an axial loading force. The force first causes compressive deformation of the intervertebral discs (*C*, a and b). As the energy input continues and maximum compressive deformation is reached, the spine flexes and buckles (*C*, c) with resulting fracture, subluxation, or dislocation (*C*, d and e). The sequence of events occurs in as little as 8.4 seconds. (From Fine KM, et al: Prevention of cervical spine injuries in football. Phys Sportsmed 19(10):56, 1991, with permission.)

10. What is the current opinion about helmet removal on the field in football players with a potential cervical spine injury?

Improper handling of an unstable neck in the prehospital setting may result in potential iatrogenically induced neurologic injury. The potential for spinal instability after cervical spine trauma, as well as the inability to access the cervical spine fully in the prehospital setting, mandates cautious handling of the injured helmeted athlete until the extent of skeletal and neurologic injury can be defined. For this reason, sports medicine professionals almost universally discourage removal of a football helmet when cervical spine injury is suspected. The unique characteristics of the properly fitted football helmet allow safe access to airway and cervical spine management, and helmets should not be removed unless absolutely necessary.[22] Current guidelines from the National Collegiate Athletic Association for helmet management for an athlete with a potential injury to the head or neck state that unless there are special circumstances such as respiratory distress coupled with an inability to access the airway, the helmet should not be removed on the field when there is a potential head/neck injury.[12]

11. Describe the technique of helmet face mask removal.

Trainers and emergency medical personnel should have the proper equipment to remove the face mask if airway access is required. Do not remove the chin straps unless necessary. The face mask is attached to the football helmet by four plastic clips. All four clips should be cut carefully to remove the face mask completely.[3] Simple retraction of the face mask by cutting only the lower clips may subject the patient to more head and neck movement than complete face mask removal.[7,8] The chin strap should remain in place. The plastic clips can be cut off easily with special tools that should be readily available during practices as well as games. The Trainers Angel is currently the most widely used tool for face mask removal, but less expensive alternatives available in most hardware stores include commercially available cutting pliers (Channel Lock no. 148-10) or anvil pruners.[7,15] Using a screwdriver to unscrew the plastic clips is not recommended because of the possibility of damaged or rusted screws, the deleterious torque associated with manual screwdrivers, and the need for charged electric screwdrivers. This helmet design enables prehospital providers to gain access to the airway without having to remove the helmet. Professionals working with football teams should be well skilled in the methods of face mask removal; it is a learned skill that needs to be practiced.

12. Why must helmet and shoulder pads be removed simultaneously?

If the helmet is removed, shoulder pads should also be removed; removal of equipment should be an all-or-none proposition.[13,14,17] With the helmet removed and shoulder pads in place, the head tends to hyperextend, with a significant increase in the amount of cervical lordosis. Currently, there is no effective immobilization device for the athlete's helmetless head without simultaneous shoulder pad removal. It is recommended that any attempt at helmet removal be delayed until the helmet and shoulder pads can be removed together in a controlled setting such as the locker room or emergency department.[22]

13. Describe the technique for helmet and shoulder pad removal.

When equipment removal is required, it should be performed only by personnel trained in the procedure. The neck with potential cervical spine injury should be stabilized on a backboard with helmet and shoulder pads in place and face mask removed[7] (as previously discussed). Careful placement of a rigid collar should be attempted. If possible, proper radiographs should be obtained before removal of the helmet. Manual in-line stabilization should be maintained throughout the procedure. Helmet and shoulder pads should be removed simultaneously. The helmet's chin strap is cut just before helmet removal. The helmet is removed by first unsnapping the cheek pads and then expanding the helmet laterally to clear the ears. It is helpful to remove glasses before helmet removal if possible. Shoulder pads can be removed by cutting away the jersey, the lacing on the front and back of the shoulder pads, and the straps under the player's arms. While manual stabilization of the cervical spine is maintained, the pads can be carefully separated and slid off.[3,4,15]

14. When should you recommend helmet and shoulder pad removal in the field by prehospital personnel?

Equipment removal in the field may be considered when the face mask or visor cannot be removed safely and interferes with adequate airway management; the helmet is so loose that adequate spinal immobilization cannot be obtained with the helmet in place; a head injury or chest wound requires direct inspection; or shoulder pads interfere with the delivery of adequate chest compressions. In athletes requiring airway management and equipment removal on the field, protocols have been established.[3,4,15]

15. Is respiratory compromise requiring intubation common in helmeted football players with cervical spine injury?

Cervical spine injuries in helmeted football players tend to occur anatomically in the vertebrae from C5 to C7, and respiratory compromise is uncommon at these levels.[20] If intubation is required, practitioners should choose the method with which they have the greatest experience and skill.

16. How can we prepare for the clinical scenario of a football player with cervical spine injury?

There is a need for greater communication between the sports medicine team and local emergency providers about neck management in the helmeted football player. Prehospital and sports medicine teams should formulate a plan in advance to prepare for unexpected clinical scenarios such as cervical spine injuries, and skills such as facemask and helmet removal should be practiced.

17. What is a "stinger" or "burner"? How is it managed?

Burners or stingers are the most frequent nerve injury in football players. The most common mechanism in football is thought to be traction or compression of the brachial plexus, causing traumatic neurapraxia of the involved nerve roots. The general trend is that such injuries are more common in defensive players and occur more often in games than in practice.

The athlete may report unilateral symptoms such as burning or stinging pain, numbness, and tingling radiating down the affected arm from the supraclavicular area into the fingers. These signs are frequently accompanied by weakness, with a relative absence of associated neck pain or stiffness. The athlete may try to relieve the discomfort by shaking the arm, holding the involved arm with the other hand, and bending the waist to the involved side. The upper part of the brachial plexus containing the nerve roots C5 and C6 is usually involved. The most common motor deficit is deltoid weakness; thus shoulder abduction should be checked routinely in all athletes with burners. Mild biceps and serrati muscle weakness may also be present. Symptoms usually resolve within several minutes. The athlete with full active range of motion without pain and a normal neurologic examination may return to competition.

Cervical spine radiographs to investigate spinal disease are recommended for athletes who exhibit persistent symptoms or findings 24 hours after injury as well as athletes with recurrent episodes.[10] An electromyogram (EMG) is not an appropriate guide for return to competition because abnormalities may persist for years despite clinical recovery. Preventive measures include a neck and shoulder conditioning program, instruction on proper tackling technique, a neck roll, and properly fitting equipment.

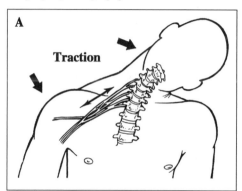 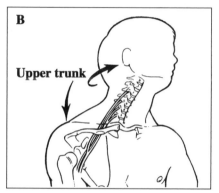

A blow to the head causing lateral flexion and shoulder depression may cause a traction injury (A) to the upper trunk of the brachial plexus. A compression injury (B) may occur when a blow to the supraclavicular region causes lateral flexion with rotation and extension of the cervical spine away from the blow. (From Nissen SJ, et al: Burner syndrome: Recognition and rehabilitation. Phys Sportsmed 24(6):58, 1996, with permission.)

18. What is transient quadriplegia? How is it managed?

Transient quadriplegia is an episode of cervical cord neurapraxia that occurs after forceful hyperextension, hyperflexion, or axial loading of the cervical spine. Symptoms include burning, numbness, tingling, or complete loss of sensation, with accompanying motor weakness or complete paralysis in all four extremities. There may be no associated neck pain, and the episode is transient, with complete recovery within 10–15 minutes, although some cases gradually resolve over 36–48 hours. Note that symptoms are bilateral, which often differentiates this clinical entity from "stingers" or "burners."

A complete work-up, including a magnetic resonance imaging (MRI) scan of the cervical spine, should be performed because transient quadriplegia has been associated with spinal stenosis, congenital fusion, cervical instability, and disc disease. Further participation in a contact sport such as football should be strongly discouraged in a case of transient quadriplegia associated with the following:

- Structural cervical abnormality
- Ligamentous laxity
- Intervertebral disc disease
- Degenerative disc disease
- MRI evidence of cord defects or swelling
- Symptoms or positive neurologic findings lasting longer than 36 hours
- More than one occurrence

If a player sustains a one-time episode of cervical cord neurapraxia without the findings noted above, the decision to return to contact sports is made on an individualized basis. No strong evidence indicates that an athlete who experiences such an episode is predisposed to future permanent neurologic injury.[18] Careful thought must be taken before returning such athletes to contact sports.

19. How do you diagnose and manage a clavicular fracture?

Clavicular fractures are common fractures in young football players and occur during a fall on the point of the shoulder or a direct blow to the clavicle. Visible and palpable clavicular deformity with marked swelling, ecchymosis, and pain is present. On-the-field management includes a thorough upper extremity neurovascular examination and chest auscultation to rule out the rare complication of ipsilateral pneumothorax due to posterior displacement of one of the fragments. Clavicular fractures are generally treated nonoperatively, and athletes may return to full contact sports as soon as full range of motion, normal strength, and clinical union are demonstrated. A padded donut worn under the shoulder pads may decrease discomfort upon return to play. Because of the high incidence of clavicular refractures, care must be taken to ensure clinical union before resumption of contact activities.

20. Discuss the management of acute anterior shoulder dislocation.

Over 95% of acute shoulder dislocations are anterior dislocations of the glenohumeral joint. In football, they occur when a runner or tackler gets his arm forced into excessive abduction, external rotation, and extension. When a young athlete sustains an acute first-time dislocation on the field, relocation can be attempted, depending on the physician's level of comfort with the diagnosis and skill with relocation. When radiographs are available, documentation of the dislocation without fracture can be obtained before attempted reduction. Note the neurovascular status before and after reduction, and obtain radiographic confirmation of relocation with views in two different planes, preferably an anteroposterior view and either an axillary or scapular Y-view.

The frequency of recurrent instability in school-aged athletes after a primary dislocation is high (50%) regardless of the treatment. First-time dislocations can be immobilized initially for comfort, but range of motion with external rotation to the neutral plane is begun as soon as tolerated. An aggressive functional rehabilitation and strengthening program can be instituted. Athletes may return to sports when they have attained painless full range of motion with at least 90% strength compared with the contralateral shoulder. Limitation shoulder harnesses are available to wear during play and may help to stabilize the shoulder and prevent redislocations.

Recurrent anterior-inferior subluxations and dislocations are often resistant to rehabilitation programs owing to the presence of injury to the labral-ligamentous complex. Often, relocation of the recurrent dislocated shoulder can be accomplished easily on the field. A young player with recurrent anterior instability may elect to finish the season after a program of strengthening exercises. Surgical stabilization in the off-season is usually advisable for such athletes if they wish to continue to participate in contact sports such as football.

21. Does posterior shoulder instability occur in football players?

Symptomatic posterior shoulder instability[9] is seen mainly in offensive linemen and other blockers as a result of the recent rule changes that permit extension of arms from the body during pass blocking. The shoulder girdle is pushed posteriorly, and with repetitive trauma the shoulder may sublux or dislocate posteriorly. The treatment of posterior instability centers on flexibility and muscle-strengthening exercises, specifically the rotator cuff muscles and scapular stabilizers. Players who have posterior instability should adjust weight training exercises that stress the shoulder posteriorly, such as the bench press. Offensive linemen who lock elbows at the time of contact during blocking have noted an associated increased occurrence of posterior shoulder problems, and a modification of blocking technique that uses bent elbows at the time of initial contact has been associated with decreased posterior instability complications.

One should start with physical therapy, instituting posterior cuff-strengthening exercises. No posterior stabilization surgical procedures have been proved effective, but preliminary studies suggest that newer techniques may be beneficial in selected patients.[6] The occurrence and recognition of this entity have recently increased; therefore, the natural history and success of various management strategies are presently unclear.

22. What is jersey finger?

Jersey finger is an avulsion of the flexor digitorum profundus tendon. It is commonly seen in a football player who attempts to tackle an opponent by grabbing his jersey. The ring finger is most commonly involved, followed by the middle finger. It presents as an inability to flex the distal interphalangeal joint independently. The athlete reports the feeling of a "pop" as the tendon ruptures. Pain and ecchymosis can be palpated at the base of the finger. Often the retracted ruptured tendon also can be palpated. Delayed diagnosis may lead to a worse surgical outcome; thus early diagnosis and surgical reattachment are the treatment of choice.

23. What is blocker's or tackler's exostosis?

Blocker's exostosis is an area of painful bony prominence that results from direct blows to the anterolateral humerus distal to the edge of the shoulder pads. Bone forms in continuity with the cortex, grows by accretion, and results from periosteal damage at the insertion of the deltoid or at the origin of the brachialis. Early recognition and treatment are important because the localized pain and swelling may be disabling. Initial treatment consists of ice, rest, compression dressing, and hematoma aspiration if necessary. Local padding is usually sufficient to allow play, and surgical excision is rarely required if the area remains painful despite conservative management. Improvements in prophylactic padding have significantly decreased the incidence of this problem.

24. Discuss the management of thigh contusions.

Thigh contusions are extremely common in football secondary to direct blunt trauma to the quadriceps muscle. Severe contusions may lead to myositis ossificans, which has been reported in 9–20% of thigh contusions that have been treated inadequately. It is unclear exactly why some thigh hematomas form ossification and others do not. However, the use of aggressive physical therapy[16,22] and nonsteroidal antiinflammatory drugs (NSAIDs) has been shown to decrease the incidence. Treatment strategies are aimed at limiting the hemorrhage and edema in the muscle itself, treating the loss of motion at the knee joint, and maintaining muscular strength. Some advocate initial strapping of the knee in 120° of flexion to limit hemorrhage in severe contusions. Therapeutic modalities such as massage and ultrasound should be avoided early in the course of treatment. Athletes may return to competition when full range of motion is present and 90% of contralateral leg strength returns.

25. Prophylactic knee bracing: fact or fiction?

Present studies do not conclusively support or disprove the use of routine bracing. Conditioning and strengthening as well as rule changes outlawing improper blocking techniques appear to have been more important in the prevention of knee injuries. Some athletes may benefit simply from the proprioceptive benefits of bracing. The decision to wear a brace should be left to the individual athlete.

26. What is a hip pointer? How is it managed?

Hip pointers result from either a contusion to the iliac crest or a separation of muscle fibers pulled from the crest. A bruised iliac crest may result in marked local pain and swelling, causing considerable disability to the athlete. Tenderness and lameness may persist for days or weeks, and injuries should be treated as early as possible. An x-ray film may be taken to rule out iliac crest fracture, especially in the high school athlete who may have avulsion or fracture of the iliac crest apophysis. However, radiographs are not necessarily required if the clinician is confident with the diagnosis. A fluctuant hematoma may be aspirated if present. The acute application of compression dressings, ice, rest, and NSAIDs may be instituted early. In physically mature athletes, injection of the acute hematoma with a small amount of local anesthetics and corticosteroid may decrease morbidity. Return to play with protective hip padding is generally allowed when the pain is tolerated and the gait has returned to normal. Such injuries can be prevented by wearing properly positioned hip pads.

27. What are the causes of back pain in football players?

Low back pain is a common problem in football players. In treating school-aged athletes with low back pain, common conditions to consider include sprains and strains, apophyseal fractures, and discogenic pain.[1] Although most low back pain in young athletes is related to trauma, developmental, infectious, neoplastic, or visceral conditions also must be considered.

Spondylolysis appears to be the most common cause of recalcitrant low back pain.[11] Interior linemen have been identified as susceptible to this disorder, but it may develop in players at any position. Other factors such as weight training errors or congenital predisposition may contribute. The usual presentation for a young athlete with a spondylolytic injury is chronic low back pain that is unilateral and nonradicular. The pain is exacerbated with hyperextension and twisting and relieved in the supine position. Tight musculature with decreased flexibility is usually noted.

In players with clinical symptoms highly suggestive of an isthmic pars lesion and normal radiographs, a bone scan with single-photon emission computed tomography (SPECT) gives a detailed topographic evaluation of the vertebrae in question. CT scanning may give additional information to help determine the type of fracture and treatment course.[2] Restricting vigorous activity and bracing may allow this process to heal, thus preventing a subroentgenographic stress reaction from becoming a radiographically detectable defect. If a defect of the pars interarticularis consistent with spondylolysis is noted on plain radiographs, the prospect for bony healing is small.

Patients may be treated conservatively with NSAIDs and a temporary reduction in activity level. Rehabilitation involves generalized strengthening and flexibility exercises, with special attention to the hip extensors, abdominal and back musculature, and dynamic lumbar stabilizers. Players may return to play when they can tolerate the discomfort and perform functionally.

28. What is turf toe?

Turf toe is a sprain of the plantar capsular-ligament complex with damage to the articular cartilage of the metatarsal heads or the base of the proximal phalanx. It occurs most often in the large toe, although all toes are susceptible. The mechanism is commonly a hyperextension injury at the metatarsophalangeal (MTP) joint as another player falls on the elevated heel. It also may occur in football linemen as they push off. Firm, artificial playing surfaces and lightweight, flexible shoes are predisposing factors. One of the hallmarks of diagnosis is increasing pain at the MTP joint beginning several hours after the initial injury, with ecchymosis, swelling, and plantar tenderness beneath the metatarsal head. Radiographs are negative, and initial treatment includes rest, ice, compression, elevation, NSAIDs, and antiinflammatory modalities. Protective aids with donut padding, special taping techniques, orthotics, and rigid steel inserts stabilize the joint during motion and facilitate return to play. Turf toe injuries may be temporarily disabling, and full athletic participation may begin as soon as the player can tolerate full weight-bearing. Properly fitting shoes with a rigid forefoot are recommended to prevent recurrence. The probability of developing long-term sequelae, including hallux rigidus and metatarsalgia, can be decreased with proper management.

BIBLIOGRAPHY

1. Barton B, Hough DO, Barnes RP, Micheli LJ: Low back pain in athletes. Sports Sci Exchange 6(1):1–4, 1995.
2. Congeni J, McCulloch J, Swanson K: Lumbar spondylosis: A study of natural progression in athletes. Am J Sports Med 25:248–253, 1997.
3. Denegar C, Saliba E: On the field management of the potential cervical spine injured football player. Athl Train J NATA 24:108–111, 1989.
4. Feld F: Management of the critically injured football player. J Athl Training 28:206–212, 1993.
5. Fine KM, Vegso JJ, Sennett B, Torg JS: Prevention of cervical spine injuries in football. Phys Sportsmed 19(10):54–64, 1991.
6. Hardy P, Thabit G, Fanton GS, et al: Arthroscopic management of recurrent anterior shoulder dislocation by combining a labrum suture with antero-inferior holmium: YAG laser capsular shrinkage. Orthopade 25:91–93, 1996.

7. Kleiner DM: Football helmet face mask removal. Athl Ther Today 1:11–13, 1996.
8. Kleiner DM: Face mask removal vs. mask retraction [abstract]. J Athl Train 31(2):S32, 1996.
9. McFarland EG, Campbell G, McDowell J: Posterior shoulder laxity in asymptomatic athletes. Am J Sports Med 24:468–471, 1996.
10. Meyer SA, Schulte KR, Callaghan JJ, et al: Cervical spinal stenosis and stingers in collegiate football players. Am J Sports Med 22(2):158–166, 1994.
11. Micheli LJ, Wood R: Back pain in young athletes. Significant differences from adults in causes and patterns. Arch Pediatr Adolesc Med 149:15–18, 1995.
12. NCAA 1997–1998 Sports Medicine Handbook, 9th ed. Overland Park, NCAA, 1997, pp 67–68.
13. Nissen SJ, Laskowski ER, Rizzo TD: Burner syndrome: Recognition and rehabilitation. Phys Sportsmed 24(6):57–64, 1996.
14. Palumbo MA, Hulstyn MJ, Fadale PD, et al: The effect of protective football equipment on alignment of the injured cervical spine. Radiographic analysis in a cadaveric model. Am J Sports Med 24:446–453, 1996.
15. Prinsen RKE, Syrotuik DG, Reid DC: Position of the cervical vertebrae during helmet removal and cervical collar application in football and hockey. Clin J Sports Med 5:155–161, 1995.
16. Segan RD, Cassidy C, Bentkowski J: A discussion of the issue of football helmet removal in suspected cervical spine injuries. J Athl Train 28:294–305, 1993.
17. Steidl L, Ditmar R: Soft tissue calcification treated with local and oral magnesium therapy. Magnes Res 3(2):113–119, 1990.
18. Swenson TM, Lauerman WC, Donaldson WF, et al: Cervical spine alignment in the immobilized football player—Radiographic analysis before and after helmet removal. Am J Sports Med 25:226–230, 1997.
19. Torg JS: Cervical spinal stenosis with cord neurapraxia and transient quadriplegia. Sports Med 20(6):429–434, 1995.
20. Torg JS: Epidemiology, pathomechanics, and prevention of football-induced spinal cord trauma. Exerc Sport Sci Rev 20:321–338, 1992.
21. Torg JS, Ramsey-Emrhein HA: Management guidelines for participation in collision activities with congenital, developmental, or post-injury lesions involving the cervical spine. Clin J Sports Med 7:273–291, 1997.
22. Torg JS, Vegso JJ, O'Neill MJ, Sennett B: The epidemiologic, pathologic, biomechanical, and cinematographic analysis of football-induced cervical spine trauma. Am J Sports Med 18:50–57, 1990.
23. Waninger KN: On-field management of potential cervical spine injury in helmeted football players: Leave the helmet on! Clin J Sports Med 8:124–129, 1998.
24. White MD, Cabanac M: Physical dilatation of the nostrils lowers the thermal strain of exercising humans. Eur J Appl Physiol 70:200–206, 1995.
25. Wieder DL: Treatment of traumatic myositis with acetic acid iontophoresis. Phys Ther 72:133–137, 1992.
26. Winter FD, Snell PG, Stray-Gundersen J: Effects of 100% oxygen on performance of professional soccer players. JAMA 262:227–229, 1989.

83. VOLLEYBALL

E. Lee Rice, D.O., FAAFP, and Stephen R. Steele, D.O.

1. Is aerobic fitness critical for volleyball training?

Yes. In volleyball, power and agility are important to achieve success, but without aerobic fitness a player's ability to maintain his or her intensity throughout the game is impaired. Also, a player's recovery time from a match is much quicker if aerobically fit, which is crucial in tournament situations where many matches are played in condensed periods of time.

2. Which method of training improves and hones players' skills the best—court drills or practice scrimmages?

Neither. A well-balanced training program that includes weight training, aerobic fitness, ability/court drills, scrimmaging, and psychological preparation is the most successful. Time should be devoted to each of these issues.

3. What other types of training are essential for volleyball players?

Upper and lower body strength is important, with alternating days of weight training and jump drills. Daily aerobic training along with practice of basic skills is important. Players also perform better with proper psychological preparation. Deep relaxation and positive imagery are well established as helpful skills for competitive athletes in general. They have been helpful for individual volleyball players and entire teams.

4. Name the most common chronic ailment of volleyball players.

Patellar tendinitis. This is defined specifically as inflammation and pain of the inferior pole of the patella at the patellar tendon attachment. Patellofemoral pain syndrome, chondromalacia patella, and Osgood-Schlatter's disease are also quite common. These are distinct problems that must be properly diagnosed and treated. Localization of the site of pain and proper diagnosis are essential elements to assure proper care and rapid return to the court.

5. Is there a common ailment of volleyball players that mimics a lateral knee injury?

Iliotibial band (ITB) friction syndrome is most commonly felt at the superior lateral aspect of the knee over the lateral femoral epicondyle or lateral tibial condyle. It is the end result of a chronically tight ITB associated with repetitive microtrauma and inflammation of the fascia. A history of gradual worsening of discomfort and lack of history of trauma are important features of ITB syndrome. Treatment consisting of stretching, ice, relative rest, antiinflammatory medication, and physical therapy may also be helpful. The athlete should be evaluated and treated for excessive pronation and other biomechanical faults, all of which can be exacerbating factors.

6. Discuss the important historical features that help differentiate patellofemoral disorders from intraarticular pathology.

Of course a sudden onset of pain, deformity, or effusion is important. The history of a painful clicking sensation or locking of the knee is indicative of meniscal tear or loose body. A loud "pop" at the time of the injury followed by dysfunction, swelling, and later "giving way" of the knee are important historical features of an anterior cruciate or posterior cruciate ligament tear. The mechanism of the injury is also very helpful to elucidate the pathology. A loaded twisting maneuver is often associated with meniscal injury. A history of a traumatic event with an anterior blow to the tibia (hyperextension) is often associated with a posterior cruciate ligament (PCL) injury. A posterior lateral blow to the knee can cause an anterior cruciate ligament (ACL) disruption.

7. What are the diagnostic maneuvers used in differentiating knee injuries?

Observe the general appearance, active range of motion, and gait. Inspect for possible effusion or deformity. Palpate for effusion, patellar mobility, and tenderness of the medial and lateral patellar facets or of the superior or inferior poles. Palpate for tenderness of the medial, lateral, or posterior joint lines and for tenderness of the medial and lateral collateral ligaments. Varus and valgus stress can elicit laxity of the collateral ligaments. The Lachman test for anterior translation of the tibia on the femur is the most sensitive test for ACL laxity. In experienced hands, the Lachman and pivot shift tests are very sensitive for ACL disruption and rotational instability. The anterior drawer test also is used when looking for ACL laxity. McMurray's test is used to feel and listen for a click of the medial or lateral meniscus. See pages 307–311 for descriptions of these various tests.

8. When the diagnosis is not clear, what imaging techniques are used?

Plain films of the knee are the first level. Anteroposterior (AP) and lateral views are the basics. If looking for patellofemoral problems, a Merchant view is preferred. Sometimes a tunnel view will help to see free-floating fragments from osteochondritis dissecans (OCD) or other loose bodies in the intercondylar notch. Other osteochondral lesions can sometimes be seen with this view.

Magnetic resonance imaging (MRI) has become very helpful in difficult diagnostic cases. It is most useful in cases where cruciate ligament ruptures or meniscal tears are suspected but are not clear cut. OCD is often appreciated with the MRI. Computed tomographic (CT) scans may help to elucidate unclear osseous pathology.

9. What is the length of recovery after an ACL reconstruction?

It depends on your definition of recovery. Most competitive athletes are able to return to their sport in 6–9 months. The patients are usually on crutches for 2–3 weeks and doing straight leg raises immediately. They usually reach 90° of flexion by 7–10 days and are able to strengthen the knee with closed-chain kinetic exercises such as step machines by 1 month. They usually return to running by 5–6 months.

10. Name some other lower extremity injuries occurring frequently in volleyball.

Acute ankle sprains, metatarsal or tibial stress fractures, Achilles tendinitis, Morton's neuroma, plantar fasciitis, tarsal tunnel syndrome, calcaneal contusions, and retrocalcaneal bursitis.

11. Name the three anatomic soft tissue structures in the shoulder that are typically involved in shoulder impingement syndrome.

1. Subacromial bursa
2. Supraspinatus tendon
3. Biceps tendon

12. Name four conditions that often contribute to shoulder impingement.

1. Acromioclavicular arthritis
2. Glenohumeral instability
3. Acromial spurring
4. Weak rotator cuff musculature

13. Discuss the factors that contribute to shoulder impingement syndrome and its treatment.

This is an inflammatory condition caused by repetitive overuse, generally from the overhead activities of hitting and blocking. It is extremely common in volleyball and can lead to significant time lost from the sport. Ice, stretching, rotator cuff muscle strengthening, physical therapy, and selective use of corticosteroid injections can all be of benefit. Occasionally, those patients who do not respond to conservative care, especially those with hypertrophic spurring of the distal clavicle or acromion seen on the radiograph with outlet (scapular Y) view, can be relieved with decompression arthroscopy, which involves an acromioplasty, bursectomy, and lysis of the coracoacromial ligament. Additionally, debridement and/or resection of the distal clavicle may be necessary. Instability of the glenohumeral joint capsule secondary to repetitive stretching of the capsular ligaments or from a glenoid labral injury can also contribute to this syndrome.

14. How are shoulder rotator cuff tears diagnosed and treated in the modern sports medicine office?

Shoulder rotator cuff tears are not uncommon in volleyball. The history of either traumatic injury or prolonged symptoms of impingement associated with muscular weakness of the rotator cuff usually provides a good clinical impression of a partial or complete rotator cuff tear. Routine shoulder radiographs (AP with internal and external rotation views and a lateral view with outlet views) are performed to rule out fractures, calcific tendinitis, or secondary degenerative changes. An MRI can be ordered if the pathology is unclear. Arthrogram can be helpful but is less frequently necessary. The physician then can advise conservative management with rest, limited range of motion, rotator cuff strengthening exercises, and slow return to activity. It may be necessary either for full-thickness or for partial-thickness tears that fail to respond to conservative management to undergo open or arthroscopic surgical repair.

15. Name the most common stress fractures in volleyball players.

Metatarsal shaft fractures. The third or fourth digits are most common. This is often a clinical diagnosis, because radiography may not show the acute fracture and only picks up the callus formation 2–4 weeks later. If not managed properly, these can become difficult management problems. A non–weight-bearing or partial weight-bearing short leg cast or cast brace is suggested. When the athlete shows clinical and radiographic evidence of healing, weight bearing is progressed as tolerated without pain. Appropriate strengthening and range-of-motion exercises are used throughout the healing process to minimize atrophy and allow return to play in the shortest possible time.

16. What type of injury occurs fairly frequently to the thoracic region in volleyball players?

Thoracic facet joint sprain. Because althletes frequently make quick lateral movements involving twisting of the trunk and reaching with the upper extremity, the thoracic facets are subject to shear forces. This can acutely sprain the joint or can often cause overuse and inflammation associated with muscular pain, spasm, and limited range of motion.

17. Are there common injuries that result from blocking in volleyball?

Mallet finger, metacarpal fractures, and phalangeal fractures frequently result from front row blocking, particularly when the blocking technique is faulty because of improper hand position.

18. What biomechanical mechanism predisposes volleyball players to sacroiliac ligament sprains?

Players who flex forward at the waist with extended knees to reach for a ball, especially if trunk twisting or side bending is involved, are at increased risk for sacroiliac sprain. This is a common position when receiving and passing a serve. Sacroiliac stress is minimized by flexing the knees and keeping the lumbar spine in the neutral position. Acute sacroiliac injuries also are seen when players land unevenly and forcefully from a jump.

19. How much fluid do volleyball players require during a match?

It is not uncommon for players to lose 6–8 pounds or more during a long match. Because this is more fluid loss than athletes can replace during competition, it is necessary to prehydrate as well as to consume 5–7 ounces of fluid approximately every 15 minutes during the match. Water is the best replacement fluid and is absorbed most rapidly if it is slightly chilled (about 40° F).

20. Are any injuries relatively unique to volleyball players?

Isolated infraspinatus muscle atrophy due to injury to the suprascapular nerve has become an increasingly identified problem among competitive volleyball players. Isolated infraspinatus atrophy has been found in 12–33% of elite volleyball players. Atrophy may result from impingement of the suprascapular nerve by ganglion cysts at the spinoglenoid notch. Traction neuropathy is another possible etiology; rapid deceleration during both serve and spike has been proposed as a causative factor. Symptoms may include pain over the suprascapular notch. Examination and testing reveal paresis and atrophy of the supraspinatus and/or infraspinatus muscles. Electromyography is helpful in diagnosis. If rest and conservative treatment are not successful, surgical decompression of the nerve has yielded promising results.

21. What is "sand toe"?

Plantarflexion injury to the metatarsophalangeal joint of the great toe in beach volleyball players has been described as "sand toe." This injury may result in significant functional impairment of push-off, running, and jumping motions. Recovery commonly takes up to 6 months and is often accompanied by loss of dorsiflexion. Conservative care includes rest, taping, ice, NSAIDs, physical therapy, and shoe modification.

BIBLIOGRAPHY

1. Antoniadis G, Richter HP, Rath S, et al: Suprascapular nerve entrapment: Experience with 28 cases. J Neurosurg 85:1020–1025, 1996.
2. Broom MJ, Fulkerson JP: The plica syndrome: A new perspective. Orthop Clin North Am 17:279–281, 1986.
3. Burk LD: Rotator cuff tears: Prospective comparison of MR imaging with arthrography, sonography and surgery. Am J Radiol 153:87–92, 1989.
4. Clark JM: Tendons, ligaments and capsule of the rotator cuff. J Bone Joint Surg 74A:713–725, 1992.
5. Donaldson WF, Warren RF: A comparison of acute anterior cruciate ligament examination. Am J Sports Med 13:5–10, 1985.
6. Frey C, Andersen GD, Feder KS: Plantarflexion injury to the metatarsophalangeal joint ("sand toe"). Foot Ankle Int 17:576–581, 1996.
7. Hankin FM, Peel SM: Sport-related fractures and dislocations i the hand. Hand Clin 6:429–453, 1990.

8. Holzgraefe M, Kukowski B, Eggert S: Prevalence of latent and manifest suprascapular neuropathy in high-performance volleyball players. Br J Sports Med 28:177–179, 1994.
9. Jacobson KE, Flandry FC: Diagnosis of anterior knee pain. Clin Sports Med 8:179–195, 1989.
10. Katz JW, Fingeroth RJ: The diagnostic of ruptures of the ACL comparing Lachman, anterior drawer and pivot shift test in acute and chronic knee injuries. Am J Sports Med 14:88–91, 1986.
11. Lindenburg BS, Pinshaw R: Iliotibial band friction syndrome in runners. Phys Sportsmed 12(15):118–130, 1984.
12. Micheli LJ, Smith AD: Injury recognition and evaluation: Upper extremity. In Cantu RC (ed): ACSM's Guidelines for the Team Physician. Philadelphia, Lea & Febiger, 1991.
13. Wang DH, Koehler SM: Isolated infraspinatus atrophy in a collegiate volleyball player. Clin J Sport Med 6(4):255–258, 1996.

84. SOCCER

Warren B. Howe, M.D.

1. Is "heading" the ball dangerous?

Possibly. The cumulative effect of repeated head trauma is well known in boxers and may be present in soccer players as well. The first recorded head-injury death in soccer was due to subdural hematoma after heading the ball. However, at least one recent study indicates that any symptoms suggesting encephalopathy in soccer players relate more to history of acute head injury than repeatedly heading the ball.

2. How can heading be made safer?

It is unlikely that heading will disappear as a soccer technique; thus the emphasis must be on maximizing safety. Use of waterproof soccer balls (a leather ball may increase 20% in weight from absorbed water) has proved helpful. Careful instruction in and use of proper technique are critical. Strengthening of neck and shoulder musculature and coaching players in careful selection of appropriate times to employ heading are other important means to improve safety.

3. Are some field positions in soccer more injury-prone than others?

Center-midfielders seem most injury-prone, followed by center-forwards and goalkeepers. In general, players most directly involved in attack or defense are at greatest risk. Most injuries are to the lower extremities and tend to be relatively minor injuries to soft tissue. Goalkeepers are at high risk for collision with other players or with the fixed and unpadded goalposts; some have recommended that goalkeepers in soccer wear head protection. Padding the goalposts is mentioned with increasing frequency as a means of reducing the likelihood and severity of injury to goalkeepers, but many object to this strategy as a significant alteration of the game itself.

4. Does gender influence soccer injury rates?

Apparently yes, in at least a few studies. One recent study shows an incidence of injury in elite female players that is two times the incidence in elite male players. Another study has shown that female players are more prone to traumatic injury during the premenstrual and menstrual period than during the rest of the menstrual cycle and that players using oral contraceptives had a lower rate of injury than players not on birth control pills. The incidence of anterior cruciate ligament injury in female soccer players is approximately twice that in males.

5. How far does a soccer player run in the course of a game?

Studies show wide variation, depending on competitive level, position played, and method by which distance run is recorded and/or measured. It seems clear that elite midfielders may run 8–10 km during the course of a game, with frequent alterations in tempo, direction, and speed.

6. What is the best treatment for skin abrasions?

Careful cleansing of the wound with soapy water removes foreign material. To allow continued competition, dressings held in place with elastic wraps supported by tape are satisfactory for commonly abraded parts. Second Skin can soothe small abrasions, but greasy ointments generally should be avoided in favor of letting the wound dry and form an eschar. Any skin break must be observed for infection. An athlete should not participate with a wound that is actively bleeding, and the so-called universal precautions should be used when treating any open wound.

7. Can blisters be prevented?

Definitely. Careful break-in and accustomization to new shoes are important. Wearing two pair of socks (the innermost should be thin and of fine weave, whereas the outer should be standard, well-fitting tube socks) allows friction to occur between socks rather than between socks and skin. Skin lubricant or petroleum jelly can be applied to potential blister sites to minimize friction and sometimes is applied to socks. Moleskin or tape pads at "hot-spots" also help, as does skin treatment with benzoin or collodion.

8. How should one treat established foot blisters?

Small blisters should be left unbroken as long as possible. The longer one can delay in opening a blister, the more infection-resistant the underlying skin will become. Large blisters may require unroofing to permit comfort. The use of a moleskin donut applied with the hole over the blister and the material secured to skin coated with tincture of benzoin adequately treats small blisters or hot spots where irritation indicates that a blister may soon form. For large blisters and after unroofing, Second Skin is an excellent dressing, held in place with Micropore tape. Once the skin is open, maintain careful surveillance for infection.

9. How should a player control callus formation on the foot?

Callus formation is common and may lead to problems with deep-seated blisters, foot pain, and even mechanical problems. Callus is best prevented by the use of tape and/or padding on vulnerable places on the feet. Once present, calluses should be trimmed with a specially-designed callus trimmer or a pumice stone. Razor blades and other "free" blades can easily cause serious injury and should be avoided except in the hands of a physician or podiatrist.

10. What is the usual mechanism of ankle sprain in soccer?

Forced supination, adduction, and inversion of the foot leading to injury to the anterior talofibular ligament.

11. What factors can be modified to prevent ankle sprains?

The field should not have holes or be significantly uneven; turf should be in good condition. Shoes should fit well, have cleats of uniform length (observe for cleat wear and replace worn cleats when possible, or replace the shoes early if molded soles have worn cleats), and be in good repair. Strengthening of the muscles that resist inversion of the ankle (peroneus brevis and longus) helps, as does work on ankle proprioception (daily balancing on one foot with eyes closed). Achilles tendon and calf muscle flexibility is important also.

12. How important are ankle taping and support for sprain prevention in soccer?

Perhaps more important than in most other sports, because such significance attaches to use of the feet and lower legs in soccer. Many soccer players do not like to tape because they feel it modifies their "touch" on the ball. Tape applications or ankle braces should be less like a boot and more like a stirrup, so that extraneous tape or brace material does not insulate the anteromedial foot border from sensitive contact with shoe and ball.

13. What are some potential dangers of hematoma formation?

Hematomas are caused by direct blows or muscle strains and tears that result in bleeding within soft tissue. They are exceptionally common in soccer, especially in the lower extremity.

Small, subcutaneous hematomas, not involving muscle, are generally of small risk and resolve with little treatment other than local ice application. Intramuscular hematomas, however, may be serious because they may organize and calcify or lead to heterotopic bone formation (myositis ossificans). Such injuries are often overlooked by player, coach, and physician but should be treated with great respect and aggressive rehabilitation.

14. How should intramuscular hematoma be treated?

Initial treatment should emphasize limitation of swelling and bleeding by resting the part, ice applications, and compression. Knee immobilization for 24–48 hours in 120° of flexion has been recommended for acute treatment of quadriceps contusion, because it minimizes intramuscular hemorrhage and preserves flexibility. Once bleeding is no longer a threat (24–48 hours), maintenance of rest and ice applications and gentle stretching return the muscle to full flexibility compared with its mate in the opposite extremity. Return to practice and competition must be delayed until the player is pain-free and has regained full range of motion in the injured muscle.

15. Is eye injury a significant risk in soccer?

Yes. One may think that the relatively large ball would help to minimize eye trauma, but it may occur, although with lesser frequency and severity than in sports using smaller missiles (hockey, lacrosse, racket sports in general). Underinflation of the ball has been implicated in eye trauma. Knees, elbows, and heads are other common eye-injuring agents. No soccer-specific eye protection has been devised, and eye protection is at present not commonly used. The use of protection similar to that used for racket sports has been advocated.

16. Is dental protection advisable for soccer players?

Yes, particularly for older and more experienced players and goalkeepers. A custom-fitted mouthguard can be fitted by a dentist, is comfortable and durable, does not interfere with speech or mouth-breathing, and can help to protect not only against dental or orofacial injury but also against cerebral concussion in some cases.

17. What is footballer's ankle?

Footballer's ankle is a condition in experienced soccer players in which osteophytes, produced by repeated ankle overload, form on the anterior talus and distal tibia. Symptoms include pain, especially anteriorly, and loss of ankle flexibility. Surgery is often required to remove the osteophytes.

18. Do shin guards really help to prevent injuries?

Yes. They not only protect against anterior leg contusion (which can have serious consequences, including development of compartment syndrome) but also diffuse the force of a kick enough to prevent tibial and fibular fractures. It is critical that the rules regarding use of shin guards be carefully enforced and that shin guards are of high quality construction, protecting the entire length of the tibia.

19. What is the significance of anterior leg pain in a soccer player?

Usually anterior leg pain is a result of minor trauma or overuse and in some cases represents a chronic exertional compartment syndrome. In such situations, the pain is usually not disabling and diminishes or disappears with rest. However, it anterior leg pain continues to increase despite rest, an acute compartment syndrome should be suspected and orthopedic consultation obtained immediately.

20. What is the differential diagnosis of groin pain in a soccer player?

The usual causes of groin pain are muscular strains and overuse injuries, particularly involving the adductor muscles of the hip. Uncommon causes of groin pain include referred pain from abdominal or genitourinary structures, hernia (femoral hernia can and does occur in males), pain of neurologic origin (including herniated lumbar disc), and various nerve entrapments. The symptom of groin pain is exceptionally common in soccer players and demands careful history-taking and physical examination by a physician familiar with the anatomy of the region. Sometimes special studies, including magnetic resonance imaging, herniography, bone scanning, and laparoscopy, may be required to elucidate the cause of long-standing groin pain.

21. What causes muscular cramps in the calf and thigh during soccer matches?

Probably a combination of dehydration, electrolyte depletion, and overstress of the musculature. Predisposing factors include tight Achilles tendon, the low-heel shoes used in soccer, insufficient conditioning, playing surface (more cramps on artificial surfaces than grass), and inadequate fluids and electrolytes before and during competition, especially in hot weather.

22. What steps should be taken to minimize risk of heat injury in soccer?

Heat injury is a distinct possibility when soccer is played under hot, humid conditions. Traditions that the game is played continuously, that substitutions are restricted at higher levels of play, and that breaks for rest and fluid replenishment are not encouraged predispose to heat injury. Prevention requires departures from these traditions. Modification of schedules to avoid games in the hottest part of the day, unrestricted substitutions, scheduled fluid breaks, free access to fluids at all times, and shorter game times can be used, depending on conditions, to decrease the likelihood of heat injury. In any setting with significant heat and/or humidity, facilities for coping with heat illness, including heat stroke, should be readily available. Coaches of teams practicing or competing in hot or humid conditions should be aware that diminished levels of performance may be an early sign that a player is developing heat injury.

23. Can ingestion of glucose or glucose polymer during a soccer match improve performance?

Probably—by slowing the rate of glycogen loss and thus delaying the onset of fatigue. If used, it should be made available shortly before the competition begins and/or at half-time to avoid the stimulation of insulin secretion and resultant fall in blood sugar, which may occur if the solution is given too far in advance of activity. Large volumes of ingested fluid should obviously be avoided immediately before game time.

BIBLIOGRAPHY

1. Arendt E, Dick R: Knee injury patterns among men and women in collegiate basketball and soccer. Am J Sports Med 23:694, 1995.
2. Aronen JG, Chronister RD: Quadriceps contusions: Hastening the return to play. Physician Sportsmed 20(7):130, 1992.
3. Daily SW, Barsan WG: Head injuries in soccer. Physician Sportsmed 20(8):79, 1992.
4. Ekstrand J, Nigg BM: Surface-related injuries in soccer. Sports Med 8:56, 1989.
5. Elias SR, Roberts WO, Thorson DC: Team sports in hot weather: Guidelines for modifying youth soccer. Physician Sportsmed 19(5):67, 1991.
6. Engstrom B, Johansson C, Tornkvist H: Soccer injuries among elite female players. Am J Sports Med 19:372, 1991.
7. Fields KB: Head injuries in soccer. Physician Sportsmed 17(1):69, 1989.
8. Garrick JG, Webb DR: Sports Injuries: Diagnosis and Management. Philadelphia, W.B. Saunders, 1990.
9. Hunt M, Fulford S: Amateur soccer: Injuries in relation to field position. Br J Sports Med 24:265, 1990.
10. Jordan SE, Green GA, Galanty HL, et al: Acute and chronic brain injury in United States National Team soccer players. Am J Sports Med 24:205, 1996.
11. Leatt PB, Jacob I: Effect of glucose polymer ingestion on glycogen depletion during a soccer match. Can J Sports Sci 14:112, 1989.
12. Mellion MB, Walsh WM, Shelton GL (eds): The Team Physician's Handbook, 2nd ed. Philadelphia, Hanley & Belfus, 1997.
13. Fehlandt A, Micheli L: Acute exertional compartment syndrome in an adolescent female. Med Sci Sports Exerc 27:3, 1995.
14. Moller-Nielsen J, Hammar M: Women's soccer injuries in relation to the menstrual cycle and oral contraceptive use. Med Sci Sports Exerc 21:126, 1989.
15. Schneider RC, Kennedy JC, Plant ML (eds): Sports Injuries: Mechanisms, Prevention and Treatment. Baltimore, Williams & Wilkins, 1985.
16. Shephard RJ: The energy needs of the soccer player. Clin J Sports Med 2:62, 1992.

17. Smodlaka VN: Medical aspects of heading the ball in soccer. Physician Sportsmed 12(2):127, 1984.
18. Torg JS, Welsh RP, Shephard RJ (eds): Current Therapy in Sports Medicine-2. Philadelphia, B.C. Decker, 1990.

85. BASKETBALL

Scott W. Eathorne, M.D., and Douglas B. McKeag, M.D., M.S.

1. What is the body part most commonly injured in basketball?

The ankle is the most frequently injured part of the basketball player's anatomy, usually succumbing to the acute sprain of the lateral compartment ligaments. Other regions involved (in decreasing frequency), based on epidemiologic data from various age and skill levels and geographic locations, are the knee; hand, wrist, and forearm; head, face, and neck; back; hip and thigh; shoulder; and elbow. Ankle injuries generally account for over 50% of basketball injuries. The nature of the sport, including the emphasis on running with frequent, sudden accelerations and decelerations, sharp cutting, pivoting, lateral movement, and jumping, often in cramped quarters, predisposes to ligamentous and bony injury of the ankle.

2. What physical tests can be used to assess ligamentous integrity in ankle sprains?

The **anterior drawer** and **talar tilt tests** are commonly used to determine ligamentous instability. Anterior drawer testing, which can be performed with the patient in various positions, assesses integrity of both the lateral and medial ligamentous structures of the ankle. The tibia and fibula are stabilized with one hand while the other hand, holding the foot in 20° of plantarflexion, applies a posterior-to-anterior force, attempting to translate the talus forward in the ankle mortise. The amount of translation reflects the degree of injury to the anterior talofibular ligament and anterolateral capsule and potentially the deltoid ligaments.

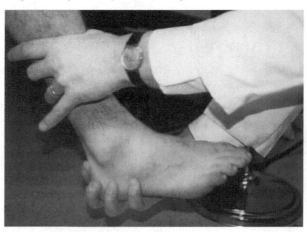

Position for anterior drawer testing.

The talar tilt or inversion stress test is used to assess integrity of the anterior talofibular (ATF) and calcaneofibular (CF) ligaments. The test is performed with the foot in neutral or anatomic position. Grasping the talus in one hand and stabilizing the tibia and fibula with the other allow application of an adduction force to test for laxity in the CF ligament, as evidenced by increased adduction compared with the unaffected side. The medial compartment (deltoid ligaments) can be evaluated by reversing the test and applying an abduction force. Applying a side-to-side force (side-to-side test) to the talus assesses the integrity of the ATF ligament and ankle mortise.

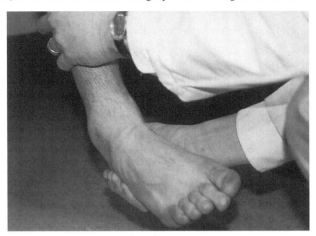

Position for talar tilt testing.

All tests should be performed with the knee in 90° of flexion to help relax the gastrocnemius and Achilles tendon. Comparison with the unaffected side improves appreciation of the degree of laxity. Such comparison also aids in the evaluation of acute injuries in athletes who have increased physiologic laxity, which initially may give the appearance of more severe ligamentous involvement.

3. What criteria should be included in determining eligibility for return to play after an acute ankle sprain?

The interval between initial injury and return to play depends on the severity (degree) of ankle sprain and how quickly and appropriately care is rendered. The factors most relevant to determining eligibility for return to play include achievement of pain-free, full range of motion (ROM), adequate functional strength, return of proprioception, and resolution of pain. Full ROM is best achieved by initiating early, pain-free ROM and stretching exercises to limit the loss of motion from nonuse. Functional strength is expressed as the ability to perform various activities (straight running, figure-of-eights, lateral movements) inherent to the sport in a pain-free manner. Proprioception, the sense of knowing the position of an extremity at any given moment, is sometimes lost and needs to be reinforced. The athlete who chooses to play with pain may be predisposed to further injury. However, some degree of mild soreness and swelling after activity may be anticipated for up to 6 weeks and can be limited by use of ice, compression, and elevation as well as other physical therapy modalities.

4. What methods are available to help lessen the incidence of initial and recurrent ankle sprains?

Both intrinsic and extrinsic factors play an important role in decreasing ankle sprains. Intrinsic factors include adequate preseason conditioning focused on strengthening and stretching lower leg muscles, which provide secondary stabilization to the ankle joint. Certainly, correction of existing deficiencies from old injuries is essential. Adherence to a daily rehabilitation program (e.g., the ankle Repac), which includes proprioceptive retraining, is critical for successful rehabilitation of players with previous injury.

Extrinsic factors include various taping and bracing techniques that provide functional support to the ankle. Commercial products include a canvas, lace-up type of brace that can be worn under or over the sock (e.g., Swede-O-Universal); a rigid, lateral stirrup-type brace utilizing air bladders for compression (e.g., Aircast); and newer, lightweight plastic posterior splints (e.g., ALP). High-top basketball shoes may provide some additional support. Another important factor in lessening the occurrence of ankle injury is maintaining a level, dry playing surface.

5. What is "jumper's knee"? What are the proposed mechanisms and contributing factors to its occurrence?

Jumper's knee refers to overuse injuries involving the soft tissue portions of the knee extensor mechanism. Commonly, it involves the patellar tendon, either at the inferior pole of the patella or at the tibial tubercle insertion. The proposed mechanism is eccentric overload from repetitive landing (jumping). Subsequent microtrauma to the tendon fibers results in an inflammatory reaction, producing characteristic pain and tenderness at the involved site.

Predisposing factors include relative weakness of the vastus medialis obliquus (VMO) muscle compared with the vastus lateralis, VMO dysplasia, increased Q-angle, abnormal patellar alignment (e.g., patella alta), poor hamstring flexibility, weakness of the ankle dorsiflexors, pes planus, and genu valgus. Jumper's knee is a common malady among basketball players, both male and female, and therapy is directed not only at relieving acute symptoms, but also at correcting underlying deficiencies.

6. What should be the initial treatment of a quadriceps contusion?

Because of the inherent nature of the sport and lack of padding in the quadriceps area, quadriceps contusions are relatively common among basketball players. Controversy surrounds the best means of treatment for preventing long-term sequelae, including loss of functional strength and range of motion and development of myositis ossificans. Despite differences in opinion about definitive management, initial care of quadriceps contusions appears to be fairly consistent.

As with all contusions, the basic pathology in impact injuries to the quadriceps ranges from cellular swelling of muscle components in mild cases to capillary disruption with localized hemorrhage in more severe injuries. The goal of initial therapy is to minimize the amount of swelling and/or extravasation of blood. This goal is best accomplished by sustaining pressure at the site of impact. One commonly advocated technique is use of an elastic bandage to immobilize the injured limb with the knee in 120° of flexion. This uncomfortable position must be maintained for 24 hours after injury with use of crutches for ambulation and application of ice for 15–20 minutes every 2–3 hours. Once initial swelling and hemorrhage are controlled, further therapy is aimed at prevention of reinjury and return of full ROM and functional strength. This goal is usually achieved by a graded rehabilitation program focusing first on pain-free stretching and progressing to more functionally oriented activities.

7. What is the differential diagnosis of heel pain in basketball players?

The differential diagnosis of heel pain in basketball players should take into account the repetitive trauma that occurs with the sport. Disorders affecting the general population also must be considered. More common causes of heel pain in basketball players are listed in the table below.

Differential Diagnosis for Heel Pain in Basketball Players

Plantar fasciitis	Contusions (fat pad)
Achilles tendinitis or rupture	Medial plantar tendinitis
Calcaneal apophysitis	Benign/malignant bone tumors
(Sever's disease)	Lacerations/foreign body
Medial calcaneal neurapraxia	Skin lesions
Bursitis	Blisters
Retro-Achilles	Calluses
Retrocalcaneal	Plantar wart
Calcaneal stress fractures	Talar dome fracture

Plantar fasciitis typically presents with heel pain localized to the medial calcaneal tubercle and often is worse on arising in the morning. Medial plantar tendinitis also may present with medial heel pain, usually localized to the medial plantar eminence (abductor hallucis muscle). Achilles tendinitis is another overuse injury characteristically presenting with pain and tenderness at the calcaneal insertion of the tendon. This highly stressed tendon should not be injected because of the risk of rupture. Radiographs of the calcaneus in both plantar fasciitis and Achilles tendinitis may show traction spur formation along the inferior and posterior borders, respectively. Calcaneal apophysitis or Severs disease occurs primarily in boys aged 8–14 years with open epiphyseal plates. Complaints are similar to those of Achilles tendinitis; pain and swelling worsen with activity. The process is self-limited and often responds to conservative therapy.

Stress fractures of the calcaneus should be suspected in players with insidious onset of localized, bony heel pain. Radionuclide studies may confirm the diagnosis. Fractures of the talar dome may occur with more severe ankle injuries and may be missed on initial radiographs. Trauma to the medial heel may result in neuropraxia involving the medial calcaneal nerve.

8. How should superficial skin lacerations and abrasions be handled according to the National Collegiate Athletic Association (NCAA)?

Specific guidelines for handling open wounds and skin lesions have been advanced by the NCAA, based on interpretation of an NCAA policy statement adopted by the Men's and Women's Basketball Rules Committees for 1992–1993. Athletes suffering a wound with oozing or bleeding or athletes with blood on their uniform must be removed from the game at the earliest possible time. For wounds, appropriate treatment and coverage must be administered away from the field of play; medical clearance must be given before return to play. Bloodied uniforms must be cleaned with fresh 1:100 dilution of sodium hypochlorite (bleach) or changed before return. This policy was developed to conform with universal precautions as directed by the Centers for Disease Control and Prevention to minimize the chances of transmitting blood-borne diseases in athletes.

9. What common eye injuries can be expected in basketball?

One prospective study of sports-related eye injuries found the highest frequency of injury (28.7%) in basketball. The table below lists the more common injuries in basketball as well as less common, but more severe injuries. Anticipation, recognition, and early referral for ophthalmologic intervention in more severe injuries are critical for the nonophthalmologist caring for athletes.

Eye Injuries in Basketball

MORE COMMON EYE INJURIES	LESS COMMON, MORE SEVERE EYE INJURIES
Corneal/conjunctival abrasions	Traumatic hyphema
Orbital/lid contusions	Vitreous/retinal hemorrhage
Lid lacerations	Blowout fracture
Traumatic iritis	Ruptured globe
Subconjunctival hemorrhage	Retinal detachment

10. Describe a Jones fracture and its relevance to basketball injuries.

A Jones fracture occurs at the base of the fifth metatarsal, generally involving a 1.5-cm segment of the proximal diaphysis just distal to the tuberosity. The mechanism of injury may be a forceful load to the forefoot, as with pivoting, or sudden dorsiflexion concentrated over the fifth metatarsal, as with a forward lunge and landing on the lateral foot. These fractures are distinguished from more proximal fractures involving the styloid, which may result from an inversion injury in which a forceful contraction of the peroneus brevis muscle avulses a portion of bone. Because of frequent lateral movements, sudden, forceful cutting, and jumping, basketball players often generate a great deal of force over the fifth metatarsal. This force tends to predispose to both acute and chronic (stress) Jones fractures.

Jones fractures are often disabling and may require surgical intervention for delayed union or nonunion after closed reduction. Controversy surrounds the ideal treatment for acute injuries, and consideration must be given to various factors, including the athlete's level of competition. Non–weight-bearing or use of an ankle-foot orthosis walking boot is usually required for athletes treated conservatively.

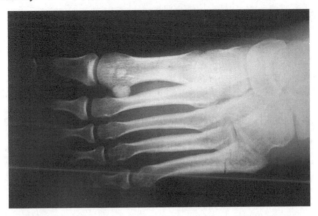

Jones fracture.

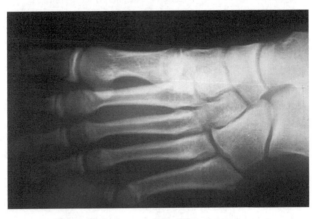

Avulsion fracture of the fifth metatarsal.

11. What is "rebound rib"?

Rebound rib is an uncommon, stress-induced fracture of the first rib thought to result from a sudden, violent contraction of the anterior scalenus muscle. Patients may present with poorly localized shoulder pain. Radiographs should confirm the diagnosis. Treatment is conservative, consisting of sling immobilization, ice, and analgesics.

12. What structures are injured in mallet finger?

A mallet finger injury involves avulsion of the digital extensor tendon insertion at the base of the distal phalanx. This common injury results most often from a direct blow to the tip of an extended finger. Provided the distal interphalangeal joint is stable and any bony avulsion fragment involves less than 25% of the joint surface, treatment includes strict use of a mallet finger splint for 3–5 weeks. Surgical repair may be required for unstable joints and fractures involving greater than 25% of the joint surface.

13. What factors have been proposed to explain the greater incidence of ACL injuries in female vs. male basketball players?

NCAA data, compiled since 1982, indicate that women are four times as likely to sustain ACL injury as men. Although numerous factors, both intrinsic and extrinsic, have been proposed to explain this difference, non has been proved. Proposed intrinsic factors include intercondylar notch size (smaller notch size is thought to be associated with greater risk for ACL injury), greater physiologic laxity of ligaments in women, and assorted biomechanical factors, including gynecoid pelvis and genu valgum leading to increased Q-angle, femoral anteversion, and external tibial torsion. Several ongoing studies focus on a possible hormonal influence, with relaxin or estrogen as the proposed culprit. Recently, women have been shown to initiate the protective neuromuscular mechanism much later than men subjected to the same stress. Specifically, the hamstring muscle recruitment lagged behind, placing more stress on the ACL complex.

Extrinsic factors potentially related to ACL injury include sport-specific mechanisms that place the ACL at risk (planting/cutting, landing on an extended leg), hamstring-to-quadriceps muscle strength imbalances, playing surface, and use of prophylactic ankle braces. Although such theories are intuitively attractive as potentially relevant factors, it is most likely that the higher ACL injury incidence in female basketball players is multifactoral. As such, efforts at prevention become more difficult.

BIBLIOGRAPHY

1. Arendt E, Dick R: Knee injury patterns among men and women in collegiate basketball and soccer: NCAA data and review of literature. Am J Sports Med 23:694–701, 1995.
2. Aronen JG, Caronister RD: Quadriceps contusion: Hastening return to play. Physician Sportsmed 20:1130–1136, 1992.
3. Davis AW, Alexander IJ: Problematic fractures and dislocations in the foot and ankle in athletes. Clin Sports Med 9:163–181, 1990.
4. Henry JH, Lareau B, Neigut D: The injury rate in professional basketball. Am J Sports Med 10:16–18, 1982.
5. Huston LJ, Wojtys EM: Neuromuscular performance characteristics in elite female athletes. Am J Sports Med 24:427–436, 1996.
6. Larrison W, Hersh PS, Kunsweller T, Shingleton BJ: Sports-related ocular trauma. Ophthalmology 97:1265–1269, 1990.
7. Magee DJ: Orthopedic Physical Assessment, 2nd ed. Philadelphia, W.B. Saunders, 1992.
8. Mellion MB: Office Management of Sports Injuries and Athletic Problems. Philadelphia, Hanley & Belfus, 1988.
9. Mellion MB, Walsh WM, Shelton GL (eds): The Team Physician's Handbook, 2nd ed. Philadelphia, Hanley & Belfus, 1997.
10. Mercier LR: Practical Orthopedics, 3rd ed. St. Louis, Mosby, 1991.
11. Moeller J, Lamb M: Anterior cruciate ligament injuries in female athletes. Physician Sportsmed 25(4):31–54, 1997.
12. National Collegiate Athletic Association Memorandum: Statement and Related Interpretations for the 1992–93 Basketball Season Concerning Bleeding and Transmission of Blood-Borne Diseases. November 1992.
13. Ray JM, McCombs W, Sternes RA: Basketball and Volleyball. In Reider B (ed): Sports Medicine: The School-Age Athlete. Philadelphia, W.B. Saunders, 1991.
14. Ryan JB, Wheeler JH, Hopkinson WJ, et al: Quadriceps contusion: West Point update. Am J Sports Med 19:299–304, 1991.
15. Sammarco GJ: Be alert for Jones fractures. Physician Sportsmed 20(6):101–110, 1992.
16. Shambaugh JP, Klein A, Herbert JH: Structural measures as predictors of injury in basketball players. Med Sci Sports Exerc 23:522–527, 1991.
17. Zelisko JA, Noble HB, Porter M: A comparison of men's and women's professional basketball injuries. Am J Sports Med 10(5):297–299, 1982.

86. WRESTLING

Warren B. Howe, M.D.

1. Compare wrestling with other sports in terms of injury incidence.
The incidence of injury is relatively high in wrestling, similar to that in tackle football and soccer. Although most injuries occur in practice, matches carry a much higher risk per minute of activity. Serious or life-threatening injuries are much less common than in tackle football. Injury incidence rises with a wrestler's increasing age and skill level. Lower extremity injuries, particularly involving the knee, predominate.

2. When is injury most likely to occur during the match?
During takedown, when the wrestler taken to the mat is relatively out of control and significant alterations in normal movement patterns may be forced on him.

3. Do any characteristics of wrestlers affect treatment results?
As with most athletes, wrestlers are highly motivated to return to action after injury. This may produce the appearance of rapid rehabilitative progress and resultant premature return to activity, which leads to a high incidence of reinjury. Wrestlers have been deemed "poorly compliant" with medical advice by some authorities, and the physician dealing with wrestlers should be highly alert for noncompliance and resist clearing the athlete for resumption of activity too soon. There is no substitute for a mutually respectful relationship between the physician and wrestler before injury, which fosters the honest communication necessary for best results.

4. What is the risk of contagion in wrestling?
Small but not absent. The uniquely close contact between wrestlers in competition makes infections, particularly skin infections, easily transmissible. Painstaking hygiene is therefore mandatory. Bleeding is not uncommon, and spread of blood-borne infections, such as HIV and hepatitis, is conceivable, although the risk is low.

5. How can the risk of contagion be reduced?
Matches must be stopped at the first sign of bleeding. The bleeding should be stopped and any visible blood cleaned up safely. The use of universal precautions is mandatory, including gloves for physicians and trainers, segregation of blood-contaminated waste and laundry, and use of appropriate disinfectant (dilute bleach in water, carefully labeled to avoid ingestion, is satisfactory) to clean up spills. Mats should be cleaned with germicide before matches, if significantly soiled during a match, and at the conclusion of the match or tournament session as well as before and after every practice and competition. Clean clothing should be used daily and laundered promptly after use. Wrestlers should shower thoroughly using soap before and after each practice session and competition. Equipment, such as headgear, should be disinfected regularly. Wrestlers with signs of contagious disease must not participate in practice or competition until such signs have resolved.

6. What is herpes gladiatorum?
A skin infection increasingly common in wrestlers, caused by the herpes simplex type I virus. It is spread by intimate skin contact between infected and uninfected wrestlers in the course of practice or competition and has assumed epidemic incidence on some teams. Once acquired, it tends to be recurrent in the affected wrestler, who may repeatedly shed the virus, especially when lesions are present.

7. How can herpes gladiatorum be prevented and treated?
Isolation of affected wrestlers until resolution of the lesions is mandatory. Wrestlers should be inspected frequently for suspicious lesions and encouraged to report lesions that they detect

themselves. Because the appearance can be deceiving, suspicious lesions should be cultured for the virus. Referees should be trained to recognize herpes gladiatorum lesions, wrestlers should be inspected for the disease at each weigh-in, and wrestlers with suspicious lesions should be barred from competition. Acyclovir, 200 mg orally every 4 hours for 5 doses daily for 10 days, has shown promise in hastening resolution. Some recommend its use for long-term suppression in affected wrestlers at a dose of 400 mg orally twice daily for 4–12 months.

8. What causes cauliflower ear?

Friction or trauma to the auricle of the ear produces cleavage of the plane between perichondrium and cartilage, and a collection of blood and serum (auricular hematoma) develops in the resulting space. Allowed to remain, the hematoma interferes with blood supply to the cartilage, and eventually new cartilage formation occurs in the space, resulting in irreversible deformity of the auricle.

9. How can auricular hematoma be treated to prevent cauliflower ear?

Prevention by use of properly fitted headgear is the best treatment. Techniques involving aspiration of fluid followed by some method of preventing reaccumulation are necessary once hematoma has occurred. Effective treatment must allow rapid return to competition, or the wrestler will not comply. Collodion casts and silicone ear molds to maintain the normal shape of the auricle after aspiration have been suggested. Probably the most effective treatment involves incision and drainage through a small incision, followed by use of cotton dental rolls or other form-fitting compressing material, cut to size and sutured through and through to either side of the auricle to achieve compression and obliteration of the cavity.[1,12]

10. Are mouth guards appropriate for use in wrestling?

Definitely. Current recommendations support the use of mouth guards in any sport in which orofacial injury is likely. For wrestling, a custom-fitted mouth protector is best, especially if the wrestler has orthodontic braces in place.

11. Why is weight control, specifically weight reduction, such an important aspect of wrestling?

Wrestlers believe that by competing in the lowest possible weight classification, they may have an advantage over other wrestlers in the same class who may not be so close to minimal weight. Because a team has only one competitor at a given weight classification per match, presence of two wrestlers at the same weight dictates a change in classification for one of them, frequently to a lower weight class.

12. Why is weight "cutting" such a concern?

Weight reduction to 5–8% body fat is not harmful if it is done gradually and with maintenance of proper nutrition and hydration; in our overnourished society, it may even be health-enhancing. Concern centers on inappropriate methods to secure rapid weight loss, including use of thermal methods (saunas, rubber sweat suits), artificial fluid elimination (spitting, induced emesis, use of diuretics and/or laxatives), or, most commonly, dehydration. Such methods may be harmful to health over the short or long term. The deaths of three collegiate wrestlers during the 1997–1998 season, apparently related to weight cutting abuses, has focused attention on such potentially unsafe practices. Some rule modifications proscribing hazardous weight-loss practices have been suggested, but the most effective regulatory action is likely a mandate that weigh-in occur within 1 hour of the match, rather than up to 24 hours preceding as has been the case. By limiting the time available to the wrestler for rehydration between weigh-in and competition, extreme dehydration to make weight will be avoided. Questions have been raised about a possible relationship between wrestling weight control and development of long-term eating disorders, but no definitive association has been proved to date.

13. How should a wrestler's minimal wrestling weight be determined?

Initially, some objective method such as anthropometry or skinfold determination of body fat should be used. Underwater weighing is difficult to administer to a significantly sized group unfamiliar with the technique. Various equations can be used to convert measurements into percent body fat.[3,6] Most authorities place the minimal weight at 5–8% body fat. Once the minimal weight for a wrestler has been determined, he should be observed as he approaches that weight, especially if significant physical growth is occurring. If he is unable to attain and hold that weight while maintaining basic nutrition, functioning properly socially and at school, avoiding illness, and practicing effectively, moving to a higher weight class may have to be considered.

A Method for Determining Minimal High School Wrestling Weight

1. Estimate body density (BD).
   $BD = 1.0982 - 0.000815 (Tsf + Ssf + Asf)$
   Tsf = triceps skinfold, Ssf = subscapular skinfold, and Asf = abdominal skinfold.

2. Use BD to estimate percent body fat (%BF):
   Postpubertal males:
   $\%BF = ([4.95/BD] - 4.5) \times 100$
   Prepubertal males:
   $\%BF = ([5.3/BD] - 4.89) \times 100$

3. Use %BF to estimate weight of body fat (FW):
   Body weight ($[BW] \times \%BF = FW$

4. Use FW to estimate fat-free weight (FFW).
   $BW - FW = FFW$

5. Decide what minimum percent body fat (M%BF) is to be allowed:
   M%BF = (literature supports 5%–8%)

6. Use (4) and (5) to determine minimum allowable weight (MAW):
   $MAW = FFW/(1.0 - [M\%BF \times .01])$

7. Assign minimum weight class, which is equal to or higher than MAW.

14. How does dehydration affect a wrestler?

Many wrestlers dehydrate 5–10% in the 24–48 hours before a match. Physicians often hospitalize patients with similar levels of dehydration for fear of complications. Acutely, dehydration produces less effective performance, especially in terms of strength and speed. Thermoregulation may be impaired; heat cramps, heat exhaustion, or heat stroke may occur. Electrolyte imbalance and the potential for disturbance in cardiac function may occur. A wrestler who has significantly dehydrated to make weight generally wrestles less well than one who made the same weight without dehydration. Chronically, it has been speculated that frequent repetition of dehydration may produce delayed renal damage, growth retardation, and problems with learning, especially if it is accompanied by malnutrition.

15. What is "injury time"? Why is it of medical significance?

During a match, an injured wrestler is allowed a maximum of two minutes to recover and be prepared to wrestle, or the match is defaulted to his opponent (unless the injury was caused by application of an illegal hold or maneuver). Injury time is not counted for bleeding, such as nosebleed, but the number of time-outs for bleeding is left to the referee's discretion. The match is terminated if bleeding is not controlled within 5 minutes. Thus, rapid decisions about the wrestler's ability to continue must be made by the physician, often under intense pressure from the wrestler and coaches. Wrestlers and coaches appreciate a physician who conserves injury time by efficient action.

16. How can the physician best use injury time?

By having a plan of evaluation in mind before the event occurs. Emphasis should be placed on determining ability to continue safely rather than definitive diagnosis. Initially check for breathing and consciousness, including orientation. If the wrestler can fully move the affected body part, has acceptable strength and sensation, can support his weight on the part and perform activity similar to that required in wrestling without evident handicap, including significant pain, and wants to return to the match, he may be allowed to do so. Signs or symptoms of significant head or neck injury preclude further competition until proved insignificant; doing so usually exceeds the two-minute limit. A conscious, oriented wrestler with a sore neck who voluntarily moves his neck through a full range of motion almost surely does not have a serious injury. In all attempts to move voluntarily, arise from the mat, or return to wrestling, the wrestler should not be assisted by the coach or any other person; if he cannot do so by himself, he has no business continuing the match. Once the match has been resumed, the prudent physician will watch for a while to ensure that the wrestler is, in fact, fully recovered and able to wrestle effectively. Current high school rules require that, in the case of a competitor rendered even briefly unconscious, a physician must certify his ability to continue in writing. A preprinted note requiring only signature will help shorten the time used in producing the note. The physician must be convinced, within injury time, that the wrestler can continue safely without a more significant risk than was present before the injury occurred, or he or she must withhold permission to continue.

17. Can medications be used during injury time?

Yes. Until 1992, the answer was no. The rule has been changed to remove the prohibition. Medications used during injury time are unlikely to be effective during the match in progress; the use of oral glucose for insulin reaction or an asthma inhaler are possible exceptions. Excessive use of inhaled sympathomimetic drugs can be dangerous, and such medications are rationally used before, not during, competition. "Banned" medications remain banned, and no medication (such as local anesthesia) should be used to camouflage pain.

18. How does one best deal with nosebleed?

Injury time is not counted for treatment of nosebleed, although the referee may terminate the match if he believes that the bleeding is excessive or uncontrollable. While preparing materials, get the wrestler off his feet; he should lie supine, depending on which position is most comfortable. Have the wrestler forcefully blow blood and clot out of nose into paper towel, then pinch the nostrils tightly until the packing is ready. Cotton is the best packing material and should be a single piece, large enough to fill the anterior nostril tightly. It is formed into an elongated strip and pushed firmly into the nostril; some is left protruding just outside the nostril to facilitate removal. Some authorities recommend coating the cotton with petrolatum or other lubricant, and some use astringents such as Nitro-tan or Germi-tan (sprayed on cotton in a zip-lock bag in advance and carried in the trainer's pocket until needed). Vasoconstrictor substances are often banned in international competition and probably are best avoided.

19. How can one handle cuts and lacerations within injury time?

After blotting off gross blood, maintain pressure on the wound to minimize further bleeding. Dry the surrounding skin to facilitate adhesive adherence, using acetone. Occlude the wound with impervious adhesive tape, or use several layers to avoid blood soaking through. Return the wrestler to action as quickly as possible. Because the adhesive may come off and bleeding recommence, conserving injury time to allow for repeated treatment is important.

20. Does suturing of lacerations require special techniques for wrestlers?

Yes. In areas where cuts are caused by tissue impact, repeated blows are likely to occur. Sutures must be placed closer together, usually require heavier suture material than ordinarily is used for maximal cosmetic effect, and are left in place longer. Meticulous technique is of major importance because of these compromises with optimal care. Skin wounds, sutured or not, must be adequately protected with bandages, which often require imaginative construction to ensure that they remain in place during competition.

21. Contrast knee injuries in wrestling with knee injuries in other sports.

The incidence is high, at or near the level in tackle football. Severity is considerably less. Meniscal injuries, especially lateral, are conspicuously more common in wrestling than other sports, probably due to the hyperflexion and torsion produced by certain holds combined with the significant and repeated knee stresses inherent in practicing and competing. Injuries may present atypically, with a minimal history of trauma.

22. What are the limitations to taping and bracing in wrestling?

Taping is legal so long as it does not significantly alter the normal range of motion of a joint. Knee and elbow pads are legal. Braces or other mechanical devices that pose the potential for injury to an opponent are illegal, as are devices that prevent application of standard wrestling holds or do not allow normal range of joint motion. Otherwise braces and taping may be used. The referee is the final authority on legality of taping or bracing.

23. How should the physician relate to the referee?

Although the referee is in total charge of the match and may stop it if he believes that a wrestler is in significant danger, he usually welcomes medical input. Introducing oneself as the on-site physician before the competition improves communication greatly. It is not appropriate to discuss a referee's decisions with him during the match, but later discussions about potentially dangerous holds or situations may educate both physician and referee. Communication with the referee during injury time is important so that he remains apprised of what is happening to the downed wrestler. The relationship between physician and referee can best be described as mutually supportive in most cases. Once a physician makes the determination that a wrestler may not continue because of illness or injury, no one, not even the referee, may overrule him or her.

BIBLIOGRAPHY

1. Dimeff RJ, Hough DO: Preventing cauliflower ear with a modified tie-through technique. Physician Sportsmed 17(3):169, 1989.
2. Garrick JG, Webb DR: Sports Injuries: Diagnosis and Management. Philadelphia, W.B. Saunders, 1990.
3. Horswill CA: When wrestlers slim to win. Physician Sportsmed 20(9):91, 1992.
4. Housh TJ, Johnson GO, Stout J, Housh DJ: Anthropometric growth patterns of high school wrestlers. Med Sci Sports Exerc 25:1141, 1993.
5. Klinzing JE, Karpowicz W: The effects of rapid weight loss and rehydration on a wrestling performance test. J Sports Med 26:149, 1986.
6. Lohman TG: Advances in Body Composition Assessment. Champaign IL, Human Kinetics, 1992.
7. Marquart LF, Sobal J: Weight loss beliefs, practices and support systems for high school wrestlers. J Adolesc Health 15:410, 1994.
8. Mellion MB, Walsh WM, Shelton GL (eds): The Team Physician's Handbook, 2nd ed. Philadelphia, Hanley & Belfus, 1997.
9. Nelson MA: Stopping the spread of herpes simplex. Physician Sportsmed 20(10):117, 1992.
10. Oppliger RA, Harms RD, Herrmann DE, et al: The Wisconsin wrestling minimum weight project: A model for weight control among high school wrestlers. Med Sci Sports Exerc 27:1220, 1995.
11. Schneider RC, Kennedy JC, Plant ML (eds): Sports Injuries: Mechanisms, Prevention and Treatment. Baltimore, Williams & Wilkins, 1985.
12. Schuller DE, Dankle SD, Strauss RH: A technique to treat wrestler's auricular hematoma without interrupting training or competition. Arch Otolaryngol Head Neck Surg 115:202, 1989.
13. Torg JS, Welsh RP, Shephard RJ (eds): Current Therapy in Sports Medicine-2. Philadelphia, B.C. Decker, 1990.
14. Webster S, Rutt R, Weltman A: Physiological effects of a weight loss regimen practiced by college wrestlers. Med Sci Sports Exerc 22:229, 1990.
15. Wroble RR, Mysnyk MC, Foster DT, Albright JP: Patterns of knee injuries in wrestling: A six-year study. Am J Sports Med 14:55, 1986.

87. SWIMMING

Paul R. Stricker, M.D., and James C. Puffer, M.D.

1. What are the most common injuries in swimmers?

Swimming injuries are more often chronic than acute and result from repetitive overuse. The most common musculoskeletal complaints involve the shoulder, knee, back, and foot.

2. Discuss the causes of foot pain in swimmers.

Slamming one's heel onto the edge of the swimming pool wall on a misjudged slip turn can certainly cause immediate heel pain. However, once beyond the beginner stage, it is hoped that this is not a regular occurrence.

The main cause of foot pain is tendinitis of the foot extensor tendons at the point where they are firmly bound by the extensor retinaculum. Repetitive motion of the foot as it goes from extreme plantar flexion to neutral in the freestyle, backstroke, and butterfly kicks causes this syndrome. Epidemiologic work has shown that overuse and acute injuries of the foot and ankle make up 15% and 30% of problems in swimmers, respectively.

3. What causes knee pain in swimmers?

Often referred to as "breaststroker's knee," knee pain in the swimmer is due to the valgus stress placed on the knee by the whip kick used in swimming the breaststroke. This can result in the development of medial collateral ligament stress, patellofemoral dysfunction, and/or medial synovial plica syndrome. Painful knees occur not only in beginners with poor breaststroke kick technique but also in elite breaststrokers as a result of the forcefulness of their kick and the high number of kick repetitions.

4. How common is shoulder pain in swimmers?

A recent survey of 1262 U.S. swimmers indicated that episodes of shoulder pain are common. Any history of interfering shoulder pain was found in 47% of age-group swimmers (13 to 14 years old), 66% of senior development swimmers (15 to 16 years old), and 73% of elite swimmers. This survey was primarily for pain that actually interfered with practice/competition. The combined incidence of interfering *and* noninterfering shoulder pain is obviously much higher and may approach 90% in selected populations.

5. What is the most common cause of shoulder pain?

Shoulder pain in swimmers is caused by a combination of overload and overuse with repetitive microtrauma and fatigue of the rotator cuff muscles and long head of the biceps. The acute process results in inflammation, and development of tendinitis, whereas a chronic process results in scarring and degenerative changes, referred to as tendinosis. Increased shoulder capsuloligamentous laxity, muscular imbalance of the cuff and weakness of scapular stabilizers contribute to fatigue, excessive glenohumeral translation, inflammation, and secondary impingement.

6. Which factors aggravate shoulder pain?

Pain is usually most prominent in the forward flexed, abducted, and internally rotated position, that is, the catch phase of the stroke. Shoulder pain is most common in freestyle, backstroke, and butterfly. Holding kickboards, certain stretches, weight training, and using hand paddles have been implicated in increasing shoulder pain.

7. Where is the vulnerable area of the supraspinatus tendon?

The distal tendon "watershed" area is approximately 1 cm from its attachment to the greater tubercle of the humerus. Microangiographic studies have shown that a "wringing out" process occurs with blood flow normal in forward flexion and abduction (catch phase) but dramatically reduced with the arm at the side of the body (recovery phase). It is thought that the high number of cycle repetitions during swimming may hasten the microscopic degenerative changes in this tendon.

8. What is impingement?

This term can be misused when describing shoulder pain in swimmers. True bony impingement rarely occurs before age 35 in swimmers, and if it does, it almost always involves a hooked acromium or some other anatomic abnormality. Impingement in swimmers less than the age of 35 is almost always secondary to instability. This results in anterior and superior migration of the humeral head with impingement of the supraspinatus under the coracoacromial arch. The "watershed" area described above is the portion of the supraspinatus tendon that is impinged on.

Symptomatic impingement can be demonstrated by passively moving the swimmer's arm into a position of forward flexion with the elbow bent to 90° and then internally rotating the arm to bring the supraspinatus tendon/greater tubercle of the humerus underneath the coracoacromial ligament. As the supraspinatus tendon (and sometimes the subacromial bursa) become inflamed, the subacromial space is decreased. This allows the tendon more easily to come in contact with the coracoacromial ligament. A positive test occurs if this maneuver causes marked pain.

9. Describe multidirectional instability.

Swimmers are noted for their highly flexible joints. Whereas some overhead athletes may have problems with unidirectional laxity or subluxation anteriorly or posteriorly, swimmers often have laxity in all directions in the absence of trauma, although the predominant directions of laxity are anteroinferior. This multidirectional instability appears to be due largely to abnormal inferior glenohumeral laxity without detachment of the glenoid labrum. This condition may cause pain during different phases of the overhead swimming strokes. Inferior instability can be demonstrated on physical examination by placing downward traction on the humerus with the resultant appearance of a sulcus between the humeral head and acromion. Anterior instability is demonstrated by positive apprehension when the arm is abducted and externally rotated with an anterior force placed behind the humeral head.

10. Should rehabilitation for shoulder pain involve only the rotator cuff muscles?

The rotator cuff muscles are significant contributors to the stability of the glenohumeral joint. A good strengthening program should definitely involve the muscles of the rotator cuff, primarily emphasizing the supraspinatus and external rotators. Unfortunately, often overlooked are the scapular stabilizers, which are important in normalizing the biomechanics of the glenohumeral joint. Swimmers often demonstrate relative strength imbalance between their internal rotators, which are strong, and their weaker scapular stabilizers and external rotators. This muscle imbalance can even cause the appearance of scapular winging. Any altered position of the scapula due to fatigue or weakness directly affects glenohumeral mechanics. Muscles involved in stabilizing the scapula against the thorax include the levator scapula, trapezius, rhomboids, and serratus anterior.

11. Does stretching do more harm than good?

Stretching before athletic activity is usually recommended, as it helps in warming up muscle-tendon units and thus helps to prevent injury. Certainly, swimmers rely heavily on good flexibility in order to train and compete well. Excessive stretching, however, has been implicated by some in increasing shoulder laxity and aggravating shoulder pain. Some swimmers feel tight if they do not stretch prior to practice or competition, whereas others rarely stretch and still compete very well at the elite level.

In reality, it is difficult to determine the actual role of stretching in the laxity/instability of swimmers' shoulders—a sort of "chicken and egg" scenario. It may be more likely that a selection process exists where the inherently more lax individuals experience greater success in this sport rather than stretching making swimmers more lax as they progress to the elite level.

12. What types of back problems do swimmers experience?

Unfortunately, **low back pain** is becoming increasingly more common in swimmers. Swimmers are at risk due to repetitive flexion, extension, and rotation of the spine with all four strokes. Changes in the backstroke turn as well as breaststroke style and hand recovery have more recently contributed to increasing torsional and hyperextension stresses on the lower spine. These various repetitive forces on the spine may lead to stress fractures of the pars interarticularis, referred to as **spondylolysis**. Very few actual reports of spondylolysis in swimmers are found in the literature, but one study reports an incidence of 7.4%. Another potential back problem is **scoliosis**. The incidence of structural scoliosis (deviation > 20° with rotation, rib hump asymmetry) in athletes has been found to be 1.6–2.0%. However, in swimmers, it has been found to be about 7%. Although controversial, it has been speculated that the muscular imbalance between the anterior and posterior musculature, repetitive torsional motion, and arm dominance of adolescent and preadolescent swimmers may cause secondary adaptation in vertebral structure leading to scoliosis.

13. Can individuals be allergic to swim goggles?

This type of allergy is quite uncommon, but actually has been seen by us. Allergy to the chemical constituents in the rubber lining of goggles, such as ethylbutylthiourea, represents a type of contact dermatitis and presents as red, swollen, pruritic, periorbital, raccoon eye-like areas. This can best be avoided by using the increasingly popular goggles that have no rubber lining or even polyvinylchloride goggles. However, some special goggles made with air-blown neoprene can be obtained directly from the manufacturers. If the reaction is severe, a short course of oral steroids is indicated.

14. What is "swimmer's ear"? How is it treated?

Swimmer's ear, or otitis externa, usually presents with pain and occasional drainage. Movement of the tragus and pinna exacerbates the pain. A contributing factor is the excessive wetness in the ear canal, which dramatically decreases the amount of cerumen protection and allows the pH to become more alkaline. As the squamous epithelium starts to break down, the lack of these protective factors provides an opportunity for infection to occur. Gram-negative bacteria predominate, with *Pseudomonas* being the most common. Fungal infections are less frequent, with *Aspergillus* being the most common cause of otomycosis.

After gentle canal cleaning, various treatment options include over-the-counter ear drops containing acetic acid for mild cases. This helps lower the pH of the ear canal. For severe cases, otic solutions that contain antibiotics (polymyxin, neomycin, or both) with or without hydrocortisone may be used.

15. Should persons with asthma or exercise-induced bronchospasm (EIB) be allowed to swim?

People with asthma or EIB should be treated with inhaled beta agonists or cromolyn sodium prior to exercise and can be allowed to participate in competitive swimming. If symptoms persist, a maintenance regimen that includes inhaled corticosteroids should be used. In fact, swimming is one of the best sports for the asthmatic child or young adult who wishes to participate in a sport. Because cold, dry air is involved in triggering bronchospasm, the warm, moist air above the surface of the water is less likely to elicit bronchospasm.

16. Are beta agonists banned drugs for swimmers participating in events at which drug testing will occur?

At present, selective aerosolized beta agonists are approved by the International Olympic Committee (IOC) for international competition, as well as other medications used in the prevention and treatment of asthma, such as cromolyn and inhaled steroids. However, the IOC requires prior written permission for athletes using inhaled beta agonists and/or inhaled steroids.

17. Should swimmers have a longer break between seasons?

If a swimmer is "overtrained," stale, and mentally overfatigued, an extra hiatus from swimming may be necessary. However, from a physiologic standpoint, the training gains made with respect to increased mitochondria and oxidative enzyme activity, glycogen utilization efficiency, and tolerance of lactate production (which requires 2–3 months of training to peak) decreases to pretraining levels in as little as 2–6 weeks.

18. Can a swimmer experience overtraining or excess fatigue?

Owing to the nature of their training patterns, swimmers become accustomed to long hours of practice at an early stage in their career. Once at the more advanced levels, swimmers are usually training twice daily for a total of 3 to 6 hours in addition to weight training. It is not difficult to see that the potential for overtraining injuries and fatigue is quite high.

Because of the duration of these training intensities and the associated short recuperation time, swimmers are at risk for glycogen depletion. Repetitive bouts of training require adequate glycogen stores for optimal performance. Diets with 70% carbohydrate content are helpful in providing necessary replacement loads for maintaining adequate glycogen stores. Glycogen resynthesis is a slow process, but there appears to be a critical window period about 30 minutes after exercising during which the muscle is most receptive to glycogen repletion. This can be accomplished by using any of the commercially available carbohydrate drinks immediately after practice (about 2 gm of carbohydrate per kilogram of body weight is needed at that time). It is also recommended that protein (0.7 gm/kg) be ingested along with carbohydrate to stimulate insulin release for better glycogen replacement. Certain sports drinks easily accomplish this goal. Inadequate nutritional status is one of the many potential factors that has been implicated in the development of chronic fatigue and overtraining in athletes.

19. Does shaving body hair for major competitions really work?

Virtually all competitive swimmers have had the experience (or danger) of "shaving down," and most would agree that it does make a difference. These competitions are usually at a time in their training when the swimmer is very rested. The swimmer feels energetic and is mentally and physically ready. These factors, coupled with the smooth feeling from shaving, give the swimmer an added mental boost. Most swimmers agree that shaving combined with other factors, such as a training taper, contributes to faster performance.

In addition to subjective reports and objective improvements in performance times, recent studies have investigated this issue scientifically. Shaving has resulted in increased distance per stroke, reduced passive drag, lower pull forces for forward propulsion, lower energy cost requirements, and faster swim times. Other observable effects seen, although not statistically significant, include lower heart rate, decreased lactate production, and less perceived exertion.

20. What are the beneficial aspects of swimming for children and adolescents?

Swimming has been shown to have many benefits for youngsters. Regular exercise such as swimming contributes to greater overall fitness. Swimmers often begin their sport at an early age, and compared with age-matched nonathlete controls ages 13–19, young swimmers have been found to demonstrate enhanced physical, cardiovascular, mental, and social skills. Although certain areas may show enhancement, these characteristics appear to follow biologic maturational patterns during normal growth and development similar to acquisition of motor skills. Endurance capacity appears to be fully developed by age 15, muscle power by age 18, and anaerobic characteristics by age 19.

BIBLIOGRAPHY

1. AAP Committee on Sports Medicine and Fitness: Chronic Health Problems. In Dyment P (ed): Sports Medicine: Health Care for Young Athletes. Elk Grove Village, IL, American Academy of Pediatrics, 1991, pp 251–256.
2. Altchek D (ed): Shoulder instability. Clin Sports Med 14:751–776, 1995.
3. Astrand PO, Rodahl K: Textbook of Work Physiology. New York, McGraw-Hill, 1977.
4. Bak K, Fauno P: Clinical findings in competitive swimmers with shoulder pain. Am J Sports Med 25:254–260, 1997.
5. Becker J: Scoliosis in swimmers. Clin Sports Med 5:139–148, 1986.
6. Dominguez RH: Water polo injuries. Clin Sports Med 5:180–181, 1986.
7. Fisher AA: Sports-related allergic dermatitis. Cutis 50:90–96, 1992.
8. Fowler PJ: Upper extremity swimming injuries. In Nicholas JA, Hershman EB (eds): The Upper Extremity in Sports Medicine. St. Louis, MO, Mosby, 1990, pp 891–898.
9. Fowler PJ, Regan WD: Swimming injuries of the knee, foot, and ankle, elbow, and back. Clin Sports Med 5:139–148, 1986.
10. Garrick JG, Requa RK: The epidemiology of foot and ankle injuries in sports. Clin Sports Med 7:29–36, 1988.
11. Hammer RW: Swimming and diving. In Mellion MB, Walsh WM, Shelton GL (eds): The Team Physician's Handbook, 2nd ed. Philadelphia, Hanley & Belfus, 1997, pp 718–728.
12. Hecker AL: Nutritional conditioning for athletic competition. Clin Sports Med 3:567–582, 1984.
13. Johns RA, Houmard JA, Kobe RW, et al: Effects of taper on swim power, stroke distance, and performance. Med Sci Sports Exerc 24:1141–1146, 1992.

14. Kennedy JC, Craig AB Jr, Schneider RC: Swimming. In Schneider RC, Kennedy JC, Plant ML (eds): Sports Injuries—Mechanisms, Prevention, and Treatment. Baltimore, Williams & Wilkins, 1985, pp 368–393.
15. Kulund DN: The Injured Athlete, 2nd ed. Philadelphia, J.B. Lippincott, 1988, pp 340–341.
16. McArdle WD, Katch FI, Katch VL: Exercise Physiology. Philadelphia, Lea & Febiger, 1981.
17. McKeag DB, Hough DO: Primary Care Sportsmedicine. Dubuque, IA, Brown & Benchmark, 1993, pp 363–367.
18. McMaster WC, Troup J: A survey of interfering shoulder pain in United States competitive swimmers. Am J Sports Med 21:67–70, 1993.
19. Middleton K: Prevention and rehabilitation of shoulder injuries in throwing athletes. In Nicholas JA, Hershman EB (eds): The Upper Extremity in Sports Medicine. St. Louis, MO, Mosby, 1990, pp 767–776.
20. Puffer JC, McShane J: Depression and chronic fatigue in athletes. Clin Sports Med 11:327–338, 1992.
21. Rathbun JB, Macnab I: The microvascular pattern of the rotator cuff. J Bone Joint Surg 52B:540, 1970.
22. Rupp S, Berninger K, Hopf T: Shoulder problems in high level swimmers—Impingement, anterior instability, muscular imbalance? Int J Sports Med 16:557–562, 1995.
23. Schuller DE, Bruce RA: Ear, nose, throat and eye. In Strauss R (ed): Sports Medicine. Philadelphia, W.B. Saunders, 1984, pp 175–179.
24. Skyhar MJ, Warren RF, Altcheck DW: Instability of the shoulder. In Nicholas JA, Hershman EB (eds): The Upper Extremity in Sports Medicine. St. Louis, C.V. Mosby, 1990, pp 181–193.
25. Troup JP: International Center for Aquatic Research Annual: 1989–1990. Colorado Springs, CO, United States Swimming Press, 1990, pp 101–105.
26. Troup JP: International Center for Aquatic Research Annual: 1991–1992. Colorado Springs, CO, United States Swimming Press, 1992, pp 3–16, 23–24.
27. USOC Drug Education and Doping Control Program. Colorado Springs, CO, United States Olympic Committee, 1990, pp 1–7.

88. SPRING BOARD AND PLATFORM DIVING

Lawrence D. Powell, M.D.

1. What are the most common injuries in diving?

Myofascial pain involving the neck and back is the most common type of injury sustained by divers. The mechanism of injury is usually hyperflexion of the neck or hyperextension of the lower back. Serious injuries involving the neck are rare in competitive divers. Treatment is usually nonoperative, with ice, NSAIDs, and physical therapy regimens that concentrate on stretching and flexibility. Any part of the body may sustain blunt trauma. Wrist and shoulder joints also may be injured as the diver enters the water. Injuries to the lower extremities are rare, but they do occur. There is at least one documented case of fracture of the talus involving the subtalar joint from forceful impact to the plantar surface of the hindfoot, which may result from the foot being struck by the spring board or from relanding on the board.

2. How common is neck pain in diving?

Injury to the neck is quite common. Diving has the highest incidence of spinal fractures. In one study from 1975–1986 at a regional spinal cord injury center, 9% of all patients admitted with suspected or proven spinal injury were involved in diving accidents. Most spinal cord injuries are associated with a closed head injury without intracranial lesion. The mechanism of injury is usually flexion/compression of the cervical spine resulting from a head-first dive with poor technique into shallow water. The head strikes the bottom of the pool or natural body of water, or a submerged object. An excessive axial load is transferred onto the cervical spine. In most cases an accompanying flexion of the cervical spine results in a fracture of the cervical spine when the force exceeds the absorbing capacity of the surrounding soft tissues and vertebral column. The athlete also may hit his or her head on the diving board or platform, causing a neck injury. Diving injuries involving the neck occur most often during recreational activities in shallow water.

3. What are other causes of neck pain associated with diving?

Less commonly rotational forces may cause subluxation of the facet joint, resulting in a locked facet joint. Another source of neck pain is atlantoaxial rotatory fixation, which may be either congenital or acquired. Most often it is associated with trauma, which is usually minimal. It is more common in children, especially females, and has been associated with fracture of the clavicle. The person may have "torticollis" and tenderness in the neck. It is diagnosed with plain radiographs of the cervical spine on the lateral and open-mouth odontoid views. CT scan may confirm widening of the odontoid-lateral mass interval. If left untreated, the associated torticollis may lead to progressive rotation of the latter mass of C1, with one documented death secondary to spinal cord transection. Initial treatment involves traction, antiinflammatory medication, and muscle relaxants. Some injuries reduce spontaneously, while others may need open reduction with atlantoaxial arthrodesis.

4. Is there a difference in the types of injuries sustained during platform and spring board diving?

In both types of diving, the cervical spine is most often injured. Spring board diving is associated with an increase in the percentage of lower extremity injuries. An example is fracture of the subtalar joint. The mechanism of injury is the board striking the plantar surface of the hindfoot or the diver relanding on the board on the hindfoot. A spring board allows the diver to reach great heights and distances. Diving from a 3-meter board may be the equivalent of diving from a 5-meter platform or 10 feet or more. The diver also may be catapulted into the shallow end of a pool, causing a neck or head injury.

5. How are spinal cord injuries treated in divers?

Unfortunately, most spinal injuries due to diving result in severe quadriplegia. In one study, only 4–9% of athletes with cervical spinal cord injuries recovered neurologic function; in another study, only 10% recovered neurologic function. The initial injury is usually a crush fracture of the cervical vertebrae, which causes dislocation of fragments toward the posterior aspect of the spinal canal. Immediate management should involve maintaining the airway, protecting the spine and spinal cord, carefully moving the diver from the water, and quick transportation to the hospital. The two most common causes of death are aspiration and shock. If possible, a history of aspiration or near drowning should be obtained so that the treating physician is aware of the development of aspiration pneumonia. A bolus of methylprednisolone (30 mg/kg) within 8 hours of spinal cord injury with neurologic deficit is followed by continuous infusion of 5.4 mg/kg/hr for 23 hours. The injured diver usually requires long-term rehabilitation and life-long assistance with activities of daily living.

6. How can diving injuries be prevented?

The general guideline that one should not dive into water shallower than twice one's height helps to prevent diving injuries. Although diving injuries are rarely fatal, they may result in serious neurologic sequelae. The injured diver is often permanently wheelchair-bound due to quadriplegia. Injuries usually result from diving into shallow water off a beach, pier, or other object into the ocean, river, lake, or private pool. Most accidents involve young males and occur during summer months. In some cases the person had been diving into an area several times before the traumatic event. Injury probably results from improvement of vertical entry into the water, which causes increased speed under water and allows the diver to obtain a greater depth than previously. The diver hits the bottom or a submerged object. One should not dive into unfamiliar water; the diver should know what is under the surface and the influence of tides on the depth. Other precautions include not diving until the area is clear of other swimmers, not engaging in horseplay in association with diving, and not mixing alcohol and diving. The American Association of

Neurological Surgeons and the Congress of Neurological Surgeons sponsor the "Think First" program. Other programs, such as "Feet First-First Time," which is sponsored by a group of Florida neurosurgeons, are geared toward education about issues such as diving head-first into water of unknown depth. Diving into above-ground pools should be prohibited. Water polo helmets help to prevent eardrum rupture. Wet suits help to prevent soft tissue damage to the back. Finally, information about safe diving should be an integral part of the regular training program of staff who teach young divers.

7. How common is back pain in divers?

Back pain is quite common. Like gymnastics, competitive diving involves tremendous stress on the vertebral column. Traumatic or congenital spondylolysis is a common cause of back pain. Continued stress to the lower back may lead to spondylolisthesis. Vertebral stress fractures and herniation of the nucleus pulposus may be caused by repeated axial stress from trampoline training, platform diving, and entry into the water. Diagnosis of back injuries is first attempted with plain radiographs of the lumbar spine and then with bone scan for osseous injuries and MRI for soft tissue pathology.

8. What is the most commonly injured vertebra?

The cervical spine is most mobile in the middle; therefore, C5 is the most commonly fractured vertebra (50% of fractures), followed by C6, C7, C4, C3, C2, and T1. Multilevel fractures occur in 10–20% of cases. Atlantooccipital fractures are rare. The most common atlantooccipital fractures are fracture dislocation of the odontoid and Jefferson fracture (compression fracture of C1).

9. What type of injuries in competitive diving involve the head?

Blunt trauma may occur as divers try to enter the water with less splash by "swimming" their arms to their side and leaving the head exposed. They also may hit their heads on the platform or diving board. Detached retinas and rupture of the tympanic membranes also may result from an awkward landing in the water from a great height. Further trauma may occur from the disorientation that accompanies such injuries, and the athlete should not be allowed to compete until the condition has been resolved. A diver with a ruptured tympanic membrane should not be allowed to enter the water because of the risk of infection. Blunt trauma also may involve the shoulders and extremities, especially when the diver attempts somersaults and twisting maneuvers. Lacerations also may result. Large scalp lacerations and facial lacerations may require referral to a plastic surgeon.

10. How are head injuries treated in diving?

Closed head trauma in diving is treated like head trauma elsewhere. One should follow the basic guidelines of cardiopulmonary resuscitation if the athlete is unconscious. Special precaution should be taken when removing the athlete from the water. If there is any risk of injury to the spine, the diver may be floated in the supine position in the water until professional help arrives. The first concern is to prevent drowning while keeping the neck stable. If possible, the athlete should be removed from the water with the neck immobilized. With any loss of consciousness a noncontrast head CT should be obtained. Return to diving should be based on established return-to-play criteria.

11. How are wrist injuries treated in diving?

Wrist injuries may be caused by hyperextension on impact with the water, often in association with "flat handing" or open hand entry technique. In this technique the hands overlap, usually with the dominant hand on top, to decrease water splash on entry by creating a "water hole" in which the rest of the body enters. The wrist is hyperextended, pronated, and radially deviated. All of the stress is directed to the posterolateral side of the wrist and hand. Such repeated trauma may result in impingement in the distal row of carpal bones that leads to periostitis or stress fractures. Ligament sprains also may occur in the wrist, especially of the triangular fibrocartilage complex. The closed-fist technique of entry into the water causes hyperextension and traction of the thumb that is held by the fist; the trapeziometacarpal ligaments are most often sprained with this technique. Treatment includes active rest and quick return to diving. On return to activity, taping or placing pads over bony prominences may help. The tape usually loosens and provides less support after getting wet; therefore, Velcro splints seem to be more effective.

12. What is the mechanism of injury for shoulder problems in divers?

Shoulder dislocations are infrequent. When they do occur, they usually result from high diving when the athlete fails to clasp the hands together before entering the water and the arms are forcibly abducted upon entry. The technique called "flat handing," in which the diver grabs one hand, hyperextending the wrist and externally rotating the arm, sometimes results in shoulder subluxation and chronic rotator cuff syndrome problems. This is more apt to happen to the young diver whose shoulders are not strong enough.

13. At what age should children and adolescents begin diving?

Adolescents may lack the strength in their hips and spinal flexor muscles to maintain proper body alignment during diving. In France, 10-m platform diving is not allowed for athletes less than 15 years old. The adolescent diver should have developed significant strength of the shoulders, which helps to prevent the arms from being forced apart upon entry into the water and exposing the head to injury.

14. What medical condition restricts participation in competitive diving?

Congenital cervical stenosis may lead to central cord compression and myelopathy. This condition may be exacerbated by repeated extreme flexion due to improper body alignment as the head enters the water or incorrectly entering the water with hands unclasped and arms shoulder width apart with the force directly on the head. Repeated microtrauma from diving also may accelerate the normal aging process of cervical spondylosis. Restricted activity and follow-up with the appropriate specialist are recommended for athletes with congenital cervical stenosis. Atlantoaxial instability, which may occur in Down syndrome, also needs further evaluation to assess the risk of spinal cord injury during diving. Any problem that causes disorientation and vertigo may affect balance and lead to significant blunt trauma; activity should be restricted until the condition has resolved.

15. Is there an association between diving and alcohol use?

A large number of diving injuries can be prevented by not drinking and diving. In three separate studies of cervical spinal injuries associated with diving injuries, physicians found that in 37–44% of recreational diving accidents, the divers had been drinking.

16. What training techniques help to prevent diving injuries?

A good conditioning program that is continued into the offseason is preventive. Because most competitive divers suffer from low back pain, aerobic conditioning is important for endurance. A fatigued muscle does not support the vertebral column as well. Aerobic conditioning is best achieved by walking or jogging. Flexibility is also important. Static stretching of major muscle groups, at least 3 times/day, helps to prevent damage to joints. Finally, strengthening the pelvic, lower back, and abdominal muscles helps to maintain proper posture and body alignment upon water entry. Athletes should dive with their eyes open to use visual cues for better control of the dive. The athlete should be taught not to double-bounce on the diving board.

BIBLIOGRAPHY

1. Albrand OW, Walter J: Underwater deceleration curves in relation to injuries from diving. Surg Neurol 4:461–464, 1975.
2. Bailes JE, Herman JM, Quigley MR, et al: Diving injuries of the cervical spine. Surg Neurol 34:155–158, 1990.

3. Damjan H, Turk PR: Prevention of spinal injuries from diving in Slovenia. Paraplegia 33:246–249, 1995.
4. Herman JM, Sonntag VKH: Diving accidents. Mechanism of injury and treatment of the patient. Crit Care Nurs Clin North Am 3:339–352, 1991.
5. Kluger Y, Jarosz D, Paul DB, et al: Diving injuries: A preventable catastrophe. J Trauma 36:349–351, 1994.
6. Le Viet DT, Lantieri LA, Loy SM: Wrist and hand injuries in platform diving. J Hand Surg 18:876–880, 1993.
7. Logan PM, O'Rourke K, Gibbey RG: Case of the month: Atlanto-axial rotatory fixation. Br J Radiol 68:93–94, 1995.
8. Marymont JV, Mizel MS: Fracture of the subtalar joint in springboard divers. A report of two cases. Am J Sports Med 24:123–124, 1996.
9. Reid DC: Sports Injury Assessment and Rehabilitation. New York, Churchill Livingstone, 1992.
10. Fu FH, Stone DA (eds): Sports Injuries: Mechanisms, Prevention, Treatment. Baltimore, Williams & Wilkins, 1994.

89. BASEBALL AND SOFTBALL

Tony C. Roisum, M.D., and James A. Whiteside, M.D.

1. What is the most common mechanism of injury in slow-pitch softball?

Sliding is the most common mechanism of injury in slow-pitch softball. The feet-first slide makes the ankle, knee, and thigh susceptible to injury. Other common injuries involve the hand, wrist, and fingers during the head-first slide. Head-first slides with arms extended may produce glenohumeral subluxation. Even with helmets, head-first slides are contraindicated.

2. How can many slow-pitch softball injuries be prevented?

Break-away or low-profile bases should be used. Sliding injuries have been shown to be preventable by using break-away or low-profile bases. It is estimated that 1.7 million sliding injuries could be prevented each year with a savings of $1.9 billion in medical costs.

3. What time-loss injuries are common in fast-pitch softball?

Injuries to the throwing shoulder, arm, and hand are common. Because of greater forces and velocities (stresses) produced from the fast pitch, the arm and shoulder are at increased risk of acute injury and overuse. Over 80% of the time-loss injuries to elite women fast-pitch softball pitchers involved the throwing arm.

4. Is the fast-pitch underhand toss a more natural motion and less susceptible to injury than the overhand throw?

Probably not. Recent investigation and biomechanical analysis of the underhand fast pitch do not support the contention that the underhand pitching motion is more natural and less injury-prone. Average shoulder distraction forces have been measured at approximately 85% body weight. The average distraction force at the shoulder in overhand baseball throwing has been estimated to be 90% body weight. It seems that more stress is applied to the fast-pitch softball thrower's shoulder and arm during the pitching act than previously considered. Certainly more scientific study is needed to clarify the biomechanics and injury types involved in the underhand pitch.

5. In fast-pitch softball, where are stress (fatigue) fractures most likely to occur?

They are likely to occur in the middle one-third of the shaft of the ulna in the pitcher. The cross-sectional area is smaller in this region and less resistant to torsion of forearm motion. In addition, the "sling" action at ball release, along with forceful contraction of the brachialis to flex the forearm, places considerable stress on the tuberosity and coronoid process of the ulna.

6. How can injuries to the throwing arm in softball be prevented?
- Learn sound pitching mechanics and engage in year-round conditioning.
- Strengthen the anterior shoulder, biceps, and flexor muscles of the throwing arm to develop ball velocity properly.
- Do not overlook eccentric strengthening of arm extensor and posterior shoulder muscles to dissipate the forces generated by the throwing arm appropriately and to help prevent overuse rotator cuff injury.
- Decrease number of innings and games pitched. Stop pitching multiple games on the same day.
- Begin and end all activity with a proper warm-up and cool-down phase.

7. In baseball, what are the most significant throwing injuries?
The injuries that cause poor performance and prevent return to the previous level of participation involve the rotator cuff, ulnar (medial) collateral ligament of the elbow, and hypertrophic spur formation of the olecranon.

8. How can baseball throwing injuries be prevented?
Learning proper body mechanics of the throwing motion is the key to injury prevention. Physical fitness must always be emphasized as a way to prevent injuries. A structured, year-round exercise program must emphasize both shoulder and elbow concentric and eccentric strengthening because a problem in one area predisposes to injury in the other. Young pitchers should learn to throw accurately and correctly only the fastball and change-up pitches. The number and frequency of mound appearances must be monitored.

For the coach, recognizing the altered mechanics of the tired pitcher and replacing the pitcher can help to avoid harmful inflammation about the shoulder and elbow. Soreness that persists or sudden, sharp pain in the throwing arm or shoulder must always be evaluated. Never play through pain.

9. During which phase of delivery does the biomechanical difference between throwing a curve ball and a fastball cause increased stress?
The throwing of a curve ball causes an increased medial elbow traction stress and lateral compression at ball release. The fastball has increased medial elbow traction stress during the early acceleration phase.

10. Does throwing the curve ball increase the risk of injury to the elbow in immature athletes?
Yes. The throwing of the curve ball may not be the culprit but rather improper mechanics while throwing the pitch. It is imperative that the athlete possess the best possible throwing technique to eliminate injury. The forearm internally rotates and pronates as the ball is released. Improper attempts to supinate when throwing the wide curve ball can cause excessive vector forces about the elbow. When learned and thrown properly, the curve ball should not produce significantly greater stress to the elbow joint than any other pitch. The increased number of pitches thrown per week at home and at practice or games is vastly more predictive of arm injury in youth. Knowledgeable coaches and parents can reduce susceptibility to acute or overuse arm impairment in immature athletes by teaching correct, safe mechanics and controlling the amount of throwing.

11. At what age can a young, male pitcher safely begin to throw the curve ball?
Because of improper mechanics, it is recommended that young pitchers be prohibited from throwing the curve ball until they begin to shave. This recommendation is based on the skeletal maturity theory that if the joints and bones are essentially mature, the increased stress applied at the shoulder and elbow is better tolerated. Ideally, before throwing the curve the player should perfect the fastball and an off-speed pitch with good velocity and control.

12. What is a major difference between men and women overhand throwers?
Elite men overhand throwers stride farther with the lead leg and push longer and harder off the back foot than elite women throwers. This difference does not explain the apparent mechanical differences in throwing between genders in children as they attempt to throw overhead.

13. What is Little Leaguer's elbow?

The purist definition is medial epicondylar apophyseal avulsion. Since its initial description other pathologic conditions, such as osteochondritis dissecans of the capitellum, have been included under this general classification in relation to medial traction and lateral compression.

14. What is Little Leaguer's shoulder?

Little Leaguer's shoulder is a Salter I fracture of the proximal humeral growth plate. The condition is manifested by shoulder pain that is aggravated by throwing or pitching. Pain is usually nonspecific and worse after activity or hard throwing. Physical examination reveals tenderness over the proximal humeral epiphysis that may be confused with rotator cuff tendinitis and impingement.

The diagnosis is made with the aid of roentgenograms that reveal widening of the proximal epiphyseal plate of the humerus owing to sheer and torque forces. Comparison roentgenograms of the opposite humerus may be necessary. Treatment includes about 6 weeks of relative rest from any form of throwing or even batting to allow the fracture to heal. Attention needs to be directed toward prevention of this overuse injury.

15. What is a SLAP lesion?

SLAP lesions are common in overhand throwers and signify a tear in the superior labrum that extends in an anterior to posterior direction (SLAP = superior labrum anterior posterior). A significant mechanism of injury is repetitive, forceful contraction that compresses the glenohumeral joint and places great stress on the biceps labral complex during the deceleration phase of the throwing motion.

16. What entity produces posterior elbow pain in extension and with valgus stress?

In valgus extension overload, after a few innings the pitches tend to rise and sail high. This loss of control is related to formation of medial olecranon osteophytes that inhibit full elbow extension. They can be identified on lateral and axial radiographs.

17. When a pitcher's arm "goes dead," what diagnosis must be considered?

"Dead arm" syndrome occurs in recurrent, anterior, transient treatment subluxation of the glenohumeral joint of the shoulder when the arm is abducted and externally rotated, as in the cocking position. Forceful repetitive throwing in this lax condition may produce a compression fracture of the posterior humeral head (Hill-Sacks lesion) or detachment of the glenoid labrum or fracture of the glenoid rim (bony—Bankart lesion).

18. What is one of the fastest human motions?

When filmed in biomechanical laboratories, professional pitchers have exhibited arm speeds greater than 7000°/sec during delivery as the arm moves from external to internal rotation.

19. What field position in baseball or softball demands the least amount of stress on the throwing arm?

First base. This position can be used by a player who is rehabilitating a throwing arm injury but still wants to participate in other aspects of the game. Playing first base along with strengthening, flexibility, and rehabilitation allows a graduated, step-wise return to full play.

20. What is the difference between the pitcher's and catcher's overhand throw?

The catcher's throw is short-armed with little transfer of energy because of reduced cocking and abbreviated follow-through. The force of this reduced motion must be absorbed by the shoulder musculature to stabilize the humeral head in the glenoid fossa and prevent instability during deceleration.

21. What specific injury is related to the lead shoulder in batting?

Baseball players may develop recurrent posterior shoulder instability of the lead shoulder while batting as a result of increased posterior glenoid shear forces and repetitive microtrauma to the posterior capsular restraints. Susceptibility to develop posterior shoulder instability increases during the checked swing, hitting the outside pitch, or trying to pull the outside pitch.

22. What is thrower's exostosis?
Heterotopic calcification adjacent to the inferior border of the glenoid due to posterior capsular traction stress. The thrower may experience pain in the posterior aspect of the shoulder, but often the radiologic finding on the anteroposterior film may be incidental.

23. What are the phases of the overhand pitching motion?

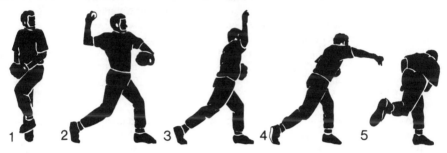

1. Windup   2. Cocking   3. Acceleration   4. Deceleration   5. Follow-through.

From Blackburn TA: Baseball and softball. In Mellion MB, Walsh WM, Shelton GL: The Team Physician's Handbook, 2nd ed. Philadelphia, Hanley & Belfus, 1997, with permission.

24. Define each phase.
The **windup** is a balance and preparation phase in which the opposite leg is cocked. The **cocking phase** begins as hands part and ends when the throwing arm is in extreme rotation. The **acceleration phase** begins when the ball moves forward with internal rotation of the humerus and ends with ball release. In **deceleration**, the elbow extends as the shoulder absorbs violent distraction forces by contraction of the rotator cuff muscles. In the **follow-through**, the body moves forward with the arm to relieve tension on the rotator cuff musculature. Strength of the opposite leg controls smooth transition to recovery as the trailing leg contacts the ground.

25. What is the best way to diagnose an injury to the thrower's shoulder or elbow?
A complete and accurate history and physical examination with ancillary radiographs and, at times, special tests, are essential. It is important to correlate symptoms to location of injury with the appropriate phase of the throwing motion. Understanding the mechanics of the throwing motion allows the examiner to categorize certain diagnoses during the history-taking process that can direct the clinical investigation and expedite management.

Phases of the Throwing Motion that Correlate with Certain Pathologic Conditions of the Elbow

1. Cocking phase	2. Acceleration phase *(cont.)*
• Strain of flexor muscles	• Olecranon posteromedial osteophyte
• Ulnar neuropathy	• Loose bodies
• Traction spurs of ulnar coronoid process	• Avulsion fracture of olecranon
2. Acceleration phase	• Olecranon apophysitis or stress reaction
• Strain of flexor muscles	3. Deceleration/follow-through phase
• Ulnar (medial) collateral ligament sprain	• Biceps strain/avulsion
• Ulnar neuropathy/subluxation	• Olecranon spurs
• Medial epicondylar apophysitis	• Chondromalacia of olecranon fossa
• Lateral epicondylitis	• Anterior capsular strains
• Deformities of the radial head	• Coronoid process spurs
• Triceps strain	

Phases of the Throwing Motion that Correlate with Certain Pathologic Conditions of the Shoulder

1. Cocking phase
   • Anterior shoulder instability or subluxation
   • Anterior inferior labral tears
   • Quadrilateral space syndrome
   • Acromioclavicular joint pathology
   • Subacromial bursitis
2. Acceleration phase
   • Anterior subluxation
   • Rotator cuff tendinitis/partial tears
   • Labral pathology
   • Subacromial bursitis
   • Proximal humeral apophysitis

3. Deceleration
   • Rotator cuff tendinitis/partial tears
   • Biceps tendinitis/rupture
   • SLAP lesion of superior labrum
   • Posterior subluxation
   • Posterior capsulitis
4. Follow-through
   • Thrower's exostosis
   • Acromioclavicular joint pathology
   • Posterior subluxation

BIBLIOGRAPHY

1. Albert MJ, Drvarie DM: Little league shoulder: Case report. Pediatr Orthop 13:779–781, 1990.
2. Andrews JR, Kupferman SP, Dillman CJ: Labral tears in throwing and racquet sports. Clin Sports Med 10:901–911, 1991.
3. Andrews JR, Schemmel SP, Whiteside JA, Timmerman LA: Evaluation, treatment, and prevention of elbow injury in the athlete. In Nicholas JA, Hershman EB (eds): The Upper Extremity in Sports Medicine, 2nd ed. St. Louis, Mosby, 1995, pp 749–788.
4. Degroot H, Mass DP: Hand injury patterns in softball players using a 16-inch ball. Am J Sports Med 16(3):260–265, 1988.
5. Duda M: Sturdy, breakaway bases would cut sliding injuries. Phys Sportsmed 16(7):123–125, 1988.
6. Fleisig GF: Biomechanics of fastball and curveball pitching. Eleventh Annual Injuries in Baseball Course Syllabus, January 21–24, 1993, Birmingham, Alabama, pp 107–110.
7. Loosli AR, Resqua RK, Garrick JG: Injuries to pitchers in women's collegiate fast-pitch softball. Am J Sports Med 20(1):35–37, 1992.
8. Loosli AR, Resqua RK, Ross W, Garrick JG: Injuries in slow pitch softball. Physician Sportsmed 16(7):110–118, 1983.
9. Mellion MB, Walsh WM (eds): The Team Physician's Handbook, 2nd ed. Philadelphia, Hanley & Belfus, 1997.
10. Nadeau MT, Boatman J, Brown T, Heaston WT, et al: The prevention of softball injuries: The experience of Yokota. Milit Med 155:3–5, 1990.
11. Tanabe S, Nakahira J, Bando E, et al: Fatigue fracture of the ulna occurring in pitchers of fast-pitch softball. Am J Sports Med 19:317–321, 1991.
12. Wheeler BR: Ankle fractures in slow-pitch softball: The army experience. Milit Med 152:626–628, 1987.
13. Zarins B, Andrews JR, et al: Injuries to the Throwing Arm. Philadelphia, W.B. Saunders, 1985.

90. TRACK AND FIELD

John P. DiFiori, M.D., and James C. Puffer, M.D.

1. In what events does a track and field athlete compete?

Track and field can be broadly classified into three types of events: running, jumping, and throwing. Because of the different nature of the running events, running athletes are usually described as sprinters, middle distance runners, distance runners, or hurdlers. The shot put, discus throw, hammer throw, and javelin throw are often referred to as the weight events because of the weighted implements involved. Decathletes and heptathletes compete in a combination of events that test speed, endurance, jumping, and throwing ability.

Track and Field Events

SPRINTS	MIDDLE DISTANCE	DISTANCE	THROWING	JUMPING	COMBINATION
100 meters	800 meters	3000 meters	Javelin throw	High jump	Long jump
200 meters	1500 meters	5000 meters	Discus throw	Triple jump	100-meter hurdles
400 meters		10,000 meters	Shot put		400-meter hurdles
		Marathon	Hammer throw		3000-meter steeplechase
					Pole vault
					Heptathlon
					Decathlon

2. What physiologic demands are placed on track and field athletes?

In running events of less than two minutes' duration, the major fuel source is glucose and the primary energy pathway is anaerobic. Oxygen debt and accumulation of lactic acid (a contributor to fatigue) are the consequences. As exercise extends beyond the initial 2–3 minutes, aerobic pathways utilizing fats and glucose derived from glycogen stores begin to provide energy. Lactic acid build-up is blunted as steady-state oxygen consumption is reached. In prolonged exercise (> 10 minutes) the ability to utilize fats and spare glycogen is an effective mechanism to provide a supply of energy to the working muscles using predominantly aerobic pathways. Thus, sprinters function primarily on anaerobic metabolism, whereas distance runners use aerobic pathways. Middle distance runners must be conditioned to utilize both anaerobic and aerobic mechanisms. Physiologic demands provide the rationale for the development of training regimens.

3. What is "hitting the wall"?

"Hitting the wall" occurs when glycogen stores have been exhausted and the shift back to anaerobic metabolism occurs. This shift causes build-up of lactic acid and onset of fatigue.

4. What special skills must the jumpers and throwers develop?

The throwing events place a premium on both strength and technique. Each throwing motion is designed to generate a maximum of momentum before the release of the implement. In the shot put, discus, and hammer throw, the different stages of the throwing motion are restricted to a 7-foot throwing circle. Thus, in addition to strength, athletes must possess precise balance and timing. Like the throwing events, the jumping events require power and technique but also demand a sprinter's speed.

5. What comprises a track and field season?

Athletes compete in an indoor season during the winter months and an outdoor season during the spring and summer months. The fall is generally a period of relative rest and conditioning. Because of the nearly year-round nature of the sport, workouts must be carefully planned to avoid injury and to provide peak performances.

6. What is overtraining?

Overtraining, often referred to as "staleness," is a syndrome characterized by fatigue, irritability, and sleep difficulty. It typically occurs in endurance athletes who have undergone an increase in training intensity or volume. Athletes who are unable to adapt to the training load manifest these symptoms along with a decrease in training and competitive performance. A psychologic assessment with the Profile of Mood States (POMS) demonstrates an increase in feelings of depression, anger, and fatigue in conjunction with a decrease in feelings of vigor. Depletion of glycogen stores is also associated with this syndrome.

7. What clinical and laboratory findings are helpful?

Physical findings are rarely significant. A focused laboratory screening should be performed to rule out other causes of fatigue, such as anemia, infection (mononucleosis), and endocrine abnormalities (hypothyroidism). The patient should also be evaluated for endogenous depression if psychological symptoms predominate.

8. How is overtraining treated?

Once the diagnosis is confirmed, a significant reduction in training load and an increase in carbohydrate intake are prescribed. Several days of complete rest are often indicated. As symptoms resolve, activity may be gradually resumed. Future training should be restructured to incorporate planned rest periods and gradual training increases to avoid a recurrence.

9. What is periodization of training?

Periodization is the systematic cycling of training sessions over time. Training volume and intensity are varied, usually progressing from high volume, low intensity to low volume, high intensity as the season develops. Periods of relative rest are built into the program in an effort to prevent injury and overtraining.

10. What are plyometrics?

Plyometric training consists of exercises in which concentric muscle action is immediately preceded by eccentric loading. Examples include hops, bounds, and depth jumps. The close coupling of eccentric and concentric muscle actions increases force development in the concentric phase. It is often used as a supplemental training technique for sprinters, jumpers, and throwers but may be accompanied by a high injury rate, particularly in nonelite athletes.

11. Which athletes incur the most injuries?

Sprinters and distance runners account for the vast majority of injuries that result in lost training days. Only a small percentage of injuries occur during competition.

12. What is the most common site of injury in track and field athletes?

The lower extremity is the most frequently injured site.

13. What etiologic process is most responsible for the development of injury in runners?

Overuse is the leading cause of injury in runners. In overuse injuries, normal tissue is subjected to repetitive stress that induces microtrauma. Over time accumulated microtrauma results in tissue injury that triggers the release of arachidonic acid and an inflammatory cascade that ends in prostaglandin formation. Prostaglandins mediate an inflammatory response that results in pain and dysfunction.

14. What are the risk factors for overuse injuries?

The strongest predictors of injury based on epidemiologic data are history of previous injury, weekly mileage, and running experience. Athletes running more than 30–40 mi/wk and novice runners are at greater risk than experienced runners who keep their mileage below 30 mi/wk. Menstrual dysfunction, which leads to a decrease in bone density, is believed to be a risk factor for the development of stress fractures. Biomechanical malalignment is also thought to be a contributor to overuse injuries. Pes planus, hyperpronation, and leg length discrepancy are examples. Worn or poorly cushioned running shoes also may lead to overuse injuries.

15. What are orthotics?

Orthotics are molded devices placed inside the athlete's shoe. They are made of plastic, foam, or a combination of materials and are designed to correct abnormal foot biomechanics such as hyperpronation and pes planus.

16. What training factors contribute to the development of overuse injuries?

Abrupt increases in training volume and/or intensity may underlie overuse injury.

17. What types of injuries are a result of overuse?
Muscle strains, tendinitis, stress fractures, and compartment syndromes may result from overuse.

18. How are overuse injuries classified?
The severity of injury is based on onset of pain in relation to onset of activity.

Overuse Injuries—Functional Classification of Pain

CLASSIFICATION	CHARACTERISTICS
Type 1	Pain after activity only
Type 2	Pain during activity, not restricting performance
Type 3	Pain during activity, restricting activity
Type 4	Chronic, unremitting pain

From Puffer JC, Zachazewski MS: Management of overuse injuries. Am Fam Physician 38:225–232, 1988, with permission.

19. How are overuse injuries treated?
Relative rest, ice massage, stretching, and progressive resistance exercises are the basis of treatment. Reduction in activity and additional measures such as antiinflammatory medications and physical therapy modalities (e.g., ultrasound, iontophoresis) depend on the severity of injury. A key point is the use of alternative activities to maintain conditioning and morale.

Guidelines for the Treatment of Overuse Injuries

I. Determine severity of injury based on functional classification.
II. Guidelines for treatment
1. Relative rest
2. Use of alternative activities to maintain aerobic conditioning (e.g., swimming, cycling, running in water with flotation vest)
3. Ice massage
4. Progressive resistance exercises
5. Flexibility program
6. Soft tissue techniques
7. Evaluation of menstrual dysfunction, if present
8. Correction of training errors and sport technique
9. Assessment of running shoes and/or sport equipment
10. Consider antiinflammatory medication, physical therapy, including modalities, modification of biomechanical abnormalities, and corticosteroid injection therapy in selected cases.

20. Which track athletes are most likely to suffer from acute muscle pulls?
Acute muscle strains are more common in sprinters and jumpers. The injury occurs when a sudden load that exceeds its tensile strength is placed on the muscle. A palpable gap is often present in the muscle belly. The hamstrings, gastrocsoleus complex, and quadriceps are common sites for such injuries.

21. Are acute muscle pulls due to overuse?
It is unclear whether the majority of acute muscle strains occur in the presence of weakness created by an overuse process.

22. What is the proper approach to the physical examination of the track and field athlete with lower extremity complaints?
The examination should begin with the patient standing in bare feet and dressed preferably in shorts. This allows gross evaluation of gait and observation of malalignment. A focused

examination of the injured area should then follow. This approach can be described as examining "from the ground up."

23. What is runner's knee?

The correct term for runner's knee is patellofemoral syndrome, which is the most common injury in runners, accounting for up to 30% of running injuries. The pain is thought to arise from nerve fibers in the subchondral bone of the patella or from synovitis.

24. What are the symptoms of patellofemoral syndrome?

The major symptom is dull knee pain "behind the kneecap." It has a gradual onset and is usually made worse with ascending or descending stairs and downhill running. The patient often experiences stiffness in straightening the knee after sitting for prolonged periods (the so-called theater sign).

25. What are the significant physical and radiologic findings of patellofemoral syndrome?

Pes planus, hyperpronation, femoral anteversion, and an increased quadriceps angle (Q angle) may be seen. As the knee is examined, pain with patellofemoral compression and palpation of patellar facets is noted. Retropatellar crepitus can be appreciated by palpating the patella during active range of motion. Radiographs are usually negative, but occasionally lateral seating of the patella is seen on Merchant views. Tight lateral structures (including the lateral retinaculum), passive patellar tilt, and vastus medialis obliquus (VMO) insufficiency may be demonstrated.

26. How is patellofemoral syndrome treated?

The guidelines for the treatment of overuse injuries should be followed, A main goal of therapy is to correct malalignment, develop the VMO, improve flexibility of the hamstrings, and stretch tight lateral structures. McConnell taping techniques are believed to be useful in promoting appropriate tracking of the patella.

27. What is jumper's knee?

This common injury is characterized by pain at the inferior pole of the patella at its attachment to the patellar tendon. The more accurate term is infrapatellar tendinitis. Treatment is similar to other overuse injuries with a focus on quadriceps strengthening.

28. A distance runner complains of lateral knee pain that is worse with downhill running and running on banked surfaces. Physical examination reveals tenderness over the lateral femoral condyle. What is the most likely diagnosis?

The history and findings are most consistent with iliotibial band (ITB) syndrome. With repeated flexion and extension of the knee during running, friction may develop as the ITB courses over the lateral femoral condyle. This friction causes inflammation of the ITB, periosteum, or bursa that lies between these structures.

29. What clinical test is helpful in making this diagnosis?

Ober's test. The patient is placed on his or her side with the affected leg uppermost. The injured leg is then flexed to 90° at the knee and fully abducted. The leg is then released and allowed to adduct. Pain or tightness, as demonstrated by the inability to adduct the leg fully is considered a positive test.

30. What are shin splints?

Shin splints is a descriptive name for what has been termed medial tibial stress syndrome (MTSS). MTSS is characterized by anteromedial or posteromedial leg pain of gradual onset. It is a type of overuse injury caused by chronic traction and inflammation of the tibial periosteum, with fibrofatty tissue filling the defect. It may involve the posterior tibialis, anterior tibialis, or soleus muscles.

31. How is MTSS different from a stress fracture?

A stress fracture occurs when periosteal resorption exceeds lamellar bone formation; it is also a result of overuse.

32. What is the most common site of stress fractures in runners?

Overall, the tibia is the site for more than 30% of stress fractures in runners; however, the prevalence appears to vary depending on the events involved. For example, the most common site in distance runners is the tibia, whereas in sprinters and hurdlers metatarsal stress fractures are more prevalent.

33. What historical clues help to distinguish between MTSS and a tibial stress fracture?

Pain from MTSS may be present at the start of running, decrease as the activity continues, and then return after the training session. Pain from a stress fracture usually does not remit during activity.

34. What are the physical findings?

MTSS is characterized by tenderness along several centimeters of the posteromedial border of the tibia, usually located near the junction of the middle and distal thirds of the tibia. Pain may increase with resisted dorsiflexion or plantarflexion and inversion. A tibial stress fracture has a focal area of tenderness along the anterior tibia. Striking the heel or passing ultrasound or a tuning fork over the site may increase the pain.

35. Which diagnostic tests are helpful?

Radiographs are negative in MTSS but may be positive in a stress fracture 2 or more weeks after the onset of symptoms. A triple-phase bone scan demonstrates a fusiform region of uptake in MTSS and a pisiform uptake pattern in a stress fracture. More recently, magnetic resonance imaging (MRI) has been used in the diagnosis of stress fractures. Findings include periosteal edema, bone marrow edema, and in some cases a fracture line.

36. How is a tibial stress fracture treated differently from MTSS?

MTSS is treated by following the general guidelines for overuse injuries. A tibial stress fracture requires an impact-free period of 4–8 weeks. If pain-free, the athlete may then begin a gradual increase in activity before resuming a full training schedule. A long pneumatic splint is often used for both injuries to provide additional support and to accelerate the return to activity.

37. A hurdler complains of the gradual onset of posterior lower leg pain, just above the heel. What is the most common injury to runners and jumpers at this site?

Achilles tendinitis, an overuse injury that occurs at the distal 5 cm of the Achilles tendon, just proximal to its insertion at the os calcis.

38. What clinical test is used to assess the integrity of the Achilles tendon?

Thompson's test, which is performed by simply placing the patient in the prone position with the feet dangling off the end of the examination table and then squeezing the calf. A positive test is one in which plantar flexion does not occur, indicating rupture of the tendon.

39. A track athlete complains of the gradual development of pain in the arch of the foot. The foot is most painful with the first several steps that the athlete takes immediately after arising each morning. What physical findings do you expect?

Tenderness of the medial calcaneal tuberosity. Pes planus and hyperpronation are also likely.

40. What is the correct name for this injury?

Plantar fasciitis, which is the most common foot injury in runners.

41. What is plantar fasciitis?

The plantar fascia is a fibrous band that originates at the os calcis and runs to the base of the proximal phalanges. It provides support to the longitudinal arch of the foot. Repetitive stress to the plantar fascia caused by running results in inflammation, tissue injury, and pain.

42. Is a radiograph necessary?

A radiograph is not necessary to make the diagnosis or to provide appropriate treatment. A radiograph may show a heel spur, which may have no significant relationship to the patient's symptoms.

43. How is plantar fasciitis treated?

In addition to the general treatment plan for overuse injuries, stretching of the heel cord and transverse friction massage may be particularly helpful. Correction of pes planus and use of supportive footwear are essential. A posterior splint worn while sleeping at night helps to prevent contraction of the plantar fascia and may speed recovery in chronic cases.

44. If a patient with plantar fasciitis does not improve with conservative management, what other options may be used?

Injection of a corticosteroid agent is often useful. Surgical release should be considered only in disabling cases that have failed all conservative treatment efforts.

45. What upper extremity injuries occur in track and field athletes?

Upper extremity injuries are typically found in the throwing athletes. Shoulder impingement syndrome, medial epicondylitis, and shoulder instability are among the most common injuries in the throwers.

46. What is runner's anemia?

So-called runner's anemia is not a true anemia. It is a dilutional pseudoanemia caused by the plasma expansion induced by chronic exercise. The process is mediated by the renin-angiotensin system.

47. What are the laboratory findings?

A mild decrease in hemoglobin, not less than 13.0 in males and not less than 11.5 in females. The mean corpuscular volume is greater than 80, and the haptoglobin, reticulocyte count, and ferritin are normal.

48. How is runner's anemia treated?

No treatment is necessary. It is an adaptive response, resulting in decreased viscosity, increased stroke volume, increased cardiac output, and increased oxygen delivery to the working muscles.

BIBLIOGRAPHY

1. Balaban EP: Sports anemia. Clin Sports Med 11:313, 1992.
2. Batt ME: Shin-splints—A review of terminology. Clin J Sports Med 5:53–57, 1995.
3. Batt ME, Tanji JL: Management options for plantar fasciitis. Physician Sportsmed 23(6):77–86, 1995.
4. Bennell KL, Malcolm SA, Thomas SA, et al: The incidence and distribution of stress fractures in competitive track and field athletes. A twelve month prospective study. Am J Sports Med 24:211–217, 1996.
5. Cook SD, Brinker MR, Poche M: Running shoes: Their relationship to running injuries. Sports Med 10:1, 1990.
6. Fredericson M, Bergman AG, Hoffman KL, Dillingham MS: Tibial stress reactions in runners: Correlation of clinical symptoms and scintigraphy with a new magnetic resonance imaging grading system. Am J Sports Med 23:472–481, 1995.
7. Hoebrings JH: Factors related to the incidence of running injuries: A review. Sports Med 13:408, 1992.
8. Mattalino AJ, Deese M, Campbell ED: Office evaluation and treatment of lower extremity injuries in the runner. Clin Sports Med 8:461, 1989.
9. Puffer JC, Zachazewski MS: Management of overuse injuries. Am Fam Physician 38:225, 1988.
10. van Mechlen W: Running injuries: A review of the epidemiologic literature. Sports Med 14:320, 1992.

91. GYMNASTICS

David J. Petron, M.D.

1. Are injury rates related to skill level in gymnastics?

Higher injury rates appear to be directly related to skill levels. Data indicate that gymnasts in the United States Gymnasts Federation (USGF) class I have an injury rate almost 5 times that of class II, 11 times that of class III, and 25 times that of class IV. This seems to be related to increased practice time and increased skill level.

2. What gymnastic event for women results in the most injuries?

Floor exercise/tumbling has the greatest number of injuries, followed by the balance beam and uneven parallel bars. The vault has the fewest injuries.

Percentage of Injuries Among Female Gymnasts by Event

REFERENCE	FLOOR (%)	BEAM (%)	UNEVEN BAR (%)	VAULT (%)	OTHER* (%)
Caine et al., 1980	35.4	23.1	20	13.8	7.7
Clarke and Buckley, 1980	39	21	25	15	0.7
Garrick and Requa, 1980[†]	38	21	10	5	18
Garrick and Requa, 1980[‡]	47	12	9	11	20
Pettrone and Ricciardelli, 1987	42.2	25.5	11.8	17.6	3.9
Vergouwen, 1986	21.9	7.4	13.9	22.2	34.6
Weiker, 1985	20.0	41.6	21.6	6.6	10.0

* Warming-up, trampoline.
[†] Interscholastic.
[‡] College, high school, club.

3. At which anatomic sites are most injuries found in female gymnasts?

50–60%   Lower extremity
25–31%   Upper extremity
12–19%   Trunk and spine[1-3]

4. What are the most common overuse injuries?

Overuse injury rates are difficult to estimate because they are frequently underreported. A partial list of common injuries includes:

Shoulder impingement syndrome
Spondylolysis
Wrist impingement
Patellar tendinitis

Anterior compartment syndrome
Tibial stress fracture
Patellofemoral dysfunction

WRIST

5. What is "gymnast's wrist"?

Excessive, repetitive compression-loading appears to result in premature closure of the radial physis and differential growth of the radius and ulna, which leads to positive ulnar variance. Thus the weight-bearing load on the ulna and triquetrium is increased, with compression of a thin, relatively unstable triangular fibrocartilaginous complex (TFCC) between the two bones. This may result in a tear of the TFCC.[4]

6. How is gymnast's wrist diagnosed?

The posteroanterior (PA) radiograph best demonstrates ulnar variance. A positive ulnar variance of 2.5 mm increases the load on the ulna by 40%. A clinical test for ulnocarpal impingement is performed by ulnar deviation with the ulnar head fixed in relationship to the triquetrium. A positive result is pain with supination and pronation.

7. How is gymnast's wrist treated?

The best treatment is to have the gymnast avoid weight-bearing on the wrist when wrist pain occurs. Once ulnar deviation is present, the usual treatment is distal ulnar resection if pain continues after prolonged rest.[5]

ELBOW

8. Name the most common stress injuries of the elbow in young gymnasts.

Avascular necrosis of the capitellar epiphysis (Panner's disease)
Osteochondritis of the capitellum
Flattening of the radial head epiphysis
Osteochondritis dissecans of the radial head
Stress fractures of the olecranon epiphysis

The principal abnormal forces experienced in the elbow joint are medial torsion, lateral compression, and extension stress, all of which ultimately may result in radiographic abnormalities.

9. How is osteochondrosis of the elbow treated?

Osteochondrosis may represent a major threat to the joint, and early diagnosis is important. If radiographic abnormalities are present, the gymnast should rest for 6–8 weeks after all symptoms have cleared and radiographic findings are stable or improving.[9]

SHOULDER

10. Do shoulder injuries occur more frequently in men or women?

Shoulder injuries occur more frequently in men. Because ring and horizontal bar exercises include movements of great amplitude and speed, an enormous amount of stress is placed on the shoulder.[1] The most frequent injuries are muscle strains and shoulder impingements. Subluxations and dislocations are also not uncommon but occur more frequently in women.

FOOT AND ANKLE

11. What is Sever's disease?

It is apophysitis due to calcaneal traction. A tight gastrosoleus complex and excessive loads can cause heel pain in young gymnasts. Treatments consist of stretching, relative rest, heel lifts, icing, and NSAIDs.

BACK

12. What is the most common cause of chronic back pain in young female gymnasts?

Spondylolysis, which is a defect in the pars interarticularis with no forward displacement. Back pain appears to result not only from single episodes of macrotrauma but also from repeated microtrauma in gymnastic movements such as vaults, twist, and hyperextension.[6] Incidence of spondylolysis is estimated to be between 15%[8] and 32%.[7]

13. What are the common findings of spondylolysis on physical examination?

Persistent back pain in an adolescent is spondylolysis until proved otherwise. The majority of patients with spondylolysis are asymptomatic. Classic presentation includes chronic midline ache at the lumbosacral junction, which is worsened by extension maneuvers. Hamstring spasm is another common finding.

14. Which radiographs are required to make the diagnosis of spondylolysis?

A 25–45° oblique radiograph is needed to see spondylolysis. If spondylolysis is suspected but not demonstrated on plain films, oblique linear tomography and computed tomography (CT) will clearly show the defect. In early acute stages radionuclide scanning with single photon emission computed tomography (SPECT) is much more sensitive than plain radiographs.

15. How are gymnasts with pars defects treated?

Treatment is controversial. Conservative measures include restriction of repetitive hyperextension of the lumbar spine and physical therapy, concentrating on abdominal and back-strengthening programs.

Micheli[7] applied a plastic lumbar flexion jacket and found that 88% of patients became symptom-free and were able to return to sports, even though only 32% demonstrated bony healing. Once the athlete's symptoms are resolved, competition is permitted.

16. How can injuries among gymnasts be prevented?

It is always difficult to draw conclusions from studies with discrepancies in factors such as definition of injury, sample size, and methodology. Reports of injury location and event at which injury occurs, however, are consistent. Upper extremities are used for weight-bearing and distributing high-impact loads across the elbow and wrist. Most back injuries also have a gradual onset from repeated microtrauma. Coaches must realize the potential seriousness of gradual onset injuries, and gymnasts with back, wrist, and elbow pain must be followed closely. Injury prevention will continue to evolve as we study maturation rate, psychological factors, technique, coaching, and training facilities.

BIBLIOGRAPHY

1. Aronen JG: Problems of the upper extremity in gymnastics. Clin Sports Med 4:61–71, 1985.
2. Caine DJ, Lindner KJ: Overuse injuries of growing bones: The young female gymnast at risk? Phys Sportsmed 13(12):51–64, 1985.
3. Ciullo JV, Jackson DW: Pars interarticularis stress reaction spondylolysis and spondylolisthesis in gymnastics. Clin Sports Med 4:95–110, 1985.
4. Garrick JG, Requa RK: Epidemiology of women's gymnastics injuries. Am J Sports Med 8:261–264, 1980.
5. Goodway J, McNaught-Davis JP, White J: The distribution of injuries among young female gymnasts in relation to selected training and environmental factors [abstract]. Proceedings of the Symposium on Paediatric Work Physiology, Leuven, 1989.
6. Micheli LJ: Back injuries in gymnastics. Clin Sports Med 4:85–93, 1985.
7. Rossi F: Spondylolysis, spondylolisthesis and sports. J Sports Med Phys Fitness 18:317–340, 1978.
8. Rossi F, Dragoni S: Lumbar spondylolysis: Occurrence in competitive athletes. J Sports Med Phys Fitness 30:450–452, 1990.
9. Singer KM, Roy SP: Osteochondrosis of the humeral capitellum. Am J Sports Med 12:351–360, 1984.

92. TENNIS AND OTHER RACQUET SPORTS

Terry L. Nicola, M.D.

1. Tennis is said to be a combination of endurance and strength. As a reflection of cardiovascular work, what percentage of maximum heart rate would be typical in a singles match? A doubles match?

In a vigorous tennis match, the player's average heart rate will reach 60–70% of maximum age-specific heart rate in a singles match and 40% of maximum heart rate in a doubles match. This is not surprising given the high number of sprints involved in an average match—on the order of 300–500 bursts of effort per match. The recommended conditioning should include repetitive anaerobic sprints or bicycle drills that reflect the large number of anaerobic periods that occur in a match, averaging 12 to 15 seconds per point with 2:1 rest periods.

2. Name three fundamental phases of any racquet stroke.

Every stroke in all the racquet sports shares the same three fundamental phases:

Preparation phase: A period of recoil for both the upper and lower extremities. Muscles such as the triceps surae, abdominal, and rotator cuff are extended to their end range of motion. The wind-up and cocking phases of the service are included.

Acceleration phase: Release of energy from the previous phase occurs serially from lower extremity drive, abdominal flexion, and finally upper extremity swing with ball contact.

Deceleration phase: Muscle contraction here is mostly eccentric, especially from all four shoulder rotator cuff muscles.

3. The shoulder rotator cuff muscle group is responsible for the stability of the glenohumeral joint during upper extremity movements. What strength deficits of the rotator cuff predispose to injury? What is coupled motion?

The four muscles of the rotator cuff muscle group (supraspinatus, infraspinatus, subscapularis, teres minor) are primarily responsible for maintaining the stability of the glenohumeral joint. However, the external rotators, the teres minor, and infraspinatus are essential for holding the humeral head in the glenoid fossa. Overuse injuries from overhead motions are reflected in a muscle strength imbalance for an external rotator:internal (subscapularis) rotator ratio less than 2:3. If the supraspinatus becomes fatigued or injured, it can no longer function as a humeral head depressor and antagonist to the cranial directional pull of the deltoid muscle. This disrupts the *coupled* motion of combined abduction between the supraspinatus and deltoid, allowing the humeral head to glide superiorly and impinge the supraspinatus tendon against the acromial arch.

4. The motion of the service and overhead strokes resembles the motion in what other sport?

The overhead motion of a service or return shot resembles that same motion as pitching. Both involve a series of movements that include the set and forward movement of the lower body, followed by 100° of scapulohumeral abduction, 30° of thoracic side tilt, and greater than 110° of humeral external rotation. This movement is shared by a number of other sports such as basketball, javelin throwing, and swimming.

5. What is "King Kong" arm?

Overdevelopment of the dominant arm in tennis players has been nicknamed King Kong arm because of the asymmetrically increased size of the dominant shoulder girdle. These factors also include a depressed scapula, protracted shoulder posture, and large forearm.

6. Name a common upper-extremity injury in which the athlete describes the arm as "feeling dead."

Injury to the glenohumeral mechanism, more specifically the rotator cuff, will give more of a dead arm feeling than pain. The athlete may also tell you about pain over the deltoid insertion. Pain can refer to the area of the deltoid tendon even though the deltoid tendon is intact.

7. In what percentage of tennis athletes with rotator cuff injuries will there be an asymmetric scapular glide abnormality?

In a recent study, Kibler[1] looked at lateral scapular glide measured from the scapula inferior angle to the thoracic spine in three positions of shoulder abduction. In almost 100% of athletes with glenohumeral injuries, there were asymmetric abnormalities of scapular glide compared with symmetric abduction of uninjured athletes.

8. In rehabilitation of upper-extremity injuries in racquet sports, what are "anchored racquet" and "windmill" exercises?

Once strength and flexibility have been restored, an injured player should perform simulated racquet swings or windmill exercises, followed by the use of an elastic band attachment to the racquet for controlled resistance exercises of racquet stroke motions called anchored racquet exercises.

9. The injury known as tennis elbow is typically a strain of the extensor carpi radialis brevis (ECRB). What is the differential diagnosis?

Symptoms of ECRB strain or lateral epicondylitis should include an examination for (1) pathology of the radial humeral joint or osteochondral lesion, (2) recurrent radial nerve entrapment or supinator syndrome, (3) C6 root injury or "stinger," and (4) epicondylar apophysitis in adolescent athletes.

10. What are the risk factors for tennis elbow?

Risk Factors for Tennis Elbow

Age of player (> 30 years old)
Improper grip size
Use of metal racquet
Duration of average practice (greater than 2 hours per day)
Tight strings
Incorrect backhand technique including snapping wrist

These risk factors cause strain to the ECRB through overly tight grip, excessive vibration through the racquet, excessive motion, or fatigue over time.

11. How would you measure racquet handle grip size?

Racquet handle grip sizes vary between 4 and 5 inches, with the exact measurement determined by the distance from the tip of the fourth digit to the proximal palmar crease, measured along the radial border of the ring finger.

12. For which stroke and in which classification of athlete will you hear complaints of medial tennis elbow?

The highly ranked competitive or professional tennis athlete maintains excellent form during the backhand motion to avoid lateral tennis elbow. The service motion, however, is forceful with heavy load to the origin of the flexor/pronator muscles during the acceleration phase.

13. Describe the location of common racquet sports-related neurologic entrapment injuries to the median, ulnar, radial, axillary, and long thoracic nerves.

The types of neurologic injury caused by repetitive entrapment between tendon, ligament, and bone are listed in the following table.

Racquet Sport-related Entrapment Neuropathies

NERVE	INJURY
Median	**Pronator teres entrapment** from the elbow/forearm combined with flexion/pronation motion during late acceleration phase **Carpal tunnel syndrome** is a rare possibility from various handle and wrist motion problems with synovitis.
Ulnar	**Cubital tunnel neuropathy** from excessive valgus elbow stresses on overhead strokes sometimes with flexor carpi ulnaris entrapment of the nerve Occasional entrapment in the wrist **Guyon's canal** from direct handle trauma
Radial	Lateral tennis elbow may be associated with **supinator** overuse and **entrapment** of the radial nerve
Long thoracic	Overuse of the dominant arm with subsequent scapular depression induces a **traction injury** to this nerve, loss of serratus anterior function, and scapular instability
Axillary	**Glenohumeral injury** to the rotator cuff or glenoid labrum leads to anterior instability and traction on the axillary nerve as it crosses anteriorly across the humeral head to the deltoid muscle

14. What is the mechanism for injury to the lower back in racquet sports?

Overhead and service strokes depend on good planning of placement on the court so that the ball remains in front of the player. Otherwise, the player may find the need to reach back for the ball causing a hyperextension and overrotation of the lower back. Poor shoulder flexibility also may prevent the needed shoulder external rotation to reach back for the ball. Once again, the lower back overcompensates to make contact with the ball. Such movements place excessive loads on the lumbar facet joints and sometimes rotation shear to the discs.

15. How does upper-extremity inflexibility cause injury to the lower back?

The overhead motion of the racquet will depend on the shoulder's capacity for scapular retraction and external rotation. Decreased flexibility of the pectoralis minor and rotator cuff muscles, respectively, will cause excessive back rotation at the T12–L1 level and excessive extension at the L4–S1 level.

16. What muscle inflexibility would be a direct cause of low back pain in racquet sports?

Most positions in all racquet sports require the player to assume a hip flexed squatting posture. This commonly leads to loss of flexibility of the key hip flexor, the iliopsoas muscle. The iliopsoas muscle, owing to its origin from the anterior lateral surface of the lumbar spine, causes pain to extend to the lumbar spine, which is sometimes alleviated by local anesthetic injection to this muscle group.

17. Given the body mechanics of movement involved in racquetball and tennis, for which muscles is flexibility the greatest concern?

The following are the specific areas of concern:

Shoulder rotator cuff:	Decreased internal rotation less than 80° in the 90° abducted positive
Lumbar spine:	Decreased sit and reach test or less than 40° flexion by inclinometer method
Hip flexors:	Decreased extension by Thomas test less than 10° extension
Hip external rotators:	Decreased internal rotation dominant vs. nondominant side
Forearm supinators and pronators:	Decreased dominant vs. nondominant side

18. Is a rehabilitation program for a racquet sport athlete with a low back injury similar to that for athletes with low back injury in other sports?

Of all sports-related injuries, 70% are extension rotation injuries. This problem is no different for tennis players. Lower lumbar facet joint injuries are the most common.

19. A racquetball player describes a mid-back pain about the level of the twelfth rib. What is the likely mechanism of injury?

The injured player is describing a rotation injury at the T12–L1 level. This level is the one area of the spine that can easily rotate owing to the frontal plane of the overlapping facets. With incorrect body mechanics, the player will twist the trunk instead of rotating the hips during the stroke or overrotate to compensate for shoulder inflexibility.

20. Abdominal wall strain to the rectus abdominis, internal and external oblique, or iliopsoas muscles may occur in aggressive racquet sports. What is the differential diagnosis for nonmuscular abdominal pain in these athletes?

Acute abdominal process	Inguinal hernia
Epididymitis	Testicular torsion
Herniated disc	Osteitis pubis
Stress fracture	Entrapped intercostal nerve

21. Tennis leg has been ascribed to the plantaris muscle. Now that we know better, what is the actual injury?

The actual injury is to the muscle tendon junction of the medial head of the gastrocnemius muscle. Abnormal stresses to this muscle from tibialis anterior/gastrocnemius soleus strength imbalance, and excessive foot and ankle pronation should be corrected.

22. In the final phase of rehabilitation of racquet sports-related injuries to the lower extremity, what other sport would share a similar protocol?

Track athletes in the sprinting events share in common with the sprinting of the tennis athlete high loads to the gastrocsoleus complex and patellar ligament insertion to the tibial tuberosity. Therefore, flexibility and strength imbalances are similar rehabilitation concerns. Plyometric drills emphasize more side-to-side movements in racquet sports.

23. Name the unique features of a good racquet court shoe that distinguishes it from a good running shoe.

Racquet sports, unlike running, stress a considerable amount of side-to-side movement. Therefore, a strong heel cup and heel counter is unique to racquet court shoes. Also, the forefoot of court shoes will be sturdier material, such as leather, to allow the trail leg to drag the toe box on the court as seen in low ground strokes.

24. Protective eyewear is considered essential equipment for racquetball and handball, possibly even tennis. What are the quality standards recommended for this type of eyewear?

Recommended eyewear must withstand impact from a handball or racquetball at speeds in excess of 100 mph. The lens should be made of polycarbonate and firmly affixed, not inserted, to the surrounding frame. Open-frame eyewear is unacceptable because studies and injury data show the ability of the ball to squeeze easily through the frame and cause severe damage and blindness. The frame should be a smooth sweep-around style with nose bridge padding.

25. When adolescent athletes describe new pains in the ankle, knee, and elbow, are these new complaints growth pains?

Young athletes entering the adolescent growth spurts are susceptible to injury of the epiphyseal and apophyseal growth plates. Particular attention should be given to girls around 12 years and boys 14 years of age, allowing for individual variations. Of particular concern in racquet sports are the greater humeral tuberosity, the patellar tuberosity, lateral elbow epicondyle, and the Achilles tendon insertion apophyses.

26. Tennis court surfaces affect the type of injury most likely to occur; for example, hard courts are associated with more stress to the lower extremity. Which type of surface is considered more forgiving to the upper extremity—hard, clay, composition, or carpeted court?

Clay court is more forgiving to the upper extremity because of the reduced speed of the ball after the return and bounce off the energy-absorbing surface.

27. Tennis service velocity, when measurable, may be considered one screening parameter for combined flexibility, strength, and coordination. Identify specific measurements in strength and flexibility that have shown a positive correlation with tennis service velocity on screening physical exam.

The following parameters have shown a significant correlation with tennis service velocity in players with a minimal score of 5.0 by the National Tennis Rating Program.

1. **Flexibility** (dominant arm)
   Shoulder flexion
   Shoulder internal rotation (neutral position)
   Wrist flexion
2. **Isokinetic strength** (dominant arm)
   Elbow extension
   Shoulder internal rotation (in 90° abduction)
   Findings are true for 60° and 180°/second testing.

The study did not attempt to correlate service velocity with muscle balance or force couple ratios.

28. Does isokinetic strengthening of the rotator cuff muscles actually translate to improved tennis service velocity in skilled tennis players (NTRP > 5.0)?

Yes—if you accept isokinetic strength testing of the shoulder in 80° abduction, 20° flexion as a reflection of rotator cuff strengthening. Improvements in eccentric and concentric strength of both internal and external rotators greater than 10% resulted in improvements in service velocity greater than 10%. The study evaluated tennis service velocity in relation to any strength ratios between internal and external rotators.

29. What is the likelihood of return to full competitive tennis after rotator cuff surgical repair and acromioplasty?

The prognosis for return to full competitive play appears to be almost 100% if the size of the rotator cuff tear was less than 5 cm. No one with a tear greater than 5 cm returns to full level of play, although 3 of 4 players were able to play at reduced intensity and performance level. The tears involved the supraspinatus, infraspinatus, or, in the case of large tears, the teres minor muscle.

BIBLIOGRAPHY

1. Bigliani LU, et al: Repair of rotator cuff tears in tennis players. Am J Sports Med 20:1992.
2. Cohen DB, Mont MA, Campbell KR, et al: Upper extremity physical factors affecting tennis serve velocity. Am J Sports Med 22:746–750, 1994.
3. Kibler WB: The role of the scapula in the overhead throwing motion. Contemp Orthop 22:525, 1991.
4. Lehman RC (ed): Racquet sports: Injury treatment and prevention. Clin Sports Med 7:1988.
5. Mont MA, Cohen DB, Campbell KR, et al: Isokinetic concentric versus eccentric training of shoulder rotators with functional evaluation of performance enhancement in elite tennis players. Am J Sports Med 22:513–517, 1994.
6. Nicola TL: Tennis. In Mellion MB, Walsh WM, Shelton GL (eds): The Team Physician's Handbook, 2nd ed. Philadelphia, Hanley & Belfus, 1997, pp 816–827.

93. GOLF

Harry L. Galanty, M.D., and James C. Puffer, M.D.

1. Do people really get injured playing golf?

Yes. Although golf is generally not considered to be a strenuous activity, studies of amateur and professional golfers have shown that a majority of participants will suffer injuries related to golf during their lives.

2. Are injuries in professional and amateur golfers different?

The most common mechanism responsible for injury to all golfers is overuse. However, the degree to which overuse occurs differs for these two groups. Excessive practice accounts for most injuries in professional golfers. A pro may perform a swing up to 1000 times each day during practice. This repetitive stress leads to cumulative microtrauma and the subsequent development of an overuse injury. In an amateur, however, injury more likely results from poor physical condition or incorrect swing mechanics.

3. What are the most frequent injuries in golfers?

Injury surveys of professional and amateur golfers show that the back and wrist are the most common sites of injury. Amateurs also have a high incidence of elbow problems as compared with pros. This is believed to be due to faulty swing mechanics. Other common locations of injury include the shoulder and the knee.

4. Describe the four phases of the golf swing.

The golf swing can be broken down into takeaway, acceleration, impact, and follow-through. **Takeaway** consists of the setup and movement of the club to the top of the backswing. **Acceleration** begins at the end of the backswing as the club is brought back down with increasing force until ball contact. At **impact**, the club strikes the ball. The postimpact phase, or **follow-through**, occurs after ball contact to the completion of the motion.

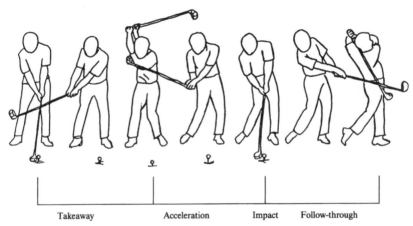

| Takeaway | Acceleration | Impact | Follow-through |

5. What occurs biomechanically during the golf swing?

Each phase can initiate stress to specific areas of the body. During **takeaway**, the shoulders, hips, and spine rotate while the head remains stationary. At the top of the backswing, hyperabduction of the left thumb, radial deviation of the left wrist, and dorsiflexion of the right wrist occurs as the wrists cock. During **acceleration**, the forces on the hands and wrists are maximal, and strain increases on the right medial elbow. At **impact**, compression of the right wrist and stress over the lateral elbow occur. **Follow-through** involves the completion of spine and hip rotation with hyperextension of the lumbar and cervical vertebrae. With the shift of weight to the left side of the body, rotation of the knees and eversion of the left ankle complete the swing.

6. Discuss the most common back injuries in golfers.

Lower back injuries account for 25% to 35% of all golf injuries. Of these, lumbar strain is the most frequent complaint. This results from the loads placed on the low back musculature from hyperrotation during takeaway and hyperextension and further rotation during follow-through. Other back problems that can be seen include herniated discs and iliolumbar ligament sprains. The majority of these injuries will improve with rest initially and are further prevented by increased flexibility and strength of the lower back, hips, and abdominal muscles. Improvement of swing mechanics also can alleviate back strain.

7. What is "golfer's elbow"?

Medial epicondylitis of the right elbow in a right-handed golfer (or the left elbow in the left-handed golfer) is referred to as golfer's elbow. This is caused by the stress placed on the wrist flexors during the acceleration and impact phases of the swing. Instead of using the legs, shoulders, and other muscles to bring the club through, the player forces the club through acceleration with the arms causing extension of the right elbow and dorsiflexion of the wrist. This eccentrically loads the wrist flexors, especially at their origin on the medial epicondyle. Possible injury to the ulnar nerve should always be considered. Treatment is symptomatic, including ice, strengthening of the muscles, and possibly counterforce bracing. It also is important for the player to correct faulty swing mechanics.

8. Are any other injuries seen in golfer's elbow?

In addition to medial epicondylitis, lateral epicondylitis similar to that seen in tennis players can occur. This is most likely seen in the left elbow of a right-handed golfer from eccentric loads applied to the wrist extensors during acceleration. The mechanism is similar to that described above for medial epicondylitis. This condition can be aggravated by gripping the handle of the club too tightly. Pain is present over the origin of the wrist extensors at the lateral epicondyle. Treatment is the same as for golfer's elbow.

9. Why is the left wrist more likely to be injured in golfers?

In a study of professional golfers, left wrist injuries accounted for 23.9% of the total, whereas right wrist injuries were only 3.1% of total injuries. This is due to the load placed on the left wrist with forceful contact with the ground at impact. At impact, the left wrist is forcibly flexed and radially deviated; this can lead to overuse of the wrist extensors. These forces are compounded by the excessive repetition in practice required of the professional. Thick playing surfaces, like the Bermuda grass found on golf courses in southern states, also can contribute to excessive force at contact. Treatment of these injuries is the same as for other overuse injuries. Other treatment considerations include decreasing practice time, or if wrist pain is more serious, rest from activity, the use of nonsteroidal antiinflammatory drugs, and the use of a wrist brace.

10. What other wrist injuries are common in golf?

De Quervain's disease, a common condition found in professional golfers, is a tenosynovitis of the extensor pollicis brevis and abductor pollicis longus in the wrist. This injury results from repeated impact between club and ground. There is pain localized to the common tendon sheath. Pain also can be elicited by forced ulnar deviation of the thumb and hand. Conservative treatment should include ice, splinting, and antiinflammatory medication. More recalcitrant cases may require injection of corticosteroid into the tendon sheath.

11. What is the shoulder's function during the golf swing?

Electromyographic analyses of shoulder activity by Jobe have shown that the rotator cuff muscles are active throughout the golf swing.[6] A golf swing is a rapid movement requiring coordinated firing of the cuff muscles to protect the glenohumeral complex. The infraspinatus and supraspinatus act together to bring the club to the top of the backswing. The subscapularis is the most active during acceleration, as it is the primary internal rotator. It remains highly active in both the left and right arms. In fact, both shoulders participate equally in the swing, whereas in the past, it was believed that the left shoulder was the driving force in the right-handed golfer. The swing does not require extremes of strength or range of motion and thus there is relatively little contribution from the deltoid to the swing.

12. How does shoulder function relate to injury?

Since the rotator cuff muscles are most active in the golf swing, it is easy to see how overuse or poor mechanics could lead to shoulder injury. In younger golfers, one will occasionally see secondary subacromial impingement of the cuff muscles due to instability but not as commonly as with the overhead motions of baseball or swimming. Injury is more likely in older golfers. With age, atrophy of the cuff occurs and the repetitive nature of the swing can lead to tendinitis or degenerative cuff tears. It is extremely important, therefore, for golfers to strengthen their cuff muscles to prevent injury.

13. What shoulder exercises will help prevent rotator cuff injury?

Prevention of rotator cuff and other shoulder injuries requires an exercise program of flexibility and strength that is performed in and out of season. The goals are to create shoulder musculature that is resistant to the wear and tear of repetitive swinging. To increase shoulder flexibility, exercises should include stretching of the shoulder capsule: anterior, posterior, and inferior regions. A weightlifting program is important not only for increasing strength but also for improved endurance. This is accomplished by a high-repetition and low-weight program. Weights heavier than 5 or 10 lb are not necessary. Exercises should include internal rotation (subscapularis), external rotation (infraspinatus and teres minor), and abduction with thumbs pointed down and arms forward flexed 30° (supraspinatus).

14. A golfer presents with pain on the ulnar side of the palm of the hand. What is the most likely diagnosis?

You should suspect a fracture of the hook of the hamate. Hamate hook fractures are thought to occur secondary to the force of trauma against the hamate bone when swinging the golf club. It will most likely occur in the hand that grasps the end of the club (the left hand in a right-handed golfer). Patients will complain of pain in the dorsal ulnar aspect of the wrist or pain exactly over the hook of the hamate. Pain is exacerbated when gripping and swinging a club. Most patients can be diagnosed with carpal tunnel view radiographs or with oblique views of the supinated wrist. CT scan can be used if the radiographs are not conclusive. Current therapy for hamate hook fractures involves surgical removal of the fractured hook, as a large number that are treated with immobilization fail to heal.

15. Can conditioning programs prevent injuries in golf?

Although the research on conditioning for golfers is limited, it is generally believed that prevention of golfing injuries requires a multistep approach that begins with a good conditioning program. Golf is a demanding activity that requires both flexibility and strength to swing the club correctly and consistently. Stretching exercises for the upper extremities, back and legs will improve the flexibility and reduce injuries during the rotational stresses that occur. Strengthening of the rotator cuff muscles has already been discussed with respect to preventing shoulder injury. Forearm and wrist strengthening also can protect the wrist from the forces associated with impact. The trunk, hips, and legs should not be forgotten, as they provide much of the power of the golf swing. Cardiovascular exercise also is necessary for improving endurance on the course. A program of jogging or bicycling can build resistance to fatigue when walking 18 holes on hot days.

16. What are other recommendations to limit golfing injuries?

The golf swing should be analyzed by a professional golf instructor. The pro can correct the deficiencies of a swing to alleviate undue stresses placed on specific anatomic regions and thereby prevent overuse injuries and also assess the player's clubs and adjust them to the proper length and weight to ensure improvement of swing mechanics. The golf professional can also assist the golfer in choosing the clubs to best fit his or her game.

17. Do special considerations need to be made for older golfers?

Unlike most sports, golf retains many of its participants throughout their lifetimes. Because the ability to recover from repetitive microtrauma decreases with age, an older golfer must be aware that he or she may more easily develop overuse injuries. This may require a reduction in the number of rounds or practices undertaken, or it may necessitate using a cart instead of walking the golf course. Appropriate conditioning in this population also is extremely important in preventing injury.

18. What conditioning is most beneficial to the older player?

A general conditioning program to improve cardiovascular fitness, strength, and flexibility is best. Specifically, with increasing age, rotator cuff degeneration appears and thus makes a strengthening program for the cuff muscles of utmost importance. This program should follow the same format stated in question 15. Degenerative arthritis also is more common with increasing age, and avid golfers may develop arthritis of the small joints of the hand owing to the stresses related to ball striking. It can be treated with grip changes and antiinflammatory medication. Special grips are available that reduce stress on the hands and wrists to help alleviate some of the problems associated with arthritis.

19. What are the "yips"?

The yips are an involuntary motor disturbance that affects some golfers. It appears to be similar to the occupational dystonias known to occur in writers and musicians. The disorder is described as jerking or spasms of the arm that primarily occur during putting. Many golfers will attempt to alleviate symptoms by changing hand preference or position with some relief. It is believed that performance anxiety contributes to the cause of this disorder. The use of benzodiazepines or propranolol have proved to be of no benefit. At this time, there are more questions than answers about this problem.

20. Is skin cancer more common in golfers?

Skin cancer is more likely to occur in individuals with fair skin, who sunburn easily, and who have increased exposure to ultraviolet light (UVL). Professional golfers spend the majority of their time in sunny locations and often play golf during the middle of the day when the UVL is most damaging to the skin. In a study of women professional and amateur golfers, the professionals had an increased incidence of basal cell carcinoma and actinic keratosis. Also, the professionals developed these lesions at a much younger age than amateurs (25.5 years compared with 51.4 years). It is recommended that golfers protect their sun-exposed skin with sunscreens and clothing that block these harmful rays.

21. What is the most unexpected injury associated with golf?

A study by Lindsay et al. found that golf was a leading cause of severe head injuries, most commonly depressed skull fractures.[8] The majority of these injuries were due to inadvertent practice swings that struck an unsuspecting bystander. Children may be at risk when playing with or swinging golf clubs in an improper or unsupervised manner. Other unusual injuries include reports of clubs acting as projectiles when they have slipped out of a golfer's hands or when the club head or shaft has broken off and hit a bystander. When around a golf course, one must always be alert for golfers who are swinging clubs.

BIBLIOGRAPHY

1. Amundson M: Golf. In Mellion MB, Walsh WM, Shelton GL (eds): The Team Physician's Handbook, 2nd ed. Philadelphia, Hanley & Belfus, 1997.
2. Batt ME: A survey of golf injuries in amateur golfers. Br J Sports Med 26:63–65, 1992.
3. Duda M: Golf injuries: They really do happen. Phys Sportsmed 15:191–196, 1987.
4. Hanke CW, Zollinger TW, O'Brian JJ, Bianco L: Skin cancer in professional and amateur female golfers. Phys Sportsmed 13:51–68, 1985.
5. Jobe FW, Moynes DR, Antonelli DJ: Rotator cuff function during a golf swing. Am J Sports Med 14:388–392, 1986.
6. Jobe FW, Perry J, Pink M: Electromyographic shoulder activity in men and women professional golfers. Am J Sports Med 17:782–787, 1989.
7. Jobe FW, Schwab DM: Golf for the mature athlete. Clin Sports Med 10:269–282, 1991.
8. Lindsay KW, McLatchie G, Jennett B: Serious head injury in sport. Br Med J 281:789–791, 1980.
9. McCarroll JR: Evaluation, treatment and prevention of upper extremity injuries in golfers. In Nicholas JA, Hershman EB (eds): The Upper Extremity in Sports Medicine, 2nd ed. St. Louis, Mosby, 1995, pp 883–890.
10. McCarroll JR, Rettig AC, Shelbourne KD: Injuries in the amateur golfer. Phys Sportsmed 18:122–126, 1990.
11. McDaniel KD, Cummings JL, Shain S: The "yips": A focal dystonia of golfers. Neurology 39:192–195, 1989.
12. Pink M, Jobe FW, Perry J: Electromyographic analysis of the shoulder during the golf swing. Am J Sports Med 18:137–140, 1990.
13. Stark HH, Chao EK, Zemel NP, et al: Fracture of the hook of the hamate. J Bone Joint Surg 71A:1202–1207, 1989.
14. Watkins RG, Uppal GS, Perry J, et al: Dynamic electromyographic analysis of trunk musculature in professional golfers. Am J Sports Med 24:535–538, 1996.

94. DOWNHILL SKI INJURIES

Alexander K. Morley, M.D., FAAFP, FACEP, and Dianne T. Morley, P.T.

Skiing continues to grow as a popular family sport. People of all ages, athletic abilities, and conditioning are going skiing. Skiing is a relatively safe sport, but injuries do occur. Severe problems are first evaluated at the ski area clinic. Many patients will then return home, often far away from the ski resort, to have their injuries treated; or they may not seek any medical attention until they consult with their physician at home. Therefore, it is important for all primary care physicians to understand common ski injuries.

1. What are the most common ski injuries?

Knee injuries are the most serious injuries commonly seen at ski area clinics. Thumb injuries are probably the most frequent, but evaluation and treatment are often delayed. The classic thumb injury is a sprain of the ulnar collateral ligament. Shoulder injuries also are prevalent and include dislocations, acromioclavicular sprains, and fractures. Studies have shown a general decrease in the total number of ski injuries per skier days. However, there has been a gradual increase in the number of upper-extremity injuries and a decline in lower leg fractures. Less experienced and fatigued skiers are more likely to be injured.

2. What are the most common knee injuries?

The most prevalent knee injury is the **medial collateral ligament sprain**, closely followed by the **anterior cruciate ligament sprain**. Patients often have multiple ligament injuries in the knee. **Tibia plateau fractures** are unfortunately common in skiing. **Tibia spine avulsion fractures** also are seen frequently. This is an avulsion of the attachment of the anterior cruciate ligament into the tibia spine.

3. How do knee injuries occur when skiing?

Skiing is a sport that combines speed with control. Many factors are involved when control is lost. The ski attached to the ski boot acts as a giant lever arm and transmits tremendous forces up through the boot to the leg and knee. Ski bindings have improved greatly and are designed to release so that these forces do not cause injury, but they are still far from perfect. Bindings do not release in every direction; they allow torsional release and forward heel ejection but not side lateral release. This is, after all, how the skier controls the ski—side pressure and angulation.

The most common mechanism causing a knee injury is a twisting motion as the inside edge of the ski catches on the snow, and the ski does not come off. It twists the leg outward, transmitting a valgus stress to the knee. This may result in a medial collateral ligament or anterior cruciate ligament sprain. Another mechanism for anterior cruciate injuries is falling backward, especially after jumping or coming over a bump. As the skis slap down against the snow, the tibia levers forward from the femur and the anterior cruciate gives way. With this mechanism the lateral collateral ligament is stressed and may rupture, but the medial collateral ligament remains intact. With the gradual introduction of upper-releasing toe bindings, it is hoped there will be a decline in this type of anterior cruciate injury.

Jumping is another way to damage the knee. Sometimes a skier is propelled in the air unintentionally and comes down with dire consequences. The forces of landing from height, combined with twisting, can force the femoral condyles down hard into the tibia plateau resulting in a tibia plateau fracture. At busy ski area clinics, this is an unfortunately prevalent problem.

4. How is the knee examined?

First, obtain the history. It is important to determine whether the patient was able to ski down or had to be rescued by the ski patrol. Ask if the knee was too painful to ski on or if it was unstable—possibly indicating ligament damage. Was a pop heard? Did the binding release? Is there a previous knee injury complicating the examination?

After obtaining the history of the injury, undress the legs. It is essential to be able to examine both knees. Inspect the knee for bruising or lacerations (a frequent problem from sharp ski edges). It is important to be gentle and reassuring. An accurate examination is impossible if the patient is apprehensive. Palpate for effusion by placing the thumb and index fingers of one hand on the lower medial and lateral patellar pouches. Use the other hand on each side of the upper patella and gently squeeze synovial fluid out of the upper patellar pouches. A large synovial effusion in the injured knee usually indicates an anterior cruciate ligament injury due to hemarthrosis. Next, palpate the knee for joint line tenderness that may indicate a meniscus injury or a collateral ligament injury.

Lachman's test is probably the single most important part of the knee examination for ski injuries because it tests for anterior cruciate ligament injuries that are so prevalent. With the knee flexed at 15° to 20°, hold the femur with your outside hand and the tibia with the other. Hold the femur in a stable position and try to displace the tibia forward from the femur. Normally, there should be a solid stop as the anterior cruciate ligament tightens. The test is positive if the tibia moves anteriorly more than the noninjured knee or if there is a soft end point.

Test stability of the medial and lateral collateral ligaments by using valgus and varus stresses on the knee and moving the joint from extension to 30°. Compare both knees to assess what is normal for each individual. In downhill skiing, collateral ligament injuries are often associated with anterior cruciate ligament sprains.

5. What is a lateral capsule sign?

This is a radiographic finding. It is a small avulsion of bone from where the lateral capsule of the knee attaches to the tibia. It is associated with anterior cruciate ligament injury, and it may be caused by the backward falling force on the knee described above in question 3.

6. How have lower leg injuries changed with new ski equipment?

There has been an evolution in ski equipment through the years. In the 1940s and 1950s, ankle fractures were common. Ski boots were soft and allowed some movement of the ankle in the boot. Ski boots gradually evolved to be stiffer and hold the ankle tightly. The classic ski injury in the 1960s and 1970s was a spiral boot-top tibia fracture. Ski equipment has again changed the pattern of injury. Today even higher, stiffer boots lock the ankle and leg in and give excellent edge control. But in so doing, they direct rotational forces up the leg to the knee. Now the knee is often injured instead of the lower leg. Bindings do release most of the time when they should, and there has been a decrease in the incidence of injury. However, as the number of skiers increases, knee injuries have become a common daily occurrence at ski areas.

The type of leg fracture seen most often now is a simple boot-top tibia or fibula fracture rather than the spiral fracture. A simple hairline fibula fracture can be treated with weight-bearing according to tolerance. The other fractures are more complicated. Most tibia fractures need referral to an orthopedic surgeon. Nondisplaced tibia fractures may be splinted or placed in a long leg cast to get the patient home for orthopedic care. Displaced or open fractures require immediate hospitalization and often need surgical stabilization.

7. When should a knee effusion be tapped?

Knee effusions may have several different etiologies. In ski injuries, the effusion is most often bloody. The hemarthrosis is usually due to anterior cruciate ligament rupture but may also occur with a meniscus injury or a fracture. Controversy surrounds the need to tap an acute hemarthrosis. It may afford some comfort, but the blood tends to reaccumulate. The knee should first be radiographed to rule out a fracture. Do not tap the knee if a fracture is obvious on radiography. This in theory turns it into an open fracture, and if it is large, the blood will quickly reaccumulate. If none is found, and there is a tense painful effusion, arthrocentesis will be of diagnostic and therapeutic benefit. It is diagnostic because blood indicates a traumatic effusion. If the synovial fluid is straw colored, there may be another reason for the effusion; it should be analyzed for cells and crystals. After removing blood, put it in a basin to look for small fat globules rising to the surface, indicating a fracture. This often suggests an anterior cruciate ligament tear that has avulsed off part of the tibial spine. The arthrocentesis is therapeutic because bloody synovial effusions of the knee are painful, and removing blood gives the patient relief. It also is difficult to evaluate knee ligaments if a large tight synovial effusion is present. Drain the knee and then reexamine the ligaments. Use ice and elevation. Advise all patients to avoid heat—many will want to go in the hot tub after hurting their knee.

8. How are medial collateral ligament sprains treated?

Grade III (complete) ligament sprains should be immobilized, remain non–weight-bearing, and be referred to an orthopedic surgeon. Grades I and II (partial) medial collateral ligament sprains should be treated aggressively. If there is pain, any instability, or if the patient cannot lift the leg keeping the knee straight (extension lag), apply a knee immobilizer. Some patients will still need crutches.

It is important to send these patients to physical therapy quickly and stress range of motion, strength, proprioception, soft tissue healing, and endurance. Medial collateral ligament sprains are very painful and stiffen quickly with immobility. The best way to improve range of motion is by riding a stationary bicycle with low or no resistance. Patients should start peddling back and forth with progression to spinning. Before allowing the patient full weight-bearing ambulation, he or she must exhibit good quadriceps control. Progress the patient from the knee immobilizer to a hinged knee brace with a 10° extension stop. The extension stop prevents forced hyperextension of the knee that could result in an anterior cruciate ligament injury.

Depending on the level of medial collateral ligament injury and return of range of motion and function, these patients can return to skiing anywhere from 2 days to 8 weeks. Consider recommending that the patient wear the hinged knee brace for 6 months after injury for skiing and any sport that requires planting the foot on the ground with a pivot, such as tennis, basketball, or softball. It takes this long for complete healing.

9. How are anterior cruciate ligament (ACL) sprains treated?

In most cases, these injuries are immobilized and made non–weight-bearing. Athletic patients with an isolated ACL injury and strong muscles may be able to walk. All ACL injuries should be referred to an orthopedic surgeon. If surgery is delayed, refer these patients to physical therapy to maintain range of motion, strength, proprioception, and decrease effusion. It takes only 2 days of immobilization for atrophy to set in. Decreasing effusion is essential, as it accelerates atrophy.

10. Who needs crutches?

Most fractures of a lower extremity should be non–weight-bearing. An exception is a mid-shaft isolated fibula fracture. Medial collateral ligament sprains, if painful in an immobilizer, should be helped along with crutches. Most ACL sprains should be non–weight-bearing acutely because they are often combined with other knee structure damage and will tend to be unstable. Of course, tibia plateau fractures must be non–weight-bearing—there is a fracture of the platform that the femur sits on. Weight on the fracture, even if small, may make it worse. Patients with ankle sprains may walk with an Ace or Aircast splint, but some injuries are unstable or painful enough to require crutches.

11. How do you sprain an ankle in a ski boot?

Ankle sprains are common. How can they happen with modern ski boots? Because ski boots are stiff and high, it is thought that the skier has the boots buckled too loosely. But many skiers with ankle sprains claim that their boots were snug. Ankle sprains may be caused by hard twisting forces without a valgus or varus stress. Rotational forces twist the tibia and fibula on the talus, ripping ankle ligaments. This may explain why Maisonneuve's fracture is seen more frequently in skiing than in most sports. It is a sprain of the deltoid ligament of the ankle associated with a proximal fibula fracture, which is probably caused by hard gyration in the leg and ankle. It is an unstable sprain with a widened ankle mortise, and it requires surgery. If a skier or any patient has a medial ankle sprain, always be sure to check for tenderness at the proximal fibula, and radiograph that area.

Treat skiing-related ankle sprains the same as any ankle sprain. Grade I sprains (in which about 25% of the ligament fibers are torn) should be treated with ice and elevation, and patients may need crutches if it is painful to walk. Grade II sprains (in which 25–75% of the ligament fibers are torn) also benefit from ice and elevation and crutches. An Ace wrap may help with the swelling. Early referral to physical therapy will greatly speed healing time. The treatment of third-degree sprains (75% to complete rupture) is controversial, and these patients should be referred to an orthopedic surgeon. Put the lower leg in a posterior plaster splint, and have the patient use crutches, ice, and elevation.

12. What happens to the thumb when it is injured while skiing—"skier's thumb"?

As the skier falls, the hand reaches out instinctively to break the fall. Because the hand is gripping a ski pole, the thumb is in a vulnerable position. The pole catches in the snow, often at high speed, forcing the thumb back into abduction and extension. This stresses the ulnar collateral ligament of the thumb. The ligament will tear. **The physician should always obtain a radiograph of an injured thumb before stressing the ulnar collateral ligament**. An avulsion fracture may be present. If the fracture is in proximity to the bone, it will heal. By stressing the ligament, the fragment might be pulled farther away from the bone. To examine the thumb, firmly grasp the metacarpal bone and stress the metacarpophalangeal joint by trying to displace the thumb in the radial direction.

First- and second-degree sprains are painful, but the ligament is still intact, and these will mend without surgery. The thumb should be splinted or casted. If the patient wants to ski, the thumb **must** be casted to prevent further injury. The use of a short-arm light-weight Fiberglass thumb cast is appropriate for skiing. If it is not a third-degree sprain, the ligament will heal in 4 weeks.

A third-degree sprain is a total separation of the ligament. The thumb metacarpophalangeal joint has laxity with stress. If the ulnar collateral ligament tears completely, it will not heal owing to the anatomy of the thumb. This requires surgical repair to maintain normal opposition strength for the thumb. Third-degree ligament sprains need to be referred for orthopedic repair promptly. Delayed repair may result in poorer outcome.

13. What other upper-extremity injuries result from ski falls?

Separations of the acromioclavicular joint (AC sprains) are common. First- and second-degree sprains do not have noticeable deformity and heal quickly. Third-degree sprains show a large stepoff that may not be cosmetically acceptable to the patient but rarely result in dysfunction to the shoulder. Consider orthopedic evaluation of third-degree AC separations. Treat all AC sprains with a sling and ice, and refer to physical therapy for early rehabilitation.

Clavicle fractures are frequent and are treated conservatively with a sling and figure-of-eight braces, ice, and pain medication. Most of them will heal even if displaced or comminuted. Distal clavicle fractures should be referred to an orthopedic surgeon.

Rotator cuff injuries and supraspinatus impingement problems are due to falling on an outstretched arm. Greater tuberosity fractures and other humerus fractures occur from direct falls on the arm and shoulder. Most of these are treated with immobilization in an sling for comfort, ice, pain medication, and early referral for physical therapy.

Any elbow, wrist, or hand injury can result from a fall on the hand. Among the more common wrist injuries are Colles' fractures and navicular fractures. In the hand, the skier's thumb (ulnar collateral ligament sprain) described above is by far the most common injury, but finger dislocations are not uncommon. Other fractures include metacarpal and phalangeal fractures.

14. How do you reduce a shoulder dislocation?

This is a common ski injury. The majority of shoulder dislocations are anterior. If a shoulder dislocation is treated soon after occurring, often it can be quickly reduced without force or medication. A shoulder dislocation takes priority above all injuries except, of course, life-threatening problems. It demands the physician's immediate attention and constant attendance.

First, have the individual sit down. Assess the total patient to rule out other immediate injuries, such as cervical spine or head injury. Take off the ski boots. Undress the upper body. Most patients are in a great deal of distress and will be hyperventilating. Try to have the patient take slow deep breaths. Expeditiously obtain a radiograph to rule out a fracture. If a fracture is present, it may be impossible to reduce the shoulder and you can make the fracture worse; for example, a surgical neck fracture of the humerus. An exception to this is greater tuberosity fractures, which will come back together after reduction. Try to assess axillary nerve function by testing sensation at the deltoid area. Assess neurovascular function to the hand.

Position the patient supine. Hold the patient's arm and reassure that the reduction will be done slowly. Have the patient try to relax the shoulder and arm muscles. Talk in a gentle, reassuring voice. Hold the elbow out horizontally with the shoulder at 45° abduction with one hand and support the patient's wrist with your other hand. Slowly externally rotate the shoulder by bringing the hand backward toward the floor. The elbow stays in the same position 45° out and level. Keep reminding the patient to relax. As the hand falls back and the shoulder is in full external rotation, apply more traction—gently and slowly—for a few minutes until it goes back in. About one third of the dislocations will reduce at this point—5 to 10 minutes after starting.

If the shoulder is still dislocated, begin unhurriedly moving the arm and elbow upward in shoulder abduction toward the patient's head maintaining full shoulder external rotation until the arm is abducted to the patient's head. If necessary, you can then gradually increase pull on the arm and hold it for a few minutes. This approach will reduce another 50% of dislocations.

After the shoulder is in, bring the elbow down over the body, in front of the face, until the forearm is in a comfortable position over the abdomen, with the elbow flexed at 90°. This technique is successful at our clinic and reduces the risks of intravenous pain medication and sedation.

The remaining 25% in whom the shoulder is still dislocated will need pain control or sedation. After this is done, repeat the previous maneuvers. If you are still unsuccessful, the traditional technique of pulling out the arm, using sheets, weights while prone, and so forth, should be attempted.

Be sure to continually evaluate the patient for other injuries. Check for neck pain. Do a secondary survey from head to toe.

After reduction, reassess the axillary nerve, including sensation at the deltoid, and test for injury to all the other nerves coming through the brachial plexus to the arm and hand. Place the arm in a shoulder immobilizer or in a sling with an Ace bandage wrapped around the arm and body. Refer the patient to an orthopedic surgeon and to physical therapy.

Two to five percent of shoulder dislocations will be posterior, and routine shoulder radiographs may not show the dislocation. Clinically, the victims act just as if they have a dislocation—they will not move the shoulder and have to support the arm. If you suspect a dislocation, order an additional axillary radiographic view. It may take a while to get the patient's arm extended enough to do this. The physician should be present to help. Posterior dislocations may be more difficult to reduce, and the traditional techniques described should be used.

15. How do snow conditions affect ski injuries?

When a skier falls on hard, icy snow, the shoulder and upper extremities are susceptible to **impact injury**. Common shoulder injuries include shoulder dislocations, AC sprains, clavicle fractures, greater tuberosity fractures, and other humerus fractures. Impact injuries may also cause lower-extremity problems such as hip fractures, greater trochanter fractures, and even patella fractures.

Head injuries are also more prevalent with icy conditions. The skier simply falls and strikes the head on the hard surface. The damage ranges from simple contusions to scalp lacerations to more serious problems such as skull fractures and cervical spine injuries. Follow the routine ABCs of trauma in evaluating all ski injuries.

Powder and soft snow cushions falls nicely but can lead to rotational injuries such as tibia and fibula fractures, knee injuries, and ankle sprains. Skiers searching for powder snow may wander off the main runs and hit trees and rocks, resulting in any number of injuries.

With groomed slopes, skiers are moving faster. Racers and recreational skiers going rapidly also can have collisions with obstacles such as trees, picnic tables, or other skiers. These impact injuries include fractures and internal injuries.

16. Why do skiers get altitude illness at some ski areas?

Acute mountain sickness (AMS) begins at altitudes greater than 7000 feet above sea level. It will occur in 25% to 30% of subjects who ascend rapidly. Patients with AMS present with headache, lethargy, insomnia, nausea, and mild shortness of breath. In most cases, it is a nuisance and people can go about their activities without trouble. It usually resolves within a few days. Occasionally, the symptoms become severe enough to decrease activity. A small percentage of victims will progress on to high-altitude pulmonary edema (HAPE). This is a noncardiogenic form of pulmonary edema that usually develops within 24 to 72 hours and presents with a cough. The cough becomes productive; first the sputum is clear, but it may progress to appear blood streaked or pink and frothy. Dyspnea and severe headache are present. The patient may have progressive confusion and lethargy. Rales are present and edema is seen on the chest radiograph. The percentage of oxygen saturation in the blood drops.

The higher in elevation one goes, the greater the likelihood of developing AMS. In addition, the altitude at which one sleeps is significant—it is one of the most important factors in the illness. There is a common saying at high altitude, "play high, sleep low." Sedatives may aggravate AMS by decreasing respiration. Alcohol and sleeping medications are discouraged.

High-altitude cerebral edema (HACE) may occur at ski areas, but is more commonly seen at more extreme altitudes above 12,000 feet. Some of the confusion that occurs in patients with HAPE at moderate altitude may be due to HACE. The headache of AMS is possibly caused by mild cerebral edema.

17. How do you treat altitude illness?

Ascend slowly, drink plenty of fluids, and avoid alcohol for the first few days and until the headache and other symptoms have resolved. Engage in moderate, not strenuous, activity; eat small frequent meals rather than large rich dinners; and try to avoid salt and fat. The majority of people will have little or no problems if these recommendations are followed. Obviously smoking and the hypoxia at altitude do not mix well. Consider acetazolamide for patients who have suffered previously from altitude illness; the appropriate dose to prevent AMS is 125 mg, starting the day before ascent and continuing for 3 or 4 days after arrival at altitude. Nifedipine has been proved to prevent HAPE in patients who have had the illness previously.

Even if a person gets mild AMS, the symptoms can be treated with rest, fluids, and if severe, acetazolamide. Be sure to warn all patients to seek medical care for a cough or worsening headache, lethargy, shortness of breath, or any other unusual symptoms, as these could signify HAPE, HACE, or perhaps another non–altitude-related condition. Consider exercise testing on your patients with heart or lung disease before they ascend above 7000 feet.

BIBLIOGRAPHY

1. Bartsch P, et al: Prevention of high-altitude pulmonary edema by nifedipine. N Engl J Med 325:1284–1289, 1991.
2. Burns TP, Steadman JR, Rodkey WG: Alpine skiing and the mature athlete. Clin Sports Med 10:327–342, 1991.
3. de Clari F, von Albertini M: High-altitude pulmonary edema. N Engl J Med 335:207, 1996.
4. Deibert MC, Aronsson DD, Johnson RJ, et al: Skiing injuries in children, adolescents, and adults. J Bone Joint Surg Am 80:25–32, 1998.
5. Downhill ski fatalities: The Vermont experience [published erratum appears in J Trauma 28:561, 1988]. J Trauma 28:95–100, 1988.
6. Feagin JA Jr, Lambert KL, Cunningham RR, et al: Consideration of the anterior cruciate ligament injury in skiing. Clin Orthop 216:13–18, 1987.
7. Freeman JR, Weaver JK, Oden RR, Kirk RE: Changing patterns in tibial fractures resulting from skiing. Clin Orthop 216:19–23, 1987.
8. Fritschy D: An unusual ankle injury in top skiers. Am J Sports Med 17:282–285, 1989.
9. Higgins RW, Steadman JR: Anterior cruciate ligament repairs in world class skiers. Am J Sports Med 15:439–447, 1987.
10. Hill SA: Incidence of tibial fracture in child skiers. Br J Sports Med 23:169–170, 1989.
11. Hultgren HN: High-altitude pulmonary edema: Current concepts. Annu Rev Med 47:267–284, 1996.
12. Hultgren HN: High-altitude pulmonary edema: Hemodynamic aspects. Int J Sports Med 18:20–25, 1997.
13. Hultgren HN, Honigman B, Theis K, Nicholas D: High-altitude pulmonary edema at a ski resort. West J Med 164:222–227, 1996.
14. Johnson RJ, Ettlinger CF, Shealy JF, Meader C: Impact of super sidecut skis on the epidemiology of skiing injuries. Sportverletz Sportschaden 11:150–152, 1997.
15. Kocher MS, Dupre MM, Feagin JA Jr: Shoulder injuries from alpine skiing and snowboarding. Aetiology, treatment and prevention. Sports Med 25:201–211, 1998.
16. Kristiansen TK, Johnson RJ: Fractures in the skiing athlete. Clin Sports Med 9:215–225, 1990.
17. Matter P, Ziegler WJ, Holzach P: Skiing accidents in the past 15 years. J Sports Sci 5:319–326, 1987.
18. McConkey JP, Meeuwisse W: Tibial plateau fractures in alpine skiing. Am J Sports Med 16:159–164, 1988.
19. Mellion M: Office Management of Sports Injuries & Athletic Problems. Philadelphia, Hanley & Belfus, 1988.
20. Moller-Madsen B, Jakobsen BW, Villadsen I: Skiing injuries: A study from a Danish community. Br J Sports Med 24:123–124, 1990.
21. Oden RR: Tendon injuries about the ankle resulting from skiing. Clin Orthop 216:63–69, 1987.
22. Pliskin M, D'Angelo M: Atypical downhill skiing injuries. J Trauma 28:520–522, 1988.
23. Reeves J, Schoene R: When lungs on mountains leak. N Engl J Med 325:1307, 1991.
24. Rothenberg MH, Graf BK: Evaluation of acute knee injuries. Postgrad Med 93:75–86, 1993.
25. Sahlin Y: Alpine ski injuries. Br J Sports Med 23:241–244, 1989.
26. Schoene R: High-altitude pulmonary edema: Pathophysiology and clinical review. Ann Intern Med 16:987–992, 1987.
27. Sherry E, Fenelon L: Trends in skiing injury type and rates in Australia. A review of 22,261 injuries over 27 years in the Snowy Mountains. Med J Aust 155:513–515, 1991.
28. Thomas P: Avoiding ski injuries. Practitioner 233:90–94, 1989.
29. Warme WJ, Feagin JA Jr, King P, et al: Ski injury statistics, 1982 to 1993, Jackson Hole Ski Resort. Am J Sports Med 23:597–600, 1995.
30. Weaver JK: Skiing-related injuries to the shoulder. Clin Orthop 216:24–28, 1987.

95. NORDIC SKIING

Margot Putukian, M.D., FACSM, and Douglas B. McKeag, M.D., M.S.

1. How popular is Nordic skiing?

Nordic, or cross-country, skiing is very popular in Scandinavian countries, where it origi-
nated almost 5000 years ago. It is becoming more popular in the United States as well, although
its history here is only 70 years old. It is estimated that around the time of the 1932 Winter
Olympics in Lake Placid, NY, 10,000 Americans participated in the sport. By the year 1980, this
number reached 3 million, and by 1988, approximately 7.2 million enthusiasts enjoyed the sport
in the United States. In the 1990s the popularity of the sport has continued to grow, and the
number surely exceeds 8 million.

2. What makes Nordic skiing so enjoyable?

Nordic skiing is an excellent sport that combines aerobic conditioning, a relatively low basic
skill level in order to participate, and an opportunity to exercise comfortably outdoors and enjoy
the solace of natural surroundings. Unlike alpine skiing, it does not entail costly equipment, lift
lines, or exorbitant fees, and does not significantly alter the environment. It also has a relatively
low injury rate, although it is not completely risk free. Finally, skiers of all levels can participate
together, making it an excellent family activity.

3. What benefits, if any, does Nordic skiing have over other aerobic sports?

Nordic skiing is similar to other endurance exercise in that it is primarily an aerobic exercise,
although with competitive racing, there is certainly a large anaerobic component to consider. The
potential for increasing aerobic fitness is immense, with the highest recorded aerobic capacity—
> 80 ml/kg/min—being measured in a cross-country skier. It also is an exercise involving both
the upper and lower extremities and is an excellent exercise for improving the muscle tone and
strength of the entire body musculature. Cross-country skiing is associated with maintaining bone
mineral density in 70- to 81-year-olds when compared with nonactive controls, and participants
even have higher bone mineral density levels compared with runners. Yet, cross-country skiing has
less pounding forces than many other sports, with only forces of 1.5 times body weight during
the "kick" phase of skiing compared with running, which entails forces 3.5 times body weight.
This decreases some of the overuse injuries that are so prevalent in other endurance sports.

4. Is Nordic skiing safer than alpine skiing?

Unfortunately, all sports appear to entail some kind of risks for injury, and Nordic skiing is
no exception. It has an injury rate of 0.15–0.72%, depending on the study looked at, which is
about 10 times less than the injury rate for alpine skiing. Additionally, at higher levels of competition, the injury rate is almost nonexistent for Nordic skiers compared with alpine skiers, where
79–85% have suffered a serious injury (missing all or part of a season) at some point in time.

5. What kinds of injuries occur in Nordic skiing?

In a prospective control-matched 2-year study of cross-country skiers in Vermont, an incidence of 0.72 injuries per 1,000 skier days was reported. This compares with an incidence of
3.4–7.4 injuries per 1,000 skier days in alpine skiers. Forty-nine percent of the injuries were to
the lower extremity, 41% were to the upper extremity, and the remaining 10% were to the face
and head or trunk. Of the injuries, 88.4% occurred on downhill terrain. The number of lessons
taken did not alter the incidence of injuries, although the number of years of experience *did* have
an effect (the more experience, the fewer injuries). Data from the National Ski Patrol state that
66% of injuries are musculoskeletal, 20% are hypothermia-related problems, and 14% "other."

As skiers gain experience, most of the injuries that occur are overuse injuries, with fractures and other acute injuries being less common.

6. What kinds of musculoskeletal injuries are the most common in Nordic skiers?

Of the musculoskeletal injuries that occur, lower-extremity injuries predominante, with internal knee derangements, ankle sprains, and overuse injuries being the most common. The ankle is fixed only at the toe, and therefore the increased mobility leads to a decrease in stability and an increase in potential injuries compared with alpine skiing. The injuries to the knee and hip occur secondary to twisting motions and torque occurring throughout the body, which increase as the length of the skis increases. Upper-extremity injuries usually occur secondary to a fall or the catching of the poles on surrounding trees or bushes. Wrist and forearm fractures, "skier's thumb" (ulnar collateral ligament injuries), acromioclavicular separations, and even glenohumeral subluxation or dislocations can occur. Low back pain is a common musculoskeletal complaint. In a recent study, 64% of competitive male and female Nordic skiers complained of backache that affected skiing ability. Finally, the head and face injuries include concussions and lacerations, as well as corneal damage secondary to the cold weather and dehydration, which are not uncommon. The following table summarizes some of the most common injuries seen in Nordic skiing.

Common Injuries in Nordic Skiing

INJURY	COMMENTS
Lower Extremity Injuries	
Internal knee derangements	Often due to catching tip of ski with external
Anterior cruciate ligament	rotation and valgus stress
Medial collateral ligament	
Meniscal injuries	
Ankle sprains, tibial/fibular fractures; hip	Ski acts as a lever and increases forces acting on long
dislocations; proximal femur fractures	bones and joints
"Skier's toe" (first metatarsophalangeal	Increased with skating technique
joint inflammation)	
Upper Extremity Injuries	
"Skier's thumb" (ulnar collateral ligament)	Made worse by strap of pole levering against pole
sprain or rupture	
Colles' fracture; navicular fracture	Fall on outstretched hand
Acromioclavicular separation; clavicle	Fall directly on shoulder
fracture	
Glenohumeral subluxation or dislocation	Catching pole on ground or trees while going forward
Extensor digitorum synovitis	Increased by strap pressure
Triceps tendinitis	Increased with longer poles, skating technique
Head/face/trunk Injuries	
Low back pain	Increased with double-poling technique, weak
	abdominals
Lacerations; head concussions	Often due to fall on hard ground or into trees
Cold Injuries	
Hypothermia	Dehydration, caloric intake, and clothing important;
Frostbite	avoid alcohol

7. What types of techniques are used in Nordic skiing?

Various techniques are used in cross-country skiing. The three classic techniques, all of which involve skiing in parallel tracks, are differentiated by poling techniques. In the 1980s three skating techniques became popular. Skating does not make use of tracks but is done on packed snow. It is associated with an increase in speed. Classic diagonal pole techniques may lead to speeds of 6 meters/second compared with 8–9/second for double poling with the skating technique. In the skating technique one ski is alternately placed in a V pattern, as in ice skating. Other modifications have included a longer pole length and a more rigid heel fixation to increase the edging capabilities of the skier when the heel is on the ski. These modifications may change the types of injuries that occur.

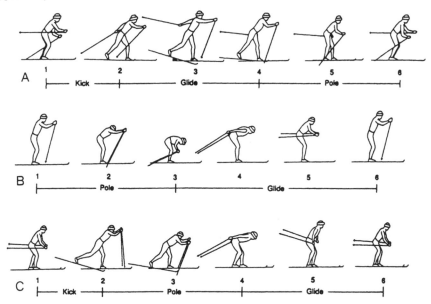

General movement pattern for (A) the classic or diagonal stride, (B) the double pole technique, and (C) the kick-double pole technique. (From Elmquist LG, Johnson R, Kaplan MJ, Renstrom PA: Alpine skiing. In Fu, FH, Stone DA (eds): Sports Injuries. Baltimore, Maryland, 1994, pp 481–500, with permission.)

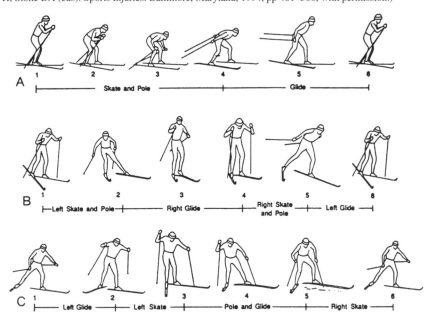

General movement patterns in the recently evolved skiing techniques, including (A) the marathon skate, (B) the V2 skate, and (C) the V1 skate. (From Elmquist LG, Johnson R, Kaplan MJ, Renstrom PA: Alpine skiing. In Fu, FH, Stone DA (eds): Sports Injuries. Baltimore, Maryland, 1994, pp 481–500, with permission.)

8. In what ways do these modifications affect the injuries seen in Nordic skiing?

With the development of skating techniques, speeds that are 10–30% faster than with classic techniques are possible. The skating technique uses longer poles and a more rigid heel fixation so that the skier can use the edges to control the ski better. The longer poles increase the incidence of triceps tendinitis, and the more rigid heel fixation makes injuries at the knee and hip more devastating, especially because the skis act to increase the torque that occurs. Double-poling is associated with low back overuse syndromes, as well as triceps tendinitis. The skating technique also puts more stress on the adductors and internal rotators of the hip, as well as the toe extensors, and is commonly implicated as a cause for the "skier's toe," an overuse injury of the first metatarsophalangeal (MTP) joint. A recent study assessed anterior compartment pressures of the leg during skating techniques on either skating or classic skis. The average compartment pressure increase was higher for the classic ski trials, but this difference was not significant. Therefore, although the techniques may be different, the ski used does not affect compartment pressure in the lower leg.

9. Is any Nordic skiing technique superior to the other in terms of efficiency?

Although the data have only recently been generated, the double-pole technique appears to be the most efficient, and the diagonal-stride techniques (classic) the least efficient. Diagonal-stride techniques induce greater demands physiologically than skating techniques, with 19% higher oxygen consumption, 5% higher heart rates, and 36% higher ventilation rates, as well as higher ratings of perceived exertion and respiratory exchange ratios. In another study on flat terrain, double-poling techniques had a 24% lower VO_2 requirement and a 10% lower heart rate than the diagonal-stride technique, and a 15% lower VO_2 and 6% lower heart rate than the skating techniques.

10. Are there any techniques for training in Nordic skiing during the summer?

There has been more and more information regarding the usefulness of sport-specific training, and this has made "dry-land" training important for competitive cross-country skiers, as well as for recreational athletes trying to prepare for the winter season. Roller skiing and in-line skating have been used for this purpose. Interestingly, data on the various techniques again reveal that double-poling techniques induce a lower VO_2 requirement than other techniques on flat terrain, with diagonal-stride and skating techniques having similar VO_2 requirements. Thus, for dry-land training, all techniques can be used to increase aerobic performance, and this may potentially decrease some of the overuse injuries that may occur if only one technique is used.

11. What kinds of cardiovascular adaptive changes occur with Nordic skiing activity?

As in other exercise programs, cross-country skiing can cause adaptive changes to occur, including an increased aerobic capacity, an increase in the lean body mass, an improvement in the lipid profile, a decrease in the resting heart rate, an increase in the left ventricular end-diastolic diameter and volume, and an increase in the left ventricular wall thickness. Because of the isometric activity of the arms in cross-country skiing, there is an increased pressure load that also can increase left ventricular wall thickness. Noninvasive testing often reveals these changes, with radiographic, electrocardiographic, and echocardiographic changes being consistent with "athlete's heart." These changes may be misinterpreted as abnormal if an exercise history is not taken or one is not familiar with the normal findings seen in the "athlete's heart."

12. What kinds of cold injuries occur in Nordic skiing?

Cold injuries account for 20% of the injuries seen in Nordic skiing. Cold injuries include frostnip and frostbite but also can progress to hypothermia, which can be life threatening. The best treatment is prevention. Adequate caloric intake and protective clothing will allow for proper maintenance of body temperature. Heat loss occurs through radiation, convection, conduction, and evaporation, and with increasing speeds, the wind-chill is increased. Ways to decrease heat loss include avoiding dehydration (adequate fluids, avoiding caffeine, alcohol), avoiding exposure (wear hat, mittens, face protection), and wearing layers of clothing that wick moisture (so that wet clothes are not on the body surface) and protect from the wind.

13. What risks are involved in skiing at altitude?

Skiing at altitude is usually well tolerated, even in those with mild cardiovascular disease, at moderate altitudes (9,000 to 10,000 feet) and as long as the altitudes are reached gradually (over 1–2 days). The forms of altitude illness that occur include acute mountain sickness, high-altitude pulmonary edema (HAPE), and high-altitude cerebral edema (HACE). The symptoms of acute mountain sickness include headache, nausea and vomiting, fatigue, and anorexia. Symptoms occur in roughly 20–25% of individuals who travel rapidly to altitudes of 9,000 to 9,500 feet, and abate in 1–2 days. A small subset of these individuals (0.01–0.05%) will progress to HAPE and HACE, where the symptoms are more severe and the consequences can be life threatening. Individuals at particular risk for altitude illnesses include those who quickly ascend (if fly to altitude), those with uncontrolled hypertension, and those individuals who are unconditioned. These risks can usually be identified and avoided by a careful screening examination.

14. What are the other special concerns in Nordic skiing?

Avoiding hypoglycemia and exercise-induced bronchospasm are special concerns to consider. Adequate nutrition is imperative, especially given the long treks and increased caloric demands because of the cold weather. Exercise-induced bronchospasm can usually be avoided by premedicating with sodium cromolyn or beta-agonists.

Additionally, one always needs to ensure safe participation in an exercise activity, and for cross-country skiing, this is especially important. Not only can it be a very demanding aerobic activity, it often occurs in cold weather and at high altitudes, far from an organized medical support system. Skiers should not venture out alone; if an injury occurs, whether it be cold induced, musculoskeletal, or cardiac, having a companion can avoid significant problems. The preparticipation examination should assess cardiovascular risks and musculoskeletal demands, as well as medications and other medical illnesses. With a thoughtful approach, most individuals will be able to participate safely and enjoy cross-country skiing.

BIBLIOGRAPHY

1. Boyle JJ, Johnson RJ, Pope MH: Cross-country injuries: A prospective study. Iowa Orthop J 1:41, 1981.
2. Eriksson K, Nemeth G, Eriksson E: Low back pain in elite cross-country skiers: A retrospective epidemiologic study. Scand J Med Sci Sports 6(1):311–315, 1996.
3. Grover RF, Tucker CE, McGroarty SR, et al: The coronary stress of skiing at altitude. Arch Intern Med 150:1205, 1990.
4. Hoffman MD: Physiological comparisons of cross-country skiing techniques. Med Sci Sports Exerc 24:1023, 1992.
5. Hoffman MD, Clifford PS: Physiological responses to different cross country skiing techniques on level terrain. Med Sci Sports Exerc 22:841, 1990.
6. Hoffman MD, Clifford PS, Foley PJ, Brice AG: Physiological responses to different roller skiing techniques. Med Sci Sports Exerc 22:391, 1990.
7. Houston CS: Trekking at high altitudes: How safe is it for your patients? Postgrad Med 88:56, 1990.
8. Johnson RJ: Skiing and snowboarding injuries: When schussing is a pain. Postgrad Med 88:36, 1990.
9. Lawson SK, Reid DC, Wiley JP: Anterior compartment pressures in cross-country skiers. A comparison of classic and skating skis. Am J Sports Med 20:750–753, 1992.
10. Renstrom P, Johnson RJ: Cross-country skiing injuries and biomechanics. Phys Sportsmed 8(6):346, 1989.
11. Stray-Gunderson J, Denke MA, Grundy SM: Influence of lifetime cross-country skiing on plasma lipids and lipoproteins. Med Sci Sports Exerc 23:695, 1991.
12. Street GM: Technological advances in cross-country ski equipment. Med Sci Sports Exerc 24:1048, 1992.
13. Suominen H, Rahkila P: Bone mineral density of the calcaneus in 70–81-yr-old male athletes and a population sample. Med Sci Sports Exerc 23:1227, 1991.

96. ROWING

Razib Khaund, M.D., and John M. Henderson, D.O.

1. Where did rowing originate as a sport?

Almost 300 years ago in England, race rowing was performed on the River Thames. In the early 19th century English colleges used rowing as part of their educational curriculum. The first boat race between Oxford and Cambridge was in 1829. In the United States the first intercollegiate rowing competition was between Harvard and Yale in 1852.

2. What are the two types of rowing competition?

Sweep rowing and sculling. Sweep rowing refers to the use of one oar 4 meters long. In sculling two oars 3 meters long are used. Sweep rowing employs crews of 2, 4, or 8 people. Sculling employs 1, 2, or 4 people.

3. What is the role of the coxswain?

The coxswain (pronounced *coksun*) is an extra member of the sweep rowing crew who serves as coach and navigator. The coxswain may be male or female. He or she uses a rudder to steer the boat and voiced cadence to organize the rhythmic rowing by the crew. Sculling does not employ a coxswain. Sweep rowing with crews of 2 and 4 rowers has the option of using a coxswain, whereas crews of 8 always use a coxswain.

4. How many boat classes are there?

There are a total of eight boat classes. Sweep oaring accounts for five: coxless pair, coxed pair, coxless four, coxed four, and coxed eight. There are three sculling classes: single, double, and quadruple. There are lightweight and heavyweight modifications to these classes.

5. How long and fast are rowing races?

The typical competition covers 2000 meters, approximately 1.25 miles. Some high school courses are 1500 meters. The approximate time elapsed is 6–8 minutes. The speeds attained by various boat classes range from 10–13 miles per hour.

6. Is rowing an aerobic or anaerobic sport?

Studies of energy provided for work demands reveal that two-thirds of rowing energy is derived aerobically and one-third anaerobically. Other studies reveal that the overall contribution of anaerobic capacity is approximately 10–20%. About 70% of the rower's muscle mass is involved in rowing. About 70–80% of involved muscles are slow-twitch fibers. The maximum oxygen uptake recorded among elite rowers is quite high; however, when expressed relative to body dimensions, oxygen uptake is lower than in elite runners, cyclists, or skiers.

7. What type of training is beneficial in rowing?

Training should be directed at increasing both aerobic and anaerobic power. Several studies suggest that endurance training is of chief importance. During season (spring to fall), approximately 70–80% of training is spent on the water. Rowing at about 65–75% maximum effort helps to build aerobic power, whereas short periods of all-out effort help to build anaerobic power. Off-water training includes stretching, running, and weight training. During the off-season, a rowing ergometer is commonly used in training to simulate rowing on water.

8. What medical problems commonly occur in rowers?

Extreme fatigue is not uncommon in rowers, given the high demands of training and competition. Chronic low back pain is another common problem. Other common injuries include various muscle strains, tendinitis, and blisters. There is growing recognition of eating disorders in rowers. Competitive rowers are under pressure to keep within a certain weight range and thus are at risk for disordered eating habits. Overall, with proper technique and training programs, rowing is a relatively safe sport.

The common soft tissue problems include bursitis and tendinitis. Bursitis may be due to compression or lateral friction at the ischial tuberosity or greater trochanter and subacromial muscles. Tendinitis may be due to overuse or exceeding the tensile properties of the muscle-tendon junction. Commonly involved sites include the rhomboid major/minor muscles at the medial border of the scapulae; erector spinae muscle at the sacroiliac crevice; tensor fascia lata muscle at the hip; iliotibial band at the lateral distal thigh; popliteus muscle at the lateral joint line of the knee.

9. Who should row?

Given the wide variety of rowing from recreational to competitive, some form of rowing is available to everyone. People should understand that rowing can be demanding and is excellent exercise to develop muscular strength as well as aerobic health. Given the various types of boats, one can row as an individual or part of a crew or team. Before beginning to row, a general physical examination by a physician is prudent. People with cardiovascular and pulmonary diseases should have individually modified programs designed and monitored by a physician. All rowers should be able to swim.

10. What are the rowing organizations?

The international organization governing rowing is the Federation Internationale des Societes d'Aviron (FISA). This organization has been arranging international competitions since 1893. The United States Rowing Association (USRA) arranges national competitions. Established in 1872, its original name was the National Association of Amateur Oarsmen. The USRA can be contacted for more information about rowing at 201 South Capitol Ave., Suite 400, Indianapolis, IN 46225.

11. What is the current status of rowing?

Interest and participation in rowing are on the rise. More and more people are participating in recreational rowing, which helps to popularize the sport. In 1995 there were approximately 530 members in the USRA. Members come from rowers at the high school, college, and club levels.

BIBLIOGRAPHY

1. Brackett JW: Rowing. In Mellion M (ed): Sports Medicine Secrets. Philadelphia, Hanley & Belfus, 1994, pp 406–409.
2. Mendenhall TC: A Short History of American Rowing. Boston, Charles River Books, 1980.
3. Nelson R, MacNee MJ (eds): Rowing. In The Olympic Factbook. A Spectator's Guide to the Summer Games. Detroit, Visible Ink Press, 1996.
4. Secher NH: Physiological and biomechanical aspects of rowing: Implications for training. Sports Med 15:24–42, 1993.
5. Secher NH: Rowing. In Shephard RJ, Åstrand PO (eds): Endurance in Sport. Oxford, Blackwell Scientific, 1992, pp 563–569.
6. Steinacker JM: Physiological aspects of training in rowing. Int J Sports Med 14:503–510, 1993.
7. Steinacker JM, Secher NH: Advances in physiology and biomechanics of rowing. Int J Sports Med 14:51–52, 1993.
8. Sykora C, Grilo CM, Wilfley DE, Brownell KD: Eating, weight, and dieting disturbances in male and female lightweight and heavyweight rowers. Int J Eating Disord 14:203–211, 1993.

97. ICE HOCKEY

David Thorson, M.D.

1. When did ice hockey develop as a sport?

Ice hockey dates back to the early 1600s as a game played by Native Americans. The first recorded match in the modern form occurred in Montreal in 1875.

2. How many amateurs participate in ice hockey?

It is estimated that over 300,000 amateurs participate, including 25,000 high school players.

3. How fast do hockey players skate?

Professional hockey players skate at speeds in excess of 30 mph, whereas young skaters can reach speeds of 20 mph. Players slide on the ice at speeds up to 15 mph.

4. How fast does the puck travel?

Puck speeds range from 50 mph with young players to more than 120 mph with professionals, producing impact forces greater than 1,250 pounds.

5. How has the sport evolved?

As in other sports, the players have increased in size, strength, skill, and endurance. The proliferation of indoor rinks and "perfect" ice has allowed the sport to be played year round at higher speeds.

Equipment has also changed to enhance performance. The sticks have evolved from wood to fiberglass and the blades from straight to curved. The boots are made of plastic/leather combinations, and improved blade design allows greater speed and precision.

The protective equipment has improved to the point that hockey players now look like armored gladiators. They wear pads over all body surfaces (shin, elbow, midsection, shoulder, hands). Helmets, face shields, and mouth guards are required at all but the professional level.

Fan expectations have also changed, with fans demanding more fights and violence; the players have responded.

6. What are the common mechanisms of injury in ice hockey?

Collisions with other players or the boards account for 60–90% of all injuries. The stick contributes 12–25% of injuries. The puck is involved in only 10–15% of injuries. Less than 5% of the time is the skate involved. Overuse contributes to less than 15% of injuries.

7. What types of injuries are seen in ice hockey?

Composite injury data indicate that about 70% of all injuries are contusions; 10% strains or sprains; 14% fractures of dislocations; 2% lacerations; and less than 8%, abrasions.

8. Have injury patterns changed?

Although injury rates have not changed significantly over the past several years, there has been an alarming change in injury patterns. The incidence of dental injuries has almost disappeared with the use of mouth guards and face shields. Concussions have decreased in severity with mandatory use of helmets and improvements in design (deaths and bleeds are now rare). Facial lacerations and eye injuries are almost nonexistent when full face shields are used. However, **cervical spine injury has become more prevalent**.

9. Why has there been an increase in cervical spine injuries in hockey?

In a Canadian study, Tator was unable to document *any* hockey-related injuries of the cervical spine before 1972. One cervical spine injury was reported between 1974–1980, 5 between

1980–1981. Tator established a research advisory board that currently is tracking over 117 injuries to the cervical spine, all of which have occurred since 1980, correlating with the rules mandating face masks. The age of injured players ranges from 11–41 years, with 1 female; the majority of injured players are 15–25 years old. A review of data found that most injuries resulted from illegal checks (checking from behind).

10. What is the mechanism of cervical spine injuries in ice hockey?

The injury occurs when the neck is flexed forward and the cervical spine is straightened, receiving an axial load. An example is sliding into the boards head first. This results in failure of the column, vertebral fractures, and catastrophic injury. Various factors may be involved in the increase in such injuries. Helmeted and masked hockey players may feel indestructible and take more chances; coaches may not teach proper techniques; and most certainly officials do not enforce the rules strictly. In younger players inadequate neck strength may promote a head-down position. No data suggest that helmet design is a contributing factor, but helmet weight may contribute to muscle fatigue.

11. What are the rates of nonfatal catastrophic injury in ice hockey?

Injury statistics show 2.55 nonfatal catastrophic injuries per 100,000 player hours compared with 0.68 per 100,000 player hours in football.

12. Do concussions still occur in ice hockey?

Concussions of varying severity still occur in spite of the helmet rule, but life-threatening head injuries have become rare. Concussions are likely to be underreported, because often no care is sought for grade 1 (or less) concussions. Insurance data indicate that fewer than 15% of players suffer a concussion each year. A 1982 study by Gerberich and Finke indicates a 10% rate in high school hockey.

13. How should concussions be treated?

The players need to be educated that any loss of awareness after a head injury indicates a significant insult to the brain. To avoid second-impact syndrome, all coaches, trainers, parents, and physicians should be aware of guidelines for return to participation after head injury. Guidelines should be strictly enforced. Subdural hematomas, although rare, still occur; thus any athlete who develops a slow change in mental status after head injury needs to be evaluated appropriately.

14. How frequent are eye injuries in ice hockey?

Eye injuries have become almost nonexistent since the mandated use of full face shields.

15. Do mouth guards work?

Mouth guards not only have minimized the occurrence of dental injuries but also help to prevent concussions. The combination of mouth guards and face shields has made dental injuries almost nonexistent.

16. What are the common upper extremity injuries in ice hockey?

Shoulder: Acromioclavicular (AC) separations are graded from 1–3, with 3 being a complete separation. Radiographic studies suggest that 45% of all hockey players experience arthritic AC changes. Rotator cuff tendinitis, shoulder dislocations, and clavicle fractures also occur.

Elbow: Chronic, recurrent, and painful olecranon bursitis is a frequent injury that may be prevented by better elbow pads. When conservative treatment (e.g., ice, NSAIDs, compression, and steroid injection) fails, these injuries may need surgical treatment.

Wrist: Wrist injuries range from carpal tunnel syndrome to scaphoid fractures. Snuff-box tenderness or pain over the palmar side of the scaphoid needs to be treated as a fracture even if radiographs are normal; it is not unusual for radiographs to lag behind symptoms by 2–5 weeks. Because of the high nonunion rate for these injuries, early diagnosis and appropriate casting are indicated.

Hand: Gamekeeper's thumb (injury to the ulnar collateral ligament) occurs frequently. If stress testing yields no endpoint and radiographs do not show a bone chip, consider a Stener lesion, which may need surgery. Apply a hand-based thumb spica cast that can be molded to a hockey stick and thus allows the player to continue to participate. Jersey finger (rupture of the flexor digitorum profundus) requires surgical repair. This completely avoidable injury occurs when players drop their gloves to fight and attempt to hold on to the opponent's jersey.

17. Are there reports of significant abdominal injuries in ice hockey?

Abdominal injuries such as spleen or liver hematoma and capsular bleeds are rare but need to be considered after significant trauma (e.g., when the stick is trapped between the boards and the player, with its butt end in the player's abdomen). Kidney contusions may also occur.

18. Why does it take so long to return to play after a groin strain or hip pointer?

Hockey skating requires above-average strength of the hip adductor, and players should not be allowed to return after a groin strain until they have symmetrical strength and range of motion. A hip pointer is a contusion (possibly a strain or tear of the sartorius muscle) at the iliac crest; these injuries are exquisitely painful and difficult to rehabilitate.

19. Describe the complications of thigh contusions.

A thigh contusion can cause significant bleeding into the extensor mechanism of the lower leg. This can be minimized by placing the knee in a maximally flexed position for compression and by packing the injured area with ice. Too rapid a return to sport can result in muscle tears and myositis ossificans. Full and symmetric range of motion should be documented before return to participation.

20. Do major knee injuries occur in ice hockey?

Most knee injuries are minor. The most frequent severe injuries involve the anterior cruciate and medial collateral ligaments or the meniscus. A knee injury with intraarticular swelling (within hours of the incident) and an associated pop is an injury to the anterior cruciate ligament until proved otherwise.

21. What injuries occur at the foot and ankle in ice hockey?

Ankle sprains occur despite the supportive skate boot. Aggressive rehabilitation geared to maintaining range of motion and redeveloping proprioception minimizes time off. Casting and prolonged immobilization should be avoided.

Skaters can develop tarsal tunnel syndrome, which is similar to carpal tunnel syndrome in the wrist. A positive Tinel's sign over the posterior tibialis nerve justifies consideration of a steroid injection into the tarsal tunnel. If symptoms are present for more than 6 weeks, an EMG should be obtained; if the results are positive, surgery is recommended.

Ankle fractures can occur with inversion injuries or from impact with the puck. Forefoot injuries include Morton's neuroma, metatarsal fractures, sesamoid fractures and lace bite (tendinitis of the forefoot flexor mechanism, usually related to skate fit). Lace bite can be prevented and treated by creating a padded tunnel with orthopedic felt under the tongue of the skate.

22. What are the injury rates in ice hockey?

The data are confusing because there are no universal studies and definitions of injury change.

Professional hockey: 79 injuries/1,000 player game hours or 1 injury/7 game hours

College hockey: 1/11 game hours

High school hockey: 1/16 game hours

Youth hockey: 1/7 game hours (29% of players were injured, 1 severely, every 34 game hours).

23. What sites are most frequently injured in ice hockey?

Composite of studies:	Head and neck	20–30%
	Upper body	15–20%
	Trunk	15–25%
	Arm	8–20%
	Leg	20–30%

24. Are certain positions at increased risk for injuries?

Injury rates by position:	Forward	49–60%
	Defense	35–48%
	Goalie	3– 8%

25. Are injuries more common during games or practice?

Injuries during games account for up to 74% of all injuries. The rare injury that occurs during practice is often related to goofing off or not wearing appropriate equipment. At the professional and senior elite level, most injuries occur during the second period; the first period has the next highest injury rate. In youth hockey, rates are higher in the third period.

26. Can ice hockey be made safer by education?

Administrative changes can make hockey safer. Education of parents, coaches, and players regarding injury risk and prevention will help to reduce injury rates. Officials need to enforce the rules strictly and not to tolerate illegal activity.

27. Can equipment be further refined to make ice hockey safer?

Although equipment can be altered to promote safety, strict adherence to the rules will have a greater impact. Ongoing research in helmet design may improve shape, fit, and energy absorption. Clothing can be designed to decrease sliding speed and to reduce impact of the fallen player. The rink size can be increased to promote skating and finesse rather than hitting. An energy-absorbing rink board, although under consideration, is probably not practical.

28. Is an attitude adjustment needed?

Most importantly we need to work on attitudes. The players need to be educated in the true protective value of equipment. The coaches need to teach players the correct way to play and not to tolerate or promote intentional violence. The emphasis needs to be on skill and speed, rather than violence. The fans, parents, coaches, and players must encourage officials to enforce the rules and to prevent high-risk behavior.

29. How could rule changes affect safety?

Rule changes may enhance safety. For example, the player who injures another player through illegal activity should be suspended for the same amount of time the injured player is off, plus 1–3 games. Suspensions should be automatic for players who check from behind. Checking below the age of 16 years should be eliminated. In youth hockey, because of the great size difference among players of the same age, players should be matched by maturation age, skill, and size.

30. How does ice hockey compare with other sports in terms of danger?

According to Dr. Robert Cantu, ice hockey is "the most dangerous sport in the U.S.A. for non-fatal catastrophic injury." The equipment advances have not changed injury rates markedly over the past 20 years, but the types of injuries have changed. Severe eye injuries and toothless grins no longer characterize high school and college players. Instead, there is an increase in shoulder injuries and clavicle fractures as well as an alarming number of catastrophic cervical spine injuries. Proper rule enforcement and player education can make ice hockey a safer sport.

BIBLIOGRAPHY

1. Agre JC, Baxter TL, Casal DC, et al: Musculoskeletal characteristics of professional ice hockey players. Can J Sport Sci 12:1987.
2. Castaldi CR: Prevention of craniofacial injuries in ice hockey. Dent Clin North Am 35:647–656, 1991.
3. Castaldi CR, Sparacio L, Wood AW, Bernard J: Injury rates in amateur college and professional hockey. In Castaldi CR, Hoerner EF (eds): Safety in Ice Hockey. Philadelphia, American Society for Testing and Materials, 1989, pp 14–28.
4. Daly PJ, Sim FH, Simonet WT: Ice hockey injuries—A review. Sports Med 10(3):122–131, 1990.
5. Dyment PG: Violence in youth hockey. Phys Sportsmed 17(3):55, 1989.
6. Ganzhorn R, Toy BJ: Fractures to the fifth metatarsal. Phys Sportsmed 18(12):67–70, 1990.
7. Gerberich SG, Burns SR: Neurologic injuries in ice hockey. In Jordan BD, Tsairis P, Warren RF (eds): Sports Neurology. Gaithersburg, MD, Aspen Publishers, 1989, pp 245–255.
8. Gerberich SG, Finke R, Madden M, et al: An epidemiological study of high school hockey injuries. Child Nerv Syst 3(2):59–64, 1987.
9. Hancock LG, Ross BL, Dupont M, et al: Violence and injuries in ice hockey. Clin J Sport Med 1(2), 1991.
10. Jorgensen U, Schmidt-Olsen S: The epidemiology of ice hockey injuries. Br J Sports Med 20:7–9, 1986.
11. Lorentzon R, Wedren H, Petiela T, Gustavsson B: Injuries in international ice hockey. Am J Sports Med 16:389–396, 1988.
12. Minkoff J: Helping ice hockey players reduce injuries. J Musculoskel Med 2(2):30–39, 1985.
13. Montgomery DL: Physiology of ice hockey. Sports Med 5:99–126, 1988.
14. Pelletier RL, Montelpare WJ, Stark RM: Intercollegiate ice hockey injuries. Am J Sports Med 21:78–81, 1993.
15. Sane J, Ylipaavalniemi P, Leppanen H: Maxillofacial and ice hockey injuries. Med Sci Sports Exerc 20:202–207, 1988.
16. Sim FH, Chao EY: Injury potential in modern ice hockey. Am J Sports Med 6:378–384, 1978.
17. Sim FH, Simonet WT, Melton LJ, Lehn TA: Ice hockey injuries. Am J Sports Med 15:30–40, 1987.
18. Sim FH, Simonet WT, Scott SG: Ice hockey injuries: Causes, treatment, and prevention. J Musculoskel Med 6(3):15–44, 1989.
19. Smith MD: Violence and injuries in ice hockey. Clin J Sport Med 1(2):104–108, 1991.

98. DANCE

Marie D. Schafle, M.D.

1. At what age is it safe for a young dancer to go en pointe?

Ballet training begins with specific exercises done in soft leather slippers. The purpose of the exercises or barre is to strengthen the foot, the turnout muscles, and the torso. Over time the progression of the barre exercises teaches the symmetrical or centered movement that is essential for proper execution of the more difficult jumps, balance movements (or attitudes), and turns. When a young dancer is strong enough to perform a passe steadily, away from the barre, she probably is prepared physically to begin pointe classes. This position requires the dancer to have great strength in the foot and ankle, of course, but of equal importance, she must have excellent strength in the torso and in the turnout muscles (external rotators of the hip).

2. What is turnout?

Turnout is the amount of external rotation that is possible at the hip.

3. How is turnout measured?

The degree of turnout varies from one dancer to another. Every dancer would like to have 180° of turnout, but this is rare. In my experience, the Staheli method of measuring turnout has proved to be the most accurate, but it is important to ensure that there is no inadvertent flexion or abduction of the hip. Contract/relax stretching of the internal rotators sometimes adds a few degrees of turnout to the measurement. Most dancers who reach the stage of attending summer sessions have enough turnout to pursue a career. Surprisingly, many dancers who are seen for injuries are not strong enough to use all of the turnout that they have, especially if they are blessed with a great degree of external rotation at the hip. Apparently such dancers are not compelled to work the external rotators until they begin to dance en pointe. At this stage the friction of the foot on the floor is no longer able to keep the feet turned out and the hip musculature is forced to do the work.

4. Can turnout be increased?

Turnout can be increased by increasing the flexion at the hip and exaggerating the lordosis of the lumbar spine, while at the same time torquing the knees outward by grasping the floor with the toes and pronating the foot. There is no known, safe method of altering the amount of external rotation at the hip, which is determined genetically.

5. How do the bones of the foot respond to dance training?

The cortex of the first and second metatarsals becomes thickened over time in response to dance, especially pointe work. If pointe work is initiated prematurely or suddenly increased at any stage of a dancer's career, stress fracture of the second metatarsal can occur. In the ideal ballet foot the first and second metatarsals bear weight equally on demipointe and on pointe. If the first toe is longer than the second when the dancer begins pointe classes, the first toe is forced into a valgus position until it equals the length of the second toe. This process may contribute to bunion formation. If the second toe is longer, it assumes a shortened position to equal the length of the first toe. This position causes calluses to form on the dorsum of the proximal interphalangeal joint as it rubs against the vamp of the pointe shoe.

Insufficient articulation in the posterior tibiotalar joint may result in impingement of the posterior ankle. If this syndrome is due to a large trigonum or an unusually large posterior process on the talus, it can be corrected by operative intervention. Surgery should be reserved for serious dancers with realizable professional aspirations; it should not be done in the preadolescent or in a dancer whose talent—as judged by her teachers—does not justify a professional career.

6. What causes most dance injuries?

Most dance injuries are due to errors in technique and training. The most common error that we see is forced turnout. Forcing the feet to turn out at the floor at the expense of the knees, the hips, and the back can cause a predictable pattern of injuries, including hip flexor tendinitis, facet joint irritation, stress fractures of the pars interarticularis, chronic inflammation of the medial collateral ligament, and medial tibial stress syndrome. A common training error in both young and experienced dancers is repetition of a particular piece of choreography, usually unfamiliar, to "get it right." The repetitions unfortunately continue past the point of fatigue because of the dancer's determination to achieve perfection. It is important to question the injured dancer about the practice of new choreography or new skills.

7. When is a dancer most likely to be injured?

Most injuries occur with a sudden increase in the amount of time spent in class or rehearsal or a sudden change in technique—either advancement in class level or choreography for which a classical ballet barre does not prepare the dancer. Uneven matching of partners is also a source of injury, particularly with the introduction of partnering classes at the intermediate level. Often male dancers have not been prepared for lifting with special exercises or taught proper weight-lifting technique before the first attempt to lift a female dancer. In addition, the dancers to be lifted may be inexperienced and unskilled in active participation in the lifts.

8. Why is the incidence of scoliosis so high in the dance community?

The current thinking is that scoliosis (which is genetically determined) has more time to worsen in female dancers, because the delay of menarche retards skeletal maturation. This primary amenorrhea is thought to be related to long hours of physical exercise combined with restricted caloric intake. It is also seen in gymnasts and other young female athletes with low calorie intake.

9. What is "snapping hip"?

Snapping hip is a descriptive term for a common condition in dancers characterized by an audible or palpable "snap" in the hip during specific ranges of motion. If the condition is painless, it is usually of no consequence; if pain is experienced, however, the etiology must be determined. The iliotibial band is the most likely culprit in the painful snapping hip. Radiographic examination can determine whether the hip joint is abnormally angulated or shallow, causing recurrent subluxation, which may lead to painful snapping.

10. Are stress fractures common in dancers?

Stress fractures of the second metatarsal, tibia, fibula, and pars interarticularis are seen in dancers. Pain in these areas that is unexplained by other diagnoses should be attributed to stress fracture until proved otherwise by bone scan. Although bone scan establishes the diagnosis, it is not an accurate method for monitoring the fracture, because it remains positive long after the symptoms have disappeared. Treatment of the stress fracture may depend on the skill level or professional goals of the dancer. For example, a dancer who at the apprentice level is hopeful of being hired by a professional company will not accept a treatment of rest. It is more likely that she will need to be supported through the remainder of her apprenticeship, if possible, and rested during the summer. A student, on the other hand, although she may not be eager to rest, should not be allowed to continue to dance past the next performance. She may participate in the performance that is most important to her in the next month or so before resting the stress fracture.

11. Why can dancers not be sensible about their weight?

A ballet dancer is required to be 10–20% below ideal body weight to achieve the body habitus essential to entering a professional company. It is not practical and would be considered quite intrusive for the physician to attempt to dictate to an artistic director the proper body type for his or her company. Much more helpful is a positive attitude on the part of the physician and a willingness to help the dancer to achieve the ideal body with a balanced, nutrient-dense, low-calorie diet. Most dancers realize that their weight is not normal and think of themselves as thin compared with the general population.

12. How are eating disorders detected in dancers?

Eating disorders are serious derangements of body image. Any dancer who believes she is too fat and continues to attempt to lose weight, in spite of having a proper weight as judged by her peers and teachers, should be considered to have an eating disorder. Emotional withdrawal, frequent injuries or injuries that are slow to heal, loss of tooth enamel, foul breath, increased fine body hair, and lack of concentration and stamina are clues that should alert the teacher and the physician to a possible eating disorder. Eating disorders are complex medical and psychiatric problems and should be treated in a specifically designated facility. The therapeutic team usually includes a psychiatrist, a medical doctor, and a nutritionist. Attempts by the family practitioner to treat serious eating disorders without the assistance of a psychiatrist are to be discouraged. It must be remembered that the **mortality** rate for eating disorders is extremely high, even among patients treated in designated programs.

BIBLIOGRAPHY

1. McLain D: Artistic development in the dancer. Clin Sports Med 2:563–570, 1983.
2. Schafle MD: The child dancer: Medical considerations. Pediatr Clin North Am 37:1211–1221, 1990.
3. Solomon R, Minton SC, Solomon J (eds): Preventing Dance Injuries: An Interdisciplinary Perspective. American Alliance for Health Physical Education, Recreation and Dance.
4. Warren MP, Brooks-Gunn J, Hamilton LH, et al: Scoliosis and fractures in young ballet dancers: Relation to delayed menarche and secondary amenorrhea. N Engl J Med 314:1348–1353, 1986.
5. Whiteside PL: The teacher's role in treating dance injuries. Dance Teacher Now April:32–34, 1986.

99. BOXING

Robert O. Voy, M.D., FACSM

1. What is boxing?

Boxing is a contact sport in which two athletes within the same weight category compete against each other and score points by landing blows (punches) with force on their opponent's target areas. It is one of the oldest Olympic sports, derived from ancient military tradition as an arduous form of individual combat. There are two recognized forms of boxing—professional boxing and amateur (Olympic-style) boxing. Different scoring methods and rules govern these two types of boxing, making them, in effect, two distinctly different, although closely related, sports.

2. Explain the differences between amateur and professional boxing.

The differences are numerous. Here are some of the most noteworthy: The basic philosophies of the two forms of boxing differ. The main objective in amateur boxing is to score points. Finesse, physical conditioning, and strategy are more significant factors in determining the outcome of a bout. Equal emphasis is placed on avoiding blows and scoring blows. The force of a particular blow and its effect on one's opponent are not scoring considerations in amateur boxing. Thus, the "knockout" is a by-product rather than a primary objective in this form of the sport.

The knockout, a concussive blow that renders an individual defenseless, is the primary goal in professional boxing. As is the case with amateur boxing, the athlete who scores a knockout with a legal punch or combination of punches is declared the winner of the bout. In professional boxing only, however, added "weight" is given to a scoring blow based on its impact and effect on one's opponent. A knockdown counts for 1 point out of a total of 10 points awarded for a given round. In other words, by knocking his opponent down, a boxer can win a round 10 to 8 rather than 10 to 9, which is how most rounds are scored. In amateur boxing, on the other hand, a knockdown punch is worth no more than a clean jab, because one punch is scored as 1 point. Also in amateur boxing, a standing eight-count—a period during which a referee can evaluate a boxer's ability to continue the bout—is given to an athlete who has received a stunning blow. This count is not often used in professional bouts.

Other visible differences include the use of headgear and short tops in amateur boxing to reduce the risks of cuts and abrasions (neither is worn in professional bouts); amateur bouts are shorter (three 3-minute rounds or five 2-minute rounds) than professional bouts (a minimum of 4 3-minute rounds, and usually 10 or 12 rounds). Professional boxers use lighter gloves, thus increasing the force of blows landed. Amateurs must use thumb-attached gloves to prevent eye injury.

3. What are medical concerns in boxing?
- Acute injury, such as lacerations, fractures, and head injuries
- Chronic injury, such as neurologic dysfunction—so-called punch drunk syndrome

4. What are the acute boxing injuries?

Subdural hematomas occur when the bridging veins between the brain matter and the dura lining are ruptured. The mechanism that causes this effect is acceleration/deceleration that results from the sudden impact of a punch and secondary sudden cessation due to the impact of the brain against the skull. In the former case, stretching and tearing of veins occur. In the latter, both tearing and brain contusion may result. The bleeding and swelling that ensue create an enlarging mass lesion that may lead to symptoms of hemiparesis, seizures, pupillary changes, photophobia, nausea and vomiting, increased blood pressure, decreased pulse, and ultimately uncal herniation and death.

Epidural hematomas are also possible, but very uncommon, and rarely seen, except in cases in which skull fractures are involved. This unexpected injury is theoretically possible when a boxer is knocked out and lands outside the ring or strikes his head while falling on the mat—the typical contrecoup injury.

5. Excluding closed head injuries, what other injuries do boxers sustain?

Upper-extremity injuries are the most common injuries among boxers next to closed head injuries, accounting for roughly 32% of boxing injuries. The constant throwing of punches during extensive training and competition leads to injuries such as rotator cuff strains and tears, subdeltoid or acromial bursitis, and tendinitis of the biceps tendon. Power punches that cause explosive acceleration of the glenohumeral joint and rotator cuff may cause an acute dislocation of the shoulder. It most often happens when the punch is missed and deceleration of the structures does not occur.

The elbow joint bears the same trauma from frequent punching and hyperextension strains causing chronic ulnar collateral tearing and laxity.

Wrist injuries are more chronic than acute. The majority are sprains that, over time, lead to arthritic hypertrophy, or so-called bossing of the carpal bones dorsally.

Metacarpal fractures are easy to diagnose. Most of the force of the punch should be absorbed normally by the second and third metacarpophalangeal joint. Misdirected punches are causes for fractures of the fifth metacarpal, also known as the "boxer's" or "Saturday night" fracture.

A common and career-threatening injury is **chronic traumatic synovitis**, the inflammation and swelling of which can lead to subluxation and even tearing of the extensor hood mechanism at the metacarpophalangeal joint. This injury poses a threat to the boxer's career. An extensive rest period is required to heal this injury and surgery is often indicated.

Tears of the ulnar collateral ligament of the thumb were at one time quite common, but have been greatly reduced in boxing when thumb-attached gloves are worn.

6. Do boxers sustain injuries to the lower extremity?

Lower-extremity injuries are rare. Occasionally, knee or ankle sprains occur. Fractures of the lateral malleolus may be seen where a boxer falls unconscious and inverts his ankle. Neck and back injuries also are rare. Punches to the back of the head or neck ("rabbit punching") and punches to the lower back ("kidney punching") are illegal.

7. Name some other types of injuries seen in boxers.

Rib fractures and chest wall contusions are quite common. Ringside physicians must be particularly aware of symptoms of these injuries—boxers often try to hide these injuries in precompetition and qualifying examinations.

Cuts and eye and nose injuries are among the most evident injuries in the ring. The nose is, of course, a favorite target among boxers, and epistaxis is common. Compound fractures of the nasal bone occur, in which case the bout must be stopped to prevent penetrating injury to the cribriform plate. Septal deviations are considered an occupational hazard among boxers.

Eye injuries such as retinal detachments are of major significance and must be a serious concern for physicians conducting qualifying examinations. Hyphemas are rare, but glaucoma and traumatic cataracts do result. Corneal abrasions still occur, even in bouts where thumb-attached gloves are used.

Mandibular fractures are usually caused by an improperly fitted mouthpiece or crooked wisdom teeth that act as a wedge at the angle of the jaw.

8. What are the rules for visual acuity for boxers?

Rules for visual acuity are quite specific. An athlete totally unsighted (uncorrected vision less than 20/400) in one or both eyes is prohibited from boxing. In addition, a boxer with corrected visual acuity of less than 20/60 in either eye, regardless of the cause, is not allowed to participate in amateur boxing. Most professional boxing commissions have their own specific rules regarding vision qualifications.

9. Describe the usual location of cuts in boxing.

Cuts are less common in amateur boxing than in professional boxing, because of the use of head guards, but cuts are still seen in both forms of the sport. The general rule regarding cuts in boxing is that a cut that impairs vision is cause to stop a bout. The following outlines the usual locations of cuts:

Cut A: Rarely causes visual problems.

Cut B: May cause visual problems. If it extends medially, it may injure the supraorbital nerve.

Cut C: Caution if the cut extends medially and threatens the infraorbital nerve or the nasal lacrimal duct.

Cut D: Cuts on the upper eyelid might cause permanent damage to the tarsal plate.

Cut E: Vertical cuts through the vermilion border of lip may extend on subsequent blows. Intraoral cuts are only problematic if they produce excessive intraoral bleeding.

Cut F: Cuts on the bridge of the nose must be carefully checked for evidence of compound nasal fracture.

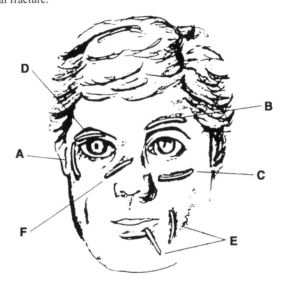

10. What must a ringside physician know about concussions?

In boxing, as in **all** contact sports, the attending physician must be aware of the basic physiologic signs of concussion. The word *concussion*, derived from the Latin "concussus," meaning "to shake violently," is a temporary disturbance of brain function that occurs without structural change to the brain.

If a concussion is suspected, baseline information, such as blood pressure, pulse rate, and quick neurologic checks of the cranial nerves and motor function tests are imperative. An extremely important measure of concussive injury is memory. Most experts use the presence or absence of post-traumatic or retrograde amnesia as early warning signs of moderate to severe concussion. In boxing, common questions asked include: "What did he hit you with?", "What do you last remember before being hit?", and "What do you first remember after coming to?" These questions are helpful in ascertaining amnesia and can indicate more exactly how long the period of unconsciousness lasted—a key factor in determining the seriousness of injury.

11. When should boxers be allowed to compete again after receiving a concussion?

The boxing rules are standard and specific in this regard; professional boxing regulations vary depending on various state commission rules. In amateur boxing, any knockout warrants a 30-day suspension. When loss of consciousness occurs, the suspension is increased to either 90 or 180 days based on the opinion of the attending physician (a notable difference from sports such as American football, where athletes are commonly evaluated on the sideline, and often sent back into the game within minutes).

12. Discuss chronic brain injury.

Traditionally, the medical profession has opposed boxing on the basis that the sport causes chronic brain dysfunction—dementia pugilistica—so-called punch-drunk syndrome. This condition is manifested by irritability, depression, slurred and monotonous speech, slow and unsteady gait, tremulousness, headaches, and seizures. The physiologic cause of dementia pugilistica is not clear, although most experts believe it is caused by microhemorrhages of the brainstem and neuronal damage.

Muhammad Ali, being one of the most popular athletes the world has ever known, and now one of the most visibly impaired ex-boxers, may sadly be the most noteworthy example of this condition. For the record, however, the exact cause of Ali's condition cannot be proved as secondary to his boxing career at this time.

Several small-scale studies have indicated that there is a connection between professional boxing and the punch drunk syndrome. There is question, however, as to whether or not amateur boxing can be associated with chronic central nervous system damage. To investigate this question, USA Boxing, the governing body for amateur boxing in the United States, in conjunction with the U.S. Olympic Committee, commissioned the Johns Hopkins University Department of Epidemiology to initiate a large-scale prospective study of this issue. The study was launched in 1986, and includes 484 boxers from six U.S. cities, which makes it the largest study of its kind ever.

The study employs 2-year intervals between examinations that determine if neuropsychologic and electrophysiologic changes are associated with competitive boxing or sparring experience. The first wave of results found: There was supporting evidence that an increased number of bouts before baseline examinations revealed a clinically insignificant change in one neurophysiologic parameter—visuoconstructional abilities. There were no changes demonstrated in attention/concentration or visual/verbal memory and some forms of motor function. No changes in any of these parameters were found during the first phase (initial 2-year follow-up), which may suggest that the safety regulations implemented in amateur boxing shortly before baseline examinations took place (including mandated use of headgear, glove size regulations, and uniform suspension periods) may have had a positive effect on improving ring safety. Continued follow-up in the second and third phases will inform us as to whether or not a minimal latency period or more exposure in the future will show any changes or progression of changes. (Interestingly, as the study has evolved, and certain subjects have turned professional, it has also become the largest prospective study of professional boxers ever.)

The bottom line is that this is a tremendously important study all physicians should monitor—certainly before formulating any opinion relating to the chronic effects (if any) of amateur boxing.

13. What is second impact syndrome?

Other than postconcussion seizures and chronic brain syndrome, second impact syndrome is the most significant—yet often unappreciated—postconcussion syndrome. Understanding of this potential sequela to head injury can lead to lifesaving action by the sports physician.

Second impact syndrome was first described by Schneider in 1973.[7] In a series of football-related head trauma, Schneider noted three cases in which moderate impact caused almost immediate lethal brain swelling. Two of these patients had earlier concussion syndromes and died after relatively minor second impacts. Saunders[6] reported in JAMA in 1984 the case of a football player who was suffering from headache after a fist fight 5 days before and stumbled off the field, collapsed, and died after receiving a minor body block. Autopsy revealed massive brain swelling.

This syndrome is clearly an important concern in boxing. Sparring and competition both involve head blows which demand medical screening for any concussive symptoms following head trauma.

Physiologic explanation is as follows: A first impact causes a cerebral vasomotor paralysis theoretically from cerebral contusion and microhemorrhages. The individual then sustains a second head injury, although remarkably minor, before symptoms of the first injury have cleared. The seemingly minor second impact on an already compliance-compromised brain vasomotor system results in vasomotor paralysis, edema leading to massive swelling, and catastrophically increased intracranial pressure. This can occur within as short a period as 2–5 minutes.

Thus, the following are extremely important responsibilities for ringside physicians:
1. Always perform as thorough a precompetition physical as possible.
2. Always perform a postcompetition examination.
3. Apply definitive suspension periods after loss of consciousness.
4. Be prepared to recognize signs of postconcussion syndromes.

14. Is HIV a concern in the sport of boxing?

The HIV virus is a concern in the sport of boxing, as it should be of concern in all contact sports where the common presence of open cuts and bleeding can theoretically lead to transmission of HIV. The risk of transmission, however, does not appear to be any more significant among boxers than, for example, football, basketball, or hockey players. Statistically speaking, the risk of transmission is considered minimal (far greater for athletes outside the ring than inside); however, safety precautions are being implemented in boxing. In fact, professional boxing, as a whole, implements some of the most thorough HIV testing regulations. Attending physicians are advised to use the same precautions against HIV as would be used in similar sports surroundings.

15. With AMA opposition to boxing clearly stated, is it responsible for a physician to be involved with this sport?

As a group, the AMA has lobbied for the sport to be banned. Many believe this was an emotional decision based more on moral/ethical dislike of a sport in which two athletes punch each other than a well-established scientific cause for disassociation.

Statistics indicate that in terms of fatalities and serious injuries per 10,000 participants, boxing is less dangerous to athletes than football or other popular athletic activities. College and high school football both experience three deaths per 10,000 participants compared with 1.3 boxing deaths per 10,000 athletes. The total injury rate (which includes concussive injuries) among boxers ranges between 1% and 4% of participants compared with as much as 46% among football players. Ice hockey, rugby, wrestling, and the martial arts also produce injury statistics that eclipse the incidence of injury in amateur boxing.

There are those who contend that boxing is wrong, because the sole intent is to injure the opponent. In amateur boxing, this is simply untrue—the object is to score points. This position was recently reinforced by Juan Antonio Samaranch, president of the International Olympic Committee (IOC), who endorsed boxing's position as a valuable element on the Olympic program. Prince Alexandre DeMerode, chairman of the IOC medical commission, clarified this common misconception by stating that boxing is as separate from fighting with intent to injure as fencing is from sword fighting with intent to run your opponent through.

Boxing is a time-honored tradition to many, and it will not disappear. It *can* be made as safe and fair as possible only with the dedicated involvement of physicians.

BIBLIOGRAPHY

1. Cantu R, Voy RO: Second impact syndrome. Phys Sports Med 23(6):27–34, 1995.
2. Jordan BD, Voy RO, Stone J: Amateur boxing injuries at the US Olympic Training Center. Phys Sportsmed 18(2):81–90, 1990.
3. Jordan B, Tsairis P, Warren R: Sports Neurology. Gaithersburg, MD, Aspen Publishers, 1989, pp 75–80.
4. McCown IA: Boxing safety and injuries. Phys Sportsmed 7(3):75–82, 1979.
5. USA Amateur Boxing Federation 1991–1993 Official Rules, 1750 E. Boulder Street, Colorado Springs, CO, 80909.
6. Voy MD, Robert O: Ringside Physician Certification Manual. Medical Responsibilities of the Ringside Physician. Colorado Springs, CO, USA Amateur Boxing Federation, 1990, pp 3–9.

7. Saunders RL, Harbaugh RE: The second impact in catastrophic contact-sport head trauma. JAMA 252:538–539, 1984.
8. Schneider RC: Head and Neck Injuries in Football: Mechanism, Treatment and Prevention. Baltimore, Williams & Wilkins, 1973.

100. MARTIAL ARTS

Leonard A. Wilkerson, D.O., M.B.A., FAAFP, FAOASM

1. What are martial arts?

The term *martial arts* describes those arts concerned with the waging of war, but in the 20th century, they no longer have a military role. It is said that the study of martial arts will develop character or higher moral standards. As a result of this change, the martial arts came to mean the "way."

2. What are some of the martial arts?

Karate (meaning the way of the empty hand), **TaeKwon-Do** (foot, hand, way), **aikido** (the way of harmony), **jiu-jit-su** (compliant techniques), **judo** (compliant way), and **Kung-fu** (Chinese martial art). **Hapkido** is a Korean martial art very similar to **aikido** (Japanese) that includes kicks and hand strikes.

3. Which are the most popular martial arts in America?

Karate and TaeKwon-Do have the most participants. The estimated number of athletes actively participating in these sports is about 1.5 million to 2 million, 20% being children. The estimated male to female ratio is 5:1.

4. Which martial arts are included in the Olympics?

Judo since 1966. TaeKwon-Do has been an exhibition sport since 1988 and is scheduled to become an official sport in the year 2000.

5. Why do people choose to study the martial arts?

In our society, there is an increased desire to know self-defense. Some join for structured exercise, improved cardiovascular fitness, flexibility, and self-esteem, whereas others want the artistic expression or have a need to compete.

6. Where are injuries associated with martial arts occurring?

Studies have shown approximately 60% of injuries are sustained in tournaments as opposed to 40% in nontournament settings. The injury rate and experience are inversely related, with punches having a higher injury ratio than kicks in karate and kicks higher than punches in TaeKwon-Do.

7. What is the tournament format for TaeKwon-Do and karate?

In TaeKwon-Do the format is 2-minute rounds. The fighter may fight a new opponent in a single or double elimination or a 3-minute single elimination. Karate has either a single or double elimination similar to TaeKwon-Do or may include three 3-minute rounds.

8. How can martial arts injuries be decreased?

Wearing protective gear will decrease morbidity. Protective gear is available for the forearms, hands, chest, shins, and feet. Also, a mouthpiece to protect teeth and groin guard to protect the testes are available.

Injury Rate per 100,000 Participants of Various Sports

Basketball	188.0	Wrestling	26.0
Football	167.0	Sledding	24.6
Aquatic activities	46.0	Dancing	18.8
Lacrosse	39.5	Martial arts	16.9

From Birrer RB, Halbrook SP: Martial arts injuries. Am J Sports Med 16:408–410, 1988, with permission.

9. What kind of injuries are seen in martial arts?
1. Injuries to the hand and face
2. Injuries to the trunk
3. Injuries to the limbs

In all studies, the most common injuries were contusions, bruises, sprains, and strains. The orthopedic injuries result from direct impact, repetitive action, or ballistic and torsional maneuvers. Serious injuries seen are concussion, paralysis, and visceral rupture.

List of Injuries at Two National TaeKwon-Do Tournaments

SITE OF INJURY	ADULT	JUNIOR
Head and Neck		
Hematoma, contusion	9	17
Laceration	6	7
Mandible, TMJ strain, R/O fracture	3	10
Epistaxis, R/O fracture	4	6
Concussion without LOC	0	8
Neck strain, R/O fracture	1	6
Nasal fracture/dislocation	3	1
Loss of consciousness	3	1
Teeth avulsion	0	2
Corneal abrasion	0	1
Diplopia, R/O orbital fracture	0	1
Totals	29	60
Upper Extremity		
Digit, hand strain, R/O fracture	5	8
Metacarpal fracture	2	3
Digit fracture/dislocation	2	0
Nail avulsion	0	2
Forearm contusion	0	1
Totals	9	14
Lower Extremity		
Foot contusion	1	2
Digit sprain, R/O fracture	1	2
Contusion, hematoma	6	2
Knee contusion/synovitis	0	2
Knee strain	1	0
Shin hematoma	0	1
Ankle strain	1	0
Foreign body	1	0
Digit fracture	0	1
Laceration	0	1
Totals	11	11

(Table continued on following page.)

Groin

Contusion, hematoma	2	5
Adductor strain	0	2
Totals	2	7

Torso

Abdominal contusion	0	1
Solar plexus concussion	0	2
Costochondral separation	1	0
Low back spasm	0	1
Lumbosacral contusion, R/O fracture	0	1
Spinal cord contusion, R/O fracture	0	1
Totals	1	6

Other

Panic reaction	0	3
Insulin reaction	0	1
Totals	0	4
Totals, all injuries	52	102
Grand total		154

From Oler M, Tomson W, Pepe H, et al: Morbidity and mortality in the martial arts: A warning. J Trauma 31(2):251–253, 1991, with permission.

Summary of Injuries by Anatomic Site (Reported as Percentages)

	PERCENTAGE OF ADULT PRESENTATIONS (n = 47)	PERCENTAGE OF JUNIOR PRESENTATIONS (n = 91)	COMBINED PRESENTATIONS (n = 138)
Head and neck	49	54	52
Upper extremity	21	14	17
Lower extremity	23	13	17
Groin	4	8	6
Torso	2	7	5
Other (systemic)	—	4	3
Totals	99	100	100
	(rounding error)		

From Oler M, Tomson W, Pepe H, et al: Morbidity and mortality in the martial arts: A warning. J Trauma 31(2):251–253, 1991, with permission.

10. What are common injuries to the head and neck in martial arts?

Lacerations, epistaxis, or periorbital hematoma can occur from an accidental strike in the face, usually with a fist or from a high kick. There have been cases of corneal abrasion as a result of a scratch from a toenail. Concussion is seen more commonly from a high kick or spinning kick. If an athlete is knocked out, it is important to consider a possible cervical spine injury.

11. Does the headgear protect against most martial arts injuries?

Headgear prevents most soft tissue injuries to the face—that is, lacerations, abrasions, and soft tissue injury to the ear or scalp. Unfortunately, headgear is not as protective to the brain as many believe in the martial arts. There now seems to be a movement in the United States toward mandatory headgear. Rhulen Insurance of New York, one of the largest insurers of martial arts in the United States, has informed its policy holders that headgear is now required if insurance is to be in force during free sparring. Because of this, mandatory headgear has reached the tournament circles and many schools and associations. From this movement, instructors and students are led to believe that they are "protected" and they can prevent serious head injuries, but this is not the case.

Studies from the neurosurgical literature have compared peak accelerations of blows to the head, with and without headgear, using punches both to the front and side of the head. These punches were with bare hand, "safety-chop hand protectors," and 10-ounce boxing gloves. Kicks also were delivered to the head, with and without headgear, using bare feet and "safety-kick" padding. These studies showed for bare or karate-style equipment-protected hand and foot blows that punches to the side of the head produced greater peak accelerations than kicks to the front and side. Kicks produced greater acceleration than did punches to the front of the head. Safety equipment failed to soften or lessen peak accelerations with or without headgear. It was perceived by the subjects in the study that safety equipment for hands or feet was protection for the wearer rather than for the opponent.

12. How does this affect the brain?

Unequivocal evidence exists that repeated brain injury of concussive or even subconcussive force results in characteristic patterns of brain damage and a steady decline in the ability to process information efficiently. Furthermore, the effects of repeated blows to the head, punch or kick, are cumulative; although some blows may be more severe than others, none is trivial and each has the potential to be lethal. Blunt head blows cause shearing injury to nerve fibers and neurons in proportion to the degree the head is accelerated, and these acceleration forces are imparted to the brain. Blows to the side of the head tend to produce greater acceleration forces than those to the face, whereas those to the chin, which acts as a lever, produce maximal forces. Shearing of blood vessels may lead to bleeding between the brain and skull (subdural hematoma) or bleeding within the brain (intracerebral hematoma) with rapid death. Headgear and protective padding to hands and feet may lessen the force of brain acceleration, which seems to decrease the chance of a fatal bleed, but increases nerve fiber shearing. Thus, extra padding may reduce the chance of death, but it will not prevent damage due to tearing of brain substance.[18]

13. What are the long-term effects of these shearing forces?

Punch drunk syndrome, or dementia pugilistica, is the medical term. Fight fans recognize the syndrome as "cuckoo," "goofy," "slug-nutty," or "cutting paper dolls." This is a traumatic encephalopathy that may occur in anyone subjected to repeated blows to the head from any cause. It has also been recognized in football players, rugby players, and wrestlers.[1]

The characteristic symptoms and signs include the slow onset of an increasingly euphoric personality; the person cries easily and has little insight into his deterioration. Speech and thought becomes progressively slower. Memory deteriorates considerably. There may be mood swings, intense irritability, and sometimes truculence leading to violent behavior. Cheerfulness is, however, the commonest prevailing mood with bouts of depression. Also, tremor and difficulty in speaking are common.

14. What kind of injuries occur in the extremities?

The injuries are numerous, with strains, sprains, fractures, dislocations, and tendon avulsions. The most common injury is hematoma to the forearm, thigh, shin, calf, and dorsum of the foot.

15. Do karate and TaeKwon-Do experts have increased incidence of osteoarthritis in their hands?

This problem was studied in Britain, where karate is an established sport. The hands and wrists of 22 karate instructors who had practiced the sport for a minimum of 5 years were examined and radiographed. There was no evidence that practice of the sport predisposed to the early onset of chronic tenosynovitis or osteoarthritis. Four activities seem to have the greatest potential for damage: doing push-ups on the knuckles, repeated punching of a firm target, sparring, and breaking objects.[5]

16. What other kinds of extremity injuries occur?

In the hands, avulsion of extensor tendons of distal fingers or dislocation of the proximal interphalangeal (PIP) joints. The metacarpophalangeal joints may have chronic synovitis from wood-breaking techniques.

Elbow dislocations have been seen, mostly posterior. Supracondylar and intercondylar fractures are rare but can occur. Tendinitis of medial/lateral epicondyles is common.

In the shoulder, 95% of dislocations are anterior, with 5% posterior. Acromioclavicular sprain is seen if a fall or roll is inaccurately executed.

17. How is the knee injured?

The knee is vulnerable in most sports. In the martial arts, especially karate and TaeKwon-Do, when ballistic and twisting moves are the rule, injury is usually from hyperextension, rotation, flexion, valgus, or varus clipping. Injuries vary from meniscus, ligament, patella tendinitis, patella subluxation or dislocation, and epiphyseal fracture to Osgood-Schlatter disease. Knee dislocation is very rare and a true emergency.

18. How about hematoma to the quadriceps from kicking?

Hematoma can occur in any of the extremities and is the most common injury, with the quadriceps the most common site. In all studies, contestants had to stop fighting secondary to the pain. A late complication is myositis ossificans.

19. What about the ankle and foot?

Ankle sprain and fracture are seen, just as in any contact or collision sport. Injury to the great toe, second toe, and fifth toe is common, and they may develop osteoarthritis in later years.

20. Why do martial arts teach mid-abdominal blows?

They are aiming at the region of the solar plexus surrounding the coeliac ganglia. This blow causes the classic winding of the opponent, leaving them vulnerable for further attack. A blow to the solar plexus produces transient inspiratory difficulty with spontaneous recovery in 20 to 40 seconds.

21. Is the chest vulnerable?

In TaeKwon-Do, chest protectors are worn to disperse the penetration of the blow. In karate, chest protectors are not worn. Karate instructors believe it decreases the student's ability to control the blow and thus decreases discipline. Damage to the chest is usually by direct kicks or punches. Costochondritis, rib fracture, or even pneumothorax have been seen. There have been three reported cases of death from anterior chest trauma.

22. What other vital organs are at risk?

The liver, spleen, kidney, and pancreas are at risk from a punch or more commonly from the roundhouse kick (round kick). Testicular injury may result from an uncontrolled kick. Groin guards decrease this risk.

23. What are the most common trunk injuries?

The ribs, mainly from punches; the solar plexus, which has the potential to cause pancreatitis; and the testicles.

24. Can the athlete with a seizure disorder participate in the martial arts?

Studies have shown that a regular exercise program may have a beneficial effect on seizure control. There are no reports of status epilepticus triggered by exercise. It is a difficult decision for physicians, parents, and the martial arts school to give permission to participate. Reservations are based on the following concerns:

1. Would a seizure during practice or a tournament predispose the athlete to a serious injury, particularly of the brain or spinal cord? Most data to date do not support this.

2. Would single or cumulative head blows adversely affect seizure control or cause an immediate or early post-traumatic seizure? To date reports suggest that this should not be a concern; however, because of inherent dangers, kicking or punching to the head should be excluded.

The Committee on Children with Handicaps and Sports Medicine of the American Medical Association recommends that children be allowed to participate in physical education and interscholastic athletics, including contact and collision sports, provided there is[14]: (1) proper medical management, good seizure control, and proper supervision; and (2) avoidance of situations in which a dangerous fall could occur.

With the studies and data given above, I allow athletes with a seizure disorder to participate, but when they are ready to participate in sparring, I do not allow any head contact. I limit the contact to the trunk (chest and abdomen) and insist that a chest protector be worn.

25. What disorders would disqualify an athlete from martial arts?

Participation in the martial arts, *including* competitive sparring is not allowed for persons with medical disorders such as carditis, severe uncontrolled hypertension, severe congenital heart disease, absence or loss of function of one eye, absence of one kidney, hepatomegaly, splenomegaly, poorly controlled seizure disorder, pulmonary insufficiency, and atlantoaxial instability. I also disqualify athletes with skin infections such as boils, herpes, impetigo, and scabies until the condition is no longer contagious. Acute illnesses need individual evaluation so as not to worsen the illness or put others at risk of being in contact with a contagious individual.[16]

If the participant wants to do martial arts for self-defense, fitness, or flexibility but *never* to participate in full contact sparring, then some of the above conditions will need individual assessment, allowing some persons to train only in a noncontact environment.

26. Does asthma prevent training?

Usually not. Asthma and exercise-induced asthma can usually be controlled with beta-agonist or cromolyn sodium. If continued breakthrough occurs, then a sustained-release theophylline can be added. A good warm-up before activity induces bronchodilation and refractoriness to exercise-induced asthma.

27. What are the physician's responsibilities at a karate or TaeKwon-Do competition?

The physician's duties are to examine competitors before the competition if requested by officials. The fighting areas should be inspected to ascertain if adequate flooring is used. The physician treats any minor injuries received, such as lacerations, strains, and sprains. In serious injuries, it is best to refer to a hospital. When requested, the physician advises the referees as to the fitness of a competitor to continue in a competition.

28. Name the injuries that would exclude further participation.

1. Fractures
2. Concussion that has resulted in disorientation and amnesia, and especially loss of consciousness
3. Ocular injuries when sight is impaired, including periorbital injuries, i.e., hematoma and lacerations
4. Certain cases of testicular injuries where recovery is not rapid and scrotal hematomas are present

29. Have there been any deaths in the martial arts?

Only three fatalities due to martial arts have been reported. All resulted from anterior chest trauma.[17]

All three of the fatally injured had been in training for less than 1 year. These deaths are inexcusable! I recommend free-sparring training only for students who have undergone a period of adequate physical conditioning and have demonstrated competence in the basic free-sparring techniques.

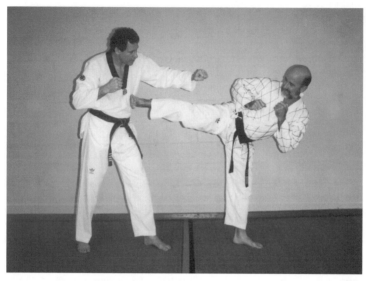

Case 1. A 26-year-old Caucasian male (Korean TaeKwon-Do stylist) was practicing kumite (free-sparring) with his instructor when he received a kick to the left lower lateral aspect of the anterior chest. The patient was seen in the emergency room with fixed dilated pupils and isoelectric EKG. By clinical history and autopsy, the suggested cause of death was aspiration and asphyxia secondary to the blow to the chest.

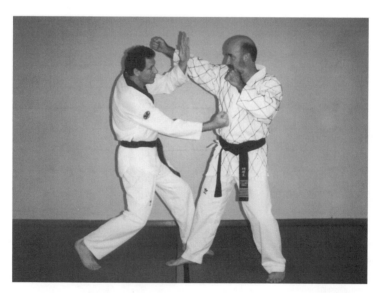

Case 2. An 18-year-old Caucasian male (kempo stylist) was participating in his fifth bout of a competitive free-sparring tournament when he received a blow, or multiple blows, to the midsection that ruptured his spleen. Later in the evening, he began to have pain and nausea and vomiting. He was transported to an emergency room, where he was admitted with diagnosis of a ruptured spleen. A laparotomy and splenectomy were performed. The patient, however, expired within 1 hour postoperatively. A microscopic diagnosis of infectious mononucleosis involved the heart, liver, and spleen.

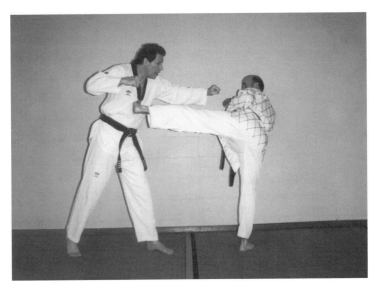

Case 3. An 18-year-old black male (Korean TaeKwon-Do stylist) was practicing kumite with an advanced student when he received light contact from a roundhouse kick to the solar plexus. The patient expired in the dojang (practice studio). Autopsy revealed hemorrhage into the soft tissue around the carotid sinus and vagus nerve at the level of the bifurcation of the innominate artery, multiple areas of ecchymoses in the liver, multiple petechial hemorrhages of all lobes of the lungs, hyperinflation of both lungs, and aspiration bronchitis.

BIBLIOGRAPHY

1. Adams WM, Bruton CJ: The cerebral vasculature in dementia pugilistica. J Neurol Neurosurg Psychiatry 52:600–604, 1989.
2. Birrer RB, Halbrook SP: Martial arts injuries: The results of a five-year national survey. Am J Sports Med 16:408–410, 1988.
3. Birrer RB, Birrer CD: Martial arts injuries. Phys Sportsmed 10(6):103–108, 1982.
4. Birrer RB, Birrer CD, Son DS, et al: Injuries in Tae Kwon-Do. Phys Sportsmed 9(2):97–103, 1981.
5. Crosby AC: The hands of karate experts. Clinical and radiological findings. Br J Sports Med 19:41–42, 1985.
6. Jaffe L, Minkoff J: Martial arts: A perspective on their evolution, injuries, and training formats. Orthop Rev 17:208–221, 1988.
7. Kurland HL: Injuries in karate. Phys Sportsmed 8(10): 1980.
8. Liebert PL, Buckley T: Providing medical coverage at karate tournaments. J Musculoskel Med 1992.
9. McLatchie GR: Recommendations for medical officers attending karate competitions. Br J Sports Med 13:36–37, 1979.
10. McLatchie GR: Prevention of karate injuries—A progress report. Br J Sports Med 11:78–82, 1977.
11. McLatchie GR: Karate and karate injuries. Br J Sports Med 15:84–86, 1981.
12. McLatchie GR, Davies JE, Caulley JH: Injuries in karate—A case for medical control. J Trauma 20: 1980.
13. McLatchie GR: Analysis of karate injuries sustained in 295 contests. Injury 8:132–134, 1976.
14. Mellion MB, Walsh WM, Shelton GL (eds): The Team Physician's Handbook, 2nd ed. Philadelphia, Hanley & Belfus, 1997.
15. Oler M, Tomson W, Pepe H, et al: Morbidity and mortality in the martial arts: A warning. J Trauma 31:251–253, 1991.
16. Preparticipation Physical Evaluation: Joint publication of American Academy of Family Physicians, American Academy of Pediatrics, American Medical Society of Sports Medicine, American Osteopathic Academy of Sports Medicine, American Orthopaedic Society for Sports Medicine, McGraw-Hill, 1996.
17. Schmidt RJ: Fatal anterior chest trauma in karate trainers. Med Sci Sports 7:59–61, 1975.
18. Schwartz ML, Hudson AR, Fernie GR, et al: Biomechanical study of full-contact karate contrasted with boxing. J Neurosurg 64:248–252, 1986.
19. Stricevic MV, Patel MR, Okazaki T, et al: Karate: Historical perspective and injuries sustained in national and international tournament competitions. Am J Sports Med 11:320–324, 1983.

101. MOUNTAINEERING AND CLIMBING

Robert B. Schoene, M.D.

1. What is different about the atmosphere at high altitude?
Although the fraction of oxygen in the atmosphere is constant from sea level to very high altitude, barometric pressure decreases the higher one goes, which results in less available oxygen.

2. What does the body do to adapt to the availability of less oxygen?
High-altitude acclimatization is a complex and not fully understood process that is a reflection of the body's resiliency under stressful conditions. The process optimizes the transfer of oxygen from the air through the lung to the blood and to the mitochondria in the tissues of the body. Each step of adaptation occurs at its own pace, and each individual has his or her inherent rate of acclimatization. These processes are briefly listed below:

Acclimatization to High Altitude

RESPONSE	MECHANISM	TIME
Ventilation	Stimulation by hypoxia	Immediate and ongoing
Gas exchange in in the lung	Better matching of ventilation and perfusion to optimize oxygen transport from the air to the blood	Immediate
Blood	Increase in red blood cells to increase oxygen-carrying capacity	Days to weeks
	Shift of the oxygen-hemoglobin dissociation curve	
Tissues	Increase in capillary density Increase in mitochondrial density	Probably weeks

3. Do some people adapt more quickly to high altitude than others?
Yes. Even though some may take longer than others, eventually almost everyone can adapt to the low-oxygen environment. Climbers must, therefore, be aware of this so as to be patient for their own and each other's rate of adaptation.

4. Does training facilitate the process of adaptation to high altitude?
Although it is always important to be physically fit when going to the mountains, physical training will not facilitate the adaptation process nor will it minimize one's chances of getting altitude illness (see below).

5. How should one prepare for high altitudes?
Of course, the best preparation is to climb; however, most working people do not have the luxury of time or mountains nearby. It is, therefore, important to undergo aerobic training that best simulates climbing such as hill running, stair climbing, or bicycling. For individuals who include rock climbing in their mountain activities, certain forms of stretching and weight training or climbing on indoor practice walls are important activities.

6. I have heard that some people become sick at high altitude. Are these maladies specific to high altitude?
Yes. All the altitude illnesses are a spectrum of syndromes from acute mountain sickness (AMS), which is an aggravating, self-limited disease, to the more severe, potentially fatal forms

462

of high-altitude pulmonary edema (HAPE) and high-altitude cerebral edema (HACE). Chronic mountain sickness (CMS) can occur in some individuals living at high altitudes for years. All occur if the person ascends too quickly.

High-altitude Illnesses

	AMS	HAPE	HACE	CMS
Location	Above 8,000 ft	Usually above 10,000 ft	Above 12,000 ft	Above 10,000 ft
Time	1–2 days after ascent	3–4 days after ascent or possibly later	4–7 days after ascent or possibly later	Months, years, generations
Symptoms	Headache, lethargy, sleep disturbances, anorexia, nausea, vomiting	Dyspnea at rest, weakness, cough, can progress to production of pink, frothy sputum	Severe headache, confusion, hallucinations	Lethargy, decreased exercise capacity
Signs	Mild tachycardia, possible mild peripheral edema	Tachycardia, tachypnea, low-grade fever, cyanosis	Ataxia, focal neurologic or visual signs, retinal hemorrhage	Plethora, peripheral edema, conjunctival injection
Laboratory findings	Possible mild arterial O_2 desaturation	Moderate-to-severe arterial O_2 desaturation, relative hypoventilation	Moderate arterial O_2 desaturation	Polycythemia, severe arterial O_2 desaturation, relative hypercapnia
Treatment	Rest at same altitude, hydration, mild analgesics; usually ascent can continue in 1–2 days; prophylaxis and treatment with acetazolamide (125 mg bid)	Immediate descent,* O_2 if available; nifedipine effective to prevent HAPE (30 mg XL qd) and HAPE and dexamethasone (4 mg q6h) (both unproven but possibly effective); hyperbaric therapy if descent impossible	Descent,* dexamethasone (8 mg bolus, 4 mg q6h) hyperbaric therapy if descent impossible	Descent, O_2, respiratory stimulants (acetazolamide, progesterone, phlebotomy)

* Descent must not be delayed to implement other modalities.

7. What is the incidence of AMS?

It varies, but two-thirds of the people who ascend Mount Rainer (over 14,000 feet) in 2 days get AMS, whereas 25% of visitors from low altitude to certain ski areas above 9,000 ft in Colorado will get AMS.

8. What are the symptoms of AMS?

The symptoms vary in severity. They almost always include headache with at least one of the following symptoms as well: loss of appetite, trouble sleeping, excessive fatigue, nausea and vomiting, and mild shortness of breath.

9. How long do the symptoms of AMS last? Can they be prevented? Can they be treated?

The best prevention for AMS is slow gradual ascent to allow time for the body to adapt. If one suffers from AMS and stays at the same altitude and rests, the symptoms usually last 24–48 hours and then abate. If they worsen, then one must descend. Additionally, if one cannot avoid a fast ascent or is predisposed to AMS, acetazolamide (Diamox) (125 mg, twice a day for several days) is quite effective in preventing AMS. This drug is also effective for treatment of symptoms once they occur. Individuals allergic to sulfa drugs should not take acetazolamide. Dexamethasone (4 mg, four times a day) also will prevent and treat AMS, although it should be reserved for more severe cases or those individuals allergic to sulfa.

10. How can I avoid the more severe forms of altitude illness?

Again, slow gradual ascent is the key to avoiding HAPE and HACE. They usually occur at higher altitudes than AMS (10,000 to 14,000 feet) and take several days to develop. They can, of course, occur at much higher altitudes even after a prolonged stay. These two diseases can be fatal and often occur together. Unless orthopedic injury or severe weather prevents descent, no one should die of HAPE or HACE.

11. Does HAPE occur only in people with underlying disease?

No. Not at all. In fact, younger people may be more susceptible to HAPE. Its symptoms may be preceded by those of AMS or may occur de novo. They include excessive shortness of breath, dry cough, cyanosis, tachycardia, crackles on chest examination, marked decrease in exercise capabilities, and eventually a cough productive of pink frothy sputum. It is important to recognize the early signs when the victim is still ambulatory. Quick descent is mandatory. Even 1,000 to 3,000 feet descent is enough to provide relief. Oxygen, if available, also is quite effective, although descent should not be delayed to wait for oxygen.

12. Are some people susceptible to HAPE?

Yes. Some people seem to get it every time they go to high altitude, which should cause them to question their need to go there. If, however, they insist, slow ascent and the use of nifedipine, which lowers pulmonary artery pressures, are helpful in preventing the development of HAPE in susceptible individuals.

13. What are some of the pathophysiologic findings associated with HAPE?

Individuals tend to have a blunted breathing response on ascent to altitude, which makes them relatively more hypoxemic than others. They also have a more accentuated degree of pulmonary hypertension, which may stress the pulmonary vascular endothelium. This may result in stretching of the endothelial barrier and allow leak of high protein fluid into the interstitium and alveoli. Bronchoalveolar lavage performed on Mount McKinley climbers with HAPE found high-protein fluid in the alveolar space. Additionally, an inflammatory response may contribute to the ongoing permeability leak. Complete understanding of the underlying mechanism is still forthcoming.

14. Is HACE as common as HAPE?

No. As mentioned, some degree of HACE may be present in individuals with HAPE, but HACE usually occurs at higher altitudes. It always includes severe headache unrelieved with analgesics and neurologic signs that may include ataxia, confusion, diplopia, hallucinations, nausea, vomiting, stupor, coma, and death.

15. HACE sounds serious. What can one do so one's companions don't die?

Again, picking up the early signs while the person is still ambulatory is the key to getting him or her down and preventing disaster. Victims who become unable to care for themselves are a greater risk to their team members and themselves. If one is ataxic at high altitude, then it is mandatory to descend as soon as possible. Additionally, dexamethasone (initially 8 mg and 4 mg four times a day thereafter) and oxygen, if available, help.

16. Are there any other conditions associated with high altitude to be aware of?

Yes. One must have some knowledge of weather and its thermal effects. Knowledge of the signs of hypothermia and the prevention thereof are important. Although it is beyond the scope of this article, it is medically important to know proper techniques of layering clothing so as not to become too hot, too cold, or most importantly, too wet. Shivering and confusion are often signs of early hypothermia, at which point it is usually treatable by getting the victim dry and in the warmest environment possible (which may mean being in a sleeping bag with you). Frostbite also is a danger of high-altitude climbing. The hands and feet are particularly susceptible, and proper use of vapor barrier boots is essential, because ignorance of how to use them may lead to worse cold injury. Remember, they do not "breathe," so feet are usually damp in the evening. It is, therefore, essential to remove the inner sock, put on dry socks, and sleep with the wet items in your sleeping bag so that by morning they are dry. This rotation is very important.

17. Are there any other therapeutic modalities available for the treatment of altitude illness?
Portable hyperbaric bags are available that can be inflated to higher pressures and simulate lower altitudes. Victims of any of the altitude illnesses can be effectively treated in this manner. Larger expeditions or high-altitude treks should have one such bag, because its use can buy one some time until descent is feasible. In the United States, the Gamow Bag is available from Chinook Medical Products in Boulder, CO.

18. Are there any other tips for keeping healthy and enjoying a climb or trek?
Remember that you are a guest in the beautiful mountains of the world; therefore, feel lucky and treat the environment respectfully. Also remember that you are there to enjoy yourself, and no trip or mountain summit is worth risking the loss of fingers and toes from frostbite or death from severe altitude illness. The leaders of the trips should be experienced and responsible. However, each individual, as he or she gains experience, should become more and more self-reliant; and although rescue may be available, never depend on being rescued by other climbers, rangers, or rescue agencies. Weather in the mountain environment can often prevent rescue, and it is not appropriate to put other people at risk because of your foolish mistake or arrogant attitudes. You are entering a risky environment and should be willing to accept some degree of risk.

BIBLIOGRAPHY

1. Bartsch PP, Maggiorini M, Ritter C, et al: Prevention of high altitude pulmonary edema by nifedipine. N Engl J Med 325:1284–1289, 1991.
2. Hackett PH, Roach RC: High altitude pulmonary edema. J Wilderness Med 1:3–26, 1990.
3. Honigman B, Theis M, Koziol-McClain J, et al: Acute mountain sickness in a general tourist population at moderate altitude. Ann Intern Med 118:587–592, 1993.
4. Houston CS, Dickinson J: Cerebral form of high altitude illness. Lancet 2:758–761, 1975.
5. Johnson TS, Rock PB: Acute mountain sickness. N Engl J Med 319:841–845, 1988.
6. Reeves JT, Schoene RB: When lungs on mountains leak: Studying pulmonary edema at high altitudes. N Engl J Med 325:1306–1307, 1991.
7. Schoene RB, Swenson E, Pizzo C, et al: The lung at high altitude: Bronchoalveolar lavage in acute mountain sickness and pulmonary edema. J Appl Physiol 64:2605–2613, 1988.
8. Singh I, Kanna PK, Srivastava MC, et al: Acute mountain sickness. N Engl J Med 280:175–184, 1969.
9. Ward MP, Millage JS, West JB: High Altitude Medicine and Physiology, 2nd ed. Philadelphia, University of Pennsylvania Press, 1995.

102. BICYCLING

Morris B. Mellion, M.D.

1. Is it more challenging for physicians to treat bicyclists than participants in other sports?
The challenge is greater because the physician must understand how problems in the configuration and fit of the bicycle can cause injury and how proper changes and adjustments are important to treat injuries. In sports medicine, injuries are generally divided into two categories, overuse and trauma. Overuse injuries in cycling are generally related to improper fit of the bicycle

and improper training techniques. Adjustments of just a few millimeters, which may be considered trivial for people who ride only 3 or 4 miles a day, may be enough to cause or prevent injury to a serious cyclist or racer.

2. What is the basic anatomy of the modern bicycle?

The bicycle consists of a frame ("frame set") with various components such as handlebars, brakes, wheels, and pedals attached.

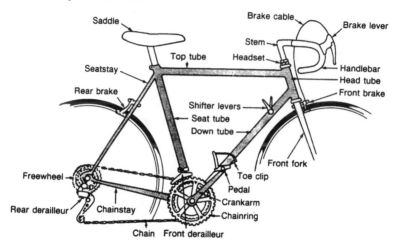

Anatomy and terminology of the modern bicycle. (From Hill JW, Mellion MB: Bicycling injuries: Prevention, diagnosis, and treatment. In Mellion MB (ed): Office Management of Sports Injuries and Athletic Problems. Philadelphia, Hanley & Belfus, 1988.)

3. What is the easiest way to understand the differences and similarities among the wide variety of bicycles currently popular?

Modern bicycles fall into two basic categories with many variations. The modern bicycle frame is shaped somewhat like a diamond lying on its side.

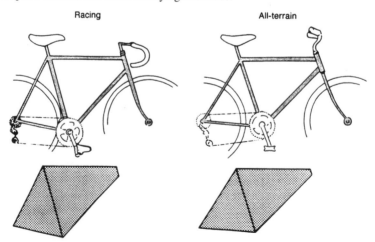

The bicycle frame is shaped like a diamond lying on its side. Racing bicycles have upright geometry with steep angles to the diamond. All-terrain bicycles have somewhat flatter geometry with more shallow angles. Touring bicycles are generally in between. (From Mellion MB: Bicycling. In Mellion MB, Walsh WM, Shelton GL (eds): The Team Physician's Handbook, 2nd ed. Philadelphia, Hanley & Belfus, 1997.)

Racing bicycles have upright geometry with steep angles to the diamond, which makes the frame stiffer and more responsive to hard pedaling and turning. They also have dropped handlebars that are generally set at a lower height than the saddle to obtain an aerodynamic riding position.

All-terrain bicycles (mountain bikes) have much flatter geometry to allow shock absorption. Mountain bikes also have sturdier frames and considerably wider tires to absorb the shock of riding on a rough surface. The racing bike is designed for high speeds, whereas the mountain bike is designed for steep hill climbing and gearing down for riding over obstacles.

The **triathlon bicycle** has aerobars for even more aerodynamic benefit. **Time trial bicycles** have a similar configuration. The **touring bicycle** has a slightly heavier frame than the racing bike but has the lower gearing that is commonly seen on all-terrain bicycles.

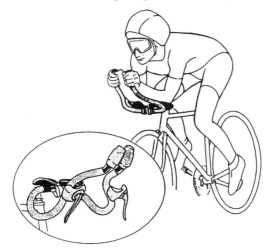

The aerobar is designed to permit the rider to maintain a highly aerodynamic position for a prolonged time. (From Mellion MB: Common cycling injuries: Management and prevention. Sports Med 11:52–70, 1991; with permission.)

Two spin-offs from the all-terrain bicycle are the **city**, or urban, **bicycle** and the **hybrid bicycle**. The city bike looks like a mountain bike but has the old-fashioned upright handlebars of the traditional one-speed bicycles. This configuration provides comfortable riding in an upright position and a good view in traffic. The hybrid has a frame that is a cross between that of the mountain bike and the racing bike. Its tubing is intermediate in strength and weight, and its tires are intermediate in size. This bicycle has increased in popularity with riders who started on all-terrain bikes but wanted a little bit more high performance without converting to dropped handlebars or aerobars.

4. What is the most efficient, accurate method to fit a bicycle for a racer or a serious rider?

A **Fit Kit** is a commercial set of measuring devices and data tables designed to determine appropriate bicycle setup from a rider's measurements. Bicycle shops that cater to racers often have a Fit Kit for the mechanics to use in setting up bicycles. A fee is usually charged for the service. The Fit Kit provides a good starting point for bicycle set up. Individual riders often make some fine tuning adjustments to suit their own physiques and riding styles. Riders using cleated shoes or step-in pedals may have their cleat adjustment checked and set using the rotational adjustment device (RAD), which is a part of the Fit Kit.

5. "Can I adjust my own bicycle properly?"

Yes. There are many systems for the individual to use. Bibliographic references at the end of this chapter preceded by an asterisk discuss bicycle fit in detail. There are six basic fit adjustments: frame size, seat height, fore and aft saddle position, saddle angle, handlebar reach, and handlebar height. Only the first three are illustrated here for the sake of brevity.

   Optimal frame size is determined with the rider straddling the frame. On a racing bike, there should be a 1–2-inch clearance between the crotch and top tube. On an all-terrain bike, this clearance should be 3–4 inches to allow the rider to get a foot down when stopping on uneven terrain.

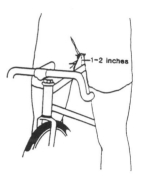

   Proper frame size. (From Hill JW, Mellion MB: Bicycling injuries: Prevention, diagnosis and treatment. In Mellion MB (ed): Office Management of Sports Injuries and Athletic Problems. Philadelphia, Hanley & Belfus, 1988, pp 257–269.)

   A reasonable estimate of proper seat height may be obtained by positioning the bicycle next to a wall or vehicle for support or by placing it in a wind trainer. The rider sits with his heels on the pedals, which are held in the 6 and 12 o'clock positions. The seat should be raised or lowered until the leg on the 6 o'clock pedal is barely straight. All seat height formulas are estimates. Consequently, after a trial of several rides, adjustments of one-fourth inch at a time may be made, usually upward.
   The bicycle saddle is built on a pair of rails that are connected to the seat post and allow approximately a 1½-inch (3.5 cm) fore and aft saddle position adjustment. With the rider in the saddle and the pedals at 3 and 9 o'clock positions, the seat should be adjusted so that a plumb line dropped from the tibial tubercle would intercept that axle of the forward pedal. This positional relationship is important to prevent or treat patellofemoral pain problems.

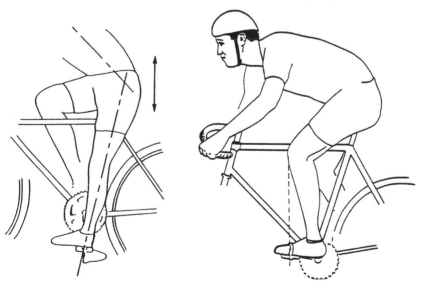

Left, Seat height estimation from leg length. (From Mellion MB: Bicycling. In Mellion MB, Walsh WM, Shelton GL (eds): The Team Physician's Handbook, 2nd ed. Philadelphia, Hanley & Belfus, 1997.)
Right, Fore and aft saddle position. (From Mellion MB: Bicycling. In Mellion MB, Walsh WM, Shelton GL (eds): The Team Physician's Handbook, 2nd ed. Philadelphia, Hanley & Belfus, 1997.)

6. Why are there so many gears on modern bicycles?

Bicyclists function most effectively and safely in a narrow range of pedal resistance to their effort. Riding with too much pedal resistance at too low a cadence (pedal revolutions per minute) magnifies patellofemoral pressure and is second only to improper bicycle fit as a cause of overuse problems in cyclists.

7. What are the sources of resistance to bicycle movement?

(1) The inertia of the bicycle and rider, (2) uphill grade (gravity), (3) wind, (4) the rolling resistance of the tires on the road surface, (5) the relative fatigue of the rider, and (6) the friction of air. The magnitude of air friction is a surprise to most people. If a cyclist is riding at 20 miles per hour on a calm day, 90% of the rider's energy expenditure will be used to overcome the friction of the bicycle and the rider against the still air.

8. Why are there so many gears on the bicycle?

The broad range of gears on the modern bicycle (from 10–24 "speeds" or gears) allows the cyclist to pedal comfortably with a relatively constant pedal resistance at a generally uniform cadence by shifting gears to meet the varying demands of hills, wind, and fatigue.

9. Is there an optimal pedaling cadence?

In terms of gross efficiency, heart rate, perceived exertion, and lactate concentration, the optimal pedal rate is 80 rpm with a range of 60–100 rpm as the optimal range for racing.

A relatively high cadence with low resistance reduces the incidence of overuse injuries. Racers and serious cyclers should begin their riding seasons with 500–1,000 miles of this kind of riding. Many overuse injuries similarly call for this approach. With some serious racers, a change to high cadence/low resistance pedaling may require changing some of the gears on the bicycle.

10. Is bicycle trauma a major problem?

There are over 500,000 bicycle injury visits each year to United States emergency rooms. Approximately half involve motor vehicles and are most often the result of the driver failing to see the bicyclist, especially in the low light conditions at dawn, dusk, and night riding. Road surface damage and obstacles are often involved.

11. What accounts for most of the serious bicycle injuries?

Head injuries account for the serious injuries and deaths. They are generally preventable by wearing a good bicycle helmet.

12. How do the modern bicycle helmets work?

Bicycle helmets are composed of crushable foam and are held together by an internal skeleton or by a firm layer of a harder condensed foam on the surface. A good bicycle helmet is a single-use device designed to absorb shock by crushing on impact. A helmet that has sustained a significant crash should be replaced.

13. Are bicycle helmets heavy and hot?

The newer bicycle helmets weight approximately ½ of a pound, are extremely aerodynamic, and have intricately designed air-flow systems that keep the head cool.

14. Are there special strategies to prevent trauma?

Use proper protective clothing and safety equipment. Maintain the bicycle in top mechanical condition, check tires and tubes frequently, anticipate the errors of others, and control speed, especially when brakes are wet.

15. What do we know about mountain bike injuries?

Although mountain bikes have recently become the most popular bicycles in the United States, there are few good published studies of mountain bike injuries. Research by Chow, who surveyed serious riders in mountain bike clubs, indicates an 84% annual injury rate. Most injuries were minor; 26% required professional care, and 4% necessitated hospitalization. Ninety percent were soft tissue injuries, and 12% were fractures or dislocations. Only 12% were head and/or neck injuries; this low incidence was attributed to 88% helmet use. Eighty-eight percent of the injuries occurred off paved road, and 74% occurred while descending a grade. Thirty-six percent of the injured riders identified excessive speed as a factor, and 35% attributed the injury to riding unfamiliar terrain; 20% admitted riding beyond their ability. Professional riders sustain a much higher rate of injuries. Pfeiffer has shown that elite male racers average over 4 injuries a year, and elite women average over 6.

16. Is there a general strategy for treating overuse injuries in cyclists?

It is important to treat the bicycle as well as the rider. Sometimes minor adjustments will be all that is necessary, but often a complete refitting is required.

17. What are the common overuse injuries and strategies for treatment?

Summary of Common Overuse Bicycle Problems with Mechanical and Technique Adjustments to Consider in Treatment

	MECHANICAL ADJUSTMENTS	TECHNIQUE ADJUSTMENTS
1. Neck and back pain	Adjust seat position (move forward) Change mirror placement Change to handlebar with less drop (randonneur) Shorten stem extension Raise stem height Switch to upright handlebars	Change hand positions frequently Ride with "unlocked" elbows
2. Ulnar neuropathy (handlebar palsy)	Wear padded gloves Add handlebar padding Adjust frame size Adjust seat and handlebar (decrease reach)	Decrease length and intensity of rides Change hand position on bar Ride with "unlocked" elbows
3. Skin problems	Use padded riding shorts Appropriate use of sunscreens Adjust seat type	
4. Pudendal neuropathy Traumatic urethritis Vulval trauma	Adjust saddle angle Change saddle width Consider padded cycling shorts Add saddle padding	
5. Hip problems	Adjust seat height Change frame size	
6. Biker's knee	Change frame size Adjust seat height and position Adjust foot and pedal position	Increase cadence Lower gear ratio Ride flatter terrain Slowly increase riding intensity and duration
7. Foot/ankle problems Paresthesia Metatarsalgia Achilles tendinitis	Adjust toe clips (decrease tightness) Change cleat position Adjust saddle height	Change foot position Change gear and cadence Adjust pedaling technique

18. Is there special safety equipment for bicycling?

Bicycle Safety Equipment

SAFETY EQUIPMENT	FUNCTION	IMPORTANT FEATURES
Helmet	High-density, expanded polystyrene (EPS) or polyurethane foam helmet crushes to absorb the shock of a severe impact.	Minimum standards are provided by American National Standards Institute (ANSI). Snell Memorial Foundation Standards are more stringent, especially the Snell Z90 Standard.
Mirrors	Allows cyclists to observe overtaking vehicles without turning head.	Various models mount on helmet, eyeglasses, sunglasses, and handlebars.
Protective eyewear	Protects rider from radiation of sun, flying objects (bugs, dust, stones, etc.) and irritants (wind, rain, cold air, allergens).	Wraparound or semi-wraparound preferred. Polycarbonate or other unbreakable material. Clear lenses for riding in rain.
Cycling gloves	Cushion hands from road shock. Protect hands in a fall. Protect from cold in winter.	Summer gloves are fingerless; winter gloves have full fingers with insulation. Palms may be padded with shock-absorbent elastopolymer or neoprene.
Handlebar tape and padding	Absorb shock on hands and enhance handlebar grip.	Special padded tape is available for extra shock absorption
Saddle pads and padded saddles	Provide extra shock absorption and relieve discomfort.	Elastopolymer or air pocket saddle covers may be added to bicycle seat but may reduce pedaling power slightly. Saddles with intrinsic padding may be as effective with less loss of performance. Titanium rails on the saddle also help to absorb shock.
Bicycle tape and reflectors	Increase visibility for dawn, dusk, and night riding.	Bicycle reflectors or bicycle tape should be used for all riding in poor lighting conditions. Wheel-mounted reflectors should be removed for riding at high speeds or in windy conditions because they contribute to bicycle vibration and instability. All reflectors are generally omitted by racers to reduce drag. Reflective tape is particularly useful on the back of bicycle shoes, on the helmet, and on the wheels. Another alternative is reflective clothing.
Lights	Enhance visibility at night, dawn, and dusk.	Halogen headlights and either flashing or strobe tail lights are best.
Bright, tight cycling clothing	Advertise presence of cyclist. Special materials keep cyclist cool in hot weather and warm in cold, windy weather.	
Cycling shorts	Protect inner thighs, groin, and buttocks from chafing and pressure trauma.	Shorts should have a virtually seamless crotch pad. Specially designed crotch pads are available for women's shorts.
Bicycle shoes	Along with toe clips or binding, fasten the foot to the pedal.	Stiff mid-sole distributes the pedaling forces over the entire foot, thus preventing many foot and ankle overuse syndromes.

BIBLIOGRAPHY

* 1. Biggar A: Women's cycling: The comfort zone. Bicycling 37(3):38–41.
 2. Burke ER (ed): Science of Cycling. Champaign, IL, Human Kinetics, 1986.
* 3. Burke ER: Proper fit of the bicycle. Clin Sports Med 13:1–14, 1994.
 4. Burke ER, Newsom MM (eds): Medical and Scientific Aspects of Cycling. Champaign, IL, Human Kinetics, 1988.
 5. Chow TK, Bracker MD, Patrick K: Acute injuries from mountain biking. West J Med 159:145–148, 1993.
 6. Coast JR, Cox RH, Welch HG: Optimal pedalling rate in prolonged bouts of cycle ergometry. Med Sci Sports Exerc 18:225–230, 1986.
* 7. Cohen GC: Cycling injuries. Can Fam Phys 39:628–632, 1993.
 8. Davis MW, Litman T, Crenshaw RW, Mueller JK: Bicycling injuries. Phys Sportsmed 8(5):88–96, 1980.
 9. Dickson TB Jr: Preventing overuse cycling injuries. Phys Sportsmed 13(10):116–123, 1985.
 10. Ellis TH, Streight D, Mellion MB: Bicycle safety equipment. Clin Sports Med 13:75–98, 1994.
 11. Fragnoli D: Women's cycling: Love your butt. Bicycling 38(2):34–37, 1997.
 12. Grisolfi CV, Rohlf DP, Navarude SN, et al: Effects of wearing a helmet on thermal balance while cycling in the heat. Phys Sportsmed 16(1):139–146, 1988.
 13. Grandjean AC, Ruud JS: Nutrition for cyclists. Clin Sports Med 13:235–247, 1994.
 14. Hankey GJ, Gubbay SS: Compressive mononeuropathy of the deep palmar branch of the ulnar nerve in cyclists. J Neurol Neurosurg Psychiatry 51:1588–1590, 1988.
*15. Holmes JC, Pruitt AL, Whalen NJ: Cycling knee injuries: Common mistakes that cause injuries and how to avoid them. Cycling Sci 3(2):11–14, 1991.
 16. Holmes JC, Pruitt AL, Whalen NJ: Iliotibial band syndrome in cyclists. Am J Sports Med 21:419–424, 1993.
 17. Holmes JC, Pruitt AL, Whalen NJ: Lower extremity overuse in bicycling. Clin Sports Med 24:187–205, 1994.
 18. Kronisch RL, Pfeiffer RP, Chow TK: Acute injuries in cross-country and downhill off-road bicycle racing. Med Sci Sports Exerc 28:1354–1355, 1996.
 19. Kyle CR: Energy and aerodynamics in bicycling. Clin Sports Med 13:137–164, 1994.
 20. Lofthouse GA: Traumatic injuries to the extremities and thorax. Clin Sports Med 13:113–135, 1994.
*21. Mayer PJ: Helping your patients avoid bicycling injuries. II. How to choose, adjust, and use a bicycle properly. J Musculoskel Med 2(6):31–38, 1985.
*22. Mellion MB: Common cycling injuries: Management and prevention. Sports Med 11:52–70, 1991.
 23. Mellion MB: Bicycling injuries: Prevention, diagnosis and treatment. In Mellion MB (ed): Office Sports Medicine, 2nd ed. Philadelphia, Hanley & Belfus, 1996, pp 355–375.
*24. Mellion MB: Neck and back pain in bicycling. Clin Sports Med 13:137–164, 1994.
*25. Mellion MB: Bicycling. In Mellion MB, et al (eds): The Team Physician's Handbook, 2nd ed. Philadelphia, Hanley & Belfus, 1997, pp 783–805.
*26. Overend N: Dirz degree: Eleven steps to a perfect fit. Bicycling 38(1):100–101, 1997.
 27. Pfeiffer RP: Off-road bicycle racing injuries—the NORBA pro/elite category. Clin Sports Med 13:207–218, 1994.
 28. Powell B: Correction and prevention of bicycle saddle problems. Phys Sportsmed 10(10):60–67, 1982.
 29. Richmond DR: Handlebar problems in bicycling. Clin Sports Med 13:165–173, 1994.
 30. Ryschon TW: Physiologic aspects of bicycling. Clin Sports Med 13:15–38, 1994.
 31. Weiss BD: Nontraumatic injuries in amateur long distance bicyclists. Am J Sports Med 13(3):187–192, 1985.
 32. Weiss BD: Bicycle-related head injuries. Clin Sports Med 13:99–112, 1994.
 33. Weiss BD: Clinical syndromes associated with bicycle seats. Clin Sports Med 13:175–186, 1994.
* = Discuss bicycle "fit" in detail.

103. WEIGHTLIFTING AND POWERLIFTING

Chris N. Christakos, M.D., C.A.Q., SpMed.,
and Karl B. Fields, M.D., C.A.Q., SpMed.

1. What is weightlifting?
The athletic exercise or competition of lifting weights to increase strength and/or muscle mass.

2. What is powerlifting?
The sport of weightlifting in which the athlete competes in three different lifts: bench press, deadlift, and squat.

3. What is the difference between powerlifting and Olympic weightlifting?
Olympic weightlifting involves two different lifts: the snatch and the clean and jerk.

4. What are the most common injuries seen in weightlifting?
Injuries involving the major joints are most common, especially the shoulders, back, and knees.

5. Is weightlifting a safe form of exercise for children?
If proper techniques, appropriate weight limitations, and recommended workout frequency are followed in performing lifting exercises, weightlifting should be safe at any age.

6. Do children gain strength and muscle mass like adolescents and adults by lifting weights?
Children make similar strength gains (percentagewise) compared with adolescents and adults in response to similar weight training programs; however, there appears to be little, if any, effect on muscle size. The increase in strength has been associated with improvements in levels of neuromuscular activation and changes in intrinsic contractile characteristics of muscle. Theoretically, strength training may improve motor coordination, which also increases strength.

7. Is weightlifting safe and effective in older men?
Studies have shown substantial increases in muscle strength and hypertrophy by weightlifting in older men. However, because of the decrease in flexibility that comes with aging, greater care must be taken to use proper technique in lifting weights.

8. What effect does weightlifting have on premenopausal women?
Studies have shown significant improvements in soft tissue lean mass and muscular strength in premenopausal women who exercise regularly with weights. The same studies also show significant but smaller gains in bone mineral density in the same women.

9. Should postmenopausal women lift weights?
Yes. One of the hallmarks to prevent osteoporosis is weightbearing exercise in addition to calcium supplementation, hormone replacement therapy, and/or other medications.

10. How can weightlifting injuries be prevented?
Through education of proper techniques for each weightlifting exercise, which includes a steady controlled lift, not locking out (hyperextending) any joints, and always lifting with a spotter.

11. What precautions need to be taken by diabetics who lift weights?
As with any form of exercise, diabetics should monitor their blood sugar (BS) before exercise. If BS is less than 120 mg/dl or greater than 240 mg/dl, levels should be returned to this range

before exercise. Care also should be taken to monitor BS after exercise. Diabetics who require exogenous insulin should plan where they administer their insulin. They should not inject insulin into a region of the body that they will be exercising, because it will be absorbed too fast. For example, they should not inject insulin into a thigh before doing squats.

12. How safe is weightlifting during pregnancy?

Using proper technique, especially breathing techniques, light weightlifting should be safe through the first two trimesters of pregnancy. Heavy lifting and weightlifting during the third trimester should be discouraged.

13. What is weightlifter's headache?

This condition is described in the literature as the sudden onset of an intense occipital, upper cervical, or parietal headache in weightlifters while they are lifting weights. The cause of weightlifter's headache is thought to be related to increased intrathoracic pressure with Valsalva or cervical muscle and ligament strain. This condition may be precipitated by holding the breath while performing a lift.

14. What is distal clavicle osteolysis? How is it related to weightlifting?

This painful condition involves the resorption of bone adjacent to the acromioclavicular (AC) joint at the distal clavicle. The cause is uncertain, but possibly related to muscle hypertrophy, which may occlude the blood supply to the distal clavicle. Precipitating factors may be repetitive overhead activity or direct trauma to the distal clavicle. Athletes often become frustrated because the treatment of choice is prolonged rest. Refractory cases may require localized steroid injections or resection of the distal clavicle.

15. What is the prevalence of anabolic steroid use in weightlifters?

No one knows. Because of the difficulty in detecting anabolic steroid use and the sophisticated methods of avoiding detection, the prevalence may never be known.

16. What effect does weightlifting have on the heart?

Limited cardiovascular adaptations result from weightlifting. In general, weightlifters have a thickened myocardial wall relative to their cavity size, but the myocardial wall thickness remains within normal limits.

17. Is weightlifting safe in patients with known cardiovascular disease?

Yes. As long as cardiovascular patients are not symptomatic and take appropriate precautions, they should be able to exercise safely with weightlifting. They should limit their maximal intensity to 60% of one repetition maximum. Studies have shown a favorable effect of weightlifting in patients with known cardiovascular disease. Some cardiac rehabilitation programs incorporate weightlifting into exercise programs.

18. What effect does weightlifting have on blood pressure?

Powerlifters have been reported to have blood pressures that average 320/250 at peak pressure measurement during the performance of maximal effort leg presses. There have been two case reports of possible cerebrovascular consequences of weightlifting—brainstem ischemia and subarachnoid hemorrhage—but the risk of stroke as a direct result of lifting weights remains speculative. The highest blood pressures are during the final repetitions of a weightlifting set. Subarachnoid hemorrhage has been reported in weightlifters with intracranial aneurysm. Patients with known or suspected intracranial aneurysm should not pursue weight training.

19. What is weightlifter's back?

A tear in the muscles and/or tendons in the lower back that results from pushing or pulling against a great resistance.

20. What is spondylolysis?

A fracture of the pars interarticularis. There may be a genetic predisposition for this condition, which is thought to be a stress-type fracture due to repetitive stresses at the pars interarticularis. One should suspect spondylolysis in patients with point tenderness on the lumbar spine and increased pain with extension of the lumbar spine (one-legged hyperextension test/flamingo test).

21. How helpful are weight belts?

Whether weight belts prevent injury and/or improve strength is controversial. Weightlifters swear by their weight belts and typically will not perform heavy lifts, especially squat or dead lift, without one. Several studies show improved support of the trunk with weight belts. Improved support is thought to be due to the increased intraabdominal pressure observed in lifters wearing a weight belt. There has been no evidence of increased strength or lifting capacity as a result of wearing a weight belt.

22. At what age does one reach maximal strength?

Strength generally improves rapidly for both men and women during childhood and adolescence, reaching a peak between the ages of 20 and 30 years.

23. What is the bench press?

The powerlifting event in which the athlete lies supine on a bench and presses a barbell vertically from the chest by extending the arms. Care should be taken not to lock out (hyperextend) the elbows and to keep the shoulders and buttocks on the bench. The feet should be planted firmly on the floor.

24. What is the dead lift?

The powerlifting event in which the athlete squats down and grasps the barbell with the arms extended and stands up, slightly hyperextending the back.

25. What is the squat lift?

The powerlifting exercise in which the athlete puts the barbell on the upper back, across the shoulders, and squats down, just breaking parallel to the ground with the thighs, and then stands upright again. Care should be taken not to lock the knees.

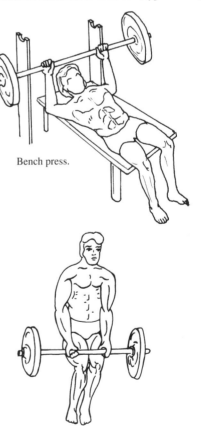

Bench press.

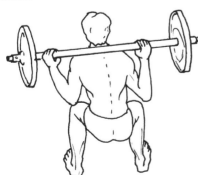

Squat press.

Dead lift.

26. How often should one lift weights?

One may lift weights daily as long as different body parts are exercised (e.g., chest and triceps on day one, shoulders and legs on day two, back and biceps on day three). Preferably the athlete should have at least 2–3 days rest between working out the same body part.

27. How can athletes tell if they are overtraining?

They typically see a plateau or decrease in performance. Other signs and symptoms of overtraining include:

1. Extreme muscle soreness or fatigue that lasts for more than 2–3 days (soreness is common for 1–2 days)
2. Elevated resting blood pressure and/or pulse
3. Inability to complete a workout that usually can be completed
4. Decreased immune system function as evidenced by frequent colds or viral illnesses
5. Symptoms of clinical depression (i.e., changes in sleep and/or appetite, depressed mood, concentration difficulties)
6. Unexplained weight loss

28. What is weightlifter's wrist?

Pain over the dorsum of the wrist that is thought to result from repetitive entrapment or trauma of the dorsal capsule by hyperextension of the wrist in the bench press. Treatment consists of rest, splinting, and nonsteroidal antiinflammatory drugs.

29. What is weightlifter's shoulder?

Impingement syndrome caused by tearing and inflammation of the tendons that form the rotator cuff (teres minor, supraspinatous, infraspinatous, and subscapularis). Repetitive overhead activities and forward flexion of the shoulder cause the humeral head to abut the acromium and coracoacromial ligament, which is rubbed by the supraspinatous tendon. Treatment consists of rest, ice, and nonsteroidal antiinflammatory drugs followed by flexibility and strengthening exercises of the shoulder girdle. Shoulder stabilization exercises may limit impingement and balance anterior and posterior muscle strength inequality.

BIBLIOGRAPHY

1. Berkow R, Fletcher MB (eds): The Merck Manual of Diagnosis and Therapy. Rahway, NJ, Merck, Sharp, & Dohme, 1992.
2. Blimkie CJ: Resistance training during preadolescence: Issues and controversies. Sports Med 15:389–407, 1993.
3. Dupler TL, Cortes C: Effects of a whole-body resistive training regimen in the elderly. Gerontology 39:314–319, 1993.
4. Haykowsky MJ, Findlay JM, Ignaszewski AP: Aneurysmal subarachnoid hemorrhage associated with weight training: Three case reports. Clin J Sports Med 6:52–55, 1996.
5. Lander JE, Hundley JR, Simonton RL: The effectiveness of weight-belts during multiple repetitions of the squat exercise. Med Sci Sports Exerc 24:603–609, 1992.
6. Lillegard WA, Rucker KS (eds): Handbook of Sports Medicine: A Symptom-oriented Approach. Boston, Butterworth-Heinemann, 1993.
7. Lohman T, Going S, Pamenter R, et al: Effects of resistance training on regional and total bone mineral density in premenopausal women: A randomized prospective study. J Bone Miner Res 10:1015–1024, 1995.
8. Mckeag DB, Hough DO (eds): Primary Care Sports Medicine. Dubuque, IA, Brown & Benchmark, 1993.
9. McKelvie RS, McCartney N: Weightlifting training in cardiac patients. Considerations. Sports Med 10:355–364, 1990.
10. Mellion MB, Walsh WM, Shelton GL (eds): The Team Physicians Handbook, 2nd ed. Philadelphia, Hanley & Belfus, 1997.
11. Reyna JR Jr, Leggett SH, Kenney K, et al: The effect of lumbar belts on isolated lumbar muscle: Strength and dynamic capacity. 20:68–73, 1995.
12. Spirito P, Pelliccia A, Proschan MA, et al: Morphology of the athlete's heart assessed by echocardiography in 947 elite athletes representing 27 sports. Am J Cardiol 74:802–806, 1994.

13. Sullivan IA, Grana WA (eds): The Pediatric Athlete. Park Ridge, IL, American Academy of Orthopaedic Surgeons, 1990.
14. Webb DR: Strength training in children and adolescents. Pediatr Clin North Am 37:1187–1210, 1990.
15. Wiecek EM, McCartney N, McKelvie RS: Comparison of direct and indirect measures of systemic arterial pressure during weightlifting in coronary artery disease. Am J Cardiol 66:1065–1069, 1990.

104. IN-LINE SKATING

Russell D. White, M.D., FAAFP, and Ravi S. Tak, M.D.

1. What is in-line skating?

In-line skating, also known as roller-blading, is a form of low-impact exercise that has become popular recently. Each in-line skate has 3–5 wheels set in line with each other. This design gives them the appearance of ice skates with the blades replaced by a sequential line of wheels.

2. What is the history of in-line skating?

The original in-line skate was created to simulate ice skating by a Dutchman in the 1700s. In 1863 angle wheels were fitted to a shoe bracket at the front and back by an American, James Plimpton, and roller skates were created. In 1884 the invention of ball-bearing wheels further revolutionized the sport. In 1980 two brothers, Scott and Brennan Olson of Minneapolis, redesigned the skate using a hockey boot and polyurethane wheels, and Rollerblade, Inc. was born. The Olson brothers were ice hockey players and recognized the cross-training capability of the in-line skate.

3. What are the different types of in-line skating sporting events?

Speed skating or racing (either on straight or curved tracks), in-line hockey, figure skating, and stunt or artistic skating are among the sports enjoyed by in-line skaters.

4. How common is the sport?

According to American Sports Data, in-line skating is the fastest growing sport in America. The marketing of skates began in 1987. It is estimated that more than 23 million Americans participate, and total equipment sales exceeded $1 billion in 1995. Between 1993 and 1995, the number increased by 79%.

5. Why has in-line skating become so popular?

The sport's popularity is due to (1) low-impact aerobic exercise, (2) relatively inexpensive equipment, (3) recreation, (4) transportation, (5) ability to cross-train for other sports (ice hockey, ice skating, roller-skating, cross-country skiing), and (6) fun.

6. What speeds can in-line skaters attain?

Skaters commonly reach speeds of 15–20 miles per hour (25–32 km/hr). Experienced skaters can achieve 50 miles per hour. Skaters may exceed 70 miles per hour with the practice of "skitching"—which is *not* recommended. These speeds are the result of improved technology and materials, including sealed systems and polyurethane wheels. Longer frames accommodate more wheels and allow greater speed. In addition, harder wheels are faster.

7. What is skitching?

Skitching is the practice of holding onto a speeding motor vehicle while skating, i.e., "skate hitching." It is also known as skimming a ride in some areas. Some authors report speeds in excess of 70 miles per hour. With any untoward event, the risk of serious injury or death is greatly increased. This practice is *not* recommended.

8. What is railing?

Railing is a skating trick in which the skater jumps onto the rail and then slides downward. The skates are placed at right angles to the rail as the skater slides down. Because the plastic runners housing the wheels wear down quickly, grind-plates (metal plates) are placed along the runners. Skaters often perform these tricks in skating parks or shopping centers where pedestrian hand rails are found. Such skaters are also called "rail sliders."

9. How do physiologic responses to in-line skating compare with running?

Melanson et al. found that in-line skating at a mean speed of 21.7 km/hr elicited a VO_2 of 42 ml/kg-1/min, which corresponded to 73–98% of maximal heart rate (HRmax). They believed that appropriate cardiovascular training effect can be achieved with in-line skating. Skating at a comfortable pace for 30 minutes expends 285 calories. These numbers compare with jogging. Interval skating—alternating hard and easy paces—can burn up to 450 calories in 30 minutes.

10. How do cardiorespiratory responses during exercise compare with competitive in-line skating?

Wallick et al. found that the physiologic responses and rate of perceived exertion with submaximal and maximal in-line skating were similar to those achieved with treadmill running. To achieve these benefits, in-line skaters had to skate 11.0–13.0 miles per hour continuously for 20–30 minutes. (This intensity level may prove dangerous in crowded urban areas). Several authors have found that the slope of the HR/VO_2 relationship is greater for in-line skating than for cycling or running. Thus, using heart rate as a guide for exercise may result in inadequate workload for aerobic training with in-line skates.

11. What is the leading cause of injury?

Inexperience. Most injured skaters are beginners. In fact, serious injuries have occurred in beginners who attached their skates and fell down before even moving. For this reason, skaters should don protective gear before putting on their skates. In 1995, 103,000 skaters required evaluation in hospital emergency departments. This total does not include self-treated injuries and those evaluated in physicians' offices.

12. What is the mechanism of injury with in-line skating?

Injuries are the result of the biomechanics of falling. The vertical vector (fall from a height) and the horizontal vector (skater's momentum) combine to create sudden, large forces. When one begins to fall, the instinctive reaction is an outstretched upper extremity. The resultant forces are transmitted to this extremity and injuries occur.

13. Describe the mechanisms (biophysics) of the common injuries.

When one falls on ice, the ice gives, and the involved forces are dissipated as the skater slides on the ice after impact. When one falls on pavement, friction and sticking of the skater to the surface are increased. The force is then absorbed by the athlete's points of contact. These points are usually the outstretched hand, elbow, and head.

14. Can death result from accidents or injuries with in-line skating?

Fatal accidents may occur; 15 deaths were reported in 1994. Most deaths were the result of accidents with motor vehicles. In contrast, there are approximately 900 bicycle deaths/year.

15. Does risk of injury increase with skill and level of competition?

No. The novice skater is most likely to be injured. Banus et al. found that the average skating experience at time of injury was 2 months. In most studies 50% of injured skaters were novices.

16. What are the main risk factors for injury?

Speed, obstacles, and hard surfaces. In addition to inexperience, risk of injury increases with high speed, hard surfaces, lack of protective gear, and competition for space with pets, pedestrians, bicycle riders, other skaters, and motor vehicles. A change in the surface coefficient of rolling friction due to water, gravel, sand, or change in skating surface (from concrete to asphalt) may produce a sudden alteration in velocity that makes control difficult. In addition, foreign objects such as twigs or grass may impede the normal rotation of the in-line wheels, producing abrupt changes in velocity and problems with balance. Finally, the art of controlled stopping is difficult to learn and may cause accidents and subsequent injuries.

17. How is deceleration/braking accomplished?
    Either by dragging the heel of one skate, which is equipped with a rubber brake, or by skating forward with one skate and dragging the other skate at right angles to the forward moving skate, forming a T and creating friction. If this technique is well-developed, the T forms a stable base and prevents falling. Other braking techniques include jumping onto grass and running, grabbing a fixed object, or pushing a slow-moving object with the hands. Braking requires practice and skill, and inexperience in deceleration is often the cause of accidents. In Calle and Eaton's study, most injured skaters had not mastered deceleration and stopping techniques.

18. Describe the common types of injuries suffered by in-line skaters.
    Common injuries include abrasions, lacerations, contusions, avulsions, sprains/strains, dislocations, closed head injuries/concussions, and fractures.

Types of Injuries Seen with In-line Skating

Fractures	40%
Avulsions/contusions	22%
Sprains/muscle strains	18%
Lacerations	13%
Other	7%
Total	100%

From Gunther SB, Gunther SF: In-line skating: A popular new sport brings risk of injury. J Musculoskel Med 13:47–50, 1996, with permission.

19. List the most common areas of injuries seen with in-line skating.
    After the wrist and lower arm, the next most commonly injured areas are the elbow, face, and ankle. Commonly, the skater falls on an outstretched arm with hyperextension of the wrist.

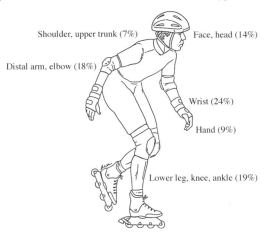

Common areas of injury. (From Gunther SB, Gunther SF: In-line skating: A popular new sport brings risk of injury. J Musculoskel Med 13:47–50, 1996, with permission.)

20. Discuss special injuries seen with the sport of railing.

Because railing involves skating down elevated hand rails or bars, the risk for injury is great if the skater falls. The perineum and genital structures are often injured with this practice.

21. What are the most common sites of fractures with in-line skating?

The most common sites include the wrist, lower arm, and elbow.

Common Fractures with In-line Skating

Wrist	46%
Lower arm	17%
Elbow	11%
Finger	8%
Shoulder	4%
Hand	3%
Lower extremity	7%
Other	4%
Total	100%

From Calle SC, Eaton RG: Wheels-in-line roller skating injuries. J Trauma 35:946–951, 1993, with permission.

22. What are the most common injuries in novice skaters?

Colles' fractures of the wrist, olecranon fractures, and head injuries.

23. How does the injury rate of in-line skating compare with skate-boarding and roller-skating?

In-line skating produces the fewest total number of injuries. For each in-line skating injury, there are 1.2 skate-boarding and 3.3 roller-skating injuries.

24. How does the in-line skating injury rate compare with other sports and recreation categories?

In 1995 in-line skating ranked 7th overall behind basketball, biking, football, baseball, skiing, and soccer.

25. Does protective gear help to prevent injuries?

Yes. In most studies fractures are uncommon in skaters who use protective equipment. In one study skaters who wore wrist guards had no wrist injuries. Because the risk of wrist injury is so great and because the wrist is easily protected, all in-line skaters should wear wrist guards. Other protective equipment includes knee pads, elbow pads, gloves, and helmets. Although many of the more serious injuries involve the head and face, only 15–20% of skaters in most studies wear helmets. Another author found that only 25% of skaters used protective equipment. Older skaters, beginners, and females were more likely to use protective devices than experienced skaters. Adolescent males were least likely to wear protective equipment.

26. How do wrist guards prevent injury?

They are designed (1) to prevent sudden wrist extension, (2) to prevent direct contact with the hard surface and to promote sliding, and (3) to dissipate the transmitted force.

27. What is the order of frequency with which protective equipment is used?

Wrist guards were the most commonly used, followed by knee pads, elbow pads, and helmets.

28. What are the stated reasons in-line skaters do not wear protective equipment?

Inadequate knowledge about benefits, discomfort, inconvenience, cost, and image/peer acceptance are reasons that skaters give for not wearing protective equipment.

29. What precautions can be taken to prevent injuries?

1. Always wear protective equipment.

2. Take lessons from experienced skaters or contact the International In-Line Skating Association (800-56SKATE).

3. Learn to stop safely.

4. Practice falling to one side, not on an outstretched upper extremity.

5. Be familiar with surfaces and terrain.

6. Be prepared for the unexpected surface objects, hills, pedestrian, or automobile.

7. Pay attention to your surroundings.

8. Avoid skating in crowded areas.

9. Know your limitations, and skate within your skill.

BIBLIOGRAPHY

1. The benefits and perils of in-line skating. Emerg Med 27:37–38, 1995.
2. Calle SC, Eaton RG: Wheels-in-line roller skating injuries. J Trauma 35:946–951, 1993.
3. Cheng SL, Rajaratnam K, Raskin KB, et al: Splint-top fracture of the forearm: A description of an in-line skating injury associated with the use of protective wrist splints. J Trauma 39:1194–1197, 1995.
4. Gunther SB, Gunther SF: In-line skating: A popular new sport brings risk of injury. J Musculoskel Med 13:47–50, 1996.
5. Hensinger RN: In-line skating: Play it safe [editorial]. Am Fam Physician 53:2430, 1996.
6. Jacques LB, Grzesiak E: Personal protective equipment use by in-line roller skaters. J Fam Pract 38:486–488, 1994.
7. Melanson EL, Freedson PS, Webb R, et al: Exercise responses to running and in-line skating at self-selected paces. Med Sci Sports Exerc 28:247–250, 1996.
8. Orenstein JB: Injuries and small wheel skates. Ann Emerg Med 27:204–209, 1996.
9. Potera C: In-line downfalls. Am Health 15:85, 1996.
10. Powell M, Svensson J: In-line skating. Champaign, IL, Human Kinetics, 1993.
11. Schieber RA, Branche-Dorsey CM, Ryan GW: Comparison of in-line skating injuries with rollerskating and skateboarding injuries. JAMA 271:1856–1858, 1994.
12. Schieber RA, Branche-Dorsey CM, Ryan GW, et al: In-line skating and the effectiveness of safety gear. Sport Med 19:427–432, 1995.
13. Schieber RA, Branche-Dorsey CM, Ryan GW, et al: Risk factors for injuries from in-line skating injuries: Epidemiology and recommendations for prevention. N Engl J Med 335:1630–1635, 1996.
14. Snyder AC, O'Hagan KP, Clifford PS, et al: Exercise responses to in-line skating: Comparisons to running and cycling. Int J Sports Med 14:38–42, 1993.
15. Wallick ME, Porcari JP, Wallick SB, et al: Physiological responses to in-line skating compared to treadmill running. Med Sci Sports Exerc 27:242–248, 1995.
16. Young CC, Mark DH: In-line skating. An observational study of protective equipment used by skaters. Arch Fam Med 4:19–23, 1995.

105. CHEERLEADING

Matthew A. McQueen, M.D., and John M. Henderson, D.O.

1. Why do cheerleaders get injured?

Improper conditioning, inadequate equipment (mats), inexperienced coaching, poor spotting techniques, and overzealous maneuvers have been implicated. Formerly, cheerleading was considered an "activity," and the resources allotted to athletic teams were not available to cheerleading squads. Squads often practiced without supervision or with untrained supervision. Regulations concerning dangerous stunts were lacking because schools and colleges had no regulatory organizations. The fact that most injuries are strains and sprains implies poor overall conditioning.

Over the past 10–15 years, cheerleading has been viewed as a true sport, likened to floor-exercise gymnastics. Organizational structure and safety have thus improved.

2. What is the most frequently injured body part in cheerleading?

Good medical data about cheerleading are scant. General correlations are made with floor-exercise gymnastics. The National Electronic Injury Surveillance System (NEISS), administered by the U.S. Consumer Product Safety Commission, provided data in the early 1980s. Emergency visits for cheerleading injury numbered 5000 in 1980 and peaked at 6900 in 1984. This number represents a gross underestimate since only emergency department data are used.

The ankle is the most frequently injured area, followed by knee, wrist, and lower trunk. This pattern also is seen in floor gymnasts. The knee is the most frequent site of serious injury.

3. What are the most dangerous maneuvers in cheerleading?

Stunts involving pyramids and minitrampolines are notoriously dangerous. Data from the National Center for Catastrophic Sports Injury Research (NCCSIR) documented 20 catastrophic injuries from 1982–1992, 10 of which involved pyramids. Spinal cord and closed-head injuries were the most common. Minitrampolines are now universally banned in gymnastics and cheerleading.

4. Who sets rules and regulations governing cheerleading?

Apparently there are four national organizations, although no single system for rules and regulations exists. The National Cheerleaders Association (NCA) and the Universal Cheerleading Association (UCA) are owned by private companies and sponsor summer instructional camps.

The American Association of Cheerleading Coaches and Advisors (AACCA), a nonprofit educational association, offers a safety certification course and manual and has contributed much to improved cheerleading safety.

Certain states have adopted guidelines that regulate cheerleading at the high school and below level. Some conferences in the National Collegiate Athletes Association also have regulatory committees.

5. Where can information about safety in cheerleading be obtained?

The AACCA can be located on the worldwide web at http:///www.aacca.com or at 1-800-533-6583. The *U.S.A. Gymnastics Safety Handbook: For Gymnastics and Other Sports Activities*, 4th ed., is a further reference for gymnastic safety.

6. What, in general, can be done to reduce injuries in cheerleading?

Cantu and Mueller propose ten guidelines based on the NCCSIR data. Of particular note is the importance of a sound preparticipation evaluation. Preexisting musculoskeletal problems, particularly inadequately rehabilitated injuries, contribute significantly to risk for injury. Overall conditioning and skeletal maturity level also should be assessed (skeletal growth spurts are thought to be a time of increased injury risk).

A sound preseason and ongoing conditioning regimen should be implemented, consisting of (1) strength training, (2) aerobic conditioning, and (3) flexibility training. Strength training is sport-specific and should emphasize quadriceps, hamstrings, calf muscles, and trunk muscles. High repetition/low weight is most appropriate. Flexibility of hamstrings, heel cords, and back are especially important. Universal rules and regulations that govern stunts, coaches, and equipment are critical.

7. What training, by specific body area, can be done to improve preparation for cheerleaders?

Ankle. Dorsiflexor strengthening, heel-cord stretching, and proprioceptive training (e.g., slide board) may reduce ankle sprains. Avoidance of off-balance or torsional landings should be emphasized.

Knee. The female knee is at particular risk for ligamentous disruption. Single-leg or wide-stanced landings should be avoided. Rotatory knee instabilities involving the anterior cruciate ligament generally require surgical reconstruction; bracing is generally inadequate. Overuse anterior knee pain is best averted by isometric and closed-chain quadriceps strengthening and diligent hamstring stretching.

Wrist. Traumatic impaction syndromes involving the distal radius and ulna and proximal carpal row are common. The radial growth plate is also at risk. Forearm flexor training and dorsiflexor "stop bracing" may provide protection.

Upper extremity. The elbow tends to hyperextend and thus is subject to fracture and dislocation. The shoulder tends to be lax. Osteochondritis dessicans also tends to occur at the elbow with repetitive loading. Shoulder girdle strengthening (especially internal and external rotators) should be emphasized. Biceps and triceps strengthening, proprioceptive training, and avoidance of hyperextension may reduce problems related to the elbow.

Trunk. Repetitive hyperextension from maneuvers such as back walkovers contributes to back pain and possible pars interarticularis stress fractures. Abdominal strengthening (crunches and leg lifts) and back/hamstring flexibility training are appropriate.

8. Besides traumatic injury, what other medical or psychological issues concern cheerleaders?

Cheerleaders are not exempt from hydrational, thermal, and nutritional problems typical of adolescent athletes. Because the cheerleading season corresponds with football, proper hydration and heat discipline are mandatory. An appropriate athletic diet should be followed.

Female athletes participating in sports in which appearance is judged are at particular risk for eating disorders. Clues to an eating disorder include weight loss, skipped meals, stress fractures, personality changes, menstrual irregularities, and dental changes.

BIBLIOGRAPHY

1. Cantu RC, Mueller FO: Cheerleading [editorial]. Clin J Sports Med 4(2):75–76, 1994.
2. DeBenedette V: Are cheerleaders athletes? Physician Sportsmed 15(9):214–220, 1987.
3. Gottlieb A: Cheerleaders are athletes too. Pediatr Nurs 20(6):630–633, 1994.
4. Grana WA, Weiker GG: Injuries in gymnastics. In Renstrom PAFH (ed): Clinical Practice of Sports Injury Prevention and Care. Oxford, Blackwell, 1994, pp 526–534.
5. Hage P: Cheerleading: New problems in a changing sport. Physician Sportsmed 9(2):140–145, 1981.
6. Hutchinson MR, Ireland ML: Knee injuries in female athletes. Sports Med 19:288–302, 1995.
7. Ireland ML, Hutchinson MR: Upper extremity injuries in young athletes. Clin Sports Med 14:533–569, 1995.
8. Lockey MW: The sport of cheerleading. J Miss State Med Assoc 32(10):375, 1991.
9. Reel JJ, Gill DL: Psychosocial factors related to eating disorders among high school and college female cheerleaders. Sport Psychol 10(2):195–206, 1996.
10. Steptoe S: The pom-pom chronicles. Sports Illust 75(28)d:38–46, 1991.
11. Whitlock S (ed): The U.S.A. Gymnastics Safety Handbook: For Gymnastics and Other Sports Activities, 4th ed. U.S.A. Gymnastics, 1998, appendix 1.2.

106. MASS PARTICIPATION SPORTS AND EVENTS

John M. Henderson, D.O.

1. Are mass participation sports approached differently from other sports?

Mass participation sports are often high-profile sporting events sponsored by large corporations for charitable causes but supported by volunteers organized by local agencies. Such events usually have a medical director—a physician identified as the focal point for medical responsibility and recommendations. Some sports by their nature require large numbers of competitors.

2. What kinds of sports involve mass participation?

Most mass participation sports involve individual athletic efforts, but a few involve team effort. Mass participation sports include the following:
- Walking: recreational and volksmarching, plus race walking
- Soccer and football tournaments/jamborees
- Running: 5-k, 10-k, half and full marathons
- Softball and tennis regional tournaments
- Cross-country (Nordic) skiing
- Cycling: century, half-century, cross-state, tours
- Triathlon: run-bike-swim combinations of varying distances
- Biathlon: cross-country skiing-riflery
- Snowmobile races
- Motorcross/supercross and enduro races
- Special Olympics track and field events

3. What are the most common concerns in mass participation events?

Heat injuries, cold injuries, altitude injuries, and lightning strikes are among the major concerns. The prevention of these problems hinges on collecting accurate climate, meteorologic, and geographic information. Prevention also includes the ability to monitor the situation and to communicate hourly changes to participants so that they can modify their responses accordingly.

4. How can the major concerns be monitored?

Heat load can be monitored with a wet bulb globe thermometer. Cold index can be measured using a wind meter and dry bulb thermometer. Altitude injuries can be anticipated by using an altimeter. Lightning strikes can be monitored through the National Weather Service's Doppler reports on AM radio frequencies.

5. What other medical concerns should be addressed?

- Playing surface problems—loose gravel on an asphalt road race course, sprinkler heads projecting above a soccer field, loose jumps on a motocross course.
- Venomous bites—fire ants, brown recluse spiders, scorpions, hymenoptera, jellyfish, snakes.
- Stands and bleachers—loose boards, exposed nails or screws, rotten wood, wobbling superstructure, sinking foundations.
- Food and beverage quality—poorly prepared food or maintained eating areas, contaminated food, ill food service workers.
- Chronobiology—ill effects of traversing several time zones.
- Air pollution—ophthalmic and respiratory effects of exposure to air polluted with disulfides, acids, and particulate matter.
- Water safety—water temperature and purity are important to monitor; capabilities for water rescue are required for water sports.

6. What minimal protection issues are involved?

Depending on the sport or event, the medical director of a mass participation event needs to consider the following basic minimal protection:

1. The participants are given a review of the course and current as well as anticipated weather conditions.

2. Each participant wears some sort of personal identification.

3. Each participant is tracked through several mileposts throughout the course of competition.

4. At least the minimal safety equipment is used by each participant (e.g., helmet use by cyclists, mouthpiece use in collision sports).

5. Water and, in certain events, carbohydrate replacement should be available in mass volumes.
   - Water requirements: 8 ounces (240 cc) of water per participant every 2 miles of a running or walking event.

- Carbohydrate replacement—events running longer than 2 hours should consider offering participants some sort of carbohydrate replacement, such as a medium-chain sugar polymer.
- No unbiased study, free from commercial influence, proves the unequivocal superiority of replacement drinks. A balance should be achieved in the volume and osmolality of replacement drinks available during an endurance sport.
  (1) Inadequate replacement results in volume contraction.
  (2) Hypertonic fluid replacement may cause gastroparesis and diarrhea.
  (3) Hypotonic fluid replacement may cause hyponatremia due to hemodilution.

7. What pre-event preparations must the medical director oversee?

The medical director supervises the medical review of applications to participate in the event. Questionnaires are used to identify participants who are possibly at risk of sustaining an injury. The common conditions inquired about include:

- Pregnancy
- Cardiovascular disease—specifically hypertension, angina, chronic congestive cardiomyopathy, and peripheral vascular diseases.
- Endocrinopathies—particularly diabetes mellitus and hypothyroidism and whether these conditions are under control.
- Past injuries—the competitor may be more susceptible to sustaining an injury because he or she has a history of injury such as heat stroke or frostbite.
- Participants who are ill-prepared—competitors are asked if they made reasonable preparations for the event, especially if it is an endurance sport such as the marathon.

8. For what other problems should the medical director plan?

There are three more concerns for which medical directors for mass participation events must plan in advance:

1. **Spectator concerns.** From past events, the anticipated attendance can be estimated. Spectators can fill a medium-size city in many cases (Indianapolis 500—2 million spectators; University of Tennessee football at Neyland Stadium—106,656 spectators; World Series Baseball at Atlanta's Fulton County Stadium—48,000 spectators; New York City Marathon—1–3 million spectators; New Year's Day Rose Bowl Football Game—120,000 spectators). The medical director of a mass event may be responsible for the health and welfare of spectators, vendors, and volunteer staff.
   - Exposure (even if the weather is good, sun and wind exposure may present problems)
   - Safety for able-bodied and handicapped patrons (ramps and emergency exits)
   - "Attractive nuisances" (e.g., swimming pools, fountains, fireworks)
   - First aid (for the most minimal care)
   - Evacuation to a fixed facility (plan for ambulance transport by ground or air routes)
   - Mass casualty plan ("mass cal")—a plan to accommodate large numbers of injured or stunned people in the shortest possible time usually involves triage and multiple transport sites.

2. **Severe weather.** The medical director must have a means to monitor the ever-changing weather and to obtain reliable reports about the possibility of thunderstorms, snow storms, hail storms, tornado, hurricane, and high winds.

3. **Litigation**
   - **Exculpatory waivers.** When the medical director for a mass participation event deems it unwise or imprudent for an at-risk athlete to participate but the athlete insists on participating, the athlete should sign an exculpatory waiver. This legal document acknowledges the risks to be taken by the athlete and absolves the medical director or the organization of responsibility in the event of mishap. These arrangements are not without loopholes and problems. Most large events maintain their own legal counsel.

• **Usual and customary practice of any reasonable practitioner.** Regardless of the festive atmosphere of any mass sporting event, the medical director should take the usual and customary precautions any reasonable physician would take in similar situations. Although there is no uniform list of preparations, common sense is a guide; for example, water events require water rescue abilities.

9. What sensitive issues may arise?

One of the most sensitive aspects of competition is gender verification or sex testing. Attempts to cheat in female-only competitions at the world-class level date back to the 1930s. Men have undergone sex-change surgery to compete as women. During the Summer Olympic Games of 1996, gender verification for women became a standard part of precompetition preparations. Chromosome analysis of buccal mucosal cells obtained by brush cytology techniques has proved superior to phenotyping from gross examination. Because athletes always strive to win, episodes at cheating should be anticipated at lower levels in the future. The medical director of a mass participation event needs to coordinate the efforts of the medical genetics technicians, cytology laboratory, and reporting system officials and to keep in mind the privacy of the female athletes who are tested.

10. Is the medical director involved in doping surveillance?

Cheating also involves the use of performance-enhancing drugs. Ergogenic drugs include stimulants, anabolic agents, and analgesics. Ergolytic drugs, such as beta-adrenergic blockers, also enhance performance in certain sports (e.g., marksmanship). The medical director of some mass participation events, such as the NCAA championships and the Olympic Games, oversees drug surveillance efforts. The selection of athletes to be tested, specimen collection techniques, chain of custody for specimens, specimen analysis, and the results reporting process are perceived as part of the medical director's responsibility (although once the specimen leaves the director's jurisdiction, much is left up to the governing body's standard operating procedures). The medical director should make sure that no banned substances are used in the training rooms or athlete first aid stations.

11. What does history teach medical directors about mass participation sports?

Since the 1972 Olympic Games in Munich, medical directors of mass participation events have had to develop a contingency plan that includes rapid reaction to unwanted and fearful possibilities:

1. **Terrorist activities**—a coordinated plan of action is developed with local law enforcement agencies.

2. **Natural catastrophies**—such as severe weather (see above).

3. **Competition venue catastrophies**—such as a roofing panel or bleachers breaking loose and falling.

12. What other preparations can help the medical director of a mass participation sporting event?

1. **Communications.** The medical director must be able to communicate with the operations headquarters of the event as well as with local emergency medical services and the different first responders, first aid stations, police, and security.

2. **Transportation.** The medical director should be able to get around the entire competition venue as well as the parking areas and support areas.

3. **Liaisons.** The medical director needs to maintain open lines of communication and excellent working relationships with the other functional areas of event support, such as security, media, and officials.

4. **Health care facilities.** The medical director should establish an understanding with local hospitals about timely transportation, treatment, and disposition of participants.

5. **Volunteer coordinator.** The medical director should interface with the person coordinating volunteers to identify volunteers who have a serious or chronic illness or who may need day-to-day monitoring.

6. **Legal responsibilities.** The medical director should check with his or her insurance carrier to be sure that professional liability insurance covers this kind of activity. In addition, the organizing committee may offer some type of legal protection.

BIBLIOGRAPHY

1. Henderson JM: Comprehensive medical support for an Olympic venue. Atlanta Committee for the Olympic Games, Atlanta, GA, 1992.
2. Hunter SC: Coverage of games and events. In Baker CL (ed): The Hughston Clinic Sports Medicine Book. Baltimore, Williams & Wilkins, 1995, pp 9–11.
3. McCormick DP: Medical coverage for Special Olympics Games. In Mellion MB, Walsh WM, Shelton GL (eds): The Team Physician's Handbook, 2nd ed. Philadelphia, Hanley & Belfus, 1997, pp 116–124.
4. McKeag DB: On-site care of the injured youth. In Kelley VC, et al (eds): Brennemann's Practice of Pediatrics, vol. 10. New York, Harper & Row, 1985, pp 1–23.
5. Roberts WO: Administration and medical management of mass participation endurance events. In Mellion MB, Walsh WM, Shelton GL (eds): The Team Physician's Handbook, 2nd ed. Philadelphia, Hanley & Belfus, 1997, pp 875–887.
6. Simon S, McKeag DB, Joy E: How to manage major event issues. Presented at Sports Medicine: An In-Depth Review. American Academy of Family Physicians, Dallas, Texas, February 3, 1997.
7. Tucher JB, Marrow JT: Fieldside management of athletic injuries. Am Fam Physician 34(2)137–142, 1986.

INDEX

Page numbers in **boldface type** indicate complete chapters.